Brain Targeted Drug Delivery Systems

Brain Targeted Drug Delivery Systems

A Focus on Nanotechnology and Nanoparticulates

Edited by

Huile Gao

Key Laboratory of Drug Targeting and Drug Delivery Systems, West China School of Pharmacy, Sichuan University, Chengdu, China

Xiaoling Gao

Department of Pharmacology and Chemical Biology, Faculty of Basic Medicine, Shanghai Jiao Tong University School of Medicine, Shanghai, China

ELSEVIER

ACADEMIC PRESS

An imprint of Elsevier

Academic Press is an imprint of Elsevier
125 London Wall, London EC2Y 5AS, United Kingdom
525 B Street, Suite 1650, San Diego, CA 92101, United States
50 Hampshire Street, 5th Floor, Cambridge, MA 02139, United States
The Boulevard, Langford Lane, Kidlington, Oxford, OX5 1GB, United Kingdom

Library of Congress Cataloging-in-Publication Data
A catalog record for this book is available from the Library of Congress

British Library Cataloguing-in-Publication Data
A catalogue record for this book is available from the British Library

ISBN: 978-0-12-814001-7

For information on all Academic Press publications visit our website at https://www.elsevier.com/books-and-journals

Publisher: John Fedor
Acquisition Editor: Glyn Jones
Editorial Project Manager: John Leonard
Production Project Manager: Sreejith Viswanathan
Cover Designer: Mark Rogers

Typeset by SPi Global, India

Dedication

We dedicate this book to our supervisor, Prof. Xinguo Jiang.

Huile Gao
Xiaoling Gao

Contents

Contributors

Rujing Chen Institute of Interdisciplinary Integrative Medicine Research, Shanghai University of Traditional Chinese Medicine, Shanghai, China

Saurabh Dhanda Department of Biochemistry, Panjab University, Chandigarh, India

Jiajun Fan Department of Microbiological and Biochemical Pharmacy & The Key Laboratory of Smart Drug Delivery, Ministry of Education, School of Pharmacy, Fudan University, Shanghai, PR China

Huile Gao Key Laboratory of Drug Targeting and Drug Delivery Systems, West China; School of Pharmacy, Sichuan University, Chengdu, China

Xiaoling Gao Department of Pharmacology and Chemical Biology, Faculty of Basic Medicine, Shanghai Jiao Tong University School of Medicine, Shanghai, China

Xiaojiao Ge Key Laboratory of Smart Drug Delivery, Ministry of Education, School of Pharmacy, Fudan University, Shanghai, China

Xiao Gu Department of Pharmacology and Chemical Biology, Faculty of Basic Medicine, Shanghai Jiao Tong University School of Medicine, Shanghai, China

Qian Guo Department of Pharmaceutics, College of Pharmaceutical Sciences, Soochow University, Suzhou, People's Republic of China

Smriti Gupta Department of Biochemistry, Panjab University, Chandigarh, India

Liang Han Department of Pharmaceutics, College of Pharmaceutical Sciences, Soochow University, Suzhou, People's Republic of China

Xiuxiu Hao Department of Pharmacology and Chemical Biology, Faculty of Basic Medicine, Shanghai Jiao Tong University School of Medicine, Shanghai, China

Kaili Hu Institute of Interdisciplinary Integrative Medicine Research, Shanghai University of Traditional Chinese Medicine, Shanghai, China

Yilan Huang School of Pharmacy, Fudan University, Key Laboratory of Smart Drug Delivery, Ministry of Education, Shanghai, PR China

Rongqin Huang Department of Pharmaceutics, School of Pharmacy, Key Laboratory of Smart Drug Delivery, Ministry of Education, Fudan University, Shanghai, China

Meng Huang Department of Pharmacology and Chemical Biology, Faculty of Basic Medicine, Shanghai Jiao Tong University School of Medicine, Shanghai, China

Yongzhuo Huang Shanghai Institute of Materia Medica, Chinese Academy of Sciences, Shanghai, China

Kai Jin School of Pharmacy, Fudan University, Key Laboratory of Smart Drug Delivery, Ministry of Education, Shanghai, PR China

Xiufeng Ju Department of Pharmaceutics, College of Pharmaceutical Sciences, Soochow University, Suzhou, People's Republic of China

Dianwen Ju Department of Microbiological and Biochemical Pharmacy & The Key Laboratory of Smart Drug Delivery, Ministry of Education, School of Pharmacy, Fudan University, Shanghai, PR China

Naveed Ullah Khan Department of Pharmaceutics, College of Pharmaceutical Sciences, Soochow University, Suzhou, People's Republic of China

Wahid Khan Department of Pharmaceutics, National Institute of Pharmaceutical Education and Research (NIPER), Hyderabad, India

G.T. Kulkarni Amity Institute of Pharmacy, Amity University Uttar Pradesh, Noida, India

Guangzhe Li School of Pharmaceutical Science and Technology, Dalian University of Technology, Dalian, China

Chengyi Li Department of Pharmaceutics, School of Pharmacy, Key Laboratory of Smart Drug Delivery, Ministry of Education, Fudan University, Shanghai, China

Cong Li Key Laboratory of Smart Drug Delivery, Ministry of Education, School of Pharmacy, Fudan University, Shanghai, China

Yubin Li Department of Microbiological and Biochemical Pharmacy & The Key Laboratory of Smart Drug Delivery, Ministry of Education, School of Pharmacy, Fudan University, Shanghai, PR China; Perelman School of Medicine, University of Pennsylvania; Corporal Michael J. Crescenz VA Medical Center, Philadelphia, PA, United States

Qingfeng Liu Key Laboratory of Smart Drug Delivery, Ministry of Education (Fudan University), Shanghai, People's Republic of China; Department of Pharmaceutics, School of Pharmacy, Fudan University, Shanghai, People's Republic of China

Ergang Liu Shanghai Institute of Materia Medica, Chinese Academy of Sciences, Shanghai; School of Chemical Engineering and Technology, Tianjin University, Tianjin, China

Kanishk Luhach Amity Institute of Pharmacy, Amity University Uttar Pradesh, Noida, India

Tongtong Miao Department of Pharmaceutics, College of Pharmaceutical Sciences, Soochow University, Suzhou, People's Republic of China

Xiaopeng Mo Shanghai Institute of Materia Medica, Chinese Academy of Sciences; Shanghai University College of Sciences, Shanghai, China

Zhiqing Pang School of Pharmacy, Fudan University, Key Laboratory of Smart Drug Delivery, Ministry of Education, Shanghai, PR China

Min Qian Department of Pharmaceutics, School of Pharmacy, Key Laboratory of Smart Drug Delivery, Ministry of Education, Fudan University, Shanghai, China

Raju Saka Department of Pharmaceutics, National Institute of Pharmaceutical Education and Research (NIPER), Hyderabad, India

Rajat Sandhir Department of Biochemistry, Panjab University, Chandigarh, India

Priyadarshini Sathe Department of Pharmaceutics, National Institute of Pharmaceutical Education and Research (NIPER), Hyderabad, India

Kun Shao State Key Laboratory of Fine Chemicals, Dalian University of Technology, Dalian, China; Julia McFarlane Diabetes Research Centre (JMDRC) and Department of Microbiology, Immunology and Infectious Diseases, Snyder Institute for Chronic Diseases and Hotchkiss Brain Institute, Cumming School of Medicine, University of Calgary, Calgary, AB, Canada

Bhupesh Sharma Amity Institute of Pharmacy, Amity University Uttar Pradesh, Noida, India

Xiaoyu Shen Department of Pharmacology and Chemical Biology, Faculty of Basic Medicine, Shanghai Jiao Tong University School of Medicine, Shanghai, China

Channakeshava Sokke Umeshappa Julia McFarlane Diabetes Research Centre (JMDRC) and Department of Microbiology, Immunology and Infectious Diseases,

Snyder Institute for Chronic Diseases and Hotchkiss Brain Institute, Cumming School of Medicine, University of Calgary, Calgary, AB, Canada

Shanshan Wang Department of Pharmaceutics, School of Pharmacy, Key Laboratory of Smart Drug Delivery, Ministry of Education; Department of Pharmacy, Zhongshan Hospital, Fudan University, Shanghai, China

Hualin Wang Department of Pharmacology and Chemical Biology, Faculty of Basic Medicine, Shanghai Jiao Tong University School of Medicine, Shanghai, China

Changyou Zhan School of Basic Medical Sciences & State Key Laboratory of Molecular Engineering of Polymers, Fudan University; Key Laboratory of Smart Drug Delivery (Fudan University), Ministry of Education, Shanghai, P.R. China

Zui Zhang School of Basic Medical Sciences & State Key Laboratory of Molecular Engineering of Polymers, Fudan University, Shanghai, P.R. China

Qizhi Zhang Key Laboratory of Smart Drug Delivery, Ministry of Education (Fudan University), Shanghai, People's Republic of China; Department of Pharmaceutics, School of Pharmacy, Fudan University, Shanghai, People's Republic of China

Yuyan Zhang Department of Pharmacology and Chemical Biology, Faculty of Basic Medicine, Shanghai Jiao Tong University School of Medicine, Shanghai, China

Xiao Zhao Institute of Interdisciplinary Integrative Medicine Research, Shanghai University of Traditional Chinese Medicine, Shanghai, China

Xiaowen Zhu School of Pharmacy, Fudan University, Key Laboratory of Smart Drug Delivery, Ministry of Education, Shanghai, PR China

Preface

Brain targeting drug delivery is a hard task for researchers due to the integrated blood brain barrier (BBB). Benefiting from the quickly developed materials science, nanotechnology and biology science, many brain-targeted drug delivery systems were developed in the past two decades. The brain-targeted drug delivery efficiency and mechanism have been extensively improved and evaluated. As a leading scientist in the field of brain-targeted drug delivery in China, Prof. Xinguo Jiang started the related research in late 1990s. From then on, Jiang's lab published many studies that were trying to improve the brain-targeted drug delivery, both intravenous and intranasal. And the mechanisms behind the brain-targeted drug delivery were also extensively evaluated. As a summary of related works both from his lab and colleagues, Prof. Jiang edited a book named "*Brain Targeted Drug Delivery Systems*", which was published in Chinese by People's Medical Publishing House Co., LTD in 2011. Although Prof. Jiang has retired, the field is still going on. To further summarize the updated progress in the field, and to provide deep discussion about the potential directions of the field, we edit the current book.

The chapters in this book were written by active researchers, mostly Prof. Jiang's students and colleagues, who dedicated their effort to enlarge the efficiency of brain-targeted drug delivery, develop nanomedicines for central nervous system (CNS) disorders, and improve the understanding of interaction of nanomaterials and CNS. We appreciate these authors for sharing their knowledge, ideas, and insights about the topic. These knowledge, ideas, and insights provide all of us, especially who work toward nanomedicines and drug delivery, with overview of the brain-targeted drug delivery and spark to think more about our research.

The book is divided into four sections, including physiology and principles for brain targeting drug delivery, nanoparticles-based brain targeting delivery strategies, nanoparticles-based brain targeting delivery for CNS disorder management, and perspective and pitfalls of nanoparticles-based brain targeting delivery. And we tried to include all the important topics and researches in the field to this book.

We heartily thank Prof. Jiang for his valuable guidance during our study and work. We greatly appreciate the individual chapter contributors for kindly sharing their knowledge and insights. It is a great pleasure and honor to collaborate with them to develop this book. We admire their contribution of outstanding work which would help researchers of nanomedicines and drug delivery benefit from this book and make greater success in their own work.

Huile Gao

Introduction and overview

1

Huile Gao
Key Laboratory of Drug Targeting and Drug Delivery Systems, West China School of Pharmacy, Sichuan University, Chengdu, China

Brain is the most important organ for human beings that is protected by blood-brain barrier (BBB) to restrict the access of harmful compounds or substrates from peripheral blood circulation. However, the BBB also restricts distribution of therapeutics drugs into diseased brain, making treatment of central nervous system (CNS) disorders a most difficult task for doctors and pharmaceutics. Over 98% of small molecule drugs and almost 100% proteins, peptides, and genes could not penetrate through BBB. Therefore, how to overcome the BBB and improve drug delivery to brain is important and has been attracting increasing attention in recent decade.

Accompanied with the development of biology and materials science, researchers developed many kinds of brain-targeted drug delivery systems (DDS) to carry the therapeutic drugs and specifically deliver them for major CNS disorders, including brain tumor, Alzheimer's disease, Parkinson's disease, stroke, CNS inflammation, etc. Although great achievement has been made, there are still many unmet concerns, and none of the brain targeting DDS was approved for clinical use.

In this book, the mechanisms for brain targeting drug delivery and various brain targeting DDS were reviewed and discussed. The book includes the following:

- The anatomy, physiology, and models of BBB;
- The mechanisms and strategies to transport through or bypass BBB;
- The brain targeting DDS for various CNS disorders;
- The neurotoxicity, intra-brain distribution, and excretion of brain targeting DDS;
- The perspective and unmet concerns in brain targeting drug delivery.

1 Is it possible to deliver drugs to brain?

To answer this question, in Chapter 2, Dr. Gupta et al. reviewed the anatomy of BBB. The BBB is consisted by specialized endothelial cells, astrocytes, pericytes, neurons along with extracellular matrix, while tight junction and cytoplasmic proteins further contribute to the function of BBB. Although the BBB considerably restricted the distribution of most compounds into brain, many nutrients, ions, and hormones could specifically penetrate through BBB. In Chapter 3, Dr. Li et al. reviewed the mechanisms to overcome BBB, which provided possible routes for delivering drugs to brain. Then, the current progress of transportation in BBB was summarized. For evaluating brain-targeted drug delivery efficiency, model is important. In Chapter 4, Dr. Sharma et al. reviewed both the in vitro and in vivo models of BBB.

Brain Targeted Drug Delivery Systems. https://doi.org/10.1016/B978-0-12-814001-7.00001-9

Brain is a nutrient-consuming organ that requires great amount of glucose and amino acids; therefore, the BBB are overexpressed with a wide range of transporters that can selectively transport nutrients to the brain, such as amino acid transporters, hexose transport system, monocarboxylate transporter system, organic anion transporter family, etc. So, the corresponding substrates could act as ligands to deliver compounds, even nanoparticles, to brain that are mediated by the transporters, which was reviewed in Chapter 6 by Dr. Han et al. Except the nutrients, a variety of endogenous peptides and proteins can penetrate through BBB by receptor-mediated transcytosis (RMT) because these peptides and proteins play necessary roles in brain functions. Therefore, in Chapter 5, Dr. Zhang and Dr. Zhan reviewed the overexpressed receptors on BBB, including insulin receptor, transferrin receptor, low-density lipoprotein receptor, low-density lipoprotein receptor-related proteins, nicotinic acetylcholine receptors, lactoferrin receptor, scavenger receptor class B type 1, leptin receptor, diphtheria toxin receptor, and single domain llama antibody receptor, and discussed the progress and concerns of utilizing ligands of these receptors for brain-targeted drug delivery. Additionally, cationic peptides and proteins could also be used as ligands for brain-targeted drug delivery due to adsorptive-mediated endocytosis through the negative-charged BBB, which was reviewed by Dr. Pang et al. in Chapter 7. Considering that the BBB could not only restrict the penetration of compounds, but also pump out substrates from brain to blood, it is applicable to improve brain-targeted drug delivery by inhibiting efflux pumps. ATP-binding cassette (ABC) transporters are overexpressed in BBB, such as ABCB1 (multidrug resistance proteins, MDR1 or P-gp), ABCC (multidrug resistance-associated protein, MRPs), and ABCG2 (breast cancer resistance protein, BCRP). Therefore, in Chapter 8, Dr. Chen et al. reviewed the current developed strategies to inhibit these efflux pumps using nanoparticles to improve brain-targeted drug delivery.

In addition to penetrating through BBB, the brain-targeted drug delivery could also be achieved by bypass BBB or temporarily open BBB. After intranasal administration, drugs and nanoparticles could be transported to brain by olfactory nerve pathway, trigeminal nerve pathway, and cerebrospinal fluid (CSF) pathway. Since the intranasal administration could avoid the BBB, it has been served as a noninvasive strategy for CNS disorders treatment. In Chapter 10, Dr. Liu and Dr. Zhang reviewed the anatomy of the nasal cavity, pathways for nose-to-brain drug delivery, and then various nanoparticles that are developed for intranasal brain-targeted drug delivery. What's more, the problems faced in nose-to-brain drug delivery were carefully discussed. Open BBB is an alternative strategy for brain-targeted drug delivery. Since BBB, especially tight junctions in BBB, restricted the penetration of compounds and particles, there are several methods that can temporarily work on tight junctions, either chemically or physically, to disrupt the function of BBB and improve drug delivery across BBB. In Chapter 9, Dr. Hu et al. reviewed the methods involved in temporarily open BBB, including pretreatment with compounds, such as hyperosmolar mannitol, borneol, lexiscan, alkylglycerols, C-type natriuretic peptide, lipopolysaccharide, bradykinin, and bradykinin analog, and physically open BBB, such as focused ultrasound, electromagnetic field exposure, photodynamic therapy, and photochemical internalization. In addition, brain local administration could directly inject drugs and nanoparticles into brain, which is also used for CNS disorders treatment, especially in clinic. In Chapter 11, Dr. Khan et al. reviewed the current developed strategies to improve the brain's local drug delivery efficiency.

Encouraged by the strategies that overcome the BBB, many DDSs were developed to diagnose and treat CNS disorders. Therefore, in Chapters 12–14, several contributors and the drug delivery strategies for brain tumor were reviewed, Alzheimer's disease, Parkinson's disease, stroke, and CNS inflammation. In these chapters, the physical and pathological characters of these diseases were reviewed, and then the drug delivery strategies were carefully reviewed and discussed.

2 What's the major concerns of brain-targeted DDS?

Although great achievement has been made, there are still many unmet concerns for brain-targeted DDS. The first one is the neurotoxicity of the DDS. In most studies, the neurotoxicity was not paid enough attention, while most neurotoxicity studies were evaluated on inorganic or metal-contained nanoparticles or cationic polymers. In Chapter 15, Dr. Li et al. reviewed the in vitro and in vivo neurotoxicity of nanoparticles to neurons, astrocytes, microglia, and other neuronal cells. Then the physical chemical mechanisms of the nanotoxicity were discussed, which was influenced by the particle size, shape, and surface charge. Furthermore, the cellular mechanism behind the neurotoxicity was discussed, including apoptosis, necrosis, autophagy, NETosis, pyroptosis, and cell cycle arrest; while the molecular mechanisms behind the neurotoxicity involved oxidative stress, DNA damage, and several signal pathways. All these mechanisms were contributed to the neurotoxicity of brain-targeted DDS, which required in-depth evaluation.

The second concern is the intra-brain distribution. In Chapter 16, Dr. Huang et al. reviewed the anatomic characteristics of brain, such as brain extracellular microenvironment, blood and lymphatics circulation, and blood-brain and blood-CSF barriers, then the diffusion in the CSF and extracellular space were reviewed and the factors that influenced the diffusion were discussed. Last one is the excretion of brain-targeted DDS from brain, which was important for the biocompatibility and safety of the brain-targeted DDS. In Chapter 17, Dr. Gao et al. further discussed the excretion of particles from brain. Three routes are involved in the brain clearance of nanoparticles: a. degradation in the brain, b. entering CSF circulation mediated by the convective bulk flow, and then cleared from the CNS to the bloodstream or the cervical lymphatics, and c. brain-to-blood efflux. After entering blood, the nanoparticles could be further excreted from body by renal and hepatic clearance pathways. During the elimination, several factors influence the behavior of nanoparticles, including particle size, shape, matrix materials, and surface properties of nanoparticles and physiological conditions of the body.

Apart from the above-mentioned three concerns, in Chapter 18, I also systemically discussed the problems faced in brain targeting drug delivery, including targeting specificity, off-target potential, BBB penetration capacity, intra-brain distribution, and brain cell type selectivity as well as neurotoxicity. The progress and things that can help in these areas were discussed.

3 Conclusion

This book is prepared with the purpose of benefiting nanomaterial and nanomedicine researchers in the following areas:

- Fundamental knowledge about physiological characters of brain and BBB, concept, main routes, and mechanisms about brain-targeted drug delivery;
- Progress in developing brain-targeted DDS for the diagnosis and treatment of various CNS disorders;
- Major concerns in preparing and evaluating brain-targeted DDS.

The valuable insights shared by chapter authors are intended to expand the fundamental knowledge about brain-targeted drug delivery, progress, and concerns in developing brain-targeted DDS. Researchers from all related fields may further develop the DDS with better brain distribution and CNS disorder selectivity and better satisfaction for human beings.

Part I

Physiology and principles for brain targeting drug delivery

Anatomy and physiology of blood-brain barrier

2

Smriti Gupta, Saurabh Dhanda, Rajat Sandhir
Department of Biochemistry, Panjab University, Chandigarh, India

1 Introduction

Central nervous system (CNS), being the most critical and sensitive organ in the human body, necessitates a highly regulated extracellular environment, wherein the concentration of ions such as Na^+, K^+, and Ca^{2+} as well as different metabolites must be maintained within a narrow range for proper neuronal functions (Rolfe and Brown, 1997). Brain constitutes only 2% of the body weight, but utilizes 20% of the total blood supply. A uniquely complex network of blood vessels extending up to 650 km and spanning a surface area of about 20 m^2 delivers blood to the CNS. However, unlike all other organs of the body where a free exchange occurs between the blood and the interstitial fluid, the capillaries of the CNS have evolved to restrain the movement of molecules and cells between blood and the brain. Hence, most of the molecules must take a transcellular route to enter the brain, as a result of which majority of small molecules, peptides, proteins, RBCs, and leukocytes cannot cross the interface between blood and the CNS (Palmer, 2010). Therefore, a dynamic regulator of ion balance, a facilitator of nutrient transport and a barrier to potentially harmful molecules, is essential that acts as an interface between the CNS and peripheral circulatory system. This homeostatic and dynamic function of cerebral microcirculation is performed by the blood-brain barrier (BBB) (Hawkins and Davis, 2005). BBB also protects CNS against various neurotoxic substances and infective agents circulating in the blood.

The site of the BBB is CNS capillaries consisting of a single, nonfenestrated, continuous layer of specialized endothelial cell. These endothelial cells are highly polarized with distinct apical (luminal) and basolateral (abluminal) compartments (Betz and Goldstein, 1978). The high polarity of the CNS endothelial cells is exhibited in their four vital barrier properties that contributes to the proper functioning and integrity of the BBB (Daneman and Prat, 2015). CNS endothelial cells present between the circumferential tight junction complexes, create a high-resistance paracellular barrier to ions and small hydrophilic molecules (Brightman and Reese, 1969; McDonald and Potter, 1951). Tight junction complexes are composed of (a) tight junction proteins such as occludin and claudin; (b) adhesion junctions like epithelial-cadherin (E-cadherin), vascular endothelial-cadherin (VE-cadherin) and (c) junctional adhesion molecules (JAMs) (Liu et al., 2012; Siegenthaler et al., 2013). These transmembrane proteins are further stabilized and connected to the

Brain Targeted Drug Delivery Systems. https://doi.org/10.1016/B978-0-12-814001-7.00002-0

adaptor proteins like zona occludens (ZOs) present inside the cytoplasm (Balda and Matter, 2009). Studies have shown that a significant crosstalk occurs between these tight junction complexes to maintain the restrictive barrier junction (Tietz and Engelhardt, 2015). Secondly, the endothelial cells of CNS exhibit minimal vesicular trafficking (transcytosis), thus limiting the vesicle-mediated transcellular movement of cargo known as transcytosis (Tuma and Hubbard, 2003). Thirdly, the formation of restricting paracellular and transcellular barrier allows endothelial cells of the CNS to employ highly polarized cellular transporters to dynamically control the influx of nutrients like glucose through glucose transporter 1 (GLUT 1) and efflux of toxins and metabolic wastes between blood and the CNS through ATP-binding cassette (ABC) transporters (Chow and Gu, 2015). Lastly, the endothelial cells of the CNS lack leukocyte adhesion molecules which prevent the entry of immune cells from the blood into the CNS, resulting in healthy brain being immune-privileged (Engelhardt and Ransohoff, 2012; Feldt Muldoon et al., 2013; Ransohoff and Engelhardt, 2012).

2 Concept of blood-brain barrier

Unlike nonneural tissues, where endothelium of the capillary walls is permeable to ions and electrolytes, neural tissues are partitioned by restrictive endothelium that is very selective for the entry of molecules from blood to the brain. This complex physiological phenomenon is known as BBB (Katzman and Pappius, 1973). BBB is a highly regulated interface between peripheral circulation and CNS. BBB affords CNS a 'privileged' microenvironment and protects it from abrupt fluctuations in plasma components that may disturb neuronal functions (Lawther et al., 2011). Controlled reversible opening of BBB in the presence of some local agents is essential for normal physiological functions, and disruption in pathological conditions lead to detrimental consequences (Lawther et al., 2011).

In 1909, Goldmann observed the failure of intravenously administered dye, trypan blue, to stain the brain and spinal cord tissue and suggested the presence of a mechanical membrane separating blood from the brain that is now known as BBB (Goldmann, 1909). In 1913, Goldmann further suggested that such a barrier did not exist between the cerebrospinal fluid (CSF) and brain (Liddelow, 2011). These pioneer experiments led to the hypothesis that there is a mechanism that protects brain from peripheral circulation. Lewandowsky for the first time in 1990, coined the term BBB for this phenomenon, but the idea of the existence of this barrier was not clear until much later (Tschirgi, 1950). BBB holds three barrier layers that isolate neural tissues from the blood: (1) highly specialized layer of endothelial cells that partitions blood and interstitial fluid, (2) choroid plexus epithelium that secretes CSF into the ventricles, and (3) arachnoid epithelium which further separates blood from CSF in the subarachnoid spaces (Abbott et al., 2006). Initial physiological studies suggested that the BBB is impermeable, whereas it is now well-established that BBB has specific transport systems that allow active transport of ions, carrier-mediated transport of glucose (Yudilevich and De Rose, 1971), and amino acids (Davson, 1976; Oldendorf, 1973); however, it prohibits the entry of plasma components, red blood cells, and leukocytes to the brain. Pathological conditions disrupt selective permeability of BBB and result in compromised CNS functions (Abbott et al., 2006; Hawkins and Davis, 2005; Zlokovic, 2005). Brain capillary endothelium provides the surface area for blood-brain exchange and complex tight junctions between adjacent endothelial cells channelize molecular trafficking through transcellular route across the BBB (Abbott et al., 2006). BBB separates the reservoir of neurotransmitters and neuroactive agents centrally and peripherally to avoid any type of crosstalk between these two systems (Abbott et al., 2006). Endothelial lining with the surface area of $\sim$20 m^2 per 1.3 kg brain plays a remarkable role in maintaining the brain microenvironment.

3 Neurovascular unit

Neurovascular unit is the building block that encompasses astrocytes, pericytes, neurons, and the extracellular matrix, which all together serve to maintaining CNS homeostasis as well as protect the underlying cells (Neuwelt, 2004; Wang et al., 2004). BBB is characterized by the presence of tight junction complexes in the inter-endothelial space that includes tight junction proteins (Vorbrodt and Dobrogowska, 2003), adhesion junctions (Schulze and Firth, 1993), JAMs (Dejana et al., 2000), and accessory proteins. The neurovascular unit helps in understanding brain responses to cerebrovascular pathology as well as multiple pathways that regulate microvascular permeability in disease conditions (Lo et al., 2004). Lining the intraluminal portion of blood capillaries, BBB is composed up of specialized endothelial cells and provides dynamic functional value to the CNS. BBB is a high-security structural as well as functional unit which refers to a closed association of endothelial cells, extracellular matrix, basal lamina, pericytes, closely juxtaposed neurons, and astrocytes (Huber et al., 2001). Intracellular communications between the building blocks of BBB regulate the maintenance and influence the permeability of BBB (Mulligan and MacVicar, 2004). Major function of neurovascular unit is to regulate the transport and diffusion through endothelial cells of brain capillaries (Staddon and Rubin, 1996). Apart from basic neurovascular unit, some other modular structures are present in the BBB that are recognized as gliovascular unit. In gliovascular unit, each astrocyte provides trophic support to neuronal population via their end feet processes. Astrocytes have different levels of organization in the CNS. Astrocytic interaction with the vasculature system comes under gliovascular network and such repeated astrocytic domains form the primary structure (Banerjee and Bhat, 2007). In between these astrocytic domains and adjacent astrocytic feet, microvessels are positioned which form the secondary organization (Banerjee and Bhat, 2007). Interspersed neurons among these astrocytic domains and glial processes provide higher level of structural complexity (Nedergaard et al., 2003; Simard et al., 2003). Initially, astrocytes were recognized as passive members of CNS that provide trophic support to the neurons, but now they are a recognized bidirectional communication partners in the CNS. Glia receives signals from neurons and releases neuroactive substances in the internal milieu (Araque et al., 2000). Moreover, astrocytes have also gained attention for their

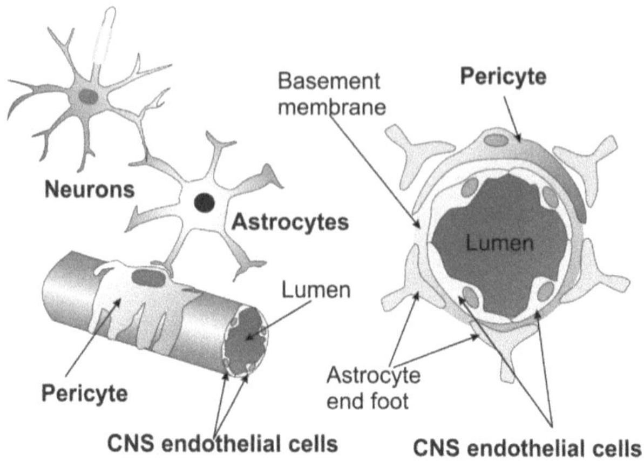

Fig. 1 Schematic representation of BBB anatomy. BBB is formed of endothelial cells that line CNS microvessels and sealed by tight junctions. The astrocytes, pericytes, and basement membranes interact with the endothelium of the BBB, providing functional and structural support.

role in brain remodelling and plasticity (Kirchhoff et al., 2001). Structure of BBB is illustrated in Fig. 1, which includes different cellular and protein components.

BBB is a complex dynamic structure that is highly regulated by transmembrane proteins (JAMs, occludin, and claudins) and cytoplasmic accessory proteins (ZO-1, ZO-2, cingulin, AF-6, and 7H6). These components glue the endothelial lining and allow polar molecules to pass through BBB. JAMs are known to regulate tight junction properties. Claudin proteins facilitate tight barrier capabilities, while occludins and ZO-1 regulate targeted signaling.

3.1 Occludin

A vast range of structural and signaling proteins have been identified at the tight junctions (Guillemot et al., 2008). Claudin family has different member proteins having differential expression at the tight junctions, while occludin is an invariably expressed in all epithelial and endothelial tight junctions (Van Itallie and Anderson, 2006). Occludin is a 60–65 kDa protein that has four transmembrane domains, with its carboxyl and amino terminals oriented to the cytoplasm and two extracellular loops traversing the intercellular cleft (Furuse et al., 1993). It is present uniformly along the margins of CNS endothelial cells (Hawkins et al., 2004). The cytoplasmic C-terminal domain of occludin is associated with the cytoskeleton of the endothelial cell via accessory proteins (Rodgers and Fanning, 2011). An increase in the paracellular permeability to low molecular weight molecules can be accounted for expression of C-terminal-truncated versions of occludin (Balda et al., 1996). Balda et al. (2000) demonstrated that occludin regulates the functions of tight junction barrier.

Occludin is known to increase the electrical resistance of BBB, a property attributed to its second extracellular loop domain (McCarthy et al., 1996; Wong and Gumbiner, 1997). Studies with null phenotypes have shown abnormalities in many organs. However, occludin knockout mouse-based study showed normal structure and function of tight junctions (Schulzke et al., 2005). Occludin is involved in endocytosis and protein trafficking (Yu and Turner, 2008). Other than its putative role in protein trafficking, occludin also interacts with the cholesterol-binding protein caveolin-1 (Lynch et al., 2007). Moreover, decreased occludin expression is associated with disrupted BBB in a number of pathological conditions (Hawkins and Davis, 2005).

3.2 Claudin

Claudins are the tight junction proteins, involved in the establishment of barrier properties (Morita et al., 1999) and help to maintain the specificity of tight junction permeability (Angelow et al., 2008). The word Claudin is derived from the Latin word "*claudere*" which means "*to stand*" (Findley and Koval, 2009). Claudins are 20–24 kDa proteins having membrane topography similar to that of occludin but do not share any sequence homology (Hawkins and Davis, 2005). All the claudins express a high-sequence homology among themselves in the first and fourth transmembrane domains and extracellular loops (Heiskala et al., 2001). It is believed that claudins form a primary "seal" of tight junction complex with occludin acting as an additional support protein. CNS endothelial cells primarily contain claudin-1, claudin-3, and claudin-5 (Hawkins and Davis, 2005). Mutagenic assays showed that extracellular loops of claudin determines the selectivity for ions (Colegio et al., 2002). Initially, claudin 1 and claudin 5 were detected in endothelial cells. Paracellular activity of tight junctions is influenced by 52 residue extracellular loop with a highly conserved signature motif [Gly-Leu-Trp-xx- Cys-(8-10aa)-Cys] (Van Itallie and Anderson, 2006). A molecular study of 16-33 residue long second extracellular loop suggested its role in claudin-claudin interactions. Epithelia has many isoforms of claudin which interact and form strands at the tight junctions (Findley and Koval, 2009). It is evident that intracellular transport through tight junctions and its stability depends on the claudin protein (Rüffer and Gerke, 2004). C-terminal domain of the claudin protein gets phosphorylated and provides the barrier function to the tight junctions (Müller et al., 2006). Cyclic AMP has been shown to phosphorylate thr-207 residue in claudin 5 and improve the barrier functions of the endothelium (Ishizaki et al., 2003). There are many kinases known to phosphorylate claudin proteins and regulate their localization and function (Gonçalves et al., 2013). Besides phosphorylation, claudins undergo several other modifications such as palmitoylation that occur at conserved di-cysteine motifs (Van Itallie et al., 2005). Palmitoylation of these motifs lodges claudin 2, claudin 4, and claudin 14 to tight junctions (Van Itallie et al., 2005). At the C-terminus, claudin has PDZ-binding motifs that interact with some cytoplasmic scaffold proteins through their PDZ domains. These cytoplasmic scaffold proteins are ZO-1/2/3 and multi-PDZ domain protein 1 (MUPP1) (Hamazaki et al., 2002). Expression of claudin subtypes varies with cell type and developmental stages which further vary in barrier properties (Krause et al., 2008). These subtypes are claudin 1, claudin 3,

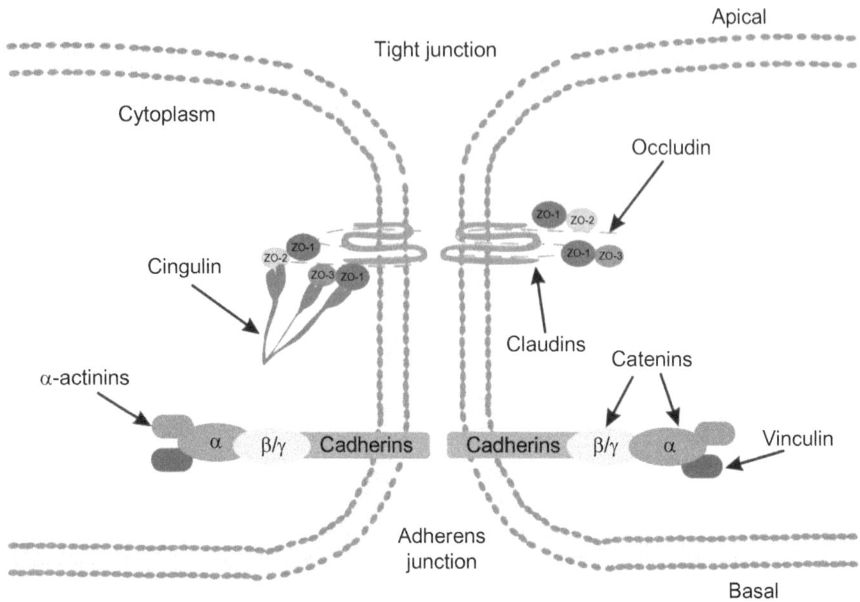

Fig. 2 Schematic representation of tight junction complexes between two adjacent endothelial cells. Tight junction complex is composed of occludin and claudin proteins, adhesion junctions (integral membrane-bound cadherins and cytoplasmic accessory proteins, i.e., α and β catenin), JAM-1, and accessory proteins (ZO-1, ZO-2, ZO-3).

and claudin 5 which are further recognized as sealing or barrier-forming claudins (Ohtsuki et al., 2008). Studies showed that claudin-11-deficient mice had myelination defects (Gow et al., 1999). Arrangement of different tight junction proteins is illustrated in Fig. 2.

3.3 *Adhesion junctions*

The adhesion of endothelial cells to each other is mediated by the presence of adhesion molecules that are ubiquitous in the vasculature. These molecules play an important role in vascular growth, remodelling endothelial polarity and to certain extent in the regulation of paracellular permeability (Bazzoni and Dejana, 2004; Hawkins and Davis, 2005). The major component of adhesion junctions is VE-cadherin, a Ca^{2+} regulated protein that facilitates cell-cell adhesion via homophilic interactions between the extracellular domains of proteins expressed in the neighboring cells (Vincent et al., 2004). The stabilization of adhesion molecules-mediated cell-cell association is dependent on the binding of the VE-cadherin to β-catenin and plakoglobin, which in turn bind to the actin cytoskeleton via α-catenin, α-actinin, and vinculin (Lampugnani et al., 1995; Watabe-Uchida et al., 1998).

3.4 Junctional adhesion molecules

JAM is the transmembrane component of the tight junctions at the BBB (Del Maschio et al., 1999). JAM-1 a 40-kDa protein is a member of the immunoglobulin G (IgG) superfamily. It is believed to facilitate the early attachment of adjacent endothelial cell membranes via homophilic interactions (Dejana et al., 2000). It consists of a single membrane traversing chain with a large extracellular domain (Martìn-Padura et al., 1998). Although the exact role of JAM-1 in mature BBB is not fully understood, it is suggested to be involved in the trans-endothelial migration of leukocytes (Del Maschio et al., 1999). First isoform of JAM, i.e., JAM-A, was identified using anti-endothelial antigen antibodies (Martìn-Padura et al., 1998). JAMs are glycosylated and primarily located at tight junctions, where they form cell-cell contact between endothelial and epithelial cell (Bazzoni et al., 2000; Liu et al., 2000). Glycosylated JAMs have two domains, an extracellular variable type Ig domain and a transmembrane domain. At its C-terminus, JAM-A contains type II PDZ-binding motif through which it interacts with cytoplasmic proteins (Bazzoni et al., 2000). Subsequently, after discovery of JAM-A, JAM-B and JAM-C have also been characterized (Aurrand-Lions et al., 2001). It is reported from human studies that null mutation of JAM-C resulted in intracerebral hemorrhages, subependymal calcification, and congenital cataracts (Mochida et al., 2010).

3.5 Accessory proteins

Several accessory proteins are associated with components of tight junction complex. These mainly include the members of the membrane-associated guanylate kinase-like (MAGUK) protein homolog family. These proteins contain multiple postsynaptic density protein-95/discs-large/ZO-1-binding domains, an Src homolog-3 domain, and a guanylate kinase-like domain enabling multiple protein-protein interactions (Chung-Kwan Shin et al., 2000). MAGUK proteins are involved in clustering of protein complexes to the cell membrane along with the creation of specialized domains within the endothelial cell membranes (Gonzalez-Mariscal et al., 2000). The major MAGUK proteins identified at the tight junction complex are ZO-1, zona occludin-2 (ZO-2), and zona occludin-3 (ZO-3). ZO-1 is a 220-kDa phosphoprotein expressed in endothelial cells and has been found to be associated with adhesion molecules and gap junction proteins (Toyofuku et al., 1998). ZO-1 links the transmembrane proteins of tight junction complex to the actin cytoskeleton of the cells which is critical for the stability and proper functioning of tight junction proteins. Dissociation of ZO-1 from the junctional complex is often associated with enhanced permeability (Fischer et al., 2002). ZO-1 can also communicate the state of the tight junction complex to the interior of the endothelial cell or vice versa, in turn acting as a signaling molecule. Moreover, under conditions of proliferation and injury, ZO-1 has also been shown to localize inside the nucleus of endothelial cells (Gottardi et al., 1996). ZO-2 is a 160-kDa phosphoprotein with a high-sequence homology to ZO-1. Apart from binding to the structural components of tight junction complexes, it can also bind to the signaling molecules such as transcription factors and localize into the nucleus during conditions of stress and proliferation (Betanzos et al., 2004). ZO-3 is a 130-kDa homolog that has been found in tight junctions in some tissues, but not in the BBB (Inoko et al., 2003).

3.6 Pericytes

Pericytes were first described by Rouget in 1870, as perivascular cells sharing the basement membrane with adjacent capillaries (Trost et al., 2016). In CNS, pericytes are considered as second line of defense and have macrophage functions. Pericytes have various functions in CNS such as they are source of BBB-specific enzymes, have potential to modulate endothelial permeability, stabilize microvessel wall, and promote angiogenic processes (Daneman and Prat, 2015). Pericytes create an interface between the circulatory system and surrounding tissue (Hirschi and D'Amore, 1996). Enveloped in the basement membrane, pericytes have intimate association with endothelial cells which demarcates them from smooth muscle cells. *In vitro* studies suggest that basement membrane is produced by pericytes and endothelial cells (Stratman and Davis, 2012). Pericytes play a key role in providing vasodynamic property as well as structural support to the microvasculature. In genetic cases of cerebral hemorrhage and amyloidosis, degeneration of pericytes has been observed that suggests its important role in structural integrity of microvessels (Verbeek et al., 1997). Besides providing structural support, pericytes also express many cell surface receptors for different endogenous chemical mediators such as catecholamines, vasopressin, and angiotensin II (Healy and Wilk, 1993; van Zwieten et al., 1988). *In vitro* studies have revealed that pericytes prevent apoptosis in endothelium and stabilize capillary-like structures present at the BBB (Ramsauer et al., 2002). A number of experimental studies suggest role of pericytes in BBB differentiation and angiogenesis (Balabanov et al., 1999). Pericytes are also known to exhibit neuroimmune function with phagocytic activity (Balabanov et al., 1996).

Loss of pericytes leads to impaired brain perfusion, disturbed vaso-reactivity, and leakiness of BBB that all together results in memory and cognitive deficits with age-dependent neuroinflammation (Bell et al., 2010). The exact role of pericytes at the BBB is yet to be elucidated however; the presence of contractile proteins suggests that they might be involved in regulating capillary blood flow (Bandopadhyay et al., 2001). In pathological conditions (hypoxia and traumatic brain injury) associated with increased BBB permeability, pericytes have also been shown to migrate away from the CNS microvessels (Dore-Duffy et al., 2000; Gonul et al., 2002). Additionally, angiopoietin derived from pericytes can induce the expression of occludin in endothelial cells of CNS, indicating that pericytes are involved in the induction and/or maintenance of barrier properties of CNS endothelium in a manner similar to that of glia (Hori et al., 2004). In addition to providing structural support to the CNS, pericytes have also functional significance in BBB. Endothelial culture-based study showed that, like astrocytes, pericytes are involved in the tightening of paracellular barrier (Dohgu et al., 2005). Deli et al. (2005) confirmed in a coculture study that barrier integrity of cerebral endothelial monolayers is strengthened by pericytes. Analogues to anatomical situation in cerebral microvessels, endothelial-pericytes, and astrocytic triple co-culture model showed maximum BBB integrity as compared to the other models of BBB (Nakagawa et al., 2007).

3.7 Neurons

The dynamic nature of neural activity and the substantial metabolic needs of nervous tissue are served by the BBB. The communication between neurons and the vasculature regulate blood flow as well as BBB permeability. This can be attributed to the fact that CNS endothelial cells in association with astrocytic processes are directly innervated by noradrenergic, serotonergic, and cholinergic neurons (Cohen et al., 1997). Neurons are critical in regulating the function of BBB, but their role in the development of the BBB phenotype is yet to be identified. BBB plays a significant role in maintaining brain neurochemical milieu and neuronal activity (Marchi et al., 2007).

3.8 Extracellular matrix

The extracellular matrix serves as an anchor for the endothelial cells via interaction of matrix proteins (laminin) with endothelial integrin receptors that can also stimulate a number of intracellular signaling pathways (Hynes, 1992). The expression of tight junction complexes can also be regulated by matrix proteins, signifying that although the tight junction complexes constitute primary impediment to paracellular diffusion, the proteins of the basal lamina are also involved in their maintenance (Savettieri et al., 2000). Moreover, disruption of the extracellular matrix is strongly associated with increased BBB permeability in pathological conditions (Rascher et al., 2002).

4 Role of astrocytes

Astrocytes play a critical role in the development and maintenance of BBB (Davson and Oldendorf, 1967). Astrocytes, alone or in combination with neurons, act as mediators in regulation of CNS microvascular permeability (Ballabh et al., 2004). Besides providing trophic support, astrocytes are involved in water and ion balance regulation at BBB interface. Astrocytic projections are known as astrocytic end feet, which is a complex gliovascular system that controls the homeostasis of the CNS. This process is carried out by a dynamic Ca^{2+} signaling between astrocytes and the CNS endothelial cells via gap junctions and purinergic transmission (Dhanda and Sandhir, 2018). The end feet process of the astrocytes tightly ensheath pericytes and endothelial cell wall and release trophic factors that are essential for the induction and maintenance of BBB. Astrocytic foot processes contain water channels (aquaporins) and under pathological conditions, are associated with brain edema (Zonta et al., 2003).

Microenvironment of the CNS induces endothelial cells to form BBB and incorporate the barrier properties to the blood vessels. Astrocytic end feet interacts with pericytes and endothelial cells (Serlin et al., 2015). Astrocytes maintain the homeostasis of transmitters, metabolites, ions, and water. Synaptic neurotransmission and neuronal plasticity is dependent upon astrocytic population in the CNS (Wong et al., 2013). Evidence from a study wherein avascular tissue from 3-day old quail brain was planted into the coelomic cavity of chick embryo and it resulted into the vascularization of the quail brain grafts forming a competent BBB (Abbott et al., 2006). In contrast, transplantation of these embryonic quail coelomic grafts in the chick brain led the endothelial cells to form leaky capillaries and venules. It was also observed that astrocytic culture implanted in the area of these leaky vessels resulted into the tightening of endothelium (Janzer and Raff, 1987). In addition to the long-term inductive signaling between endothelium and astrocytes, there are many short cell to cell signaling pathways existing in astrocytes (Berzin et al., 2000; Nicchia et al., 2004). These signaling pathways are the basis of BBB physiology which provide the evolutionary significance to the direct contact between astrocytes and endothelial cells. Astrocytes have syncytium like organization which is extensively coupled by gap junctions (Reisin and Colombo, 2002). Electron microscopical and freeze-fracture studies in mammals showed clear association between astrocytes and gap junctions (Massa and Mugnaini, 1982). Expression of various gap junctions was also observed in primary cultures of astrocytes and these findings suggested that the gap junctions are important constituents of astrocytes and play an important role in physiology of BBB (Massa and Mugnaini, 1985). Astrocytic feet function as gliovascular system and, apart from trophic support, these cell populations are involved in the regulation of water-ion balance in the CNS. This osmotic balance between astrocytes and CNS endothelial cells is maintained by gap junctions and purinergic transmission (Zonta et al., 2003). The end feet of the astrocytic cells tightly ensheath the pericytes and the endothelial cell wall and releases trophic factors that are essential for the induction and maintenance of BBB. Astrocytic foot processes also contain water channels (aquaporins) that allow for the uptake of water and, in pathological conditions, are associated with brain swelling (Zonta et al., 2003).

Astrocytes support neurons and in turn extent and architecture of astrocytes are maintained by neurons (Rouach et al., 2000). Astrocytic surface expresses receptors for various neurotransmitters and neuromodulators and their end feet processes surround synaptic buttons and collaborate with them for neuronal signal transduction (Frerking, 2004; Singh et al., 2015). Although extensive work has been done regarding functional domains of astrocytic functions, the cellular mechanisms of the interaction between endothelial cells and their environment are yet to be fully elucidated. Astrocytes have dense array of processes that are highly fibrous structures interspersed between neurons and vascular walls, where they couple with neurons and play important role in metabolic activity (Pellerin et al., 1998). Endothelial cells have BBB characteristics prior to astrocytic differentiation which showed that astrocytes are not the sole basis of establishment of BBB. As astrocytes are required for synaptic modulation and networking, their number is strikingly higher as compared to the neurons (Nedergaard et al., 2003).

5 Transportation across blood-brain barrier

BBB, choroid plexus, and arachnoid epithelium form the physical and immunological barrier of the brain. These barriers are functional in both directions from blood to the brain and vice versa. Restrictive nature of the BBB is due to the presence of tight junctions. Tight junctions positioned at the barrier allow diffusion of many gases as well as gaseous anesthetics, but restrict the entry of polar solutes. Small molecules like glucose and amino acids are transported through the respective transporters, while larger molecules are passed through receptor-mediated endocytosis (Zhang and Pardridge, 2001). It is also notable that 98% of all small molecules are not freely transported through the BBB (Pardridge, 2005). Generally, BBB is permeable to water, but lipid-soluble molecules can also pass through it by simple diffusion. BBB is also known to regulate the entry of leucocytes and is found to be involved in CNS surveillance and reactivity. Entry of leucocytes into the CNS is achieved by integrin proteins and adhesion molecules such as intercellular adhesion molecule 1 (ICAM-1), vascular cell adhesion molecule 1 (VCAM-1), and platelet endothelial cell adhesion molecule (PECAM-1) (Greenwood et al., 2003; Laschinger and Engelhardt, 2000). BBB expresses some multidrug transporters that limit the entry as well as concentration of different drugs inside the CNS. Under some cases, up-regulation of some transporters on the barrier surface leads to impaired uptake of drug by the brain and results in treatment failures (Potschka, 2010).

6 Types of transport systems at blood-brain barrier

BBB expresses tight junctions and different transport systems that serve to transport various physiological requirements to the brain such as glucose, amino acids, and ions as well as different xenobiotics included drugs and their respective metabolites (Tsuji, 2005). Fig. 3 depicts different modes of transport for various molecules from blood to the brain. Essential polar molecules that are incapable of diffusing through the cell membrane, such as glucose, amino acids, and nucleosides, may pass through BBB via passive or secondary active transport mechanisms (Serlin et al., 2015).

6.1 Amino acid transport

Amino acid transporters function at the BBB to maintain homeostasis of amino acids, neurotransmitters and peptides. All essential amino acids need to be transferred from blood to the brain through various types of transporters. Sodium dependency and the substrate specificity are two functional characteristics of amino acids and, on the basis of these criteria, transporters for amino acids have been characterized (Tsuji, 2005). System L is a specific type of sodium-independent transport system which has broad range of substrate specificity that includes large neutral amino acids, notably tryptophan, tyrosine, and branched-chain amino acids (Tsuji, 2005). The wide range of substrate selectivity of the L system makes it an important mechanism for drug delivery to

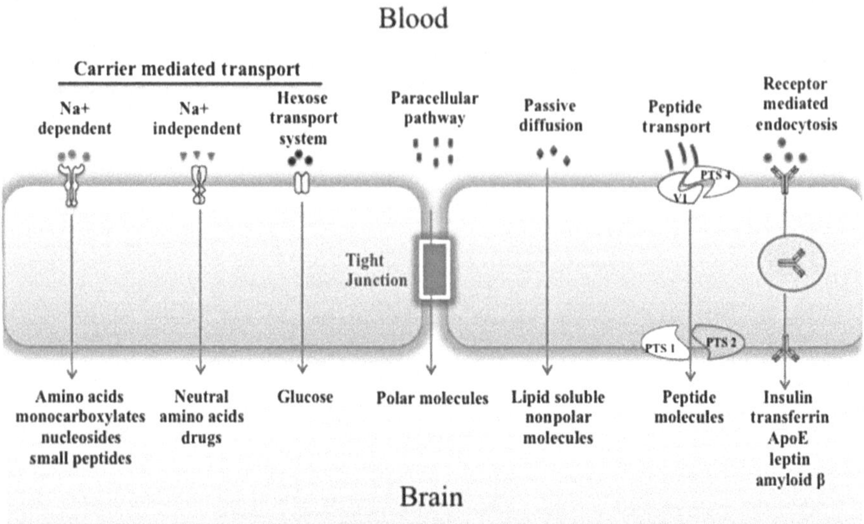

Fig. 3 Schematic representation of transport mechanisms involved in movement of molecules across the BBB.

the brain (Tsuji, 2005). Various drugs like levodopa, baclofen, and gabapentin are reported to cross through this system. Two major families of proteins are responsible for the transport of cationic amino acids (a) system y+, and (b) systems b0, +, B0,), and y+L (Barar et al., 2016a, b). Interestingly, BBB is found to be impermeable to neuroactive amino acids, aspartate and glutamate. BBB encompasses paracellular barrier capacity that limits the transport of monoamines. Homeostasis of brain neurochemical milieu and neurotransmitters levels are maintained by influx rate across BBB and synthesis of different neurotransmitters such as serotonin, dopamine, and histamine (Smith and Takasato, 1986).

6.2 Hexose transport system

Hexose transport system is a family of transporters that allows movement of structural analogous of hexose across the BBB. Glucose, the sole energy source, is transferred through these transporters. These transporters apparently have high capacity of transferring drugs due to its significantly higher capacity of transferring glucose than other transporters (Pardridge, 1983). These hexose transporters are classified under two categories: (1) Sodium-dependent transporter that is secondary active transport system. (2) Sodium-independent transporter or facilitated transporter which are molecularly classified into sodium-glucose transport proteins (SGLT)/SLC5 and GLUT/SLC2A families, respectively. It has been observed that *GLUT1* gene is selectively expressed in the brain capillary endothelial cells, where 100% of the glucose transporter-binding sites at the BBB can be attributed to the GLUT1 isoform that functions to transport glucose independent of insulin (Pardridge et al., 1990). These transporters are membrane spanning glycoproteins containing 12 transmembrane domains and play a vital role in glucose uptake in brain (Carruthers et al., 2009). Hypoglycemic conditions inside the cells leads to up-regulation of GLUT1 transporters (Devaskar et al., 1991). Transport of sugar across the BBB and brain energy status can be controlled by the regulation of surface GLUT1 expression (Simpson et al., 2001). From the clinical perspective, GLUT1 is highly upregulated at BBB in patients with seizures and downregulated in Alzheimer's disease and diabetes (Barar et al., 2016a, b). We have also observed the decreased mRNA expression of these GLUTs (GLUT1 and GLUT3) in *in vitro* and *in vivo* models of sporadic Alzheimer's disease (Gupta et al., 2018). In addition, it has been observed that mutations in GLUT1 may lead to deficiencies in the transportation of glucose in the related disorders. Other than GLUT1, GLUT4 and neuron-specific GLUT3 transporter are expressed for regulated glucose uptake inside cell. These transporters have significance in the delivery of membrane-impermeable compounds and drugs that are structural analogues of sugar. It is proposed that glycosylation of peptides helps in stabilizing the peptides which assist their penetration through BBB (Negri et al., 1998).

6.3 Monocarboxylate transporter system

Metabolic by-products and various energy substrates such as lactate, which are structurally monocarboxylates, need a regulated uptake and efflux. Presence of monocarboxylate transporters (MCTs) at BBB is suggested by many *in vivo* studies which is further demonstrated by stereospecific transport of lactate (Sankar and Sotero de Menezes, 1999). This transporter system is also common for acetate (Gerhart et al., 1997), propionate, butyrate, benzoic acid, salicylic acid, nicotinic acid, and some antibiotics (Kang et al., 1990). Eight members of MCT family have been identified in different species which are tissue specific (Enerson and Drewes, 2003). MCT1 transporters are involved in the transport of molecules with molecular weight approximately 200 Da. Of these, the MCT1, MCT2, MCT3, and MCT4 catalyze the proton-linked transport of monocarboxylates (e.g., L-lactate) across the plasma membrane. MCT8 and MCT10 are involved in the transportation of thyroid hormones and some aromatic aromatic amino acids through the BBB respectively. MCT1 is expressed in epithelium of small intestine and colon which provides the mechanism for blood to brain and brain to blood transfer of various pharmaceuticals that are structural analogues of monocarboxylates.

6.4 Organic anion transporter family

Organic anion transporters (OAT) are reported to play an important role in transport of several organic anions in brain. There are various OAT which are specific for the transport of peptides and are known as OATPs such as rOatp1 (SLC21A1) and rOtp2 (SLC21A4) in rats and hOatp-A (SLC21A3) in humans (Gao et al., 1999; Hagenbuch et al., 2002). OATPs are tissue-specific and, in intestine, Oatp-B is the predominant type (Nozawa et al., 2004). Although the role of Oatp-B in brain is not clear, some reports showed that it transports simvastatin and lovastatin that are known inhibitors of 3-hydroxy-3-methylglutaryl (HMG)-CoA reductase and are used for the treatment of sleeping disorders (Tsuji, 2005).

6.5 Organic cation transporter (OCT and OCTN) family

Organic cation transporter (OCT) is a large family of transporters and has been identified in different species such as rats, rabbits, and humans (Zhang et al., 1998). OCTs are specific for the transport of various substrates like tetraethylammonium (TEA) and choline, neurotoxic 1-methyl-4-phenylpyridinium (MPP). OCT3 (SLC22A3) is expressed in rats, while OCT2 (SLC22A2) is expressed in human brain and reported to regulate neurotransmitter release in neurons (Wu et al., 1998). Studies reported that, physiologically, OCTs are sodium ion-dependent transporter for carnitine which has an important role in fatty acid metabolism (Nezu et al., 1999). Organic zwitterions/cation transporters2 (OCTN2) has many organic cations as a substrate and, therefore, has pharmacological significance in therapy (Ohashi et al., 2001).

6.6 Transport of nucleosides

Nucleoside transporters are required at the BBB as nucleoside can not be synthesized *de novo* and are recycled/salvaged. Furthermore, since nucleosides function as second messengers, regulation of their levels is critical for proper neuronal functioning. Among the different nucleosides, adenosine is an endogenous somnogen that is maintained at physiological levels in the brain (Barar et al., 2016a). Nucleoside transporters are classified according to their Na^+ dependence. Equilibrative nucleoside transporters (ENTs) are Na^+-independent and are members of the SLC29A transporter family, whereas concentrative nucleoside transporters (CNTs) are Na^+-dependent and are members of the SLC28A transporter family. Different analogues of nucleosides synthesized as antiviral and anticancer molecules and transported across BBB through nucleotide transporters (Siccardi et al., 2004).

6.7 Transport of peptides

BBB carries transporters specific for the delivery of different peptides and their mimetic drugs to the brain and it requires sodium motive force to facilitate the process (Barar et al., 2016b). Peptide transporters are members of solute carrier (SLC) superfamily (SLC15A) that includes peptide transporter-1 (PEPT1/Pept1; SLC15A1), peptide transporter-2 (PEPT2/Pept2; SLC15A2), peptide/histidine transporter-1 (PHT1/Pht1; SLC15A4), and peptide/histidine transporter-2 (PHT2/Pht2; SLC15A3). In human, mainly two peptide transporters have been identified, PepT1 (SLC15A1) and PepT2 (SLC15A2), and these are termed as proton-coupled transporters (Sanchez-Covarrubias et al., 2014). These transporters are coupled with Na^+/H^+ exchanger, Na^+/K^+ pump and H^+ pump (Padan and Landau, 2016). Electrochemical gradient across the cellular machinery orchestrates the maintenance of solute concentration inside the brain as well as its clearance through the CSF. In addition to specific peptide transporters, the uptake and distribution of peptides in brain are also determined by transport systems that are endogenously expressed at the BBB endothelium that is involved in unidirectional (i.e., facilitate either blood-to-brain or brain-to-blood peptide transport) or bidirectional transport of peptides through peptide transport system (PTS 1–5, 73, 74). Interestingly, PTS-1 has been observed to mediate transport of tyrosinlylated analogues of the endogenous neuropeptide melanocyte inhibiting factor-1 (MIF-1), which is known to have antiopiate activity. Oatp-A)/ SLC21A3 is reported to have important role in carrier-mediated transport of opioid peptides across the BBB (Gao et al., 2000). Reduced glutathione (GSH) has been also reported to be transferred across BBB via both sodium-dependent and independent mechanisms (Kannan et al., 1996).

6.8 Transport of macromolecules

Small molecules pass through the BBB via passive diffusion or secondary active transport, but macromolecules cannot utilize these mechanisms. Therefore, for the delivery of large molecules, formation of endocytic vesicles plays a very important role. Apparently, BBB allows penetration of such macromolecules through peptide-specific transporter proteins that assist in the delivery of peptides inside the BBB (Dogrukol-Ak et al., 2009). Thrombin, plasmin, and albumin proteins have been reported to induce local effects when delivered inside the brain. Factor Xa helps in converting prothrombin to thrombin and is widely distributed in the CNS. Similarly, plasminogen activator converting plasminogen to plasmin protein is also present in the CNS. Thrombin and plasmin trigger many signaling cascades that are responsible for the glial activation, apoptosis, seizures, and cell death. Albumin extravasation was found to be associated with innate immune response and astrocytic activation (David et al., 2009).

6.9 Transport of ions

BBB has specific ion channels that are responsible for the maintenance of the ionic environment surrounding synaptic clefts (Zhang et al., 2002). However, plasma K^+ concentration is almost double the concentration in brain interstitial fluid which is maintained by ion channels (Medbø and Sejersted, 1990). The balance of these ions is required to for normal physiology and disturbance in ionic concentrations leads to conditions like epilepsy. On the other hand, BBB is impermeable to ions like Ca^{2+} and Mg^{2+} (Michalke and Nischwitz, 2010). Ion channels at BBB are in a way responsible for proper neuronal firing and neural transmission, which is associated with influx of Na^+ and Ca^{2+} as well as extracellular increase in K^+ concentration. Astrocytic end feet help to maintain the ion balance in surrounding space within the narrow limits (Simard and Nedergaard, 2004). As extracellular K^+ is higher, it enters astrocytes through electrochemical gradient and is distributed to other neighboring astrocytes through gap junctions and helps in spatial buffering for physiological function of neurons. Similarly, water is also redistributed throughout the system from perivascular space and cleared via CSF (Serlin et al., 2015). Optimal level of Ca^{2+} helps in increasing trans-endothelial resistance and maintenance of tight junction integrity (Stevenson and Begg, 1994)

6.10 Transcytosis of macromolecules

Transcytosis is the main route for the entry of macromolecules through biological barriers and is a bidirectional process where cargo molecules move from one side to the other. Brain endothelial cells have pinocytotic vesicles that can deliver macromolecules via one of the three main types of vesicles that include: (i) *Caveolae-mediated:* In this transport process, plasma membrane vesicular pits are similar to the lipid rafts and are made up of cholesterol and sphingolipids that cargo molecules like folate receptor, tetanus toxins, and alkaline phosphatase. (ii) *Clathrin-mediated*: this clathrin-coated vesicles contain adaptor protein complex-2 transport macromolecules that transport cargo molecules like low density lipoproteins (LDL), Low density lipoprotein receptor-related protein 1 (LRP1), transferrin, and insulin. (iii) *Micropinocytosis-mediated*: In this process, irregular large fluid engulfing macropinocytotic vesicles are formed that shuffles various macromolecular entities. Twenty receptors have been identified that are involved to initiate receptor-mediated transcytosis. These include receptors for epidermal growth factor, transferin insulin, and insulin-like growth factor receptors, apolipoprotein E (ApoE) and leptin (Preston et al., 2014).

7 Conclusions

In essence, BBB is a complex anatomical structure that acts as a safety guard of the CNS that tightly regulates the movement of ions, molecules, and cells between the blood and the brain. The integrity of BBB is crucial for precise control of CNS homeostasis and protects the neural tissue from toxins and pathogens. Alterations in the barrier properties of BBB are critical determinants in pathology and progression of various neurological disorders. Furthermore, understanding the transporters at BBB opens a gateway for delivery of drugs that can be effective in different neurological conditions.

References

Abbott, N.J., Rönnbäck, L., Hansson, E., 2006. Astrocyte-endothelial interactions at the blood-brain barrier. Nat. Rev. Neurosci. 7, 41–53.

Angelow, S., Ahlstrom, R., Yu, A.S.L., 2008. Biology of claudins. Am. J. Physiol. Ren. Physiol. 295, F867–76.

Araque, A., Li, N., Doyle, R.T., Haydon, P.G., 2000. SNARE protein-dependent glutamate release from astrocytes. J. Neurosci. 20, 666–673.

Aurrand-Lions, M., Duncan, L., Ballestrem, C., Imhof, B.A., 2001. JAM-2, a novel immunoglobulin superfamily molecule, expressed by endothelial and lymphatic cells. J. Biol. Chem. 276, 2733–2741.

Balabanov, R., Beaumont, T., Dore-Duffy, P., 1999. Role of central nervous system microvascular pericytes in activation of antigen-primed splenic T-lymphocytes. J. Neurosci. Res. 55, 578–587.
Balabanov, R., Washington, R., Wagnerova, J., Dore-Duffy, P., 1996. CNS microvascular pericytes express macrophage-like function, cell surface integrin αM, and macrophage marker ED-2. Microvasc. Res. 52, 127–142.
Balda, M.S., Flores-Maldonado, C., Cereijido, M., Matter, K., 2000. Multiple domains of occludin are involved in the regulation of paracellular permeability. J. Cell. Biochem. 78, 85–96.
Balda, M.S., Matter, K., 2009. Tight junctions and the regulation of gene expression. Biochim. Biophys. Acta Biomembr. 1788, 761–767.
Balda, M.S., Whitney, J.A., Flores, C., González, S., Cereijido, M., Matter, K., 1996. Functional dissociation of paracellular permeability and transepithelial electrical resistance and disruption of the apical-basolateral intramembrane diffusion barrier by expression of a mutant tight junction membrane protein. J. Cell Biol. 134, 1031–1049.
Ballabh, P., Braun, A., Nedergaard, M., 2004. The blood-brain barrier: an overview. Neurobiol. Dis. 16, 1–13.
Bandopadhyay, R., Orte, C., Lawrenson, J.G., Reid, A.R., De Silva, S., Allt, G., 2001. Contractile proteins in pericytes at the blood-brain and blood-retinal barriers. J. Neurocytol. 30, 35–44.
Banerjee, S., Bhat, M.A., 2007. Neuron-glial interactions in blood-brain barrier formation. Annu. Rev. Neurosci. 30, 235–258.
Barar, J., Aghanejad, A., Fathi, M., Omidi, Y., 2016a. Advanced drug delivery and targeting technologies for the ocular diseases. BioImpacts 6, 49–67.
Barar, J., Rafi, M.A., Pourseif, M.M., Omidi, Y., 2016b. Blood-brain barrier transport machineries and targeted therapy of brain diseases. BioImpacts 6, 225–248.
Bazzoni, G., Dejana, E., 2004. Endothelial cell-to-cell junctions: molecular organization and role in vascular homeostasis. Physiol. Rev. 84, 869–901.
Bazzoni, G., Martinez-Estrada, O.M., Orsenigo, F., Cordenonsi, M., Citi, S., Dejana, E., 2000. Interaction of junctional adhesion molecule with the tight junction components ZO-1, cingulin, and occludin. J. Biol. Chem. 275, 20520–20526.
Bell, R.D., Winkler, E.A., Sagare, A.P., Singh, I., LaRue, B., Deane, R., Zlokovic, B.V., 2010. Pericytes control key neurovascular functions and neuronal phenotype in the adult brain and during brain aging. Neuron 68, 409–427.
Berzin, T.M., Zipser, B.D., Rafii, M.S., Kuo-Leblanc, V., Yancopoulos, G.D., Glass, D.J., Fallon, J.R., Stopa, E.G., 2000. Agrin and microvascular damage in Alzheimer's disease. Neurobiol. Aging 21, 349–355.
Betanzos, A., Huerta, M., Lopez-Bayghen, E., Azuara, E., Amerena, J., González-Mariscal, L., 2004. The tight junction protein ZO-2 associates with Jun, Fos and C/EBP transcription factors in epithelial cells. Exp. Cell Res. 292, 51–66.
Betz, A.L., Goldstein, G.W., 1978. Polarity of the blood-brain barrier: neutral amino acid transport into isolated brain capillaries. Science 202, 225–227.
Brightman, M.W., Reese, T.S., 1969. Junctions between intimately apposed cell membranes in the vertebrate brain. J. Cell Biol. 40, 648–677.
Carruthers, A., DeZutter, J., Ganguly, A., Devaskar, S.U., 2009. Will the original glucose transporter isoform please stand up!. Am. J. Physiol. Endocrinol. Metab. 297, E836–E848.
Chow, B.W., Gu, C., 2015. The molecular constituents of the blood-brain barrier. Trends Neurosci. 38, 598–608.

Chung-Kwan Shin, C.K., Ui Tak Yun, U.T., Huy Kang Kim, H.K., Sang Chan Park, S.C., 2000. A hybrid approach of neural network and memory-based learning to data mining. IEEE Trans. Neural Netw. 11, 637–646.

Cohen, L.G., Celnik, P., Pascual-Leone, A., Corwell, B., Faiz, L., Dambrosia, J., Honda, M., Sadato, N., Gerloff, C., Catala´, M.D., Hallett, M., 1997. Functional relevance of cross-modal plasticity in blind humans. Nature 389, 180–183.

Colegio, O.R., Van Itallie, C.M., McCrea, H.J., Rahner, C., Anderson, J.M., 2002. Claudins create charge-selective channels in the paracellular pathway between epithelial cells. Am. J. Phys. Cell Physiol. 283, C142–7.

Daneman, R., Prat, A., 2015. The blood-brain barrier. Cold Spring Harb. Perspect. Biol. 7, a020412.

David, Y., Cacheaux, L.P., Ivens, S., Lapilover, E., Heinemann, U., Kaufer, D., Friedman, A., 2009. Astrocytic dysfunction in epileptogenesis: consequence of altered potassium and glutamate homeostasis? J. Neurosci. 29, 10588–10599.

Davson, H., 1976. Review lecture. The blood-brain barrier. J. Physiol. 255, 1–28.

Davson, H., Oldendorf, W.H., 1967. Symposium on membrane transport. Transport in the central nervous system. Proc. R. Soc. Med. 60, 326–329.

Dejana, E., Lampugnani, M.G., Martinez-Estrada, O., Bazzoni, G., 2000. The molecular organization of endothelial junctions and their functional role in vascular morphogenesis and permeability. Int. J. Dev. Biol. 44, 743–748.

Del Maschio, A., De Luigi, A., Martin-Padura, I., Brockhaus, M., Bartfai, T., Fruscella, P., Adorini, L., Martino, G., Furlan, R., De Simoni, M.G., Dejana, E., 1999. Leukocyte recruitment in the cerebrospinal fluid of mice with experimental meningitis is inhibited by an antibody to junctional adhesion molecule (JAM). J. Exp. Med. 190, 1351–1356.

Deli, M.A., Abrahám, C.S., Kataoka, Y., Niwa, M., 2005. Permeability studies on in vitro blood-brain barrier models: physiology, pathology, and pharmacology. Cell. Mol. Neurobiol. 25, 59–127.

Devaskar, S., Zahm, D.S., Holtzclaw, L., Chundu, K., Wadzinski, B.E., 1991. Developmental regulation of the distribution of rat brain insulin-insensitive (Glut 1) glucose transporter. Endocrinology 129, 1530–1540.

Dhanda, S., Sandhir, R., 2018. Blood-brain barrier permeability is exacerbated in experimental model of hepatic encephalopathy via MMP-9 activation and downregulation of tight junction proteins. Mol. Neurobiol. 55, 3642–3659.

Dogrukol-Ak, D., Kumar, V.B., Ryerse, J.S., Farr, S.A., Verma, S., Nonaka, N., Nakamachi, T., Ohtaki, H., Niehoff, M.L., Edwards, J.C., Shioda, S., Morley, J.E., Banks, W.A., 2009. Isolation of peptide transport system-6 from brain endothelial cells: therapeutic effects with antisense inhibition in alzheimer and stroke models. J. Cereb. Blood Flow Metab. 29, 411–422.

Dohgu, S., Takata, F., Yamauchi, A., Nakagawa, S., Egawa, T., Naito, M., Tsuruo, T., Sawada, Y., Niwa, M., Kataoka, Y., 2005. Brain pericytes contribute to the induction and up-regulation of blood-brain barrier functions through transforming growth factor-beta production. Brain Res. 1038, 208–215.

Dore-Duffy, P., Owen, C., Balabanov, R., Murphy, S., Beaumont, T., Rafols, J.A., 2000. Pericyte migration from the vascular wall in response to traumatic brain injury. Microvasc. Res. 60, 55–69.

Enerson, B.E., Drewes, L.R., 2003. Molecular features, regulation, and function of monocarboxylate transporters: implications for drug delivery. J. Pharm. Sci. 92, 1531–1544.

Engelhardt, B., Ransohoff, R.M., 2012. Capture, crawl, cross: the T cell code to breach the blood-brain barriers. Trends Immunol. 33, 579–589.

Feldt Muldoon, S., Soltesz, I., Cossart, R., 2013. Spatially clustered neuronal assemblies comprise the microstructure of synchrony in chronically epileptic networks. Proc. Natl. Acad. Sci. U. S. A. 110, 3567–3572.

Findley, M.K., Koval, M., 2009. Regulation and roles for claudin-family tight junction proteins. IUBMB Life 61, 431–437.

Fischer, S., Wobben, M., Marti, H.H., Renz, D., Schaper, W., 2002. Hypoxia-induced hyperpermeability in brain microvessel endothelial cells involves VEGF-mediated changes in the expression of zonula occludens-1. Microvasc. Res. 63, 70–80.

Frerking, M., 2004. When astrocytes signal, kainate receptors respond. Proc. Natl. Acad. Sci. U. S. A. 101, 2649–2650.

Furuse, M., Hirase, T., Itoh, M., Nagafuchi, A., Yonemura, S., Tsukita, S., Tsukita, S., 1993. Occludin: a novel integral membrane protein localizing at tight junctions. J. Cell Biol. 123, 1777–1788.

Gao, B., Hagenbuch, B., Kullak-Ublick, G.A., Benke, D., Aguzzi, A., Meier, P.J., 2000. Organic anion-transporting polypeptides mediate transport of opioid peptides across blood-brain barrier. J. Pharmacol. Exp. Ther. 294, 73–79.

Gao, B., Stieger, B., Noé, B., Fritschy, J.M., Meier, P.J., 1999. Localization of the organic anion transporting polypeptide 2 (Oatp2) in capillary endothelium and choroid plexus epithelium of rat brain. J. Histochem. Cytochem. 47, 1255–1264.

Gerhart, D.Z., Enerson, B.E., Zhdankina, O.Y., Leino, R.L., Drewes, L.R., 1997. Expression of monocarboxylate transporter MCT1 by brain endothelium and glia in adult and suckling rats. Am. J. Phys. 273, E207–13.

Goldmann, E.E., 1909. Die äussere und innere Sekretion des gesunden und kranken Organismus im Lichte der "vitalen Färbung" Beitr. Klin. Chir. 64, 192–265.

Gonçalves, A., Ambrósio, A.F., Fernandes, R., 2013. Regulation of claudins in blood-tissue barriers under physiological and pathological states. Tissue Barriers. 1, e24782.

Gonul, E., Duz, B., Kahraman, S., Kayali, H., Kubar, A., Timurkaynak, E., 2002. Early pericyte response to brain hypoxia in cats: an ultrastructural study. Microvasc. Res. 64, 116–119.

Gonzalez-Mariscal, L., Namorado, M.C., Martin, D., Luna, J., Alarcon, L., Islas, S., Valencia, L., Muriel, P., Ponce, L., Reyes, J.L., 2000. Tight junction proteins ZO-1, ZO-2, and occludin along isolated renal tubules. Kidney Int. 57, 2386–2402.

Gottardi, C.J., Arpin, M., Fanning, A.S., Louvard, D., 1996. The junction-associated protein, zonula occludens-1, localizes to the nucleus before the maturation and during the remodeling of cell-cell contacts. Proc. Natl. Acad. Sci. U. S. A. 93, 10779–10784.

Gow, A., Southwood, C.M., Li, J.S., Pariali, M., Riordan, G.P., Brodie, S.E., Danias, J., Bronstein, J.M., Kachar, B., Lazzarini, R.A., 1999. CNS myelin and sertoli cell tight junction strands are absent in Osp/claudin-11 null mice. Cell 99, 649–659.

Greenwood, J., Amos, C.L., Walters, C.E., Couraud, P.-O., Lyck, R., Engelhardt, B., Adamson, P., 2003. Intracellular domain of brain endothelial intercellular adhesion molecule-1 is essential for T lymphocyte-mediated signaling and migration. J. Immunol. 171, 2099–2108.

Guillemot, L., Paschoud, S., Pulimeno, P., Foglia, A., Citi, S., 2008. The cytoplasmic plaque of tight junctions: a scaffolding and signalling center. Biochim. Biophys. Acta 1778, 601–613.

Gupta, S., Yadav, K., Mantri, S.S., Singhal, N.K., Ganesh, S., Sandhir, R., 2018. Evidence for compromised insulin signaling and neuronal vulnerability in experimental model of sporadic Alzheimer's disease. Mol. Neurobiol. https://doi.org/10.1007/s12035-018-0985-0.

Hagenbuch, B., Gao, B., Meier, P.J., 2002. Transport of xenobiotics across the blood-brain barrier. News Physiol. Sci. 17, 231–234.

Hamazaki, Y., Itoh, M., Sasaki, H., Furuse, M., Tsukita, S., 2002. Multi-PDZ domain protein 1 (MUPP1) is concentrated at tight junctions through its possible interaction with claudin-1 and junctional adhesion molecule. J. Biol. Chem. 277, 455–461.
Hawkins, B.T., Abbruscato, T.J., Egleton, R.D., Brown, R.C., Huber, J.D., Campos, C.R., Davis, T.P., 2004. Nicotine increases in vivo blood-brain barrier permeability and alters cerebral microvascular tight junction protein distribution. Brain Res. 1027, 48–58.
Hawkins, B.T., Davis, T.P., 2005. The blood-brain barrier/neurovascular unit in health and disease. Pharmacol. Rev. 57, 173–185.
Healy, D.P., Wilk, S., 1993. Localization of immunoreactive glutamyl aminopeptidase in rat brain. II. Distribution and correlation with angiotensin II. Brain Res. 606, 295–303.
Heiskala, M., Peterson, P.A., Yang, Y., 2001. The roles of claudin superfamily proteins in paracellular transport. Traffic 2, 93–98.
Hirschi, K.K., D'Amore, P.A., 1996. Pericytes in the microvasculature. Cardiovasc. Res. 32, 687–698.
Hori, S., Ohtsuki, S., Hosoya, K., Nakashima, E., Terasaki, T., 2004. A pericyte-derived angiopoietin-1 multimeric complex induces occludin gene expression in brain capillary endothelial cells through Tie-2 activation in vitro. J. Neurochem. 89, 503–513.
Huber, J.D., Witt, K.A., Hom, S., Egleton, R.D., Mark, K.S., Davis, T.P., 2001. Inflammatory pain alters blood-brain barrier permeability and tight junctional protein expression. Am. J. Physiol. Heart Circ. Physiol. 280, H1241–8.
Hynes, R.O., 1992. Integrins: versatility, modulation, and signaling in cell adhesion. Cell 69, 11–25.
Inoko, A., Itoh, M., Tamura, A., Matsuda, M., Furuse, M., Tsukita, S., 2003. Expression and distribution of ZO-3, a tight junction MAGUK protein, in mouse tissues. Genes Cells 8, 837–845.
Ishizaki, T., Chiba, H., Kojima, T., Fujibe, M., Soma, T., Miyajima, H., Nagasawa, K., Wada, I., Sawada, N., 2003. Cyclic AMP induces phosphorylation of claudin-5 immunoprecipitates and expression of claudin-5 gene in blood-brain-barrier endothelial cells via protein kinase A-dependent and -independent pathways. Exp. Cell Res. 290, 275–288.
Janzer, R.C., Raff, M.C., 1987. Astrocytes induce blood-brain barrier properties in endothelial cells. Nature 325, 253–257.
Kang, Y.S., Terasaki, T., Tsuji, A., 1990. Acidic drug transport in vivo through the blood-brain barrier. A role of the transport carrier for monocarboxylic acids. Aust. J. Pharm. 13, 158–163.
Kannan, R., Yi, J.R., Tang, D., Li, Y., Zlokovic, B.V., Kaplowitz, N., 1996. Evidence for the existence of a sodium-dependent glutathione (GSH) transporter. Expression of bovine brain capillary mRNA and size fractions in *Xenopus laevis* oocytes and dissociation from gamma-glutamyltranspeptidase and facilitative GSH transporters. J. Biol. Chem. 271, 9754–9758.
Katzman, R., Pappius, H.M. (Eds.), 1973. Brain Electrolytes and Fluid Metabolism. Williams & Wilkins, Baltimore.
Kirchhoff, F., Dringen, R., Giaume, C., 2001. Pathways of neuron-astrocyte interactions and their possible role in neuroprotection. Eur. Arch. Psychiatry Clin. Neurosci. 251, 159–169.
Krause, G., Winkler, L., Mueller, S.L., Haseloff, R.F., Piontek, J., Blasig, I.E., 2008. Structure and function of claudins. Biochim. Biophys. Acta 1778, 631–645.
Lampugnani, M.G., Corada, M., Caveda, L., Breviario, F., Ayalon, O., Geiger, B., Dejana, E., 1995. The molecular organization of endothelial cell to cell junctions: differential association of plakoglobin, beta-catenin, and alpha-catenin with vascular endothelial cadherin (VE-cadherin). J. Cell Biol. 129, 203–217.

Laschinger, M., Engelhardt, B., 2000. Interaction of alpha4-integrin with VCAM-1 is involved in adhesion of encephalitogenic T cell blasts to brain endothelium but not in their trans-endothelial migration in vitro. J. Neuroimmunol. 102, 32–43.

Lawther, B.K., Kumar, S., Krovvidi, H., 2011. Blood-brain barrier. Contin. Educ. Anaesth. Crit. Care Pain 11, 128–132.

Liddelow, S.A., 2011. Fluids and barriers of the CNS: a historical viewpoint. Fluids Barriers CNS 8, 2.

Liu, J., Jin, X., Liu, K.J., Liu, W., 2012. Matrix metalloproteinase-2-mediated occludin degradation and caveolin-1-mediated claudin-5 redistribution contribute to blood-brain barrier damage in early ischemic stroke stage. J. Neurosci. 32, 3044–3057.

Liu, Y., Nusrat, A., Schnell, F.J., Reaves, T.A., Walsh, S., Pochet, M., Parkos, C.A., 2000. Human junction adhesion molecule regulates tight junction resealing in epithelia. J. Cell Sci. 113, 2363–2374.

Lo, M.-C., Aulabaugh, A., Jin, G., Cowling, R., Bard, J., Malamas, M., Ellestad, G., 2004. Evaluation of fluorescence-based thermal shift assays for hit identification in drug discovery. Anal. Biochem. 332, 153–159.

Lynch, R.D., Francis, S.A., McCarthy, K.M., Casas, E., Thiele, C., Schneeberger, E.E., 2007. Cholesterol depletion alters detergent-specific solubility profiles of selected tight junction proteins and the phosphorylation of occludin. Exp. Cell Res. 313, 2597–2610.

Marchi, N., Angelov, L., Masaryk, T., Fazio, V., Granata, T., Hernandez, N., Hallene, K., Diglaw, T., Franic, L., Najm, I., Janigro, D., 2007. Seizure-promoting effect of blood? brain barrier disruption. Epilepsia 48, 732–742.

Massa, P.T., Mugnaini, E., 1982. Cell junctions and intramembrane particles of astrocytes and oligodendrocytes: a freeze-fracture study. Neuroscience 7, 523–538.

Martìn-Padura, I., Lostaglio, S., Schneemann, M., Williams, L., Romano, M., Fruscella, P., Panzeri, C., Stoppacciaro, A., Ruco, L., Villa, A., Simmons, D., Dejana, E., 1998. Junctional adhesion molecule, a novel member of the immunoglobulin superfamily that distributes at intercellular junctions and modulates monocyte transmigration. J. Cell Biol. 142, 117–127.

Massa, P.T., Mugnaini, E., 1985. Cell-cell junctional interactions and characteristic plasma membrane features of cultured rat glial cells. Neuroscience 14, 695–709.

McCarthy, K.M., Skare, I.B., Stankewich, M.C., Furuse, M., Tsukita, S., Rogers, R.A., Lynch, R.D., Schneeberger, E.E., 1996. Occludin is a functional component of the tight junction. J. Cell Sci. 109, 2287–2298.

McDonald, D.A., Potter, J.M., 1951. The distribution of blood to the brain. J. Physiol. 114, 356–371.

Medbo, J.I., Sejersted, O.M., 1990. Plasma potassium changes with high intensity exercise. J. Physiol. 421, 105–122.

Michalke, B., Nischwitz, V., 2010. Review on metal speciation analysis in cerebrospinal fluid—current methods and results: a review. Anal. Chim. Acta 682, 23–36.

Mochida, G.H., Ganesh, V.S., Felie, J.M., Gleason, D., Hill, R.S., Clapham, K.R., Rakiec, D., Tan, W.-H., Akawi, N., Al-Saffar, M., Partlow, J.N., Tinschert, S., Barkovich, A.J., Ali, B., Al-Gazali, L., Walsh, C.A., 2010. A homozygous mutation in the tight-junction protein JAM3 causes hemorrhagic destruction of the brain, subependymal calcification, and congenital cataracts. Am. J. Hum. Genet. 87, 882–889.

Morita, K., Furuse, M., Fujimoto, K., Tsukita, S., 1999. Claudin multigene family encoding four-transmembrane domain protein components of tight junction strands. Proc. Natl. Acad. Sci. U. S. A. 96, 511–516.

Müller, D., Kausalya, P.J., Meij, I.C., Hunziker, W., 2006. Familial hypomagnesemia with hypercalciuria and nephrocalcinosis: blocking endocytosis restores surface expression of a novel Claudin-16 mutant that lacks the entire C-terminal cytosolic tail. Hum. Mol. Genet. 15, 1049–1058.

Mulligan, S.J., MacVicar, B.A., 2004. Calcium transients in astrocyte endfeet cause cerebrovascular constrictions. Nature 431, 195–199.

Nakagawa, S., Deli, M.A., Nakao, S., Honda, M., Hayashi, K., Nakaoke, R., Kataoka, Y., Niwa, M., 2007. Pericytes from brain microvessels strengthen the barrier integrity in primary cultures of rat brain endothelial cells. Cell. Mol. Neurobiol. 27, 687–694.

Nedergaard, M., Ransom, B., Goldman, S.A., 2003. New roles for astrocytes: redefining the functional architecture of the brain. Trends Neurosci. 26, 523–530.

Negri, L., Lattanzi, R., Tabacco, F., Scolaro, B., Rocchi, R., 1998. Glycodermorphins: opioid peptides with potent and prolonged analgesic activity and enhanced blood-brain barrier penetration. Br. J. Pharmacol. 124, 1516–1522.

Neuwelt, E.A., 2004. Mechanisms of disease: the blood-brain barrier. Neurosurgery 54, 131–140.

Nezu, J., Tamai, I., Oku, A., Ohashi, R., Yabuuchi, H., Hashimoto, N., Nikaido, H., Sai, Y., Koizumi, A., Shoji, Y., Takada, G., Matsuishi, T., Yoshino, M., Kato, H., Ohura, T., Tsujimoto, G., Hayakawa, J., Shimane, M., Tsuji, A., 1999. Primary systemic carnitine deficiency is caused by mutations in a gene encoding sodium ion-dependent carnitine transporter. Nat. Genet. 21, 91–94.

Nicchia, G.P., Nico, B., Camassa, L.M.A., Mola, M.G., Loh, N., Dermietzel, R., Spray, D.C., Svelto, M., Frigeri, A., 2004. The role of aquaporin-4 in the blood-brain barrier development and integrity: studies in animal and cell culture models. Neuroscience 129, 935–944.

Nozawa, T., Imai, K., Nezu, J.-I., Tsuji, A., Tamai, I., 2004. Functional characterization of pH-sensitive organic anion transporting polypeptide OATP-B in human. J. Pharmacol. Exp. Ther. 308, 438–445.

Ohashi, R., Tamai, I., Nezu Ji, J., Nikaido, H., Hashimoto, N., Oku, A., Sai, Y., Shimane, M., Tsuji, A., 2001. Molecular and physiological evidence for multifunctionality of carnitine/organic cation transporter OCTN2. Mol. Pharmacol. 59, 358–366.

Ohtsuki, S., Yamaguchi, H., Katsukura, Y., Asashima, T., Terasaki, T., 2008. mRNA expression levels of tight junction protein genes in mouse brain capillary endothelial cells highly purified by magnetic cell sorting. J. Neurochem. 104, 147–154.

Oldendorf, W.H., 1973. Carrier-mediated blood-brain barrier transport of short-chain monocarboxylic organic acids. Am. J. Phys. 224, 1450–1453.

Padan, E., Landau, M., 2016. Sodium-proton (Na^+/H^+) antiporters: properties and roles in health and disease. In: Metal Ions in Life Sciences.vol. 16. pp. 391–458.

Palmer, A.M., 2010. The blood-brain barrier. Neurobiol. Dis. 37, 1–2.

Pardridge, W.M., 1983. Brain metabolism: a perspective from the blood-brain barrier. Physiol. Rev. 63, 1481–1535.

Pardridge, W.M., 2005. The blood-brain barrier: bottleneck in brain drug development. NeuroRx 2, 3–14.

Pardridge, W.M., Boado, R.J., Farrell, C.R., 1990. Brain-type glucose transporter (GLUT-1) is selectively localized to the blood-brain barrier Studies with quantitative western blotting and in situ hybridization. J. Biol. Chem. 265, 18035–18040.

Pellerin, L., Pellegri, G., Bittar, P.G., Charnay, Y., Bouras, C., Martin, J.L., Stella, N., Magistretti, P.J., 1998. Evidence supporting the existence of an activity-dependent astrocyte-neuron lactate shuttle. Dev. Neurosci. 20, 291–299.

Pfrieger, F.W., Barres, B.A., 1997. Synaptic efficacy enhanced by glial cells in vitro. Science 277, 1684–1687.

Potschka, H., 2010. Transporter hypothesis of drug-resistant epilepsy: challenges for pharmacogenetic approaches. Pharmacogenomics 11, 1427–1438.

Preston, J.E., Joan Abbott, N., Begley, D.J., 2014. Transcytosis of macromolecules at the blood-brain barrier. Adv. Pharmacol. 71, 147–163.

Ramsauer, M., Krause, D., Dermietzel, R., 2002. Angiogenesis of the blood-brain barrier in vitro and the function of cerebral pericytes. FASEB J. 16, 1274–1276.

Ransohoff, R.M., Engelhardt, B., 2012. The anatomical and cellular basis of immune surveillance in the central nervous system. Nat. Rev. Immunol. 12, 623–635.

Rascher, G., Fischmann, A., Kröger, S., Duffner, F., Grote, E.-H., Wolburg, H., 2002. Extracellular matrix and the blood-brain barrier in glioblastoma multiforme: spatial segregation of tenascin and agrin. Acta Neuropathol. 104, 85–91.

Reisin, H.D., Colombo, J.A., 2002. Considerations on the astroglial architecture and the columnar organization of the cerebral cortex. Cell. Mol. Neurobiol. 22, 633–644.

Rodgers, L.S., Fanning, A.S., 2011. Regulation of epithelial permeability by the actin cytoskeleton. Cytoskeleton 68, 653–660.

Rolfe, D.F., Brown, G.C., 1997. Cellular energy utilization and molecular origin of standard metabolic rate in mammals. Physiol. Rev. 77, 731–758.

Rouach, N., Glowinski, J., Giaume, C., 2000. Activity-dependent neuronal control of gap-junctional communication in astrocytes. J. Cell Biol. 149, 1513–1526.

Rüffer, C., Gerke, V., 2004. The C-terminal cytoplasmic tail of claudins 1 and 5 but not its PDZ-binding motif is required for apical localization at epithelial and endothelial tight junctions. Eur. J. Cell Biol. 83, 135–144.

Sanchez-Covarrubias, L., Slosky, L.M., Thompson, B.J., Davis, T.P., Ronaldson, P.T., 2014. Transporters at CNS barrier sites: obstacles or opportunities for drug delivery? Curr. Pharm. Des. 20, 1422–1449.

Sankar, R., Sotero de Menezes, M., 1999. Metabolic and endocrine aspects of the ketogenic diet. Epilepsy Res. 37, 191–201.

Savettieri, G., Di Liegro, I., Catania, C., Licata, L., Pitarresi, G.L., D'Agostino, S., Schiera, G., De Caro, V., Giandalia, G., Giannola, L.I., Cestelli, A., 2000. Neurons and ECM regulate occludin localization in brain endothelial cells. NeuroReport 11, 1081–1084.

Schulze, C., Firth, J.A., 1993. Immunohistochemical localization of adherens junction components in blood-brain barrier microvessels of the rat. J. Cell Sci. 104 (Pt 3), 773–782.

Schulzke, J.D., Gitter, A.H., Mankertz, J., Spiegel, S., Seidler, U., Amasheh, S., Saitou, M., Tsukita, S., Fromm, M., 2005. Epithelial transport and barrier function in occludin-deficient mice. Biochim. Biophys. Acta 1669, 34–42.

Serlin, Y., Shelef, I., Knyazer, B., Friedman, A., 2015. Anatomy and physiology of the blood-brain barrier. Semin. Cell Dev. Biol. 38, 2–6.

Siccardi, D., Gumbleton, M., Omidi, Y., McGuigan, C., 2004. Stereospecific chemical and enzymatic stability of phosphoramidate triester prodrugs of d4T in vitro. Eur. J. Pharm. Sci. 22, 25–31.

Siegenthaler, J.A., Choe, Y., Patterson, K.P., Hsieh, I., Li, D., Jaminet, S.-C., Daneman, R., Kume, T., Huang, E.J., Pleasure, S.J., 2013. Foxc1 is required by pericytes during fetal brain angiogenesis. Biol. Open 2, 647–659.

Simard, M., Arcuino, G., Takano, T., Liu, Q.S., Nedergaard, M., 2003. Signaling at the gliovascular interface. J. Neurosci. 23, 9254–9262.

Simard, M., Nedergaard, M., 2004. The neurobiology of glia in the context of water and ion homeostasis. Neuroscience 129, 877–896.

Simpson, I.A., Vannucci, S.J., DeJoseph, M.R., Hawkins, R.A., 2001. Glucose transporter asymmetries in the bovine blood-brain barrier. J. Biol. Chem. 276, 12725–12729.
Singh, N., Lawana, V., Krishnan, N., Kanuri, S.H., Jin, H., Anantharam, V., Kanthasamy, A., Kanthasamy, A., 2015. Agrochemicals-Induced Dopaminergic Neurotoxicity: Role of Mitochondria-Mediated Oxidative Stress and Protein Clearance Mechanisms. Springer, Cham, pp. 171–204.
Smith, Q.R., Takasato, Y., 1986. Kinetics of amino acid transport at the blood-brain barrier studied using an in situ brain perfusion technique. Ann. N. Y. Acad. Sci. 481, 186–201.
Staddon, J.M., Rubin, L.L., 1996. Cell adhesion, cell junctions and the blood-brain barrier. Curr. Opin. Neurobiol. 6, 622–627.
Stevenson, B.R., Begg, D.A., 1994. Concentration-dependent effects of cytochalasin D on tight junctions and actin filaments in MDCK epithelial cells. J. Cell Sci. 107, 367–375.
Stratman, A.N., Davis, G.E., 2012. Endothelial cell-pericyte interactions stimulate basement membrane matrix assembly: influence on vascular tube remodeling, maturation, and stabilization. Microsc. Microanal. 18, 68–80.
Tietz, S., Engelhardt, B., 2015. Brain barriers: crosstalk between complex tight junctions and adherens junctions. J. Cell Biol. 209, 493–506.
Toyofuku, T., Yabuki, M., Otsu, K., Kuzuya, T., Hori, M., Tada, M., 1998. Direct association of the gap junction protein connexin-43 with ZO-1 in cardiac myocytes. J. Biol. Chem. 273, 12725–12731.
Trost, A., Lange, S., Schroedl, F., Bruckner, D., Motloch, K.A., Bogner, B., Kaser-Eichberger, A., Strohmaier, C., Runge, C., Aigner, L., Rivera, F.J., Reitsamer, H.A., 2016. Brain and retinal pericytes: origin, function and role. Front. Cell. Neurosci. 10, 20.
Tschirgi, R., 1950. Protein complexes and the impermeability of the blood-brain barrier to dyes. Am. J. Physiol. 163, 756.
Tsuji, A., 2005a. Small molecular drug transfer across the blood-brain barrier via carrier-mediated transport systems. NeuroRx 2, 54–62.
Tuma, P.L., Hubbard, A.L., 2003. Transcytosis: crossing cellular barriers. Physiol. Rev. 83, 871–932.
Van Itallie, C.M., Anderson, J.M., 2006. Claudins and epithelial paracellular transport. Annu. Rev. Physiol. 68, 403–429.
Van Itallie, C.M., Gambling, T.M., Carson, J.L., Anderson, J.M., 2005. Palmitoylation of claudins is required for efficient tight-junction localization. J. Cell Sci. 118, 1427–1436.
van Zwieten, E.J., Ravid, R., Swaab, D.F., Van de Woude, T., 1988. Immunocytochemically stained vasopressin binding sites on blood vessels in the rat brain. Brain Res. 474, 369–373.
Verbeek, M.M., de Waal, R.M., Schipper, J.J., Van Nostrand, W.E., 1997. Rapid degeneration of cultured human brain pericytes by amyloid beta protein. J. Neurochem. 68, 1135–1141.
Vincent, A., Buckley, C., Schott, J.M., Baker, I., Dewar, B., Detert, N., Clover, L., Parkinson, A., Bien, C.G., Omer, S., Lang, B., Rossor, M.N., Palace, J., 2004. Potassium channel antibody-associated encephalopathy: a potentially immunotherapy-responsive form of limbic encephalitis. Brain 127, 701–712.
Vorbrodt, A.W., Dobrogowska, D.H., 2003. Molecular anatomy of intercellular junctions in brain endothelial and epithelial barriers: electron microscopist's view. Brain Res. Brain Res. Rev. 42, 221–242.
Wang, L., Renault, G., Garreau, H., Jacquet, M., 2004. Stress induces depletion of Cdc25p and decreases the cAMP producing capability in *Saccharomyces cerevisiae*. Microbiology 150, 3383–3391.

Watabe-Uchida, M., Uchida, N., Imamura, Y., Nagafuchi, A., Fujimoto, K., Uemura, T., Vermeulen, S., van Roy, F., Adamson, E.D., Takeichi, M., 1998. alpha-Catenin-vinculin interaction functions to organize the apical junctional complex in epithelial cells. J. Cell Biol. 142, 847–857.

Wong, A.D., Ye, M., Levy, A.F., Rothstein, J.D., Bergles, D.E., Searson, P.C., 2013. The blood-brain barrier: an engineering perspective. Front. Neuroeng. 6, 7.

Wong, V., Gumbiner, B.M., 1997. A synthetic peptide corresponding to the extracellular domain of occludin perturbs the tight junction permeability barrier. J. Cell Biol. 136, 399–409.

Wu, X., Kekuda, R., Huang, W., Fei, Y.J., Leibach, F.H., Chen, J., Conway, S.J., Ganapathy, V., 1998. Identity of the organic cation transporter OCT3 as the extraneuronal monoamine transporter (uptake2) and evidence for the expression of the transporter in the brain. J. Biol. Chem. 273, 32776–32786.

Yu, D., Turner, J.R., 2008. Stimulus-induced reorganization of tight junction structure: the role of membrane traffic. Biochim. Biophys. Acta Biomembr. 1778, 709–716.

Yudilevich, D.L., De Rose, N., 1971. Blood-brain transfer of glucose and other molecules measured by rapid indicator dilution. Am. J. Phys. 220, 841–846.

Zhang, E.Y., Knipp, G.T., Ekins, S., Swaan, P.W., 2002. Structural biology and function of solute transporters: implications for identifying and designing substrates. Drug Metab. Rev. 34, 709–750.

Zhang, L., Brett, C.M., Giacomini, K.M., 1998. Role of organic cation transporters in drug absorption and elimination. Annu. Rev. Pharmacol. Toxicol. 38, 431–460.

Zhang, Y., Pardridge, W.M., 2001. Rapid transferrin efflux from brain to blood across the blood-brain barrier. J. Neurochem. 76, 1597–1600.

Zlokovic, B.V., 2005. Neurovascular mechanisms of Alzheimer's neurodegeneration. Trends Neurosci. 28, 202–208.

Zonta, M., Angulo, M.C., Gobbo, S., Rosengarten, B., Hossmann, K.-A., Pozzan, T., Carmignoto, G., 2003. Neuron-to-astrocyte signaling is central to the dynamic control of brain microcirculation. Nat. Neurosci. 6, 43–50.

Recent progress in blood-brain barrier transportation research

3

*Guangzhe Li**, *Kun Shao*[†,‡], *Channakeshava Sokke Umeshappa*[‡]
*School of Pharmaceutical Science and Technology, Dalian University of Technology, Dalian, China, [†]State Key Laboratory of Fine Chemicals, Dalian University of Technology, Dalian, China, [‡]Julia McFarlane Diabetes Research Centre (JMDRC) and Department of Microbiology, Immunology and Infectious Diseases, Snyder Institute for Chronic Diseases and Hotchkiss Brain Institute, Cumming School of Medicine, University of Calgary, Calgary, AB, Canada

1 Introduction

Central nervous system (CNS) disorders are some of the most prevalent, devastating, and yet poorly treated illnesses. One of the biggest challenges in the development of therapeutics for CNS disorders is achieving their sufficient blood-brain barrier (BBB) penetration (Banks, 2016). BBB is a nonfenestrated endothelium with narrow tight junctions (TJs) between the brain capillary endothelial cells (BCECs). It helps to maintain homeostasis in the cerebral microenvironment by controlling exchanges of substances between the CNS and the blood (Begley and Brightman, 2003; Banks, 2016) and serves an important role in preventing macromolecules, infectious substances, and potential neurotoxins from entering the brain (Pardridge, 2005). More than 98% of small molecular drugs and nearly 100% of larger molecular therapeutics are ineffective in treating CNS diseases since BBB strictly limits the delivery of therapeutic agents to their target site in the CNS (Pardridge, 2005, 2007). BBB is emerged as a dynamic and adaptable interface, and its highly complex function makes the drug development very difficult (Banks, 2016). However, in-depth understanding of its complex functions offers unique and diverse opportunities for therapeutics development. From the perspective of clinical application, despite enormous efforts and intensive studies on the discovery of CNS-active drugs, the number of approved drugs for treating CNS disorders is still rare (Pangalos et al., 2007). Therefore, new strategies to increase CNS delivery of the currently available therapeutics represent major pharmacological improvement in the treatment of CNS disorders.

In the last two decades, numerous drug delivery strategies have been investigated to improve the therapeutic effect in brain disorders with varying degrees of success. These strategies range from TJs modulation and drug molecule modification to targeting strategies that are based on the endogenous transcytosis and carrier-based transport systems, including nanoparticle- and cell-based deliveries (Fig. 1). This chapter will provide an overview of recent progress in the conventional and emerging strategies for improving the delivery of CNS-active therapeutics.

Brain Targeted Drug Delivery Systems. https://doi.org/10.1016/B978-0-12-814001-7.00003-2

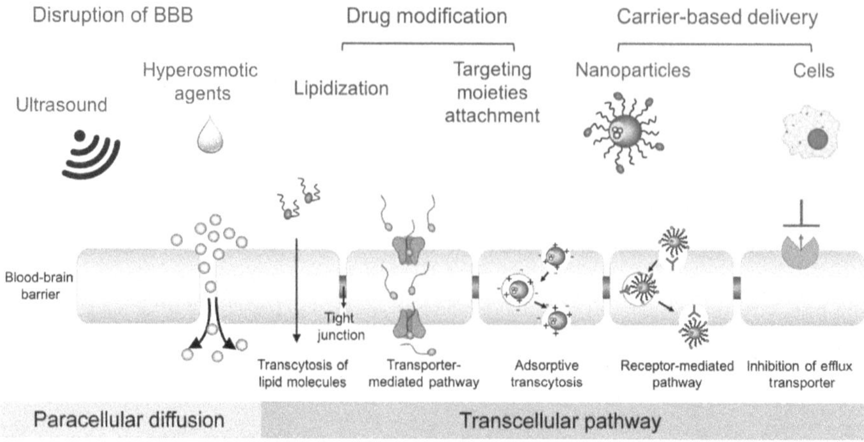

Fig. 1 Transport routes across the blood-brain barrier (BBB) and strategies for delivery of central nervous system (CNS)-active therapeutics across the BBB include physical/chemical disruption, enhanced transcytosis (e.g., drug modification, transporter-mediated, or receptor-mediated pathway), nanoparticle-based delivery, and cell-based delivery.

2 Overview of the transport mechanisms at the BBB

Different substances cross the BBB and enter CNS primarily either by paracellular or through transcellular pathway (De Boer and Breimer, 1994). Under normal physiological condition, three routes exist for small molecules to cross BBB and reach CNS parenchyma: (1) Very small hydrophilic molecules are able to diffuse to the brain *paracellularly via an aqueous pathway,* which has limited functionality due to TJs between the endothelial cells. (2) Some lipid-soluble substances, such as steroid hormones, tend to cross the BBB via *passive transcellular diffusion* (Chen and Liu, 2012). However, this pathway is only limited to certain compounds whose molecular weight is less than 500 Da and which are lipid-soluble and be either neutral or uncharged at physiologically pH with cumulative number of hydrogen bonds less than 8 (Lipinski et al., 2001; Pardridge, 2012). (3) Most of the remaining small molecular nutrients' entry to the brain relies on the *endogenous transporter- (carrier-) mediated pathway*, which is a substrate-specific process driven by the concentration gradient of the substrates with the assistance of suitable transporters.

For biomacromolecules, such as peptides and proteins, energy-dependent, receptor-mediated (e.g., for transferrin and insulin, etc.), or vesicular mechanisms (adsorptive transcytosis, e.g., for cationized albumins) are required to pass the BBB. To maintain the specific microenvironment in brain and protect neurons from toxic metabolites, many efflux transporters such as p-glycoprotein (p-gp) expressed on the BBB play important role in the externalization of various molecules, such as toxicities, metabolites, and drugs (Psimadas et al., 2015). Major molecular transport routes at the BBB are illustrated in Fig. 1. Transcytosis is a dominating approach to therapeutic agents through BBB into the CNS and consists mainly of three major mechanisms: carrier-mediated transcytosis (CMT), receptor-mediated transcytosis (RMT), and adsorptive-mediated transcytosis (AMT) (Bhaskar et al., 2010). Understanding these endogenous transport systems at the BBB considerably facilitates the development of effective strategies to deliver CNS-active biologics to the brain.

2.1 Carrier-mediated transcytosis

More than 20 endogenous carrier-mediated transporter proteins have been identified on the luminal and/or abluminal side of BCECs (Mikitsh and Chacko, 2014). CMT provides a facilitated mechanism to shuttle certain small molecules, nutrients, and hormones between the blood and the brain by stereospecific, saturable substrate systems depending on the concentration gradient of the substance (Stenehjem et al., 2009). The rate of the substrate transport depends on substrate affinity for the transporter, molecular driving force, and intracellular-binding capacity (Smith, 1993; Stenehjem et al., 2009). Many drug molecules have similar structural properties to endogenous substrates, suggesting that some membrane transporters can participate in drug transport (Tamai and Tsuji, 2000). These representative CMTs, including glucose transporter type 1 (GLUT1), large neutral amino acid transporter 1 (LAT1), and monocarboxylate transporter 1 (MCT1), are considered as the most promising transporters to be utilized for brain drug delivery.

2.1.1 Glucose transporters

Glucose transporters at the BBB have become the most prevalent targets for the delivery of neuroactive drugs to the brain due to their higher transport capacity (1420 nmol/min g tissue) than those of other nutrient transporters (91 nmol/min g tissue for monocarboxylic acid, 28 for neutral amino acid, and 11.3 for amine transport systems) (Pardridge, 1983; Guo et al., 2005). Among all the glucose transporters that have been identified in the CNS, GLUT1/SLC2A1 is the major one in terms of its location and expression levels. It has been detected in two distinct isoforms encoded by the same gene, differing in glycosylation extent. GLUT1, 55 kDa (heavily glycosylated) form, is selectively and highly expressed on both luminal and abluminal membranes of BCECs covering most neuronal area, whereas the 45 kDa form is present in other neural cells, such as astrocytes (Klepper and Voit, 2002; Farrell and Pardridge, 1991; Patching, 2017). GLUT1 provides steady transport of D-glucose and other hexoses across the BBB, ensuring a constant blood-to-brain energy supply (Patching, 2017). Another presentative substrate of GLUT1 is L-dehydroascorbic acid (L-DHA, an oxidized form of ascorbic acid). It has high structural similarity with D-glucose. Once transported, L-DHA is further reduced to L-ascorbic acid (L-AA) (Agus et al., 1997; Rumsey et al., 1997; Shao et al., 2015). The transformation of chemical structure of L-DHA makes it more attractive as a GLUT1 vector because of avoidance of pump-out by GLUT1.

2.1.2 Large neutral amino acid transporter 1

Another intensively studied transporter system is large neutral amino acid transporter 1 (LAT1) and is expressed both on the luminal and abluminal membranes of BCECs (Roberts et al., 2008; Kido et al., 2001). LAT1 mediates brain uptake of neutral L-amino acids, such as phenylalanine, leucine, and tyrosine. It is considered as an attractive drug target since it enables several prescription therapeutics transfer across the BBB. L-DOPA is an amino acid derivative transported by LAT1 and is considered as the most notable prodrug of pharmaceutical significance in the therapy of Parkinson's disease (Alexander et al., 1994; Peura et al., 2013). Similarly, an anticonvulsant drug, gabapentin is able to cross the BBB via LAT1-mediated pathway since its cyclic structure mimics that of an amino acid (Del Amo et al., 2008).

2.1.3 Monocarboxylate transporter 1

Monocarboxylate transporter 1 (MCT1) is expressed on the luminal membrane of BCECs (Gerhart et al., 1997). It is responsible for the transport of a broad range of monocarboxylate solutes, such as circulating lactate, pyruvate, and acetoacetic acid that can serve as an alternative energy source (Oldendorf, 1973; Kido et al., 2000). The functional activity of MCT1 is dependent on a proton gradient, and it facilitates the unidirectional proton-linked transport of monocarboxylates across the plasma membrane. Transport process can be stimulated by a pH gradient (low to high) as well (Broer et al., 1998). Apart from transport of endogenous substrates, earlier studies showed that acidic drugs such as valproic acid, benzoic acid, nicotinic acid, or beta-lactam antibiotics including benzylpenicillin, propicillin, and cefazolin could be transported via MCT1 into the brain in a pH-dependent manner (Kang et al., 1990; Vijay and Morris, 2014).

2.2 Receptor-mediated transport

RMT system employs the vesicular trafficking machinery of BCECs to deliver a range of proteins including transferrin, insulin, leptin, and lipoproteins to the brain (Descamps et al., 1996; Dehouck et al., 1997; Duffy and Pardridge, 1987; Golden et al., 1997). This process is initiated through a circulating ligand that first binds to a cognate transmembrane receptor expressed on the luminal BCEC membrane. Then, an intracellular vesicle containing receptor-ligand complexes forms and traffics to various final destinations. In the case of transcytosis, the vesicle is routed to the abluminal side of the BECEs and deposits the contents into the brain parenchyma (Rodriguez-Boulan et al., 2005; Brooks, 2009; Strazielle and Ghersi-Egea, 2013). Compared to the highly size-restricted stereoselective CMT, the vesicle-based RMT process allows for ferrying a wide range of large molecules, including proteins, antibodies, genes, enzymes, liposomes, nanoparticles, and drugs (Lajoie and Shusta, 2015). The three best-studied receptors include transferrin receptor (TfR), insulin receptor (IR), and low-density lipoprotein (LDL) receptor, and they have been widely investigated as the targets for CNS drug delivery.

2.2.1 Transferrin receptor

TfR is highly expressed at the BBB and is a transcytosis system that mediates iron delivery to the brain via binding and intracellular trafficking of the iron-binding protein transferrin (Tf) (Moos and Morgan, 2000; Lajoie and Shusta, 2015). Under normal physiologic conditions, TfR are mostly saturated with endogenous Tf (Stenehjem et al., 2009; Qian et al., 2002). Hence, Tf is not an ideal candidate as a targeting moiety to improve brain delivery of conjugated therapeutics or nanoparticles. Research efforts have, therefore, focused on engineering TfR monoclonal antibodies, which should target a certain sequence within the extracellular domain (ECD) of TfR, but do not interfere with the binding of endogenous Tf to TfR (Pardridge, 2015). Since there is no competition with circulating Tf in binding TfR, TfR monoclonal antibodies become attractive brain delivery vectors. Several TfR monoclonal antibodies have been engineered and shown species-specific BBB permeability (Pardridge, 2015). For example, OX26 antibody is a mouse monoclonal antibody against the rat TfR and RI7-217 or 8D3 antibody is a rat antibody against the mouse TfR (Pardridge et al., 1991; Lesley et al., 1984; Kissel et al., 1998; Lee et al., 2000). Both RI7-217 and 8D3 antibodies cross the BBB in the mouse, whereas the OX26 is transported across the BBB in the rat. Coupling these TfR monoclonal antibodies to a variety of therapeutics, including small molecules, proteins, nucleic acids, and nanoparticles, has shown some success in the delivery of drugs into the brain parenchyma.

2.2.2 Insulin receptor

IR expressed on the BBB appears to have two distinct functions: as a transporter of the circulating insulin from blood to brain (Miller et al., 1994) and as a trigger of activating intracellular signaling (Brummer et al., 2010). Since there is no source of insulin production in the CNS, the presence of insulin in the CSF is a clear evidence that insulin crosses the BBB (Blazquez et al., 2014). Studies using exogenous or radioactively labeled insulin confirmed that insulin crosses the BBB by a saturable receptor-mediated mechanism (Banks et al., 1997a, b). However, insulin is not considered as a viable RMT vector due to rapid degradation with a short serum half-life time (10 min) and a potential for inducing hypoglycemia by interfering with endogenous insulin balance (Bickel et al., 2001). The latter side effect would be less problematic with the use of insulin growth factor II (IGF-II) vector since higher concentrations of IGF are required before hypoglycemia occurs (Bickel et al., 2001). Hence, IR monoclonal antibodies have been employed as brain delivery vectors. A trifunctional fusion antibody is under development by ArmaGen for the treatment of Alzheimer's disease and it consists of (1) moieties that bind to human IR, which promotes the agent to cross the BBB; (2) the anti-Abeta peptide moiety binds to and further disaggregates the amyloid plaque; and (3) the anti-neonatal Fc receptor moiety that enables the agent to exit the brain via the BBB (Boado et al., 2007). Similarly, a BBB-penetrating form of the enzyme, NAGLU, which does not cross the BBB, was produced by reengineering of NAGLU as an IgG-enzyme fusion protein, where the IgG domain is a mAb against the human IR. The intravenous injection of the fusion protein can achieve high brain uptake of the enzyme, 1% injected dose/brain, and enables normalization of brain NAGLU enzyme activity (Boado et al., 2016).

2.2.3 Low-density lipoprotein receptor-related protein

As one major member of LDL receptor superfamily (Herz et al., 1988), low-density lipoprotein receptor-related protein (LRP1) is expressed on the BBB and participates in the transport of endogenous ligands from blood to brain (Molino et al., 2017). Instead of generating mAbs as in the case of targeting TfR or IR, for LRP1-mediated pathway, many peptide ligands have been developed as brain delivery vectors. Among these peptides, Angiopep and Angiopep-2 (ANG) have been widely used due to their greater transcytosis capacity across BBB compared to transferrin, lactoferrin, and avidin (Demeule et al., 2008a, b). There is some evidence that direct conjugation of ANG to drugs such as paclitaxel (Regina et al., 2008) and neurotensin (Demeule et al., 2014) enhances brain delivery. When used with nanoparticles in different brain disease models, ANG has shown promising results as a targeting ligand for brain delivery using nanoparticles (Shao et al., 2012, 2010; Huang et al., 2013; Ke et al., 2009; Mei et al., 2014).

2.3 Adsorptive-mediated transcytosis

AMT process is triggered by electrostatic interactions between the positively charged moieties of the proteins and negatively charged membrane surface regions on the BCECs (Kumagai et al., 1987). Upon binding of cationic molecules, such as cationic serum proteins, to the luminal surface of endothelial cells, exocytosis occurs at the abluminal surface (Herve et al., 2008). Many brain drug delivery strategies have focused on AMT due to its higher transport capacity in ferrying a range of cationized proteins into the brain when compared to RMT (Chen and Liu, 2012). However, it is still not known whether AMT is an ideal drug delivery target due to its inherent nonspecificity and random distribution that might result in undesired systemic toxicity. Basically, AMT-based drug delivery to the brain is performed using cationic proteins and cell-penetrating peptides (CPPs). The CPPs derived from natural proteins include the transcription-activating factor Tat, penetratin, and Syn-B vectors. They are heterogeneous in size (10–27 amino acid residues), positively charged and able to interact with a lipid membrane (Drin et al., 2002). Numerous studies have demonstrated that the conjugation of CPP to a potent drug can efficiently mediate drug delivery across the BBB in sufficient concentrations to elicit the desired effect in brain (Kristensen and Brodin, 2017). However, the pitfalls, such as nonspecificity, toxicity, immunogenicity, and instability of peptide vectors, need to be taken into consideration when CPP-mediated approaches are used. Apart from CPPs modification, nanoparticles which access brain parenchyma through AMT can be engineered by using biomaterials having high-density positive charge, such as chitosan (Songjiang and Lixiang, 2009), poly(ethylenimines) (PEIs) (Hwang et al., 2011), and cationized bovine serum albumin (CBSA) (Lu et al., 2005; Gao, 2016).

3 Strategies for improving CNS delivery of therapeutics

3.1 Enhanced paracellular transport

Temporary disruption of integrity of the BBB by chemical or physical approaches has long been developed as a conventional strategy for CNS biologics delivery. Chemical approach involves hyperosmotic agents, such as mannitol (Neuwelt et al., 1981, 1979; Siegal et al., 2000), arabinose (Fredericks and Rapoport, 1988), and urea (Rapoport and Thompson, 1973). These agents draw the water out of the BCECs and cause temporary shrinkage of BCECs and widening of TJs, thereby increasing the movement of drugs across the BBB via paracellular diffusion (Rapoport and Robinson, 1986; Orive et al., 2010). Studies have shown that, after the intracarotid infusion of mannitol, BBB permeability lasts 15 min to 4 h, depending on the size of the molecules being transported, with the barrier reclosing sooner to prevent larger molecules (Robinson and Rapoport, 1987). Similarly, various vasoactive agents, including alkylglycerols (Erdlenbruch et al., 2003; Lee et al., 2002), interleukin-2 (Gutman et al., 1996), leukotriene C4 (Black and Chio, 1992), bradykinin (Nakano et al., 1996), and RMP-7 (Ford et al., 1998), have been explored. These chemicals generate a temporary inflammatory reaction in the endothelial cells (Erdlenbruch et al., 2003) or cause vasodilation via signaling molecules (Nakano et al., 1996), resulting in increased vascular permeability and BBB opening. In physical approaches, different physical mechanisms such as electromagnetic wave impingement (Gao et al., 2009), magnetic nanoparticle invasion under alternating magnetic field, and microbubble-assisted focused ultrasound (FUS) are used to temporarily disrupt the BBB locally through deformation and restructuring of junction proteins (Gupta et al., 2007; Song et al., 2017). The pitfall of temporary disruption of BBB is that nonspecific components in the blood (e.g., albumin) can be transported to the CNS, resulting in neural toxicity and compromised brain function.

3.2 Improving physicochemical properties of CNS-active drugs

The physicochemical properties of small molecular drugs have a significant impact on their BBB permeability, especially via passive diffusion. As Lipinski's "rule of five", five key physiochemical parameters (molecular weight, lipophilicity, polar surface area, hydrogen bonding, and charge) require optimization to improve BBB permeability by passive diffusion (Lipinski et al., 2001). Poor BBB permeation more likely occurs when there is more than 5 H-bond donors and 10 H-bond acceptors and when MW is greater than 500 and calculated log P (C log P) is greater than 5 (or M log $P >$ 4.15) (Lipinski et al., 2001). These physiochemical parameters affect the interaction between the drug molecule and the lipophilic cell membrane on the BBB. For example, BBB permeability undergoes 100-fold reduction when the drug's MW is increased from 300 to 450 Da (Pardridge, 2012; Fischer et al., 1998). Smaller molecules have less difficulties to fill in the transient water pores formed in biological membranes (Trauble, 1971; Marrink et al., 1996). High lipid-soluble drug, which is equivalent to low hydrogen bonding and polar surface area, more readily crosses the hydrophobic phospholipid bilayer to enter the brain. It is believed that increasing the lipophilicity of a poorly permeable drug tends to increase its BBB permeability. In one report, after increasing the lipophilicity of heroin via acetylation of the two hydroxyl groups of morphine, BBB penetration rate was improved by 100-fold (Oldendorf et al., 1972). At physiological pH, lipophilic compounds with a slight positive charge favor the passive diffusion due to their enhanced interaction with the anionic cell membrane (Mikitsh and Chacko, 2014). Collectively, the physicochemical properties of the drugs need to be considered and optimized for CNS-active drug design in order to enable the passive permeation across the BBB.

For a hydrophilic CNS-active drug, lipidization via masking polar functionalities of the drug enhances more efficient CNS delivery. However, there have been only few successful cases in developing new drugs for human brain disorders by lipidization of a polar parent drug. Lipidization of the anticancer agent, chlorambucil, nicely demonstrates that increased lipophilicity and enhanced brain-to-plasma ratios of the active chlorambucil through prodrugs do not correlate with improved CNS therapeutic efficiency all the time. Compared to chlorambucil-treated group, after administration of chlorambucil-tertiary butyl ester, the brain-to-plasma ratio of the drug increased 47 folds, without showing superior anticancer activity in disease models (Genka et al., 1993; Greig et al., 1990). There are three possible reasons: (1) lipophilic modifications can lead to an increase in molecular weight of the parent drug, (2) lipophilic modifications can alter the pharmacokinetics and biodistribution of the parent drug. Instead, increased lipophilicity, while improving CNS access, also tends to increase the uptake in other tissues (Rautio et al., 2008), (3) if the hydrogen bond is blocked with a noncleavable group, prodrug cannot be effectively hydrolyzed in vivo, suggesting parent drug activity might be hindered (Pardridge, 2012). Despite several limitations, many lipidization prodrug strategies have been proposed to achieve enhanced drug brain uptake (Pavan et al., 2008; Rautio et al., 2008)

3.3 Drug modification with targeting moieties

Numerous modifications with specific ligands or targeting moieties have been applied to CNS-active therapeutics to improve their BBB permeability through transporter-mediated mechanisms. For example, several dozens of neuroactive drugs have been glycosylated in order to target GLUT1-mediated transport across the BBB. However, this approach is not consistently successful due to stringent stereochemical and molecular size requirements for GLUT1-binding and transport (Pardridge, 2003). Glucose analogues with mesylation at the 4-OH and 6-OH positions of D-glucose had slightly diminished affinity for GLUT1, while mesylation at the 3-OH position resulted in complete loss of activity (Halmos et al., 1997). Despite there is no straightforward evidence to verify whether glycosylated drugs use the same endogenous glucose transporter, GLUT1, as a way to cross the BBB, some studies indeed indicate that glycosylation improves BBB penetrability, biodistribution, and stability and reduces toxicity. Systemically delivered glycosyl derivatives of 7-chlorokynurenic acid, L-DOPA, dopamine, Ketoprofen, and Indomethacin have been shown to have pharmacological activity in the CNS of rodents (Battaglia et al., 2000; Fernandez et al., 2003; Halmos et al., 1996; Bonina et al., 2003; Gynther et al., 2009). Apart from the small molecular drugs, glycosylation has been widely applied to CNS delivery of peptides (glycopeptides) and proteins (glycoproteins). Short serum lifespan (1.3 min for dermorphin), inability to penetrate the BBB, and undesired metabolism and degradation of neuroactive peptides prevent them from reaching the receptors within the brain (Nagarajan, 1993). The strategy of appending a carbohydrate moiety through O-, N-, C-, and S-glycoside linkage to peptide backbone, or integration of "sugar amino acids" into peptides, has been broadly explored (Jones and Polt, 2015). Glycosylation of small peptides is essential for achieving brain delivery after i.v. or i.p. administration. Meanwhile, glycosylation leads to decreased lipophilicity, increased stability, altered pharmacokinetics/biodistribution, and enhanced CNS penetration. Enkephalin glycopeptides showed profound and long-lasting analgesia in mice (Polt et al., 1994). Glycosylation of opioid peptides has shown to enhance BBB penetration resulting in increased pharmacological activity (Bilsky et al., 2000; Negri et al., 1998; Elmagbari et al., 2004; Egleton et al., 2001, 2000).

3.4 Nanocarrier-based drug delivery

The distinct advantages, such as optimal size, shape, charge, stability, surface modification, biocompatibility, high drug-loading efficiency, controlled drug release as well as altered biodistribution and reduced drug side effect, allow nanoparticles to serve as potential drug delivery carriers in the treatment of different CNS diseases. Many studies have demonstrated that nanoparticles hold tremendous potential for diagnosis and therapy of brain disorders due to their capacity to cross BBB after systemic administration (Elzoghby et al., 2016). Various nanostructures, including liposomes, polymers, dendrimers, silicon, carbon, metal materials, and magnetic nanoparticles, have been tested as drug carriers in the delivery of genes, small molecules, proteins, and other macromolecules to the CNS (Ruan et al., 2017, 2016; Gao, 2017). The drug of interest can be dissolved, entrapped, adsorbed, attached, and/or encapsulated into or onto the nano-matrix (Singh and Lillard, 2009). Similar to drug modification, one of the most prevalent and attractive strategies for improving the BBB permeability is attaching targeting moieties to the nanoparticle-based delivery system via surface modification or coating. So far, plenty of ligands or substrates binding to the specific receptors (e.g., TfR, IR, LDL) (Pardridge, 2015; Clark and Davis, 2015) or transporters (e.g., GLUT1) (Shao et al., 2014, 2015; Gromnicova et al., 2013) on the BBB have been applied to the targeted nanocarriers. After coupling BBB targeting moieties, the targeted nanoparticles act as so-called "Trojan horse", transporting the cargoes across the BBB and depositing them on the brain parenchyma (Masserini, 2013). Another applied targeting approach is utilizing magnetic properties. The magnetically targeted drug nanocarriers get attracted towards the brain by magnetic fields and cross the BBB via transcytosis (Sensenig et al., 2012). Similarly, enhancement of BBB-targeted therapeutic effect can be achieved by inhibition of resistant function of efflux transporter, P-gp, expressed on the BBB. These approaches include: (1) the nanomaterials themselves at certain concentrations exhibit inhibitory effect on P-gp or its up-regulation (Wei et al., 2013; Zhou et al., 2015); and (2) encapsulation of P-gp inhibitors (Kaur et al., 2014) or silencing agents (Malmo et al., 2013) in the nanocarriers. The combination of different strategies described above for the nanocarriers design may help in achieving optimized therapeutic effect.

3.5 Cell-based drug delivery

Healthy CNS has an immune-privileged environment since BBB greatly restricts the migration of inflammatory cells into brain under normal physiological conditions (Daneman and Prat, 2015). However, brain infections, traumatic injuries, cancers, or degenerative processes can alter the BBB function and naturally recruit immune cells and stem cells towards inflamed or damaged area (Imitola et al., 2004; Larochelle et al., 2011). Theoretically, these cells that traffic to the pathological sites may serve as a targeted carrier for delivering therapeutics into the CNS.

The use of immune and stem cells, including neural stem cells (NSCs) and mesenchymal stem cells (MSCs), is one of the most exciting frontiers in the CNS drug delivery research. It has been studied extensively as a novel strategy to deliver therapeutics for cancer patients with primary or metastatic brain tumors (Aboody et al., 2000; Bagci-Onder et al., 2015; Hersh et al., 2016). Recent investigations demonstrated that cell-based drug delivery systems can be successfully applied to deliver a variety of therapeutic cargoes, ranging from gene (Ryu et al., 2011), cytokine (Ahmed et al., 2010), enzymes/prodrug (Aboody et al., 2013), and adenoviruses (Castleton et al., 2014) to nanoparticles (Steinfeld et al., 2006) across the BBB. The inherent advantages of cell-based drug delivery systems include improved targeting efficiency, controlled drug release, decreased drug immunogenicity, and enhanced drug effect. Although these encouraging findings make the cell-based carriers a very attractive avenue for potential CNS-active biologics delivery, many challenges have been encountered in their applications (Hersh et al., 2016; Batrakova et al., 2011): (1) potential cytotoxic effects of the cargo toward the cell carrier itself; (2) low level of drug loading on to cell carriers; (3) poor spatial and temporal control over the release of the therapeutic cargoes; and (4) insufficient number of cell carriers arrival to the site of action or disease. To overcome these, as a better alternative, the advantages of nanoparticle-based strategies are considered to combine with cell-based delivery strategies. Incorporation of the therapeutic cargoes into the protective nanoparticles can temporarily shield the drug cytotoxicity towards cell carriers. The drug-loaded nanoparticles can be attached to the cell carriers by cell-surface functionalization or internalization within the cell carriers (Steinfeld et al., 2006), resulting in improved drug loading efficiency, controlled disintegration, and release. Moreover, loading of cell carriers with magnetic nanoparticles enables higher therapeutics accumulation in the CNS, driven by the magnetic responses (Jain et al., 2003). Despite some progresses have been achieved, extensive studies are still necessary to optimize surface characteristics, multivalent attachment, controlled release, and biocompatibility.

4 Future perspectives

Insights into the complex and dynamic nature of the BBB paved the way for improving CNS-active therapeutics delivery strategies. In all strategies, from conventional to emerging, various novel approaches have been attempted, including increasing paracellular/transcellular diffusion, enhancing favorable pharmacokinetics, exploiting transport system's principles, and even drawing support from the vehicle trafficking.

The ultimate goal in all these approaches is efficient delivery of drugs to the CNS with optimized therapeutic but minimized untoward side effects.

Disruption of the BBB with pharmacological agents or ultrasound has shown some effects in the clinic. However, such disruption requires careful management to prevent excessive stress on TJs, leading to entry of circulating nonspecific substances and brain dysfunction. Altering physicochemical or targeting properties of a drug via chemical modification, such as lipidization and insertion of a glucose or D-amino acid moiety, is a promising but difficult approach. These modifications often influences drug's permeability and makes the mechanism of crossing the BBB less predictable, which sometimes even leads to opposite results upon drug entry to brain. At present, carrier-based delivery strategy offers effective CNS-active therapeutics delivery. The combination of endogenous transport systems on the BBB with nanoparticle-mediated delivery systems represents a powerful method for enhancing drug entry to the brain. Transporter proteins (e.g., GLUT1, LAT1, and MCT1), specific receptors (e.g., TfR, IR, and LDL), or adsorptive endocytosis (e.g., CPP) can be used to achieve drug delivery. However, some key parameters, such as BBB selectivity, safety, biocompatibility, and stability, need to be taken into consideration for designing brain-targeted nanoparticle-based delivery systems. Recently, efforts have been directed towards cell-based delivery that possesses distinct advantages including intrinsic targeting to sites of inflammation and its ability to carry drug and transport to CNS upon systemic administration. Nevertheless, further understanding is needed in terms of migration of immune cells or stem cells in different conditions of different brain disorders. This could improve the development of brain disease-specific cell-based delivery systems. Since the number of cells reaching site of action is directly proportional to the drug concentration in the brain, nanotechnology (e.g., magnetic nanoparticles and targeted nanoparticles grafting on the cell surface) can be exploited synergistically with cell-based delivery to improve targeting efficiency of cell carriers and hence drug entry to brain.

In sum, all these strategies discussed and even novel strategies development can overcome the challenges in the CNS-active therapeutics development. Although it is important to achieve high targeting efficiency, any given CNS-targeted delivery strategy must be assessed for their safety, risk, and benefits for patients, especially in the case of long-term therapy.

References

Aboody, K.S., Brown, A., Rainov, N.G., Bower, K.A., Liu, S., Yang, W., Small, J.E., Herrlinger, U., Ourednik, V., Black, P.M., Breakefield, X.O., Snyder, E.Y., 2000. Neural stem cells display extensive tropism for pathology in adult brain: evidence from intracranial gliomas. Proc. Natl. Acad. Sci. U. S. A. 97, 12846–12851.

Aboody, K.S., Najbauer, J., Metz, M.Z., D'apuzzo, M., Gutova, M., Annala, A.J., Synold, T.W., Couture, L.A., Blanchard, S., Moats, R.A., Garcia, E., Aramburo, S., Valenzuela, V.V., Frank, R.T., Barish, M.E., Brown, C.E., Kim, S.U., Badie, B., Portnow, J., 2013. Neural stem cell-mediated enzyme/prodrug therapy for glioma: preclinical studies. Sci. Transl. Med. 5184ra59.

Agus, D.B., Gambhir, S.S., Pardridge, W.M., Spielholz, C., Baselga, J., Vera, J.C., Golde, D.W., 1997. Vitamin C crosses the blood-brain barrier in the oxidized form through the glucose transporters. J. Clin. Invest. 100, 2842–2848.

Ahmed, A.U., Alexiades, N.G., Lesniak, M.S., 2010. The use of neural stem cells in cancer gene therapy: predicting the path to the clinic. Curr. Opin. Mol. Ther. 12, 546–552.

Alexander, G.M., Schwartzman, R.J., Grothusen, J.R., Gordon, S.W., 1994. Effect of plasma levels of large neutral amino acids and degree of parkinsonism on the blood-to-brain transport of levodopa in naive and MPTP parkinsonian monkeys. Neurology 44, 1491–1499.

Bagci-Onder, T., Du, W., Figueiredo, J.L., Martinez-Quintanilla, J., Shah, K., 2015. Targeting breast to brain metastatic tumours with death receptor ligand expressing therapeutic stem cells. Brain 138, 1710–1721.

Banks, W.A., 2016. From blood-brain barrier to blood-brain interface: new opportunities for CNS drug delivery. Nat. Rev. Drug Discov. 15, 275–292.

Banks, W.A., Jaspan, J.B., Huang, W., Kastin, A.J., 1997a. Transport of insulin across the blood-brain barrier: saturability at euglycemic doses of insulin. Peptides 18, 1423–1429.

Banks, W.A., Jaspan, J.B., Kastin, A.J., 1997b. Selective, physiological transport of insulin across the blood-brain barrier: novel demonstration by species-specific radioimmunoassays. Peptides 18, 1257–1262.

Batrakova, E.V., Gendelman, H.E., Kabanov, A.V., 2011. Cell-mediated drug delivery. Expert Opin. Drug Deliv. 8, 415–433.

Battaglia, G., La Russa, M., Bruno, V., Arenare, L., Ippolito, R., Copani, A., Bonina, F., Nicoletti, F., 2000. Systemically administered D-glucose conjugates of 7-chlorokynurenic acid are centrally available and exert anticonvulsant activity in rodents. Brain Res. 860, 149–156.

Begley, D.J., Brightman, M.W., 2003. Structural and functional aspects of the blood-brain barrier. Prog. Drug Res. 61, 39–78.

Bhaskar, S., Tian, F., Stoeger, T., Kreyling, W., De La Fuente, J.M., Grazu, V., Borm, P., Estrada, G., Ntziachristos, V., Razansky, D., 2010. Multifunctional nanocarriers for diagnostics, drug delivery and targeted treatment across blood-brain barrier: perspectives on tracking and neuroimaging. Part. Fibre Toxicol. 7, 3.

Bickel, U., Yoshikawa, T., Pardridge, W.M., 2001. Delivery of peptides and proteins through the blood-brain barrier. Adv. Drug Deliv. Rev. 46, 247–279.

Bilsky, E.J., Egleton, R.D., Mitchell, S.A., Palian, M.M., Davis, P., Huber, J.D., Jones, H., Yamamura, H.I., Janders, J., Davis, T.P., Porreca, F., Hruby, V.J., Polt, R., 2000. Enkephalin glycopeptide analogues produce analgesia with reduced dependence liability. J. Med. Chem. 43, 2586–2590.

Black, K.L., Chio, C.C., 1992. Increased opening of blood-tumour barrier by leukotriene C4 is dependent on size of molecules. Neurol. Res. 14, 402–404.

Blazquez, E., Velazquez, E., Hurtado-Carneiro, V., Ruiz-Albusac, J.M., 2014. Insulin in the brain: its pathophysiological implications for states related with central insulin resistance, type 2 diabetes and Alzheimer's disease. Front. Endocrinol. 5, 161.

Boado, R.J., Lu, J.Z., Hui, E.K., Lin, H., Pardridge, W.M., 2016. Insulin receptor antibody-alpha-N-acetylglucosaminidase fusion protein penetrates the primate blood-brain barrier and reduces glycosoaminoglycans in sanfilippo type B fibroblasts. Mol. Pharm. 13, 1385–1392.

Boado, R.J., Zhang, Y., Zhang, Y., Xia, C.F., Pardridge, W.M., 2007. Fusion antibody for Alzheimer's disease with bidirectional transport across the blood-brain barrier and abeta fibril disaggregation. Bioconjug. Chem. 18, 447–455.

Bonina, F., Puglia, C., Rimoli, M.G., Melisi, D., Boatto, G., Nieddu, M., Calignano, A., La Rana, G., De Caprariis, P., 2003. Glycosyl derivatives of dopamine and L-DOPA as anti-parkinson prodrugs: synthesis, pharmacological activity and in vitro stability studies. J. Drug Target. 11, 25–36.

Broer, S., Schneider, H.P., Broer, A., Rahman, B., Hamprecht, B., Deitmer, J.W., 1998. Characterization of the monocarboxylate transporter 1 expressed in Xenopus laevis oocytes by changes in cytosolic pH. Biochem. J. 333 (Pt 1), 167–174.

Brooks, D.A., 2009. The endosomal network. Int. J. Clin. Pharmacol. Ther. 47 (Suppl 1), S9–17.

Brummer, T., Schmitz-Peiffer, C., Daly, R.J., 2010. Docking proteins. FEBS J. 277, 4356–4369.

Castleton, A., Dey, A., Beaton, B., Patel, B., Aucher, A., Davis, D.M., Fielding, A.K., 2014. Human mesenchymal stromal cells deliver systemic oncolytic measles virus to treat acute lymphoblastic leukemia in the presence of humoral immunity. Blood 123, 1327–1335.

Chen, Y., Liu, L., 2012. Modern methods for delivery of drugs across the blood-brain barrier. Adv. Drug Deliv. Rev. 64, 640–665.

Clark, A.J., Davis, M.E., 2015. Increased brain uptake of targeted nanoparticles by adding an acid-cleavable linkage between transferrin and the nanoparticle core. Proc. Natl. Acad. Sci. U. S. A. 112, 12486–12491.

Daneman, R., Prat, A., 2015. The blood-brain barrier. Cold Spring Harb. Perspect. Biol. 7A020412.

De Boer, A.G., Breimer, D.D., 1994. The blood-brain barrier: clinical implications for drug delivery to the brain. J. R. Coll. Physicians Lond. 28, 502–506.

Dehouck, B., Fenart, L., Dehouck, M.P., Pierce, A., Torpier, G., Cecchelli, R., 1997. A new function for the LDL receptor: transcytosis of LDL across the blood-brain barrier. J. Cell Biol. 138, 877–889.

Del Amo, E.M., Urtti, A., Yliperttula, M., 2008. Pharmacokinetic role of L-type amino acid transporters LAT1 and LAT2. Eur. J. Pharm. Sci. 35, 161–174.

Demeule, M., Beaudet, N., Regina, A., Besserer-Offroy, E., Murza, A., Tetreault, P., Belleville, K., Che, C., Larocque, A., Thiot, C., Beliveau, R., Longpre, J.M., Marsault, E., Leduc, R., Lachowicz, J.E., Gonias, S.L., Castaigne, J.P., Sarret, P., 2014. Conjugation of a brain-penetrant peptide with neurotensin provides antinociceptive properties. J. Clin. Invest. 124, 1199–1213.

Demeule, M., Currie, J.C., Bertrand, Y., Che, C., Nguyen, T., Regina, A., Gabathuler, R., Castaigne, J.P., Beliveau, R., 2008a. Involvement of the low-density lipoprotein receptor-related protein in the transcytosis of the brain delivery vector angiopep-2. J. Neurochem. 106, 1534–1544.

Demeule, M., Regina, A., Che, C., Poirier, J., Nguyen, T., Gabathuler, R., Castaigne, J.P., Beliveau, R., 2008b. Identification and design of peptides as a new drug delivery system for the brain. J. Pharmacol. Exp. Ther. 324, 1064–1072.

Descamps, L., Dehouck, M.P., Torpier, G., Cecchelli, R., 1996. Receptor-mediated transcytosis of transferrin through blood-brain barrier endothelial cells. Am. J. Phys. 270, H1149–58.

Drin, G., Rousselle, C., Scherrmann, J.M., Rees, A.R., Temsamani, J., 2002. Peptide delivery to the brain via adsorptive-mediated endocytosis: advances with SynB vectors. AAPS PharmSciTech. 4E26.

Duffy, K.R., Pardridge, W.M., 1987. Blood-brain barrier transcytosis of insulin in developing rabbits. Brain Res. 420, 32–38.

Egleton, R.D., Mitchell, S.A., Huber, J.D., Janders, J., Stropova, D., Polt, R., Yamamura, H.I., Hruby, V.J., Davis, T.P., 2000. Improved bioavailability to the brain of glycosylated met-enkephalin analogs. Brain Res. 881, 37–46.

Egleton, R.D., Mitchell, S.A., Huber, J.D., Palian, M.M., Polt, R., Davis, T.P., 2001. Improved blood-brain barrier penetration and enhanced analgesia of an opioid peptide by glycosylation. J. Pharmacol. Exp. Ther. 299, 967–972.

Elmagbari, N.O., Egleton, R.D., Palian, M.M., Lowery, J.J., Schmid, W.R., Davis, P., Navratilova, E., Dhanasekaran, M., Keyari, C.M., Yamamura, H.I., Porreca, F., Hruby, V.J., Polt, R., Bilsky, E.J., 2004. Antinociceptive structure-activity studies with enkephalin-based opioid glycopeptides. J. Pharmacol. Exp. Ther. 311, 290–297.

Elzoghby, A.O., Abd-Elwakil, M.M., Abd-Elsalam, K., Elsayed, M.T., Hashem, Y., Mohamed, O., 2016. Natural polymeric nanoparticles for brain-targeting: implications on drug and gene delivery. Curr. Pharm. Des. 22, 3305–3323.

Erdlenbruch, B., Schinkhof, C., Kugler, W., Heinemann, D.E., Herms, J., Eibl, H., Lakomek, M., 2003. Intracarotid administration of short-chain alkylglycerols for increased delivery of methotrexate to the rat brain. Br. J. Pharmacol. 139, 685–694.

Farrell, C.L., Pardridge, W.M., 1991. Blood-brain barrier glucose transporter is asymmetrically distributed on brain capillary endothelial lumenal and ablumenal membranes: an electron microscopic immunogold study. Proc. Natl. Acad. Sci. U. S. A. 88, 5779–5783.

Fernandez, C., Nieto, O., Fontenla, J.A., Rivas, E., De Ceballos, M.L., Fernandez-Mayoralas, A., 2003. Synthesis of glycosyl derivatives as dopamine prodrugs: interaction with glucose carrier GLUT-1. Org. Biomol. Chem. 1, 767–771.

Fischer, H., Gottschlich, R., Seelig, A., 1998. Blood-brain barrier permeation: molecular parameters governing passive diffusion. J. Membr. Biol. 165, 201–211.

Ford, J., Osborn, C., Barton, T., Bleehen, N.M., 1998. A phase I study of intravenous RMP-7 with carboplatin in patients with progression of malignant glioma. Eur. J. Cancer 34, 1807–1811.

Fredericks, W.R., Rapoport, S.I., 1988. Reversible osmotic opening of the blood-brain barrier in mice. Stroke 19, 266–268.

Gao, H., 2016. Progress and perspectives on targeting nanoparticles for brain drug delivery. Acta Pharm. Sin. B 6, 268–286.

Gao, H., 2017. Perspectives on dual targeting delivery systems for brain tumors. J. NeuroImmune Pharmacol. 12, 6–16.

Gao, J., Gu, H., Xu, B., 2009. Multifunctional magnetic nanoparticles: design, synthesis, and biomedical applications. Acc. Chem. Res. 42, 1097–1107.

Genka, S., Deutsch, J., Shetty, U.H., Stahle, P.L., John, V., Lieberburg, I.M., Ali-Osman, F., Rapoport, S.I., Greig, N.H., 1993. Development of lipophilic anticancer agents for the treatment of brain tumors by the esterification of water-soluble chlorambucil. Clin. Exp. Metastasis 11, 131–140.

Gerhart, D.Z., Enerson, B.E., Zhdankina, O.Y., Leino, R.L., Drewes, L.R., 1997. Expression of monocarboxylate transporter MCT1 by brain endothelium and glia in adult and suckling rats. Am. J. Phys. 273, E207–13.

Golden, P.L., Maccagnan, T.J., Pardridge, W.M., 1997. Human blood-brain barrier leptin receptor. Binding and endocytosis in isolated human brain microvessels. J. Clin. Invest. 99, 14–18.

Greig, N.H., Genka, S., Daly, E.M., Sweeney, D.J., Rapoport, S.I., 1990. Physicochemical and pharmacokinetic parameters of seven lipophilic chlorambucil esters designed for brain penetration. Cancer Chemother. Pharmacol. 25, 311–319.

Gromnicova, R., Davies, H.A., Sreekanthreddy, P., Romero, I.A., Lund, T., Roitt, I.M., Phillips, J.B., Male, D.K., 2013. Glucose-coated gold nanoparticles transfer across human brain endothelium and enter astrocytes in vitro. PLoS One. 8E81043.

Guo, X., Geng, M., Du, G., 2005. Glucose transporter 1, distribution in the brain and in neural disorders: its relationship with transport of neuroactive drugs through the blood-brain barrier. Biochem. Genet. 43, 175–187.

Gupta, A.K., Naregalkar, R.R., Vaidya, V.D., Gupta, M., 2007. Recent advances on surface engineering of magnetic iron oxide nanoparticles and their biomedical applications. Nanomedicine (London) 2, 23–39.

Gutman, M., Laufer, R., Eisenthal, A., Goldman, G., Ravid, A., Inbar, M., Klausner, J.M., 1996. Increased microvascular permeability induced by prolonged interleukin-2 administration is attenuated by the oxygen-free-radical Scavenger dimethylthiourea. Cancer Immunol. Immunother. 43, 240–244.

Gynther, M., Ropponen, J., Laine, K., Leppanen, J., Haapakoski, P., Peura, L., Jarvinen, T., Rautio, J., 2009. Glucose promoiety enables glucose transporter mediated brain uptake of ketoprofen and indomethacin prodrugs in rats. J. Med. Chem. 52, 3348–3353.

Halmos, T., Santarromana, M., Antonakis, K., Scherman, D., 1996. Synthesis of glucose-chlorambucil derivatives and their recognition by the human GLUT1 glucose transporter. Eur. J. Pharmacol. 318, 477–484.

Halmos, T., Santarromana, M., Antonakis, K., Scherman, D., 1997. Synthesis of O-methylsulfonyl derivatives of D-glucose as potential alkylating agents for targeted drug delivery to the brain. Evaluation of their interaction with the human erythrocyte GLUT1 hexose transporter. Carbohydr. Res. 299, 15–21.

Hersh, D.S., Wadajkar, A.S., Roberts, N., Perez, J.G., Connolly, N.P., Frenkel, V., Winkles, J.A., Woodworth, G.F., Kim, A.J., 2016. Evolving drug delivery strategies to overcome the blood brain barrier. Curr. Pharm. Des. 22, 1177–1193.

Herve, F., Ghinea, N., Scherrmann, J.M., 2008. CNS delivery via adsorptive transcytosis. AAPS J. 10, 455–472.

Herz, J., Hamann, U., Rogne, S., Myklebost, O., Gausepohl, H., Stanley, K.K., 1988. Surface location and high affinity for calcium of a 500-kd liver membrane protein closely related to the LDL-receptor suggest a physiological role as lipoprotein receptor. EMBO J. 7, 4119–4127.

Huang, R., Ma, H., Guo, Y., Liu, S., Kuang, Y., Shao, K., Li, J., Liu, Y., Han, L., Huang, S., An, S., Ye, L., Lou, J., Jiang, C., 2013. Angiopep-conjugated nanoparticles for targeted long-term gene therapy of Parkinson's disease. Pharm. Res. 30, 2549–2559.

Hwang, D.W., Son, S., Jang, J., Youn, H., Lee, S., Lee, D., Lee, Y.S., Jeong, J.M., Kim, W.J., Lee, D.S., 2011. A brain-targeted rabies virus glycoprotein-disulfide linked pei nanocarrier for delivery of neurogenic microrna. Biomaterials 32, 4968–4975.

Imitola, J., Raddassi, K., Park, K.I., Mueller, F.J., Nieto, M., Teng, Y.D., Frenkel, D., Li, J., Sidman, R.L., Walsh, C.A., Snyder, E.Y., Khoury, S.J., 2004. Directed migration of neural stem cells to sites of CNS injury by the stromal cell-derived factor 1alpha/CXC chemokine receptor 4 pathway. Proc. Natl. Acad. Sci. U. S. A. 101, 18117–18122.

Jain, S., Mishra, V., Singh, P., Dubey, P.K., Saraf, D.K., Vyas, S.P., 2003. Rgd-anchored magnetic liposomes for monocytes/neutrophils-mediated brain targeting. Int. J. Pharm. 261, 43–55.

Jones, E.M., Polt, R., 2015. CNS active O-linked glycopeptides. Front. Chem. 3, 40.

Kang, Y.S., Terasaki, T., Tsuji, A., 1990. Acidic drug transport in vivo through the blood-brain barrier. A role of the transport carrier for monocarboxylic acids. Aust. J. Pharm. 13, 158–163.

Kaur, V., Garg, T., Rath, G., Goyal, A.K., 2014. Therapeutic potential of nanocarrier for overcoming to P-glycoprotein. J. Drug Target. 22, 859–870.

Ke, W., Shao, K., Huang, R., Han, L., Liu, Y., Li, J., Kuang, Y., Ye, L., Lou, J., Jiang, C., 2009. Gene delivery targeted to the brain using an angiopep-conjugated polyethyleneglycol-modified polyamidoamine dendrimer. Biomaterials 30, 6976–6985.

Kido, Y., Tamai, I., Okamoto, M., Suzuki, F., Tsuji, A., 2000. Functional clarification of MCT1-mediated transport of monocarboxylic acids at the blood-brain barrier using in vitro cultured cells and in vivo bui studies. Pharm. Res. 17, 55–62.

Kido, Y., Tamai, I., Uchino, H., Suzuki, F., Sai, Y., Tsuji, A., 2001. Molecular and functional identification of large neutral amino acid transporters LAT1 And LAT2 and their pharmacological relevance at the blood-brain barrier. J. Pharm. Pharmacol. 53, 497–503.

Kissel, K., Hamm, S., Schulz, M., Vecchi, A., Garlanda, C., Engelhardt, B., 1998. Immunohistochemical localization of the murine transferrin receptor (TFR) on blood-tissue barriers using a novel anti-TFR monoclonal antibody. Histochem. Cell Biol. 110, 63–72.

Klepper, J., Voit, T., 2002. Facilitated glucose transporter protein type 1 (GLUT1) deficiency syndrome: impaired glucose transport into brain—a review. Eur. J. Pediatr. 161, 295–304.

Kristensen, M., Brodin, B., 2017. Routes for drug translocation across the blood-brain barrier: exploiting peptides as delivery vectors. J. Pharm. Sci. 106, 2326–2334.

Kumagai, A.K., Eisenberg, J.B., Pardridge, W.M., 1987. Absorptive-mediated endocytosis of cationized albumin and a beta-endorphin-cationized albumin chimeric peptide by isolated brain capillaries. Model system of blood-brain barrier transport. J. Biol. Chem. 262, 15214–15219.

Lajoie, J.M., Shusta, E.V., 2015. Targeting receptor-mediated transport for delivery of biologics across the blood-brain barrier. Annu. Rev. Pharmacol. Toxicol. 55, 613–631.

Larochelle, C., Alvarez, J.I., Prat, A., 2011. How do immune cells overcome the blood-brain barrier in multiple sclerosis? FEBS Lett. 585, 3770–3780.

Lee, H.J., Engelhardt, B., Lesley, J., Bickel, U., Pardridge, W.M., 2000. Targeting rat anti-mouse transferrin receptor monoclonal antibodies through blood-brain barrier in mouse. J. Pharmacol. Exp. Ther. 292, 1048–1052.

Lee, H.J., Zhang, Y., Pardridge, W.M., 2002. Blood-brain barrier disruption following the internal carotid arterial perfusion of alkyl glycerols. J. Drug Target. 10, 463–467.

Lesley, J., Hyman, R., Schulte, R., Trotter, J., 1984. Expression of transferrin receptor on murine hematopoietic progenitors. Cell. Immunol. 83, 14–25.

Lipinski, C.A., Lombardo, F., Dominy, B.W., Feeney, P.J., 2001. Experimental and computational approaches to estimate solubility and permeability in drug discovery and development settings. Adv. Drug Deliv. Rev. 46, 3–26.

Lu, W., Zhang, Y., Tan, Y.Z., Hu, K.L., Jiang, X.G., Fu, S.K., 2005. Cationic albumin-conjugated pegylated nanoparticles as novel drug carrier for brain delivery. J. Control. Release 107, 428–448.

Malmo, J., Sandvig, A., Varum, K.M., Strand, S.P., 2013. Nanoparticle mediated P-glycoprotein silencing for improved drug delivery across the blood-brain barrier: a sirna-chitosan approach. PLoS One. 8E54182.

Marrink, S.J., Jahnig, F., Berendsen, H.J., 1996. Proton transport across transient single-file water pores in a lipid membrane studied by molecular dynamics simulations. Biophys. J. 71, 632–647.

Masserini, M., 2013. Nanoparticles for brain drug delivery. Isrn Biochem. 2013238428.

Mei, L., Zhang, Q., Yang, Y., He, Q., Gao, H., 2014. Angiopep-2 and activatable cell penetrating peptide dual modified nanoparticles for enhanced tumor targeting and penetrating. Int. J. Pharm. 474, 95–102.

Mikitsh, J.L., Chacko, A.M., 2014. Pathways for small molecule delivery to the central nervous system across the blood-brain barrier. Perspect. Med. Chem. 6, 11–24.

Miller, D.W., Keller, B.T., Borchardt, R.T., 1994. Identification and distribution of insulin receptors on cultured bovine brain microvessel endothelial cells: possible function in insulin processing in the blood-brain barrier. J. Cell. Physiol. 161, 333–341.
Molino, Y., David, M., Varini, K., Jabes, F., Gaudin, N., Fortoul, A., Bakloul, K., Masse, M., Bernard, A., Drobecq, L., Lecorche, P., Temsamani, J., Jacquot, G., Khrestchatisky, M., 2017. Use of LDL receptor-targeting peptide vectors for in vitro and in vivo cargo transport across the blood-brain barrier. FASEB J. 31, 1807–1827.
Moos, T., Morgan, E.H., 2000. Transferrin and transferrin receptor function in brain barrier systems. Cell. Mol. Neurobiol. 20, 77–95.
Nagarajan, R., 1993. Structure-activity relationships of vancomycin-type glycopeptide antibiotics. J. Antibiot. (Tokyo) 46, 1181–1195.
Nakano, S., Matsukado, K., Black, K.L., 1996. Increased brain tumor microvessel permeability after intracarotid bradykinin infusion is mediated by nitric oxide. Cancer Res. 56, 4027–4031.
Negri, L., Lattanzi, R., Tabacco, F., Scolaro, B., Rocchi, R., 1998. Glycodermorphins: opioid peptides with potent and prolonged analgesic activity and enhanced blood-brain barrier penetration. Br. J. Pharmacol. 124, 1516–1522.
Neuwelt, E.A., Frenkel, E.P., Diehl, J.T., Maravilla, K.R., Vu, L.H., Clark, W.K., Rapoport, S.I., Barnett, P.A., Hill, S.A., Lewis, S.E., Ehle, A.L., Beyer Jr., C.W., Moore, R.J., 1979. Osmotic blood-brain barrier disruption: a new means of increasing chemotherapeutic agent delivery. Trans. Am. Neurol. Assoc. 104, 256–260.
Neuwelt, E.A., Hill, S.A., Frenkel, E.P., Diehl, J.T., Maravilla, K.R., Vu, L.H., Clark, W.K., Rapoport, S.I., Barnett, P.A., Lewis, S.E., Ehle, A.L., Beyer Jr., C.W., 1981. Osmotic blood-brain barrier disruption: pharmacodynamic studies in dogs and a clinical phase I trial in patients with malignant brain tumors. Cancer Treat. Rep. 65 (Suppl. 2), 39–43.
Oldendorf, W.H., 1973. Carrier-mediated blood-brain barrier transport of short-chain monocarboxylic organic acids. Am. J. Phys. 224, 1450–1453.
Oldendorf, W.H., Hyman, S., Braun, L., Oldendorf, S.Z., 1972. Blood-brain barrier: penetration of morphine, codeine, heroin, and methadone after carotid injection. Science 178, 984–986.
Orive, G., Ali, O.A., Anitua, E., Pedraz, J.L., Emerich, D.F., 2010. Biomaterial-based technologies for brain anti-cancer therapeutics and imaging. Biochim. Biophys. Acta 1806, 96–107.
Pangalos, M.N., Schechter, L.E., Hurko, O., 2007. Drug development for cns disorders: strategies for balancing risk and reducing attrition. Nat. Rev. Drug Discov. 6, 521–532.
Pardridge, W.M., 1983. Brain metabolism: a perspective from the blood-brain barrier. Physiol. Rev. 63, 1481–1535.
Pardridge, W.M., 2003. Blood-brain barrier drug targeting: the future of brain drug development. Mol. Interv. 3, 90–105, 51.
Pardridge, W.M., 2005. The blood-brain barrier: bottleneck in brain drug development. NeuroRx 2, 3–14.
Pardridge, W.M., 2007. Blood-brain barrier delivery. Drug Discov. Today 12, 54–61.
Pardridge, W.M., 2012. Drug transport across the blood-brain barrier. J. Cereb. Blood Flow Metab. 32, 1959–1972.
Pardridge, W.M., 2015. Blood-brain barrier drug delivery of IgG fusion proteins with a transferrin receptor monoclonal antibody. Expert Opin. Drug Deliv. 12, 207–222.
Pardridge, W.M., Buciak, J.L., Friden, P.M., 1991. Selective transport of an anti-transferrin receptor antibody through the blood-brain barrier in vivo. J. Pharmacol. Exp. Ther. 259, 66–70.

Patching, S.G., 2017. Glucose transporters at the blood-brain barrier: function, regulation and gateways for drug delivery. Mol. Neurobiol. 54, 1046–1077.

Pavan, B., Dalpiaz, A., Ciliberti, N., Biondi, C., Manfredini, S., Vertuani, S., 2008. Progress in drug delivery to the central nervous system by the prodrug approach. Molecules 13, 1035–1065.

Peura, L., Malmioja, K., Huttunen, K., Leppanen, J., Hamalainen, M., Forsberg, M.M., Gynther, M., Rautio, J., Laine, K., 2013. Design, synthesis and brain uptake of LAT1-targeted amino acid prodrugs of dopamine. Pharm. Res. 30, 2523–2537.

Polt, R., Porreca, F., Szabo, L.Z., Bilsky, E.J., Davis, P., Abbruscato, T.J., Davis, T.P., Harvath, R., Yamamura, H.I., Hruby, V.J., 1994. Glycopeptide enkephalin analogues produce analgesia in mice: evidence for penetration of the blood-brain barrier. Proc. Natl. Acad. Sci. U. S. A. 91, 7114–7118.

Psimadas, D., Tsotakos, T., Fragogeorgi, E., Loudos, G., 2015. Nanomedicinal approach of getting across the brood-brain barrier with nanomedicinal nanoparticles. Curr. Med. Chem. 22, 4257–4270.

Qian, Z.M., Li, H., Sun, H., Ho, K., 2002. Targeted drug delivery via the transferrin receptor-mediated endocytosis pathway. Pharmacol. Rev. 54, 561–587.

Rapoport, S.I., Robinson, P.J., 1986. Tight-junctional modification as the basis of osmotic opening of the blood-brain barrier. Ann. N. Y. Acad. Sci. 481, 250–267.

Rapoport, S.I., Thompson, H.K., 1973. Osmotic opening of the blood-brain barrier in the monkey without associated neurological deficits. Science 180, 971.

Rautio, J., Laine, K., Gynther, M., Savolainen, J., 2008. Prodrug approaches for CNS delivery. AAPS J. 10, 92–102.

Regina, A., Demeule, M., Che, C., Lavallee, I., Poirier, J., Gabathuler, R., Beliveau, R., Castaigne, J.P., 2008. Antitumour activity of ANG1005, a conjugate between paclitaxel and the new brain delivery vector angiopep-2. Br. J. Pharmacol. 155, 185–197.

Roberts, L.M., Black, D.S., Raman, C., Woodford, K., Zhou, M., Haggerty, J.E., Yan, A.T., Cwirla, S.E., Grindstaff, K.K., 2008. Subcellular localization of transporters along the rat blood-brain barrier and blood-cerebral-spinal fluid barrier by in vivo biotinylation. Neuroscience 155, 423–438.

Robinson, P.J., Rapoport, S.I., 1987. Size selectivity of blood-brain barrier permeability at various times after osmotic opening. Am. J. Phys. 253, R459–66.

Rodriguez-Boulan, E., Kreitzer, G., Musch, A., 2005. Organization of vesicular trafficking in epithelia. Nat. Rev. Mol. Cell Biol. 6, 233–247.

Ruan, S., Hu, C., Tang, X., Cun, X., Xiao, W., Shi, K., He, Q., Gao, H., 2016. Increased gold nanoparticle retention in brain tumors by in situ enzyme-induced aggregation. ACS Nano 10, 10086–10098.

Ruan, S., Xiao, W., Hu, C., Zhang, H., Rao, J., Wang, S., Wang, X., He, Q., Gao, H., 2017. Ligand-mediated and enzyme-directed precise targeting and retention for the enhanced treatment of glioblastoma. ACS Appl. Mater. Interfaces 9, 20348–20360.

Rumsey, S.C., Kwon, O., Xu, G.W., Burant, C.F., Simpson, I., Levine, M., 1997. Glucose transporter isoforms GLUT1 and GLUT3 transport dehydroascorbic acid. J. Biol. Chem. 272, 18982–18989.

Ryu, C.H., Park, S.H., Park, S.A., Kim, S.M., Lim, J.Y., Jeong, C.H., Yoon, W.S., Oh, W.I., Sung, Y.C., Jeun, S.S., 2011. Gene therapy of intracranial glioma using interleukin 12-secreting human umbilical cord blood-derived mesenchymal stem cells. Hum. Gene Ther. 22, 733–743.

Sensenig, R., Sapir, Y., Macdonald, C., Cohen, S., Polyak, B., 2012. Magnetic nanoparticle-based approaches to locally target therapy and enhance tissue regeneration in vivo. Nanomedicine (London) 7, 1425–1442.

Shao, K., Ding, N., Huang, S., Ren, S., Zhang, Y., Kuang, Y., Guo, Y., Ma, H., An, S., Li, Y., Jiang, C., 2014. Smart nanodevice combined tumor-specific vector with cellular microenvironment-triggered property for highly effective antiglioma therapy. ACS Nano 8, 1191–1203.

Shao, K., Huang, R., Li, J., Han, L., Ye, L., Lou, J., Jiang, C., 2010. Angiopep-2 modified PE-PEG based polymeric micelles for amphotericin B delivery targeted to the brain. J. Control. Release 147, 118–126.

Shao, K., Wu, J., Chen, Z., Huang, S., Li, J., Ye, L., Lou, J., Zhu, L., Jiang, C., 2012. A brain-vectored angiopep-2 based polymeric micelles for the treatment of intracranial fungal infection. Biomaterials 33, 6898–6907.

Shao, K., Zhang, Y., Ding, N., Huang, S., Wu, J., Li, J., Yang, C., Leng, Q., Ye, L., Lou, J., Zhu, L., Jiang, C., 2015. Functionalized nanoscale micelles with brain targeting ability and intercellular microenvironment biosensitivity for anti-intracranial infection applications. Adv. Healthc. Mater. 4, 291–300.

Siegal, T., Rubinstein, R., Bokstein, F., Schwartz, A., Lossos, A., Shalom, E., Chisin, R., Gomori, J.M., 2000. In vivo assessment of the window of barrier opening after osmotic blood-brain barrier disruption in humans. J. Neurosurg. 92, 599–605.

Singh, R., Lillard Jr., J.W., 2009. Nanoparticle-based targeted drug delivery. Exp. Mol. Pathol. 86, 215–223.

Smith, Q.R., 1993. Drug delivery to brain and the role of carrier-mediated transport. Adv. Exp. Med. Biol. 331, 83–93.

Song, Y., Du, D., Li, L., Xu, J., Dutta, P., Lin, Y., 2017. In vitro study of receptor-mediated silica nanoparticles delivery across blood-brain barrier. ACS Appl. Mater. Interfaces 9, 20410–20416.

Songjiang, Z., Lixiang, W., 2009. Amyloid-beta associated with chitosan nano-carrier has favorable immunogenicity and permeates the BBB. AAPS PharmSciTech 10, 900–905.

Steinfeld, U., Pauli, C., Kaltz, N., Bergemann, C., Lee, H.H., 2006. T lymphocytes as potential therapeutic drug carrier for cancer treatment. Int. J. Pharm. 311, 229–236.

Stenehjem, D.D., Hartz, A.M., Bauer, B., Anderson, G.W., 2009. Novel and emerging strategies in drug delivery for overcoming the blood-brain barrier. Future Med. Chem. 1, 1623–1641.

Strazielle, N., Ghersi-Egea, J.F., 2013. Physiology of blood-brain interfaces in relation to brain disposition of small compounds and macromolecules. Mol. Pharm. 10, 1473–1491.

Tamai, I., Tsuji, A., 2000. Transporter-mediated permeation of drugs across the blood-brain barrier. J. Pharm. Sci. 89, 1371–1388.

Trauble, H., 1971. The movement of molecules across lipid membranes: a molecular theory. J. Membr. Biol. 4, 193–208.

Vijay, N., Morris, M.E., 2014. Role of monocarboxylate transporters in drug delivery to the brain. Curr. Pharm. Des. 20, 1487–1498.

Wei, Z., Yuan, S., Hao, J., Fang, X., 2013. Mechanism of inhibition of P-glycoprotein mediated efflux by pluronic P123/F127 block copolymers: relationship between copolymer concentration and inhibitory activity. Eur. J. Pharm. Biopharm. 83, 266–274.

Zhou, Y., Zhang, G., Rao, Z., Yang, Y., Zhou, Q., Qin, H., Wei, Y., Wu, X., 2015. Increased brain uptake of venlafaxine loaded solid lipid nanoparticles by overcoming the efflux function and expression of P-gp. Arch. Pharm. Res. 38, 1325–1335.

In vitro and in vivo models of BBB to evaluate brain targeting drug delivery

4

Bhupesh Sharma, Kanishk Luhach, G.T. Kulkarni
Amity Institute of Pharmacy, Amity University Uttar Pradesh, Noida, India

List of Abbreviations

ABC	ATP-binding cassette protein
AMT	adsorptive-mediated transcytosis
ANG	angiopoietin
AUC	area under the curve
BBB	blood-brain barrier
BCEC	brain capillary endothelial cells
CNS	central nervous system
EBA	Evans blue albumin
FITC	fluorescein isothiocyanate
GLUT	glucose transporter
hCMEC	human cerebral microvasculature endothelial cells
hiPSC	human-induced pluripotent stem cell
HPLC	high performance liquid chromatography
HRP	horseradish peroxidase
IAM	immobilized artificial membrane
JAM	junctional adhesion molecules
LC-MS	liquid chromatography-mass spectrometry
MRI	magnetic resonance imaging
NVU	neurovascular unit
PAMPA	parallel artificial membrane permeability
PET	positron emission tomography
P-gp	permeability glycoprotein
PVDF	polyvinylidene difluoride
QAR	quantitative autoradiography
RMT	receptor-mediated transcytosis
SLC	solute carrier
TEER	trans-endothelial electric resistance
VEGF	vascular endothelial growth factor
ZO	zonula occludens

Brain Targeted Drug Delivery Systems. https://doi.org/10.1016/B978-0-12-814001-7.00004-4

1 Introduction

Blood-brain barrier (BBB) is a complex, selectively permeable barrier which encapsulates the central nervous system (CNS) and separates it from rest of the body (Bicker et al., 2014; Patel and Patel, 2017). Thus, BBB provides physiological protection to the brain against an aberrant exposure from toxic substances (Patel and Patel, 2017). The major component of the BBB is the brain capillary endothelial cell (BCEC). A BCEC prevents most of the large molecules, i.e., more than 500 Da, to enter the brain freely (Pardridge, 2007, 2016) and, along with other cells such as astrocytes, pericytes, tight junctions, etc., it forms both an active and a passive mechanism to preserve the microvasculature and restrict the amount of drug nanoparticle that can be delivered into the brain (Azad et al., 2015; Daneman and Prat, 2015a). Restrictions to drug transport across the BBB make drug delivery and assessment of delivery into the brain especially challenging (Larsen et al., 2014).

As the BBB acts as a formidable opponent in drug delivery, majority of the drug molecules do not reach therapeutic levels inside the parenchyma (Pardridge, 2007). Thus, models which best replicate the anatomical and functional features of the BBB are being used to increase chances of a "hit" compound in the preclinical developmental process of drug discovery. Several models have been identified till date; this chapter is going to focus on in vitro and in vivo models of BBB and how they can be used to assess and improve drug nanoparticle delivery to the brain (Helms et al., 2016). In order to understand these models used to assess drug delivery through BBB, we must first take a look at the structural and functional characteristics of the BBB.

2 The neurovascular unit

Components of the BBB include the presence of endothelial cells and basement membrane. The tight junction proteins are present adjacent to the endothelial cells with pinocytic vesicles and specific transport mechanism. Surrounding the endothelium are cellular elements, which include pericytes and astroglial foot processes. These form another continuous layer of cells, which separate blood vessels from the brain tissue. This coexistence and codependency of neurons, astrocytes, microglia, pericytes, and blood vessels in a dynamically functioning unit is known as the neurovascular unit (NVU) (Oldendorf et al., 1977; Abbott, 2013; Serlin et al., 2015).

The BBB is thus formed by endothelial cells that line the capillaries in the spinal cord and the brain and by various other cells, such as, pericytes, microglial cells, and astrocytes (Begley, 2004; Bernacki et al., 2008). All of these possess a challenge of their own, when it comes to drug delivery and nanoparticle delivery; considering this, each cell type is briefly discussed.

2.1 Endothelial cells

Endothelial cells are modified simple squamous cells originating from the mesoderm; they form the walls of all the blood vessels. The CNS microvascular endothelial cells are 61% thinner than the ones found in muscle and have more mitochondria and less fenestrations (pinocytotic vesicles) anywhere along the BBB (Oldendorf et al., 1977; Coomber and Stewart, 1985; Kniesel and Wolburg, 2000; Thomsen et al., 2015). The endothelial cells form a monolayer in the innermost luminal spaces; these exhibit greater volume of mitochondria in order to maintain and operate the selective molecular permeability of BBB, which results in reduced drug delivery (Oldendorf et al., 1977). Basement membrane is 30–40 nm in thickness, made of collagen type IV, heparin sulfate proteoglycans, laminin, fibronectin, and other extracellular matrix proteins. The basement membrane ensheaths the pericytes and endothelial cells (Hawkins and Davis, 2005).

Junctional adhesion molecule-1 (JAM), occludin, and claudins1/3, 5 are transmembrane proteins and, along with cytoplasmic accessory proteins (zonula occludens-1 and -2, cingulin and AF-6), form the tight junctions between each adjacent endothelial cells (Abbott et al., 2010; Chen and Liu, 2012). Endothelial cells along with transporter molecules play a pivotal role in keeping drug molecules out of CNS and into the blood.

The BCEC express two main categories of transporters. The first are called efflux transporters; these are polarized to the luminal surface, thus transporting lipophilic molecules across the cell membrane and toward blood, e.g., ATP-binding cassette (ABC) family of transporters and the permeability glycoprotein (P-gp); these not only provide barrier function, but also restrict the amount of drugs being delivered to the CNS (Cordon-Cardo et al., 1989; Thiebaut et al., 1989; Borges-Walmsley et al., 2003; Loscher and Potschka, 2005; Shen and Zhang, 2010; Sharom, 2011). The second are nutrient influx transporters and waste efflux transporters; their polarization is variable and may be influenced by nearby astrocytes (Hawkins et al., 2006; Mittapalli et al., 2010; Banks, 2016). BCECs are also known for being richly endowed with enzymes such as monoamine oxidase, acid and alkaline phosphatases, and CYP450 enzymes; these tend to metabolize and breakdown any ligand (natural or artificial) at the surface of the BCEC (Cucullo et al., 2011; Ghosh et al., 2011).

Shear stress, a tangential force that is applied to the vascular endothelium because of the flow of blood across the luminal surface of the BCEC, plays a major role in drug delivery as it affects the physiology of the cell and the adsorptive transcytosis process (which is discussed later in Section 3 of this chapter) (Cucullo et al., 2011).

Due to these structural and functional aspects, the BCECs are considered to be of utmost importance when modeling any cell-based in vitro models of BBB to assess the extent of nanoparticle delivery.

2.2 Pericytes

Pericytes are the cells present between the basement membrane and astrocytes, thus they seem to be embedded between endothelial cell, basement membrane, and astrocytes (Sims, 1986; Daneman and Prat, 2015b). They incompletely cover the endothelial walls, about 22%–33% of it, but are somehow correlated to BBB permeability as it has been demonstrated that their deficiency leads to increase in permeability of the BBB (Peppiatt et al., 2006; Hall et al., 2014; Daneman and Prat, 2015a). Pericytes also contain contractile proteins which have the ability to control the diameter of a capillary, thus directly effecting blood flow and amount of drug nanoparticles delivered to the BBB junction (Daneman et al., 2010a, b).

Along with regulation of blood flow and BBB permeability, pericytes are also known to synthesize elements necessary for development and maintenance of BCECs. These elements include various factors such as platelet-derived growth factor—brain, angiopoetin-1 (ANG1), sphingosine 1-phosphate, and transforming growth factor β (Shepro and Morel, 1993; Armulik et al., 2005; Wolff et al., 2015). Their importance in BCEC maintenance and survival can be assessed by the fact that, when BCECs are cultured in the presence of pericytes, they show greater resistance to apoptosis (Rascher et al., 2002; Azad et al., 2015). Thus, pericyte and BCEC interactions have been implicated in certain BBB dysfunction and neuroinflammations (Daneman et al., 2010a, b)

As pericytes are known to modulate BBB permeability, they have become the target for improving drug delivery to the brain, e.g., a nano-drug carrier molecule, targeting pericytes such as membrane-associated proteases which show improved drug delivery than its conventional counterparts (Kang and Shin, 2016).

2.3 Astrocytes

Astrocytes are major glial cells in the NVU, which are responsible for extending their polarized processes to cover the entire neuronal processes, including pericytes and endothelial cells. They serve to maintain the BBB and support the endothelial cells in their function (Abbott et al., 2006; Azad et al., 2015; Serlin et al., 2015).

Astrocytes exhibit a number of different morphologies, which have a direct consequence on drug transport and delivery into the CNS. There is evidence that astrocytes can regulate BBB features which lead to tighter junctions and lesser transfer of drug from the lumen into the brain parenchyma (Dehouck et al., 1990; Rubin et al., 1991). Astrocytes also result in polarization and expression of transporters such as P-gp and glucose transporter-1 (GLUT1), which are responsible for efflux of xenobiotic and transporting glucose to the brain parenchyma, respectively (McAllister et al., 2001). Apart from these transporters, astrocytes are also actively involved in regulating vessels around them. Astrocytes are known to produce vascular endothelial growth factor (VEGF), which promotes angiogenesis (Lee et al., 2007; Argaw et al., 2009) and ANG1 and protects the BBB from VEGF's damaging effects but only when both VEGF and ANG1 are co-expressed (Shen et al., 2011).

When BCECs are cocultured with astrocytes, it is observed that the cells go under dramatic structural reorganization and produce a better BBB model (Rubin et al., 1991). Interactions between the BCECs and astrocytes are known to regulate the morphology of BCECs, affecting the rate of angiogenesis and the condition of BBB itself (Prat et al., 2001). In summary, astrocytes along with BCECs perform functions which are necessary to regulate blood flow and BBB permeability, thus affecting drug delivery inside the CNS.

2.4 Molecular structure of the junction

Proteomic and genomic studies of the BCEC have led us to identify important structural and transport components of the BBB and several differences in molecular structure of endothelial cells are present in CNS and those found elsewhere. The

BCECs present with specialized tight junctions and adhere junctions (Li et al., 2001; Ohtsuki et al., 2014; Daneman and Prat, 2015b).

2.4.1 Tight junctions

Tight junctions form the foremost seal between the lumen and abluminal spaces (Wilhelm and Krizbai, 2014). This seal prevents paracellular diffusion by creating a high resistance paracellular barrier to several ions and molecules, thus polarizing the luminal surface in process (Tajes et al., 2014; Daneman and Prat, 2015b). These tight junctions are transmembraneous and tetraspanin protein structures, made up of molecules such as claudins, occludins, and JAMs (Furuse, 2010; Wilhelm and Krizbai, 2014). Here, claudin-3, claudin-5, and claudin-12 potentially contribute to the BBB's restriction of small ions (Wolburg and Lippoldt, 2002), as the lack of claudin-5 in a transgenic mice model has shown to produce a leak toward such small ions (Nitta et al., 2003). Occludins are also highly enriched in BCECs and are very important for maintenance of the resistance (Balda et al., 1996; Saitou et al., 2000). These occludins are bound to zonula occludens protein (ZO–1/2) (Tajes et al., 2014); ZO proteins form the cytoskeletal components of the junction along with Cingulin (implicated in expression of claudins), junction-associated coiled-coil protein (anchors the junctional complex to the cytoskeleton), and membrane-associated guanylate kinase (Abbott et al., 2006; Van Itallie and Anderson, 2013). The third major component of the tight junctions are the proteins belonging to the immunoglobulin family called JAMs. JAMs are responsible for leukocyte extravasation and also restrict the paracellular permeability (Martin-Padura et al., 1998; Johnson-Leger et al., 2002; Ludwig et al., 2005).

All these factors combined together give the tight junctions the property of size selective permeability and high resistance; the measurement of these two parameters is used as a benchmark while establishing BBB models for testing drug delivery (Wilhelm and Krizbai, 2014).

2.4.2 Adherens junction

In addition to the presence of tight junctions, CNS endothelial cells also have the adherens junction (Daneman and Prat, 2015b). The transmembrane protein of endothelial adherens junctions is made of vascular endothelial (VE)-cadherin, a single span transmembrane protein capable of homophilic Ca^{2+}-dependent binding and platelet endothelial cell adhesion molecule-1 (Tajes et al., 2014; Daneman and Prat, 2015b). Adhrerens junctions are linked to the cytoskeleton through catenins (α, β and γ) and another major protein complex found in the adherence junctions, consisting of the nectins linked to afadin/AF6 (Daneman et al., 2010a, b; Wilhelm and Krizbai, 2014). The function of adherens junction is still unclear, but they play a crucial role in BBB permeability and drug delivery as experimental phosphorylation of adherens junction protein β-catenin and has demonstrated a significant enhancement in permeability and drug delivery (Farkas et al., 2005; Tajes et al., 2014; Laksitorini et al., 2015).

3 Movement through the blood-brain barrier

The BBB is poised as a significant barrier toward drug delivery as the passage into the brain is tightly regulated by the BBB (O'Keeffe and Campbell, 2016). There are two ways of passing through the BBB and into the brain. These are paracellular pathways and transcellular pathways (Tajes et al., 2014). Paracellular pathways are being protected by the presence of tight junction and the transcellular pathways are being protected by the presence of molecular transporters and efflux pumps (O'Keeffe and Campbell, 2016). We will now discuss the possible pathways for permeation through the BBB.

3.1 *Passive diffusion*

Passive diffusion can be through both paracellular pathways and transcellular pathways. It is the diffusion of the low molecular mass solute depending on the electrochemical, osmotic, and hydrostatic gradient (Tajes et al., 2014). This mechanism is mediated by the presence of tight junctions, adherens junction, and the presence of the phospholipid membrane of endothelial cells. Many lipid-soluble molecules can enter the brain passively (Liu et al., 2004). Molecules with mass in excess of 450 Da, high polar surface area (Clark, 2003), and rotatable bonds are all restricted to enter the brain (Abbott et al., 2010). The movement of gases such as oxygen and carbon dioxide is totally dependent on blood flow and is allowed to diffuse passively in both directions. Paracellular diffusion plays a very minor role in drug nano-particulate delivery to the brain (Abbott et al., 2010).

3.2 *Carrier-mediated transport*

It is a known fact that polar molecules are prohibited to diffuse freely through the BBB (Abbott et al., 2010). Many polar nutrients such as glucose, amino acids (Mann et al., 2003), small peptides, organic ions, etc. are delivered to the brain via carrier-mediated transport (Tamai and Tsuji, 2000; Brasnjevic et al., 2009; Abbott et al., 2010). Here, specialized solute carrier (SLC) transporters are utilized to transport such molecules through the BBB. The SLC are polarized and localized to both luminal and abluminal membrane (Tamai and Tsuji, 2000). As described earlier in Section 2.3, these are selective carriers, e.g., glucose is transported by GLUT1 (SLC2A1), a bidirectional transporter (Betz et al., 1983; Farrell and Pardridge, 1991; Tamai and Tsuji, 2000; Abbott et al., 2010; Patel and Patel, 2017).

The understanding of how such transporters work have led to the development of molecules which show increased brain concentrations in comparison to their predecessors, e.g., dopamine cannot cross the BBB, but levodopa was found to be transported by facilitative amino acid transporter (L1) (Mena and Cotzias, 1975; Hawkins et al., 2005) and GLUT1 has shown to carry the prodrugs nipecotic acid and 7-chlor-onokynurenic acid into the brain (Bonina et al., 1999, 2000). So far so good, but the use of these transporters is limited because they can only carry molecules which are structurally and chemically akin to their natural ligands, so researchers had to develop semisynthetic carrier molecules, e.g., ApoE, a synthetic peptide carrier molecule used for delivering anticancer drug cetuximab, which otherwise showed very poor brain uptake (Sarkar et al., 2014).

3.3 Active efflux pumps

The CNS endothelial cells express several ATP-driven efflux pumps, thus the name active. They take part in actively removing substrates from the CNS and into the blood so as to avoid accumulation of undesirable xenobiotic in the CNS (Loscher et al., 2005; Newton, 2006; Patel and Patel, 2017). They potentially remove endogenous and exogenous (those who have gained entry from elsewhere) substances; an example of such an efflux pump is the multidrug resistant-associated protein (MRP) (Dallas et al., 2006). However, the archetype for this category is the P-gp, a member of the ABC transporter, expressed on the luminal side of the membrane (Tajes et al., 2014). P-gps are notorious in removing several drugs and making them potentially useless in CNS disorders, e.g., verapamil, paclitaxel (Cannon et al., 2012), and cediranib (Wang et al., 2012). The delivery of such drugs is very poor inside the CNS, but inhibition of P-gp efflux pumps has shown to increase CNS concentrations (Cannon et al., 2012; Wang et al., 2012). Another example is the Na(+)-dependent pumps, as discussed in Section 3.2. L1 transporter system is responsible for transport of levodopa from the luminal surface, but Na(+)-dependent pumps are responsible for its removal from the abluminal surface, thus reducing its concentration in the brain (Hawkins et al., 2005).

3.4 Transcytosis

Transcytosis is a process by which large molecules cross the BBB into the CNS. This is an active, saturable, and pH- and temperature-dependent process (Scherrmann, 2002). Now, transcytosis can be achieved in two ways, receptor-mediated transcytosis (RMT) or adsorptive-mediated transcytosis (AMT) (Abbott et al., 2010; Tajes et al., 2014; Patel and Patel, 2017). AMT molecules or nanoparticles which are electrostatically charged and polycationic in nature, e.g., protein and peptides, bind to the anionic molecules of the luminal surface of the endothelial cells. These bounded molecules are then internalized in vesicles and transported across the membrane (Kamalinia et al., 2015; Patel and Patel, 2017). In RMT, there are specific receptors for specific molecules on the luminal surface of the endothelial cells. These receptors, unlike any other receptors, bind to a set of highly specified ligands and, upon binding these receptor molecules, are internalized and the ligand is then transported into the brain (Abbott, 2013). This is the primary mechanism by which macromolecules such as insulin, low density lipoproteins, transferrins, and growth factors cross the BBB (Tajes et al., 2014).

There have been many advancements in the area of drug delivery when it comes to RMT; many receptors have been utilized to increase delivery into the brain. For instance, transferrin receptors transporting antibodies and conjugated dopamine

(Yu et al., 2011; Niewoehner et al., 2014; Kang et al., 2016), folate receptor-mediated transport of anticancer and Alzheimer's medication (Yamamoto et al., 1997; Dong et al., 2014), and insulin receptor targeted increased delivery of insulin in Alzheimer's disease (Dieu et al., 2014). These are only few examples of how RMT processes can be piggybacked to deliver therapeutic nanoparticles inside the CNS.

3.5 Cell-mediated transport

Many immune system cells, such as monocytes, leukocytes, and macrophages, can be recruited into the CNS by the microglia, but still the neutrophil infiltration is very low in CNS. Under normal circumstances, immune system cells cross the BBB via a process called diapedesis, through the CNS endothelial cells without disrupting the tight junctions (Abbott, 2013; Patel and Patel, 2017). Although no drug molecules naturally pass through the BBB in this manner, this process is also used to deliver drug molecules in the CNS, e.g., supermagnetic iron oxide delivery by monocytes (Batrakova et al., 2011; Tong et al., 2016).

Therefore, understanding these pathways can give us tools in designing new molecules which can then be tested for improved drug delivery in a system. Now, these systems can be divided into the in vitro systems/models and the in vivo systems/models. In our forthcoming sections, we will be discussing these.

4 In vitro models of BBB for assessing drug delivery

The BBB has proven to be a major road block in testing drugs that might have CNS-based therapeutic actions (Stanimirovic et al., 2015). Considering our understanding about the working of the BBB, it is safe to say that the oldest and best-known models that replicate the structural and functional complexity of the BBB are in vivo models. The main advantage being the use of a live brain in its natural habitat (Wolff et al., 2015). However, using in vivo methods as a high to medium throughput screening process is difficult and very expensive; therefore, their usage in early drug developmental stages is limited (Wilhelm and Krizbai, 2014). The scientific community has now recognized the utility of in vitro experiments when it comes to the sheer number of samples that can be tested in a given amount of time (Naik and Cucullo, 2012). Although almost 50% of all compounds tested cannot be translated into humans, they still are cheaper and faster than in vivo models (Perel et al., 2007). A useful BBB model should be reproducible and have a realistic design, functional expression of transporters, and ease of setup (Wilhelm et al., 2011).

All in vitro models virtually follow the same structural design and have the following common elements to them. The common structural features are:

a. A barrier either synthetic or grown from extracted brain cells on a semipermeable membrane dividing two fluidic compartments. For sake of simplicity, we are going to call the upper chamber as the donor chamber and the lower compartment as the receiver chamber.

b. In between cells and the semipermeable substrate, extracellular matrix (Kangwantas et al., 2016) is deposited to incorporate tight junctions like functioning.

c. Establishing brain microenvironment (Nakagawa et al., 2009; Ogunshola, 2011).

A donor chamber where the drug/nanoparticle can be introduced, separated from the second receiver chamber. The fluid from the receiver chamber can be utilized for timely assessment of drug delivery. Anywhere from 6-96 wells can be prepared for such an experiment (Booth and Kim, 2012; Griep et al., 2013). The most common platform for in vitro models today is created using "Transwell" plates made by Corning, USA. Also, majority of publications use 10 μm thick polystyrene or polycarbonate membranes with a 108 pores/mm^2 pore density (Zenker et al., 2003; Brown et al., 2007; Colgan et al., 2008).

Now, to mimic the shear stress aspect of an animal model, a flow mimicking system can be utilized. So, microfluidic systems have been created and tested for this purpose (Cucullo et al., 2008, 2013).

Accomplishing these should result in a structurally and functionally sound BBB model for testing permeability through the BBB. So, for the BBB model to be considered useful or viable for testing drug delivery, it should fulfill certain functional requirements and these are;

a. Expression of tight junctions like properties between BCECs, which would confer the reduction in paracellular diffusion characteristics.
b. In vivo like distribution of relevant transporters, e.g., P-gp, GLUT-1, etc. (Roberts et al., 2008).
c. Presence and function of efflux mechanism and metabolic enzymes (Betz and Goldstein, 1978; Cox et al., 2001; Kusuhara and Sugiyama, 2005; Dutheil et al., 2010; Ghosh et al., 2010; Shen and Zhang, 2010).

Furthermore, in recent time, haemodynamically stable in vitro models have also been created for studying BBB changes in conditions such as Alzheimer's, epilepsy, or multiple sclerosis (Kalaria, 1992; Poduslo et al., 2001; Ujiie et al., 2003; Tomkins et al., 2008; Kim et al., 2011).

4.1 Methods for measuring permeability

After setting up of a BBB model, it must be made sure that the model is viable and doesn't show increased permeability to large molecules. Now, permeability assessment is necessary from a drug development and drug delivery point of view because this will predict the viability of the membrane otherwise; we could be testing the compounds in an unsuitable highly porous membrane and we wouldn't know. So, after the membrane is produced, it must be tested for permeability. All these measurement methods can be applied to any in vitro BBB model for testing paracellular leaks in cell lines or the artificial membrane that is being used.

4.1.1 TEER (trans-endothelial electric resistance) measurement

TEER measures the tightness of the membrane (Wilhelm et al., 2011) by measuring the electrical resistance between the donor chamber and the receiver chamber; the TEER value is expressed in Ω cm^2 (Wolff et al., 2015). A TEER value of at least

150–200 Ω cm^2 is considered to be ideal for testing (Deli et al., 2005). TEER value can be measured in real time, as they do not harm any cells present in the culture medium and thus allow us to assess the change in permeability of the layer continuously (Crone and Olesen, 1982; Lippmann et al., 2012, 2014). TEER value of a rat brain is around 2000 Ω cm^2 (Butt et al., 1990).

Recommended TEER values represent the presence of restricted passive diffusion, a marker of normal BBB, and it can be used for both artificial and live cell cultures.

4.1.2 FITC-dextran and sodium fluorescein

FITC (fluorescein isothiocyanate) conjugated with dextran has a molecular weight of 4000–40,000 Da and, for sodium fluorescein, the molecular weight is around 376 Da (Wilhelm et al., 2011). Both of these compounds show fluorescence and are hydrophilic in nature; the excitation wavelength is between 490 and 520 nm. Assessment of fluorescence is done by fluorescent microscopy and concentration of the conjugate is measured by a fluorescent plate reader (Hoffmann et al., 2011a; Watson et al., 2013). So, after introducing the FITC-dextran conjugate in the donor chamber, the fluorescence can be measured in the receiver chamber and the apparent permeability (P_{app}) can be determined using the following formula (Gaber et al., 2004; Takeshita et al., 2014).

$$P_{app} = \frac{dQ}{dT^{*}A^{*}C_0} \tag{1}$$

Here, dQ is the transported amount; dT is the incubation time; A is the surface area of the membrane; and C_0 is the initial concentrations in the donor chamber.

As FITC dextran conjugates vary from low to high molecular weight molecules, depending on their molecular size, apparent permeability to an ion (low molecular weight) and protein (high molecular weight) can be assessed.

4.1.3 Lucifer yellow

Lucifer yellow is a small, hydrophilic molecule that moves across the BBB through passive paracellular diffusion (Omidi et al., 2003; Watson et al., 2013). Thus, Lucifer yellow acts as a marker for the establishment of proper tight junctions. Similar to the FITC-dextran conjugate method, the fluorescence can be determined at given time points by measuring fluorescence intensities in both the donor and receiver chambers. The excitation and emission wavelengths were 485 and 529 nm, respectively. After this, calculation of permeability coefficient is done by substituting data into Eq. (1) (Qosa et al., 2016). As Lucifer yellow is a hydrophilic small molecule, it will again chemically test the presence of functional tight junctions.

4.1.4 Evans blue dye

A synthetic dye with a molecular weight of 67,000 Da is a nonspecific albumin binder forming Evans blue albumin (EBA) complex, but because of the size and binding affinity to albumin, it is used to assess the permeability of molecules which bind to albumin or are of Evans blue size equivalents (Dohgu et al., 2007; Saunders et al., 2015; Takata et al., 2015). Similar to the Lucifer yellow experiment methodology, the EBA concentration in the receiver chamber can be measured after adding the Evans blue dye to the receiver chamber, at fixed time point by determining the absorbance of samples at 630 nm with a microplate reader (Dohgu et al., 2007; Takata et al., 2015). Calculation of apparent permeability is done by substituting data in Eq. (1). Evans blue shows natural fluorescence and it is cheap which is the only reason for using it. According to one review, it is not a suitable marker for permeability measurement as better and more sensitive methods are available (Saunders et al., 2015).

4.1.5 Horseradish peroxidase (HRP)

HRP was introduced for electron microscopy-based structural analysis (Straus, 1959) because it is possible to make the reaction product an electron dense material (Brightman and Reese, 1969), thus allowing for microscopic examination of the BBB structure as the HRP antibody will bind to the walls of the endothelial cells and tight junctions (Brightman and Reese, 1969). In an in vivo study, HRP is usually injected and, in an in vitro system, it is usually introduced in the donor chamber. Once introduced into the in vitro system, the cells are then dissected out and can be used visualized using electron microscopy. The assessment, in this case, is purely visual or based on image analysis software. The main advantage with HRP is that it requires a highly scarce quantity of antibody and is highly specific to a particular cell type.

4.1.6 Mannitol/sucrose/inulin (radiolabeled)

All three (mannitol/sucrose/inulin) follow the same principle and tell the same tale about BBB permeability. Sucrose, a water-soluble molecule with less parenteral metabolism, shows limited permeability through the BBB (Saunders et al., 2015). A radiolabelled version, i.e., [^{3}H] Sucrose, is used and added to the donor chamber. After certain fixed time points, samples can be obtained from the receiver chamber to measure the counts of radiation by a liquid scintillation system (Schiera et al., 2005).

Mannitol (^{3}H-mannitol is used in the measurements of BBB permeability) is a low molecular weight marker (182.17 Da) used to measure BBB permeability with the same process as that of sucrose (On et al., 2013). Inulin (^{11}C-Inulin) can also be used in a similar fashion (Hara et al., 1988). It has been noted that the in vivo permeability of sucrose and mannitol is 3×10^{-8} and 1.4×10^{-7} cm/s, respectively (Ohno et al., 1978).

These are considered to be more sensitive than HRP, EBA, and Lucifer yellow. As they require very less amount of starting material, they utilize compounds which are naturally found in the body and produce the least amount of changes in the existing BBB integrity. Another major advantage with these molecules is that they can be coupled with any major imaging technique such as Positron Emission Tomography (PET) or MRI (magnetic resonance imaging) to give visual evidence of the extent of permeation (Hara et al., 1988; On et al., 2013).

All of these methods will tell us whether our models can reproduce the necessary conditions we would like to replicate. In all these methods, fluorescein and Evans blue are the cheapest and most widely used methods, but certainly not the most precise (Saunders et al., 2015). One of the major drawbacks of these studies is that they do not account for transport via the active and efflux proteins. So, to measure the effect on these, each unique subphenotype of the particular transporter must be identified individually, isolated, and then quantified (Cardoso et al., 2010).

4.2 *In vitro models*

Despite the knowledge that no known in vitro model can replicate the NVU of an in vivo system, the in vitro models have been accepted for certain investigations, as mentioned in Section 4 of this chapter (Nielsen et al., 2011). In general, the scope of in vitro models is to provide a highly malleable and controllable environment, allowing us to generate a system slightly comparable to the living system so as to assess the pathophysiological response toward external stimuli, which otherwise might be deemed too difficult to reproduce and characterize in vivo at an early phase of drug discovery (Lundquist and Renftel, 2002; Lundquist et al., 2002; Abbott, 2004; Liu et al., 2011).

Several models have been developed to study the role of BBB in drug delivery over the years; these can be broadly classified into noncell-based and cell-based in vitro models. These models and some key aspects of them have been briefly highlighted in Table 1. In the upcoming sections, we shall discuss the role of both of these models in assessing drug delivery.

4.2.1 *Noncell-based (synthetic) in vitro models*

4.2.1.1 Immobilized artificial membrane (IAM) chromatography

IAM membrane attempts to replicate the membrane lipid environment found in a live cell. Thus, they can be considered as stationary phase representatives of a more fluidic system (Naik and Cucullo, 2012). This technique initially was utilized to separate out compounds, but since then it has been used to study drug permeability across the BBB (Reichel and Begley, 1998). Here, modified high performance liquid chromatography (HPLC) columns have been prepared out of covalently bound phospholipid molecules to a silica base, showing a linear relationship between an aqueous phase and liposomes (Ong et al., 1995; Salminen et al., 1997). These phospholipid molecules form a sort of an artificial cell membrane and this membrane has gained acceptance in predicting the extent of permeability for small molecules and to measure lipophilicity (Ong et al., 1996; Reichel and Begley, 1998; Giaginis and Tsantili-Kakoulidou, 2008). However, IAM when coupled with another analytical technique such as LC (Reichel and Begley, 1998; Russo et al., 2017) has shown great promise, predicting extent of permeation through BBB for PDE-4 inhibitors (Yoon et al., 2006), steroids, and biogenic amines (Reichel and Begley, 1998) in comparison to in vivo studies.

Thus, IAM gives the researcher the flexibility to couple an analytical technique, screen multiple compounds in a short time, and effectively predict permeability of

Table 1 A brief about in vitro models of BBB

S. no.	Model type	Material/ source cell	Transport studied	Features	Advantages	Limitations	Reference
1. Noncell based models							
a.	IAM chromatography	Modified HPLC membrane, covalently bound to a silica membrane	Passive diffusion assessment	Small and lipophylic molecules	Cost-effective, high-throughput screen. Overall predictability is good	Lateral diffusion cannot be studied. Replication of cellular bi-layer functions such as metabolic and transport mechanisms	(Reichel and Begley, 1998; Russo et al., 2017; Shen and Zhang, 2010)
b.	PAMPA	Artificial membrane impregnated with lipids/cells on a polycarbonate support		Effect of pH, temperature and changes in lipids on BBB permeability	Versatility, automation, reproducibility and lower costs. Compatible with nano-based drug delivery systems	Inability to reflect on the role of various transporters, enzymes, and shear stress. No active transport processes	(Avdeef, 2005; Mensch et al., 2010; Naik and Cucullo, 2012; Avdeef et al., 2015; Dagenais et al., 2009; Passeleu-Le Bourdonnec et al., 2013; (Di et al., 2008a, b, 2009)
	PAMPA	PVDF membrane with 10% w/v egg lecithin in *n*-dodecane	Passive diffusion assessment	First PAMPA created. Replicating the cholesterol-rich BBB.	First PAMPA model used for understanding		

Continued

Table 1 Continued

S. no.	Model type	Material/ source cell	Transport studied	Features	Advantages	Limitations	Reference
	DOPC-PAMPA	PVDF membrane with DOPC in *n*-dodecane	Passive diffusion assessment	Improved Standard PAMPA	Better results in lipid soluble compounds		
	HDM-PAMPA	PVDF membrane with *n*-hexadecane	Passive diffusion assessment	No lipid membrane	Good for studying highly lipophilic compounds	Longer incubation times. Difficult to measure permeability of low permeable compounds	
	DS-PAMPA	PVDF membrane with a 20% mix of lipids and *n*-dodecane	Passive diffusion assessment	Double sink condition	Short incubation time. Measurement of low permeable compounds possible because of imitation of a biological sink condition	Specialized conditions are required to maintain the sink condition	
	BM-PAMPA	PVDF membrane with phospholipids resembling biological membrane	Passive diffusion assessment	A biomimetic PAMPA model. Replicating the brush-border membrane conditions			

	BBB-PAMPA	PVDF membrane with 2% w/v porcine brain tissue in *n*-dodecane	Passive diffusion assessment	A biomimetic PAMPA. Highly used in CNS drug delivery research	Sample amount required is very small	Presence of UWL altering fluid dynamics and drug permeabilities	
2. Cell based models							
a.	Mono cell cultures	BCECs from rat/mice/porcine/bovine/human origin	Passive transport and active transport. Metabolic enzymes. Presence of Tight Junctions and adherens junction	Live biological cells used for high-throughput screen. TEER value of 9–1800 Ω cm^2. Porcine cells show highest TEER values. Replication of molecular features	Presence of molecular features makes it a more robust model than noncell type models	Only 0.1% of the brain is endothelial cells. bovine shows large variation in TEER values. Fails to replicate the complete NVU	(Demeuse et al., 2002; He et al., 2014; Coisne et al., 2005; Fischer et al., 1999, 2000; Patel et al., 2017)
b.	Cocultures	BCEC and astrocytes/pericytes from rat/mice/porcine/bovine/human origin	Passive transport and active transport. Metabolic enzymes. Presence of Tight Junctions		Better replication of the NVU. Reduced loss of cellular activity. Improved stability over mono-cultures	Doesn't incorporate the shear stress parameters at the BBB	
	Endothelial cells and astrocytes	BCEC and astrocytes from rat/mice/porcine/bovine/human origin	Useful in studying nano-crystal solutions and SMEDDS.	TEER value of 200–900 Ω cm^2. Lucifer yellow permeability at $0.26 \pm 0.11 \times 10^{-3}$ cm/min. P-gp/ABC transporter expression			(Passeleu-Le Bourdonnec et al., 2013; Smith et al., 2007; Berezowski et al., 2004a)

Continued

Table 1 **Continued**

S. no.	Model type	Material/ source cell	Transport studied	Features	Advantages	Limitations	Reference
	Endothelial cells and pericytes	BCEC and pericytes from rat/mice/ porcine/bovine/ human origin		TEER values of up to 200 Ω cm^2 in case of rodent cells. Reduction in accumulated sodium fluorescein from 68.6% to 22.1%			(Nakagawa et al., 2007; Hatherell et al., 2011; Dohgu et al., 2005)
c.	Triple cultures	BCEC cocultured with two different cell type combination of astrocytes/ pericytes/ neurons	Passive, active, and carrier-mediated transport.	Rat cell-based BBB shows a TEER value of 400 Ω cm^2 and permeability coefficient for sodium fluorescein in the range of 3×10^{-6} cm/s	More complete replication of NVU than that of mono and cocultures	Doesn't incorporate the shear stress parameters at the BBB	(Wolff et al., 2015; Helms et al., 2016; Nakagawa et al., 2009)
d.	Microfluidic design model	Polycarbonate porous membrane and two channels allowing flow of fluid. Coculturing BCEC and astrocytes	Transcytosis and effect of shear stress on other processes	Built-in Ag/AgCl electrodes for TEER measurement. TEER values can rise to $\geq$250 $\Omega \cdot cm^2$	Incorporates shear stress. It is able to respond to mechanical and biochemical stimuli	Usually incorporates two cell types	(Booth and Kim, 2012)

ABC, ATP-binding cassette protein; BBB, blood-brain barrier; BCEC, brain capillary endothelial cell; DOPC, diolenylolphosphatidylcholine; DS, double sink; HDM, hexadecane; HPLC, high performance liquid chromatography; IAM, immobilized artificial membrane; NVU, neurovascular unit; PAMPA, parallel artificial membrane permeability; P-gp, Permeability glycoprotein; PVDF, polyvinylidene difluoride; SMEDDS, self-micro emulsifying drug delivery system; TEER, trans endothelial electric resistance; UWL, unstirred water layer.

a drug in CNS (Pidgeon et al., 1995; Reichel and Begley, 1998; Russo et al., 2017). As it is with anything, there are limitation to IAM and its validity in monitoring drug delivery, such as, failure to incorporate lateral diffusion (only possible with live cells); extrapolating data generated on lipid monolayer IAM to predict cellular bilayer model is difficult and it also fails to replicate metabolic and active transport mechanisms of BBB (Cox et al., 2001; Ghosh et al., 2010; Shen and Zhang, 2010).

Another such model that is based on a synthetic approach to overcome some of the shortcomings of the IAM model is the parallel artificial membrane permeability assays (PAMPA) models, the details of which will be discussed in the next section.

4.2.1.2 Parallel artificial membrane permeability assay

Passive diffusion is a vital and one of the most important entry routes into the brain and this model is used to test for passive diffusion through the BBB. In the beginning, PAMPA was developed as a high throughput screen for predicting gastrointestinal permeability (Avdeef, 2005; Avdeef et al., 2015). PAMPA also follows the same "sandwich like configuration", as the other cell-based in vitro models do (Palmiotti et al., 2014), where the drug diffused in the receiver compartment is then measured and quantified (generally by ultraviolet-visible spectroscopy or liquid chromatography-mass spectrometry) (Naik and Cucullo, 2012; Palmiotti et al., 2014). The original model involved impregnating a highly porous microfilter membrane with an oily-based solution of 10% w/v egg lecithin dissolved in *n*-dodecane (Avdeef, 2005), all of this is supported on a polycarbonate support structure, creating the receiver and donor compartments (Naik and Cucullo, 2012). PAMPA can utilize several different lipid-based models, based on different types of lipids that are used, the type of solvent, and membrane it uses (Sinkó et al., 2009). For instance, the Lecithin: Egg PAMPA contains 10% egg lecithin dissolved in *n*-dodecane and then fixed on a polyvinylidene difluoride (PVDF) membrane, DOPC-PAMPA uses dioleyoylphosphatidylcholine in *n*-dodecane on a PVDF membrane (Avdeef et al., 2001; Huque et al., 2004), HDM-PAMPA uses only *n*-hexadecane and no lipid (Avdeef and Tsinman, 2006), and DS-PAMPA uses a 20% mixture of lipids in *n*-dodecane on a PVDF membrane (Avdeef et al., 2005). Similarly, two other PAMPA models have been used for measuring drug permeability across the BBB such as, biomimetic (BM)—PAMPA using a mixture of phospholipid molecules closely resembling the biological membrane (Sugano et al., 2001a, b, 2003) and (BBB)—PAMPA which uses 2% w/v porcine brain tissue extracted in *n*-dodecane on PVDF membrane (Avdeef et al., 2015). The outcomes predicted by BBB-PAMPA model are considered as good predictions in the CNS class of drugs; here, the drugs can be classified as CNS+ (high penetration through BBB) and CNS− (low penetration through BBB). Although when a study measured the outcome of in situ brain perfusion technique versus the PAMPA model, the correlation coefficient calculated came out to be $r^2 = 0.47$; but upon closer inspection, the hit rate came out to be almost 83%, thus it can be safely said that PAMPA could act as good screening tool in early drug development stages (Di et al., 2008a, b, 2009).

PAMPA has shown a great degree of versatility, automation, and reproducibility (Avdeef, 2005), when it comes to modeling pH and temperature changes. PAMPA models have successfully replicated the pH range of 1.0–2.5 and 6.6–7.0 (Balogh et al., 2013) and temperature variations to study their possible effect on drug delivery or permeation through the BBB (Palmiotti et al., 2014; Vizseralek et al., 2014). Because of this, it is possible to check for the effect of pH, temperature, and changes in lipids on BBB permeability and thus nanoparticle delivery (Dagenais et al., 2009; Mensch et al., 2010).

Thus, over a period of years in development, PAMPA has developed into a low cost and flexible alternate to cell-based in vitro methods (Avdeef, 2005; Palmiotti et al., 2014). But, it is also plagued with the same major problems as its predecessor IAM was, the inability to reflect on the role of various transporters, enzymes, and shear stress present in the BCE, thus significantly affecting the predictability of the extent of drug delivered in the CNS.

4.2.2 Cell-based in vitro models

In 1974, for the first time ever, bovine cerebral cortex endothelial cells were successfully cultured on nylon sieves (Brendel et al., 1974). In their life span of 30 years, many in vitro models have been developed in order to facilitate and expedite the development of novel BBB crossing therapeutic molecules. However, none of these models are able to fully mimic the complexities of an in vivo system; their usage is limited to only throughput screening of compounds (He et al., 2014). Nonetheless, all in vitro models bear a few desirable advantages such as, (1) cost effectiveness—when compared to animal experimentation, they provide a relatively and significantly higher throughput for testing drug delivery; (2) simplified working environment—allowing us to study and manipulate the BBB without worrying about the organism; (3) versatility—providing highly controllable environment and the coculturing of four types of cells in a single system (Naik and Cucullo, 2012; He et al., 2014; Wolff et al., 2015; Appelt-Menzel et al., 2017). It should be noteworthy that, in vitro cell-based models can be established with any type of source CNS endothelial cells, e.g., human, animal, and cell line-derived. As these models make use of live cells originating from the brain, it becomes possible to replicate some of the molecular features as well as maintaining a tight BBB. Features such as expression of specific BBB transporter, e.g., GLUT1 transporter, ABC transporter efflux protein molecules, and enzymes such as MAO and ALP, have all been well-established (Garberg et al., 2005; Pardridge, 2005). Also, these models provide TEER values in the range of in vivo values of 1000–2000 Ω cm^2 (Gumbleton and Audus, 2001) and greater or equal to 0.03×10^{-6} cm/s permeability of sucrose (Bickel, 2005). But, these models are also not without some drawbacks of their own. For instance, cells undergoing replication tend to go under dedifferentiation because of lack of exposure to certain physiological factors available in vivo, thus affecting expression and potentially altering BBB normal physiology (Naik and Cucullo, 2012) and prompting a cautious approach (He et al., 2014).

Considering all factors in mind, several culturing techniques have been developed to produce the desired level of testing required or the number of features a researcher wants to incorporate into the model. So, on the basis of number of unique cells used for developing a model and the configuration achieved of the final model, we have classified the cell-based in vitro models.

These models also follow certain guidelines; they dictate that endothelial cells of animal CNS origin (all monocultures are basically CNS endothelial cells cultures) are always grown on a semipermeable microporous synthetic membrane in the donor compartment of the transwell system; this compartment replicates the blood vessel lumen portion of the in vivo system. All the other cells, astrocytes, pericytes, and neurons, depending on the culture type are grown in the receiver compartment mimicking the ablumenal surface of the BBB (Naik and Cucullo, 2012; He et al., 2014).

4.2.2.1 Primary mono-cell cultures

Mono cell cultures are cultures of only one type of cell from the NVU, the CNS endothelial cells. Endothelial cells can be isolated from any mammalian brain, e.g., rat BCEC culture (Demeuse et al., 2002), mouse BCEC (Sahagun et al., 1990; Imaizumi et al., 1996), Pig BCEC culture (Fischer et al., 1999, 2000), and human endothelial cells culture (Muruganandam et al., 1997; Megard et al., 2002; Wilhelm et al., 2011). These endothelial cell cultures follow the same basic protocol as discussed in Section 4. Isolation and culturing of BCEC is a difficult task as only 0.1% of the brain is endothelial cells, thus each brain produces a low quantity of endothelial cells (Perriere et al., 2007). Therefore, porcine and bovine are the most preferred monoculture type cells, as they produce the largest number of cells per animal in comparison to rat or murine models (He et al., 2014). Also, rat and murine endothelial cells express fewer BBB characteristics in comparison to bovine and porcine endothelial cells, such as TEER values between 9 and 150 $\Omega\ cm^2$; in contrast, TEER value for primary porcine culture is 150–200 $\Omega\ cm^2$ (Rubin et al., 1991; Abbruscato and Davis, 1999; Wang et al., 2001) and a P_{app} (sucrose) of approximately 7.5×10^{-6} cm/s (Coisne et al., 2005). Therefore, rodent endothelial cells result in the poor development of BBB characteristics (Coisne et al., 2005). Few studies have pointed toward the use of puromycin in cell culturing to enable healthier and functional endothelial cells culture (Perriere et al., 2005, 2007; Yao and Tsirka, 2011). Considering all this, porcine models exhibit the best TEER values of 70–1800 $\Omega\ cm^2$, a sucrose permeation value of $0.2–25 \times 10^{-6}$ cm/s, and expression of tight junction proteins claudin-5, occludin, and ZO-1 and enzymes like alkaline phosphatase (Schulze et al., 1997; Fischer et al., 1999, 2000; Yamagata et al., 2003). The immortalized variant of porcine cells is PBMEC/C1-2 and it is being used nowadays in creating a 3-D vascular model involving shear stress of BBB, which will be discussed later in Section 4.2.2.4 (Neuhaus et al., 2006). In case of bovine epithelium, the TEER value in mono-cultures is up to averages around 800 $\Omega\ cm^2$ and, in cocultures with astrocytes (averages often exceeding 1000 $\Omega\ cm^2$ up to 2500 $\Omega\ cm^2$), with values on single filters up to 3000 $\Omega\ cm^2$. Small molecule permeability measured via sucrose/mannitol is reported in the range of $0.4–15 \times 10^{-6}$ cm/s (Garberg et al., 2005; Helms et al., 2014, 2016). The major drawback of using a bovine origin cell line is the large variation that happens in TEER value (range of 30–150 $\Omega\ cm^2$) and expression of both ABC and SLC-transporters (Helms et al., 2016). Cell cultures of bovine and porcine origin are labor-intensive and reproducibility between and even within labs is a major concern (Culot et al., 2008; Hersom et al., 2016).

All these problems are observed in a nonhuman model, so to tackle all these issues human cell lines were created, in a hope that they would serve as a better model for BBB-related drug delivery measurement. Human cerebral microvasculature endothelial cell line (hCMEC/D3) and immortalized human pluripotent stem cells lines have been used so far and are now considered as the gold standard in in vitro modeling. The hCMEC/D3 BBB cell line can be prepared from cerebral micro-vessel of endothelial cells extracted form dead epilepsy patients (Helms et al., 2016). The hCMEC/D3 BBB cell line, when assayed, confirmed the presence of active transporters (GLUT1) (Sajja et al., 2014; Prasad et al., 2015), efflux transporters, tight junction (ZO-1 and claudin-5), adherence junction (VE-cadherin) proteins, and inflammatory markers (vascular cell adhesion molecule-1) (Markoutsa et al., 2011; Ma et al., 2014). Also, the TEER value for monoculture is in the range of 30–50 Ω cm^2 and permeability for sucrose, mannitol, sodium fluorescein, and Lucifer yellow in the range of 20–90 $\times$ 10^{-6} cm/s has been reported (Weksler et al., 2005; Forster et al., 2008; Poller et al., 2008; Carl et al., 2010). The Mean TEER values were between 20 and 40 Ω cm^2 which positively increased under applied shear stress to 120 Ω cm^2 (Griep et al., 2013). Larger molecules have lower permeabilities; hence, the model in its basic state presents a barrier for large molecules, whereas small molecules relatively easily permeate the barrier.

The human-induced pluripotent stem cells (hiPSCs)/PSCs have shown that they present barrier properties better than hCMEC/D3 monolayers and are nonspecific in nature (Choi et al., 2009; James et al., 2010; Patel et al., 2017). However, the use of human primary cells is also restricted by the unavailability of experimental material. Brain tissue is usually isolated from surgical material which usually is not viable for culturing (Wilhelm et al., 2011).

All in all, these models allow for high throughput screening of probable molecules CNS, testing binding affinities, and it is an ideal system to study the Michaelis-Menten kinetics as there is fixed volume on both sides (Berezowski et al., 2004b). All monocultures suffer from the same drawback, cell to cell communication or communication between different cell types, which we have established in an earlier segment (Stewart and Wiley, 1981; Hori et al., 2004).

4.2.2.2 Cocultures

Following the establishment of a variety of monoculture models, it has been realized that BCECs alone, whatever their origin be, do not express the appropriate BBB properties and show a loss in characteristic upon removing from their original environment (Cecchelli et al., 1999; Demeuse et al., 2002). So, to better replicate the anatomy and structure of the in vivo BBB, BMECs are cocultured with other cells that directly contribute to the barrier properties of BBB and are part of the NVU (Dehouck et al., 1994; Simard et al., 2003; Abbott et al., 2006; Armulik et al., 2010; Daneman et al., 2010a, b). Further, these models can be organized into two departments on the basis of the position of the supplementary cell in the culture medium. As in monocultures, all cocultures are cultured the same way and only the type of supplementary cell would change, along with their location of culture. So, according to the placement of the molecules, there are two possible arrangements; they are:

Noncontact coculture models: The endothelial cells are seeded in the donor compartment, while astrocytes (or other cell types, often pericytes) are seeded in the receiver chamber away from the abluminal membrane. Any effect the nonendothelial cell has is through the chemical gradient only (Takeshita et al., 2014).

Contact coculture models: Astrocytes (or other cell types) are seeded in the receiver chamber attached to the abluminal surface. This allows nonendothelial cells (nonendothelial cells) to directly affect the endothelial cells in the donor chamber (Pardridge, 1998; Nakagawa et al., 2009; Takeshita et al., 2014)

There is one thing that is to remember in any form of coculturing scenario, the endothelial cells will always be cultured in the donor compartment and the non-endothelial cells will always be cultured either in a contact state or a noncontact state, in the receiver compartment. Now, based on the pair of cells selected, the cocultures can be further divided into the following types of cocultures.

a. *Endothelial cells and astrocytes*:

It is recognized that many BBB features could be established partly if not completely, by just coculturing them with astrocytes (DeBault and Cancilla, 1980). These cocultures can be established with either primary cells or cell lines (Passeleu-Le Bourdonnec et al., 2013). Also, these cocultures have shown increase in TEER values and decrease in permeation of paracellular tracer molecule with the upregulation of tight junctions is observed (Fenart et al., 1998).

Also, interaction between endothelial cells and astrocytes increases the expression of transporters and tight junctions in endothelial cells, thus establishing a more robust BBB model (Arthur et al., 1987; Janzer and Raff, 1987). At par with the previous reports, higher values of TEER and lower permeability of tracer molecules were noted in endothelial cell-astrocyte coculture model (Dehouck et al., 1990; Rubin et al., 1991). Different endothelial cells could be used in this, e.g., mouse endothelial cell cocultured with astrocytes generated TEER of 200–300 Ω cm^2 and bovine cocultures produced a higher TEER of around 500–600 Ω cm^2 (Dehouck et al., 1990). Also, a TEER value of 900 Ω cm^2 can be achieved in a porcine coculture model (Lippmann et al., 2012); TEER value of 860 Ω cm^2 can be achieved when coculturing hSPC cells with astrocytes (Smith et al., 2007). In a rat BCEC and astrocyte model, the TEER value reached 300 Ω cm^2 and the permeability coefficients (Pe) for Lucifer yellow were at a very manageable $0.26 \pm 0.11 \times 10^{-3}$ cm/min. Along with increased TEER values, coculturing of endothelial cells with astrocytes also upregulated the P-gp/ABC transporters in several studies (Gaillard et al., 2001; Zenker et al., 2003; Berezowski et al., 2004a; Calabria et al., 2006; Smith et al., 2007). All these results indicate the establishment of a robust BBB model, one that is suitable to test molecules for permeability across the BBB such as, brain uptake of nano crystal solutions, inclusion compounds solution, and self-microemulsifying drug delivery systems (Yi et al., 2017).

b. *Endothelial cells and pericytes*:

It is now clear from the above sections that not only astrocytes but pericytes also play an important role in dynamically regulating the BBB behavior (Daneman et al., 2010a,b). This claim can be quantified by the study in which the permeability of sodium fluorescein was greatly reduced in coculture of mouse endothelial cells and rat pericyte (Dohgu et al., 2005); another study (Nakagawa et al., 2007) revealed an increase in TEER value to 200 Ω cm^2 for coculture with pericytes. When compared to astrocyte coculturing with hCMEC/D3 cells, TEER value increased from 39 to 60 Ω cm^2, whereas when hCMECE/D3 cells are cultured with pericytes the TEER is raised from 39 to 46 Ω cm^2 (Hatherell et al., 2011). Similarly, in an experiment when three different combinations were tried, namely only endothelial monolayer, endothelial monolayer with pericyte in noncontact condition, and that in contact condition, the TEER value in contact condition was noted as 97.5 ± 8.5 Ω cm^2 and in the noncontact condition 19.8 ± 2.6 Ω cm^2. Also, when accumulation of sodium fluorescein was measured in both conditions, noncontact showed almost 68.6% and contact showed almost 22.1% accumulation (Hayashi et al., 2004), thus clearly indicating the benefits of pericyte coculturing while testing for drug permeabilities as it clearly provides with a tighter barrier.

4.2.2.3 Triple cultures

Although it is accepted that the BCEC forms the basis of the BBB and introducing other cells into the culture improves its stability and performance (Wolff et al., 2015). This configuration includes BCEC seeded in the donor compartment of the support and pericytes or astrocytes or neurons are seeded in the receiver compartment in a contact or noncontact culture scheme. This configuration mimics the cell arrangement at the NVU and allows for interactions between all three cell types (Helms et al., 2016). The coculture of endothelial cells, pericytes, and astrocytes mimics the anatomical situation of an in vivo cell. In the presence of all three cells, rat endothelial cells-based model showed a staggering 400 Ω cm^2 TEER reading, while the permeability coefficients P(e) for sodium fluorescein were in the range of 3×10^{-6} cm/s (Nakagawa et al., 2009). In comparison to rat endothelial cells, neurons, and astrocytes, triple cultures also present with a TEER value of 268 Ω cm^2, a nine fold increase in enzyme gamma-glutamyl transpeptidase (aids in influx of amino acids) (Hawkins et al., 2006). Based on previous observations, it is clear that coculturing all three cells together brings the culture one step closer to the in vivo model.

4.2.2.4 Microfluidic design BBB model

To address the limitations of in vitro BBB model, microfluidic device-based in vitro BBB models have been developed to incorporate the factor of shear stress in modeling BBB (Booth and Kim, 2012). The microfluidic BBB (μBBB) model is one of the first such models. It contains two channels crossing at right angle to each other, allowing a dynamic flow and generate shear stress; a polycarbonate porous membrane at the intersection of these channels, which enables coculture of endothelial cells and astrocytes; and multiple built-in Ag/AgCl electrodes for TEER measurement (Booth and Kim, 2012). These channels have a height of 200 μm and widths of 2 (luminal) and 5 mm (abluminal). In this model, endothelial cells and astrocytes are seeded on the luminal and abluminal side of the membrane, respectively. A pump connected to a gas tubing contained CO_2 and O_2, which is used to generate a sheer stress of 0.023 dynes/cm^2 (lower than the physiological condition). When cocultured with astrocytes, the TEER values can rise to $\geq 250\ \Omega \cdot cm^2$ (Booth and Kim, 2012). Without shear stress, hCMEC/D3 cells show a TEER of $\approx 40\ \Omega \cdot cm^2$. With only 18 hours of physiological shear stress (5.8 dynes/cm^2), the TEER was increased to 120 $\Omega \cdot cm^2$. Just as it is seen in a normal physiological response, the presence of Tumor necrosis factor—α, a known inflammatory cytokine, dramatically decreased the TEER to 12 $\Omega \cdot cm^2$. The above-mentioned data suggest that this improved model is able to respond to mechanical and biochemical stimuli and thus can be used in permeability studies. These microfluidic-based models can only incorporate two cell types, given that the membrane and pillars have only two sides, so only a coculture can be achieved.

5 In vivo models of BBB

In vivo models make use of a live and dynamic system, thus their predictive values of permeation in brain can be directly translated to human studies. These models are thus considered as the best models to predict the behavior of a molecule in crossing BBB (Passeleu-Le Bourdonnec et al., 2013). As the BBB of all mammals is relatively same, with minor species-related differences, it has all the NVU present and functioning under normal circumstances. A number of in vivo techniques and models have been used to assess the brain uptake of drugs (Stanimirovic et al., 2015). Following are some of the models used by the industry to assess drug delivery in the brain.

5.1 Rodent model

Rodents as an in vivo model for drug delivery across the BBB have been extensively used in drug development for their ease of handling and model development. They are a natural candidate for assessing the factors that can influence drug delivery across the BBB.

Being mammalian in nature, rat and mice brain closely exhibit similar morphological, physiological, and pathological features as that of human brain. As in vitro studies have concluded the presence of tight junction proteins (claudin-3 and -5, ZO-1 and occluding) (Perriere et al., 2007) and as in humans rodent brain express two genes (Mdr1a and Mdr1b) encoding for two subtypes of P-gp (Schinkel et al., 1996; Syvanen et al., 2009), similar expression is seen for GLUT-1 (Devaskar et al., 1991); also, performing similar function as of human BBB.

The assessment of extent of penetration of a compound in the cerebral hemisphere can be achieved through several techniques, e.g., MRI-based studies (Hoffmann et al., 2011a, b; Orunoglu et al., 2017), radiolabelled ligand-binding assay, e.g., radioiodine I^{131} (Feng et al., 2017; Patnaik et al., 2017), and fluorescent assays (Xie et al., 2012; Ulapane et al., 2017). These would provide a rough idea of the quantity, but are important for having visual conformation of the event. Although they are visual models, radiolabelled assays and MRI have been used for quantifying exact concentration of compounds that have been delivered to the brain.

So, to make an absolute measurement about the quanta of drug delivered to the brain, several techniques are used, such as LC-MS/MS or spectrophotometrically generated concentration-time profiles including pharmacokinetic parameter such as area under the curve (AUC), elimination constant (K_{el}), maximum concentration of drug in blood plasma (C_{max}), time to the peak of drug in plasma (T_{max}), half-life ($T_{1/2}$), volume of distribution (V_d) and clearance (Cl), brain-to plasma partition coefficient (K_p), and it can be calculated as ratio of AUC (AUC_{brain}/AUC_{plasma}) (Zhou et al., 2011; Tan et al., 2017; Ulapane et al., 2017; Unno et al., 2017; Yamamoto et al., 2017). Also, ex vivo studies including histopathological studies and immunohistochemical studies are used in tandem with image analysis to analyse the extent of drug delivery (Schoknecht et al., 2014; Orunoglu et al., 2017). The main disadvantage of LC-MS/MS or spectrophotometrical studies is that isolated brain sample is needed as it cannot be performed in a live animal unlike the imaging studies.

The rodent models can be used to assess molecules or techniques which would induce a permeability change and thus enhance drug delivery through BBB, e.g., HAV(His-Ala-Val) and cyclic ADT(Ala-Asp-Thr) peptides (Laksitorini et al., 2015; Ulapane et al., 2017) and focused ultrasound (FUS)-guided MRI (Etame et al., 2012; Yang et al., 2014; Samiotaki et al., 2015), and to develop and assess the efficacy of newly developed carrier systems and enhance the drug delivered to the brain, e.g., Dopamine, ziconotide, and chemotherapeutic agents (Kiener et al., 1986; Aryal et al., 2013; Aliev et al., 2015; Anand et al., 2015; Pahuja et al., 2015; Tan et al., 2017). Also, rat model of BBB has been used to decipher and add to the known physiology of BBB and disease pathology, so as to exploit this knowledge in creating molecules with improved concentrations in brain, e.g., glutamate-induced bidirectional effect on BBB permeability (Vazana et al., 2016), identifying and probing disease pathology (Verwilst et al., 2017).

A wide selection of transgenic and wild-type mice/rats phenotypes is available to study drug delivery in any condition. Rodent models are the most common model used and are easily available. Human and rodent ABC transporters are slightly different and thus nonrodent models are considered (Mazur et al., 2012).

5.2 Zebrafish model

One of the smallest vertebrates, the zebrafish (*Danio rerio*) has recently been indicted as one of the reliable in vivo BBB models. The Zebrafish model has been established to be, functionally and structurally, akin to higher vertebrates (Jeong et al., 2008; Eliceiri et al., 2011; Yang et al., 2015). This is because the barrier present in a zebrafish, just like that in other vertebrates such as mice and rats, expresses HRP restriction, Sulfo-NHS-Biotin diffusion, claudin-5, claudin-3, ZO-1/TJP-1 (Furuse et al., 1999, 2001; Morita et al., 1999; Nitta et al., 2003; Jeong et al., 2008; Zhang et al., 2012), Evans blue restriction (Eliceiri et al., 2011), and pharmacological similarities (Zheng et al., 2010; Umans and Taylor, 2012b; Fleming et al., 2013). The zebrafish BBB is not just a physical barrier, but possesses chemical similarities as well with rodent models (Tam et al., 2012); thus, making the zebrafish an important model for conducting experiment which focuses on analyzing and improving drug delivery across vertebral BBB (Yang et al., 2015).

Modeling of a BBB in a zebrafish requires incubation and production of viable zebrafish embryos by mating of adults (Westerfield et al., 1997; Eliceiri et al., 2011; Fleming et al., 2013; Yang et al., 2015). In order to be considered as a viable in vivo BBB model for assessing drug delivery, the zebrafish model should present as a structurally and functionally similar barrier to drug delivery as it is in the larger vertebrate. Features of vertebral BBB limit the extent of drug delivered to the cerebral hemispheres, as the presence of drug efflux pumps, e.g., ABC efflux pumps (Lowrence et al., 2016; Zhang et al., 2016; Cunha et al., 2017; Li et al., 2017) and P-gp system (Fischer et al., 2013; Machado et al., 2014; Zhang et al., 2016), presence of metabolizing enzymes, e.g., CYP450 family (Bresolin et al., 2005; Diotel et al., 2011), and monoamine oxidase (Anichtchik et al., 2006; Arslan and Edmondson, 2010). Although it is not completely similar to the human BBB, the zebrafish BBB model has proved to be a very reliable homologue to the human BBB for studying drug delivery.

As zebrafish are structurally dissimilar to the frequently used rodent models, the method of sample collection and drug quantification in the central chamber is fast and easy (Li et al., 2017). In a zebrafish model, the accumulation of drug formulation to the brain can be visualized via confocal microscopy (Eliceiri et al., 2011). However, by using fluorescence resonance energy transfer (FRET), quantification of drug can be made in the brain. The extent of FRET occurring can be quantified by using the FRET ratio

$$\text{FRET ratio} = \frac{I_{DiI}}{I_{C6} + I_{DiI}} \tag{2}$$

here I_C is the intensity of concentrate and I_{DiI} is the intensity of diluted are the fluorescence intensities of concentrate and diluted fraction measured at 510 and 675 nm, respectively (Turner et al., 2012; Yang et al., 2015; Chen et al., 2017).

The development of a fully functional BBB in zebrafish is completed in 96 h postfertilization, thus the turnaround time from development to execution will be short (Umans and Taylor, 2012a; Li et al., 2017). Adult zebrafish are useful in providing detailed information on bio-distribution, especially in brain (Li et al., 2017). Analysis of large number of live samples is possible at any given point of time (Eliceiri et al., 2011) and real time cell imaging is possible (Jim et al., 2016) to study the transport of tagged molecules across the BBB. Other models are time-consuming and usually expensive.

5.3 Nonhuman primate models

Rhesus macaques or *Macaca Mulatta/fascicularis* model is the most accurate and the closest representation of a human system (Harvilchuck et al., 2013). Thus, the Nonhuman primate models is best suited for drug development and assessment of drug delivery, as they most closely replicate the human BBB physiology (Thorne et al., 2008; Rosenberg et al., 2017). The measurement of drug delivery parameters is similar to the ones that are followed in humans. The Pharmacokinetic/pharmacodynamics

(PK/PD) is usually obtained by drawing blood at fixed intervals and then measuring maximum concentration (C_{max}), time to C_{max} (T_{max}), and plasma concentration of any given substance (ng/mL) (Harvilchuck et al., 2013; League-Pascual et al., 2017). Also, CSF sampling can be done to measure the amount of free compound that has actually crossed BBB and into the brain (Thorne et al., 2008; League-Pascual et al., 2017). Comparing both data, it can be calculated exactly how much drug was delivered to the cerebral compartment in given time.

5.4 *Drosophila model*

Drosophila melanogaster BBB differs anatomically from the one found in vertebrates. The open circulatory system of drosophila is separated from its CNS by a layer of glia-derived epithelial cells (Carlson et al., 2000; Stork et al., 2008). Thus, the BBB or humoral brain barrier is much simple than vertebrates. However, certain common features such as presence of junctional complexes and protein complexes which create a septate junctional and adherens junctional barrier against diffusion (Edwards et al., 1993; Tepass and Hartenstein, 1994; Wu and Beitel, 2004; Hindle and Bainton, 2014), ABC transporter, and presence of MDR/Pgp (multi drug resistant/ P-glycoprotein) transporters, e.g., Mdr65 (Mayer et al., 2009; Geldenhuys et al., 2012) are found to exist in a drosophila model. It has been shown that endothelial cells grown in vitro do not maintain their complete BBB properties, e.g., down regulation of P-glycoprotein (Calabria and Shusta, 2008; Hindle and Bainton, 2014), and rodent models are quite costly, so there is need for nonvertebrate BBB model for assessing drug delivery kinetics.

5.5 *Canine model*

The dog is an important animal model for drug discovery and development, especially for safety evaluations. Recently, the presence of transporters such as SLC transporters, GLUT1, ABC transporters, P-glycoprotein, and even PEPT2 (mediates the transport of drugs such as ACE inhibitors and few antibiotics) has been confirmed (Braun et al., 2017).

5.6 *Techniques for studying extent of drug delivery to CNS*

5.6.1 *Invasive techniques*

5.6.1.1 In situ brain perfusion

Among other techniques, in situ brain perfusion is a sensitive means of studying drug delivery through BBB (Smith, 1996). The original method was developed by Takasato et al. (1984). In this method, anesthetized rats undergo retrograde infusion of HCO_3/ heparinized saline and a test compound occurring via the exposed right/left/both carotid arteries (Gynther et al., 2016). Drug infusion takes place via a catheter, inserted into the carotid artery, and the rate of perfusion is controlled so as to maintain 120 mmHg of mean arterial pressure (Takasato et al., 1984). At the end of perfusion time, brain is isolated, homogenized, and then homogenate is isolated (Takasato et al.,

1984; Jampilek et al., 2015). This technique allows us to quantitatively measure brain uptake of solutes. Cerebral hemispherectomy is used to isolate brain tissue and measure the test and reference compounds by the following formula:

$$\mathrm{PS} = \frac{V_d - V_0}{T} \tag{3}$$

Here, PS is the permeability-surface area product, T is the duration of the perfusion period (min), V_d is the brain volume of test compound, and V_0 is the brain volume of distribution of reference compound (Takasato et al., 1984; Jampilek et al., 2015)

There is no change in BBB permeability when perfusion is done for 60 s. This technique allows total control over perfusate composition, perfusion rate, and total time for perfusion. Also, it allows us to avoid errors brought upon by peripheral metabolism (Takasato et al., 1984; Dagenais et al., 2000).

In this technique, because of longer duration of perfusion, the integrity of BBB may become compromised which might skew the results (Takasato et al., 1984; Mensch et al., 2009). Metabolism within the brain microcirculation cannot be avoided (Pardridge, 2012) and requires specialized surgical skills and is labor-intensive, time-consuming, and costly.

5.6.1.2 Intravenous injection technique

Some reviewers have considered this technique as the gold standard for assessing BBB permeability (Nicolazzo et al., 2006). This is because of the simple and efficient nature of the model.

This technique involves intravenously injecting the animal with the test compound labelled with a traceable compound (Zhou et al., 2011; Tian et al., 2012) or the drug can be injected directly without any tracer conjugated with it (Azadi et al., 2013; Shityakov et al., 2016). Site of injection can be a cannulated femoral vein or a tail vein may be used (Nicolazzo et al., 2006). Blood samples are drawn at regular intervals (or as per the protocol); after this, the animals are euthanized (Mensch et al., 2009; Shityakov et al., 2016) or can be kept alive based on the type of drug quantification method used (Tian et al., 2012). Following euthanasia, brain is isolated, homogenized, and then tested for drug quantities, all the while comparing plasma and CNS levels of a drug, thus giving an accurate representation of drug delivered in the brain (Tian et al., 2012; Xie et al., 2012; Azadi et al., 2013; Shityakov et al., 2016).

The amount delivered to the cerebral compartment can be analyzed by single time point analysis (Ohno et al., 1978) or by multiple time uptake data. In single time point analysis, the formulae for C_{br} is the concentration in brain is as follows:

$$Cbr = Kin \times \mathrm{AUC}_0^T \tag{4}$$

In the above equation, K_{in} is the organ clearance, AUC_0^T is the area under the curve from time = 0 to time = T. C_{br} in that equation should represent tissue concentration after correction for intravascular content (Ohno et al., 1978; Bickel, 2005).

In multiple time points, Patlak mastered a method for estimating K_{in} from the graph of experimental data. The equation that follows is a representation of that,

$$\frac{C_{br(total)}(T)}{C_p(T)} = K_{in} \times \frac{\mathrm{AUC}_0^T}{C_p(T)} + V_i \tag{5}$$

Here, V_i is the ordinate intercept and represents the initial volume of distribution (Bickel, 2005).

Several quantification techniques can be used to quantify levels of test compounds in brain, e.g., in vivo imaging (Tian et al., 2012; Xie et al., 2012) and HPLC-MS/MS (Fan et al., 2014; Shityakov et al., 2016). The major advantage of this technique is that both plasma and brain kinetics can be obtained, thus accurately pharmacokinetics of drug delivered to the brain can be calculated (Nicolazzo et al., 2006; Mensch et al., 2009). This technique is simple to execute; an intact BBB physiology is obtained and the cells experience greater exposure to cerebral microvasculature.

5.6.1.3 Microdialysis

This technique is widely used to study drugs within the brain and also levels of neurotransmitters, inflammatory markers, and metabolites (Kendrick, 1990; Sopasakis et al., 2004). Upon injecting the test compound, the microdialysis probe is guided into the brain and perfused with CSF or physiological solution. It utilizes a specially designed probe, which has a semipermeable fiber membrane in it. So, when artificial CSF or physiological solution is pushed/perfused into the brain, this is termed as the perfusate. Molecules which are present in the brain (upon administration) can freely pass the membrane and are continuously collected; this collected fluid is called the dialysate (Mensch et al., 2009) The concentration of the test compound is measured by HPLC/UPLC/LC-MS/MS (Hammarlund-Udenaes, 2000; Bundgaard et al., 2007). It can provide us with unbound drug concentration-time profiles in brain extracellular fluid (ECF) and in blood. The extent of drug absorption is also a factor that can be measured with the help of this technique (Hammarlund-Udenaes, 2000) and allows an evaluation of the influence of efflux transporters in the passage through the BBB. As continuous collection of the dialysate is happening, the measurement of metabolites and original compound can be done at multiple time points, thus giving a complete metabolic profile of the test compound. This method suffers from several drawbacks such as biofouling and clogging of micro-dialysis membranes (Wisniewski et al., 2001; Anderson et al., 2008).

Cerebral open flow microperfusion (cOFM): This is a new microdialysis technique which doesn't require a membrane. The cOFM probe combines the use of both push and pull perfusion, resulting in mixing of perfusate with interstitial brain fluid. As this technique doesn't require any membrane, it is suitable for a wide range of molecules regardless of their size and lipophilicity (Ghosh et al., 2014).

5.6.1.4 Brain uptake index (BUI)

The BUI is a brain tissue sampling technique, which is used to study the uptake of drugs in the brain. It's one of the oldest techniques to study uptake of drugs by the brain and was originally described by Oldendorf (1970).

It is a single pass technique and requires injection of two labelled compounds, i.e., test compound (^{3}H labeled) and reference compound (^{14}C labeled) or vice versa, to anesthetize animals. Here, the reference compound would work as an internal standard, as it penetrates freely in the brain. Test compound bolus is injected via the carotid artery and it is allowed to diffuse into the brain for about 15 s, after which the animal is decapitated and brain is isolated (Oldendorf, 1970; Bonate, 1995; Mensch et al., 2009).

Now, the brain concentrations of both test and reference are measured and then the BUI can be calculated with the following formulae

$$\mathrm{BUI} = \frac{\left(\frac{[^3H]dpm}{[^{14}C]dpm}\right)(brain)}{\left(\frac{[^3H]dpm}{[^{14}C]dpm}\right)(injectedsolution)} \tag{6}$$

Here, *dpm* is the disintegration per minute.

This method is highly suitable for measuring compounds which have or are predicted to have moderate to high BBB permeability (Bonate, 1995).

Exposure time to brain for the drug is very short. Thus, BUI cannot reconcile for factors such as blood flow, brain region, and time duration between injection and sampling. Also, due to this short duration of the test, no complete drug is able to reach the cerebral compartment. This method requires the need for having radioactive labels available for the test compound (Bonate, 1995; Mensch et al., 2009).

5.6.1.5 Cerebrospinal fluid (CSF) sampling

The CSF also is bound by the BBB, thus the measurement of concentration of compounds in ventricular CSF serves as an indirect measure of unbound drug in the brain. Additionally, convectional transfer of drug from CSF to interstitial space is allowed, but because these are two separate compartments, similarities in drug concentrations are unlikely (Abbott, 2004; Palmer and Alavijeh, 2013). Nonetheless, studying CNS-active molecules provides with a rough estimate of the quantity.

CSF collection can be done by cannula placed in the lateral ventricles in cisterna magna or by directly puncturing. In humans, CSF is collected via lumbar puncture (Palmer and Alavijeh, 2013; Bicker et al., 2014). It cannot provide concentration–time profiles in humans (i.e., limited clinical application). This technique alters the CSF volume and affects pressure equilibrium. The timing and sampling site determines/influences the results (Bicker et al., 2014).

5.6.1.6 Blood/plasma (B/P) ratio determination

It is defined as the equilibrium ratio, or the ratio of concentration of drug in brain to the concentration of drug in the plasma. From the following equation, we can calculate the log BB value (Liu et al., 2008; Mensch et al., 2009).

$$\log(\mathrm{BB}) = \log\left(\frac{C_{brain}}{C_{plasma}}\right) \quad (7)$$

The *B*/*P* ratio determination was a gold standard in drug delivery assessment in the brain for a long time. This ratio measures the total amount of drug present in the brain and plasma at a given time point (Kalvass and Maurer, 2002; Di et al., 2008a, 2008b; Mensch et al., 2009). This ratio depends on the molecules' passive diffusion characteristics at BBB; also, the interactions with the transporter molecules (uptake and efflux) and drug metabolizing enzymes at the BBB. The number of sampling time points, dose, route of administration, and species investigated are not fixed, thus providing the investigator with flexibility to modify the protocol according to the need (Mensch et al., 2009). This technique fails to provide any indication for the free unbound drug that is responsible for pharmacological effect (Bourasset et al., 2005).

5.6.1.7 Quantitative autoradiography

Quantitative autoradiography (QAR) method was developed by Sokoloff's (Sokoloff et al., 1977; Sakurada et al., 1978). This technique is used to determine the quantity of radioactive-labeled test compound in a specified brain region, such as area affected by stroke (Knight et al., 2009) or brain tumor (Asotra et al., 2003). This can be achieved through various administration routes such as oral, intravenous, or subcutaneous in the chosen model animal. Blood is sampled at multiple time points; period between each sampling and start/end of sampling is protocol-dependent. After the end point of sampling, the brain is isolated for further study. Subsequently, fine 20-μm section of brain is obtained and this sample is exposed to X-ray film along with the standard (Gregoire et al., 1983). The strength of QAR lies in the high spatial resolution, which is in the micrometer range. It is not cheap, but it is very simple to perform (Bickel, 2005; Mensch et al., 2009). In QAR, there is no differentiation between parent compound and its metabolite or any other protein showing affinity to the radiotracer (Mensch et al., 2009).

5.6.2 Noninvasive imaging techniques

These techniques are generally used to determine the extent of BBB opening and presence of drug in various brain regions, but not the exact quantity of drug substance present in them. The in vivo setting of these experiments aids us in imaging an intact live biological system (Rao et al., 2007). There are three basic techniques for executing noninvasive imaging using a fluorophore such as, (1) planar technique fluorescence reflectance imaging—the intensity of reflected radiation from the object is measured against the intensity of incident radiation on the object; (2) transillumination fluorescence imaging—in this, the intensity of transmitted radiation is measured against the incident radiation; and (3) fluorescence-mediated tomography—this technique is capable of generating a three-dimensional image, as the transmitted radiation from multiple sources is analyzed by multiple detectors (Stemmer et al., 2012).

The in vivo fluorescence imaging technique generally involves labeling of nanoparticles with a fluorophore. The fluorescence thus emitted upon excitation of the fluorophore is detected by the aid of a detector/detectors (Van Rooy et al., 2011). Several studies have pointed to the fact that a very low fluorophore concentration of only 10^{-11} moles or even less is sufficient to be detected in a live mice brain (Stemmer et al., 2012); techniques such as, near-infrared fluorescence, where the test nano-formulation is labelled with an infrared wavelength sensitive dye and viewed for fluorescence upon exposure to near-infrared or infrared wavelengths (Alaofi et al., 2016; Ulapane et al., 2017). The use of an infrared-sensitive fluorophore is preferred as it tends to limit tissue auto-fluorescence, gives better resolution because of deeper tissue penetration, can also incorporate the effect of time on fluorescence easily, and is biologically safe (Abulrob et al., 2008; Van Rooy et al., 2011). Frequently used near-infrared fluorophores are pentamethine and heptamethine cyanines comprising benzoxazole, benzothiazole, and indolyl, 2-quinoline or 4-quinoline (Rao et al., 2007). Another form of fluorescence measurement technique that has emerged uses the measurement of fluorescence lifetime as the index of measurement (Bloch et al., 2005). The fluorescence lifetime (τ) is the time spent by the fluorophore in the exited state before returning to the stable ground state (Abulrob et al., 2008). The fluorescence lifetime measurements would yield the energy transfer rate from the exited to the ground state of the molecular label. Factors such as change in pH, blood flow, tissue oxygenation levels, temperature changes, and nutrient supply can alter the fluorescence lifetime. Thus, fluorescence lifetime measurement is becoming a valuable tool in elucidating the extent of nanoparticles that have crossed the BBB (Bloch et al., 2005). The main shortcoming of fluorescence measurement is limited tissue penetration, tissue auto-fluorescence, and low resolution three-dimensional data. To overcome the above-mentioned shortcomings of fluorescence imaging, more powerful tools such as MRI were introduced to better understand the dynamics of nanoparticle delivery in the brain.

The MRI, however, is a more sensitive but expensive tool for quantification of the BBB opening volume (V_{BBB}) and permeability mapping, i.e., transfer rate of gadolinium from blood plasma to the extravascular, extracellular space (K_{trans}), as well as comparing pregadolinium images and postgadolinium images, to get an estimate of drug delivered to the brain from the difference in image intensity (Marty et al., 2012; Fan et al., 2014; Samiotaki et al., 2015; Alaofi et al., 2016; Ulapane et al., 2017). Also, recently ultra-small superparamagnetic iron oxide nanoparticles were used as cell-specific MRI contrast agent for macrophage activity assessment in the brain (Abulrob et al., 2008).

Similarly, PET—tracer studies are also conducted to have a quantitative approach (Dishino et al., 1983; Josserand et al., 2006; Potschka and Luna-Munguia, 2014). PET is performed by injecting a positron emitting compound or a test compound labelled with one. Three most common PET tracers in use are mostly nutrient analogues like 18F-deoxy-glucose and several amino acid analogues (e.g., ^{11}C-methionine, ^{18}F-DOPA) (Lauenstein et al., 1987; Miletich et al., 1993; Roelcke et al., 1995; Borbely et al., 2006; Patel and Gill, 2007), tracers for detection of BBB damage (e.g., ^{68}Ga-EDTA) (6432806, 1835848), and ligands for neurotransmitter receptors or transporters. Evaluations are performed graphically and with the aid of compartment modeling (Brooks et al., 1984; Schmidt and Turkheimer, 2002).

The main advantage of noninvasive techniques is the real-time visualization of the extent of permeability being achieved by the nano-formulations and without having to euthanize the test animal.

6 Conclusion and perspective

Molecules targeting CNS disorders are in abundance, but due to the presence of the BBB, it is difficult to utilize them in therapy. Such molecules seldom reach therapeutic levels inside CNS. So, in order to test new formulations and new compounds targeting CNS-based pathologies, it is essential that a large number of molecules be tested in vitro, in conditions that mimic the action and function of BBB. The development of cell-based models to overcome the limitations of the noncell-based models was the silver bullet against the delayed development in CNS drugs. But, the cell-based models of BBB are not suitable enough to predict the clinical outcome of a molecule, even though they are very cheap and fast. Soon, several cell-based models were developed based on animal of origin (rodent, bovine or human) and culturing techniques used. Since no in vitro model factored in the dynamics of blood flow and completed the complex nature of the NVU, the hit ratio was still very low. Therefore, quadruple culture models and microfluidic models were a direct result of innovation aimed at filling these gaps, where the quadruple culture models utilized four different cells of the NVU. The microfluidic models also incorporated the complex stress associated with the dynamics of blood flow. All these modifications and advancements are now used in drug development and to test novel drug delivery tools at a medium to high throughput rate.

To reach the clinical stage, in vitro data is not sufficient and had to come up with in vivo models of BBB to assess drug delivery and further refine the pipeline reaching clinical phase. As in vivo models use a live animal, it has obvious advantages over in vitro models. One such advantage being the presence of an intact and fully functioning mammalian BBB. Now, there are few dissimilarities between human BBB and BBB of other animals. These dissimilarities originate from minor genomic variations between cells of human origin to those originating from other animals. These minor variations lead to major change in how a drug will behave at the BBB junction. Various animals have been used till date to best replicate the clinical condition and rodents are the most widely used animals; large number of pathological models (including transgenic variety) already exist. So, it becomes easy to study behavior of BBB under different pathological conditions. The extent of drug delivery can also be assessed in an in vivo model, where in vitro models made use of only two compartment modeling, and studying peripheral drug metabolism was difficult; the in vivo models can be used to factor in several compartments, and thus, will provide a complete picture of the drugs interaction with the BBB.

The development has been immense in case of BBB modeling, but still many drugs fail after reaching the clinical phase of development. As no model completely represents the human BBB, researchers are using a combination of both in vitro and in vivo models to achieve higher efficiency in preclinical studies.

References

Abbott, N.J., 2004. Prediction of blood-brain barrier permeation in drug discovery from in vivo, in vitro and in silico models. Drug Discov. Today Technol. 1 (4), 407–416.

Abbott, N.J., et al., 2010. Structure and function of the blood-brain barrier. Neurobiol. Dis. 37 (1), 13–25.

Abbott, N.J., 2013. Blood-brain barrier structure and function and the challenges for CNS drug delivery. J. Inherit. Metab. Dis. 437–449.

Abbott, N.J., Rönnbäck, L., Hansson, E., 2006. Astrocyte-endothelial interactions at the blood-brain barrier. Nat. Rev. Neurosci. 7 (1), 41–53.

Abbruscato, T.J., Davis, T.P., 1999. Combination of hypoxia/aglycemia compromises in vitro blood-brain barrier integrity. J. Pharmacol. Exp. Ther. 289 (2), 668–675.

Abulrob, A., et al., 2008. Dynamic analysis of the blood-brain barrier disruption in experimental stroke using time domain in vivo fluorescence imaging. Mol. Imaging 7 (6), 248–262.

Alaofi, A., et al., 2016. Comparison of linear and cyclic His-Ala-Val peptides in modulating the blood-brain barrier permeability: impact on delivery of molecules to the brain. J. Pharm. Sci. 105 (2), 797–807.

Aliev, G., et al., 2015. Nanoparticles as alternative strategies for drug delivery to the Alzheimer brain: electron microscopy ultrastructural analysis. CNS Neurol. Disord. Drug Targets 14 (9), 1235–1242.

Anand, P., et al., 2015. Tailored delivery of analgesic ziconotide across a blood brain barrier model using viral nanocontainers. Sci. Rep. 5, 12497.

Anderson, J.M., Rodriguez, A., Chang, D.T., 2008. Foreign body reaction to biomaterials. Semin. Immunol. 20 (2), 86–100.

Anichtchik, O., et al., 2006. Distinct structure and activity of monoamine oxidase in the brain of zebrafish (*Danio rerio*). J. Comp. Neurol. 498 (5), 593–610.

Appelt-Menzel, A., et al., 2017. Establishment of a human blood-brain barrier co-culture model mimicking the neurovascular unit using induced pluri- and multipotent stem cells. Stem Cell Rep. 8 (4), 894–906.

Argaw, A.T., et al., 2009. VEGF-mediated disruption of endothelial CLN-5 promotes blood-brain barrier breakdown. Proc. Natl. Acad. Sci. U. S. A. 106 (6), 1977–1982.

Armulik, A., et al., 2010. Pericytes regulate the blood-brain barrier. Nature 468 (7323), 557–561.

Armulik, A., Abramsson, A., Betsholtz, C., 2005. Endothelial/pericyte interactions. Circ. Res 97 (6), 512–523.

Arslan, B.K., Edmondson, D.E., 2010. Expression of zebrafish (*Danio rerio*) monoamine oxidase (MAO) in Pichia pastoris: purification and comparison with human MAO A and MAO B. Protein Expr. Purif. 70 (2), 290–297.

Arthur, F.E., Shivers, R.R., Bowman, P.D., 1987. Astrocyte-mediated induction of tight junctions in brain capillary endothelium: an efficient in vitro model. Brain Res. 433 (1), 155–159.

Aryal, M., et al., 2013. Multiple treatments with liposomal doxorubicin and ultrasound-induced disruption of blood-tumor and blood-brain barriers improve outcomes in a rat glioma model. J. Control. Release 169 (1–2), 103–111.

Asotra, K., Ningaraj, N., Black, K.L., 2003. Measurement of blood-brain and blood-tumor barrier permeabilities with [14C]-labeled tracers. Methods Mol. Med. 89, 177–190.

Avdeef, A., et al., 2001. Drug absorption in vitro model: filter-immobilized artificial membranes. 2. Studies of the permeability properties of lactones in *Piper methysticum* Forst. Eur. J. Pharm. Sci. 14 (4), 271–280.

Avdeef, A., et al., 2005. Caco-2 permeability of weakly basic drugs predicted with the double-sink PAMPA pK_a (flux) method. Eur. J. Pharm. Sci. 24 (4), 333–349.
Avdeef, A., 2005. The rise of PAMPA. Expert Opin. Drug Metab. Toxicol. 1 (2), 325–342.
Avdeef, A., Deli, M.A., Neuhaus, W., 2015. In vitro assays for assessing BBB permeability: artificial membrane and cell culture models. In: Blood-Brain Barrier in Drug Discovery: Optimizing Brain Exposure of CNS Drugs and Minimizing Brain Side Effects for Peripheral Drugs.pp. 188–237.
Avdeef, A., Tsinman, O., 2006. PAMPA—a drug absorption in vitro model 13. Chemical selectivity due to membrane hydrogen bonding: in combo comparisons of HDM-, DOPC-, and DS-PAMPA models. Eur. J. Pharm. Sci. 28 (1–2), 43–50.
Azad, T.D., et al., 2015. Therapeutic strategies to improve drug delivery across the blood-brain barrier. Neurosurg. Focus. 38 (3), E9.
Azadi, A., Hamidi, M., Rouini, M.-R.R., 2013. Methotrexate-loaded chitosan nanogels as 'Trojan Horses' for drug delivery to brain: preparation and in vitro/in vivo characterization. Int. J. Biol. Macromol. 62, 523–530.
Balda, M.S., et al., 1996. Functional dissociation of paracellular permeability and transepithelial electrical resistance and disruption of the apical-basolateral intramembrane diffusion barrier by expression of a mutant tight junction membrane protein. J. Cell Biol. 134 (4), 1031–1049.
Bloch, S., et al., 2005. Whole-body fluorescence lifetime imaging of a tumor-targeted near-infrared molecular probe in mice. J. Biomed. Opt. 10 (5), 54003.
Balogh, G.T., Muller, J., Konczol, A., 2013. pH-gradient PAMPA-based in vitro model assay for drug-induced phospholipidosis in early stage of drug discovery. Eur. J. Pharm. Sci. 49 (1), 81–89.
Banks, W.A., 2016. From blood-brain barrier to blood-brain interface: new opportunities for CNS drug delivery. Nat. Rev. Drug Discov. 15 (4), 275–292.
Batrakova, E.V., Gendelman, H.E., Kabanov, A.V., 2011. Cell-mediated drug delivery. Expert Opin. Drug Deliv. 8 (4), 415–433.
Begley, D.J., 2004. Delivery of therapeutic agents to the central nervous system: the problems and the possibilities. Pharmacol. Ther. 104 (1), 29–45.
Berezowski, V., et al., 2004a. Contribution of glial cells and pericytes to the mRNA profiles of P-glycoprotein and multidrug resistance-associated proteins in an in vitro model of the blood-brain barrier. Brain Res. 1018 (1), 1–9.
Berezowski, V., et al., 2004b. Transport screening of drug cocktails through an in vitro blood-brain barrier: is it a good strategy for increasing the throughput of the discovery pipeline? Pharm. Res. 21 (5), 756–760.
Bernacki, J., et al., 2008. Physiology and pharmacological role of the blood-brain barrier. Pharmacol. Rep. 60 (5), 600–622.
Betz, A.L., Bowman, P.D., Goldstein, G.W., 1983. Hexose transport in microvascular endothelial cells cultured from bovine retina. Exp. Eye Res. 36 (2), 269–277.
Betz, A.L., Goldstein, G.W., 1978. Polarity of the blood-brain barrier: neutral amino acid transport into isolated brain capillaries. Science (New York, N.Y.) 202 (4364), 225–227.
Bickel, U., 2005. How to measure drug transport across the blood-brain barrier. NeuroRx J. Am. Soc. Exp. NeuroTherap. 2 (1), 15–26.
Bicker, J., et al., 2014. Blood-brain barrier models and their relevance for a successful development of CNS drug delivery systems: a review. Eur. J. Pharm. Biopharm. 409–432.
Bonate, P.L., 1995. Animal models for studying transport across the blood-brain barrier. J. Neurosci. Methods 56 (1), 1–15.

Bonina, F.P., et al., 1999. Synthesis, stability, and pharmacological evaluation of nipecotic acid prodrugs. J. Pharm. Sci. 88 (5), 561–567.

Bonina, F.P., et al., 2000. Synthesis, pharmacokinetics and anticonvulsant activity of 7-chlorokynurenic acid prodrugs. Int. J. Pharm. 202 (1–2), 79–88.

Booth, R., Kim, H., 2012. Characterization of a microfluidic in vitro model of the blood-brain barrier (muBBB). Lab Chip 12 (10), 1784–1792.

Borbely, K., et al., 2006. Optimization of semi-quantification in metabolic PET studies with 18F-fluorodeoxyglucose and 11C-methionine in the determination of malignancy of gliomas. J. Neurol. Sci. 246 (1–2), 85–94.

Borges-Walmsley, M.I., McKeegan, K.S., Walmsley, A.R., 2003. Structure and function of efflux pumps that confer resistance to drugs. Biochem. J. 376 (Pt 2), 313–338.

Bourasset, F., et al., 2005. Neuropharmacokinetics of a new alpha-amino-3-hydroxy-5-methyl-4-isoxazole propionic acid (AMPA) modulator, S18986 [(S)-2,3-dihydro-[3,4]cyclopentano-1,2,4-benzothiadiazine-1,1-dioxide], in the rat. Drug Metab. Disposit. 33 (8), 1137–1143.

Brasnjevic, I., et al., 2009. Delivery of peptide and protein drugs over the blood-brain barrier. Prog. Neurobiol. 87 (4), 212–251.

Braun, C., et al., 2017. Quantification of transporter and receptor proteins in dog brain capillaries and choroid plexus: relevance for the distribution in brain and CSF of selected BCRP and P-gp substrates. Mol. Pharm. 449.

Brendel, K., Meezan, E., Carlson, E.C., 1974. Isolated brain microvessels: a purified, metabolically active preparation from bovine cerebral cortex. Science (New York, N.Y.) 185 (4155), 953–955.

Bresolin, T., de Freitas Rebelo, M. and Celso Dias Bainy, A. (2005) Expression of PXR, CYP3A and MDR1 genes in liver of zebrafish, Comp. Biochem. Physiol. Toxicol. Pharmacol., 140 (3–4), pp. 403–407.

Brightman, M.W., Reese, T.S., 1969. Junctions between intimately apposed cell membranes in the vertebrate brain. J. Cell Biol. 40 (3), 648–677.

Brooks, D.J., et al., 1984. Quantitative measurement of blood-brain barrier permeability using rubidium-82 and positron emission tomography. J. Cereb. Blood Flow Metabol. 4 (4), 535–545.

Brown, R.C., Morris, A.P., O'Neil, R.G., 2007. Tight junction protein expression and barrier properties of immortalized mouse brain microvessel endothelial cells. Brain Res. 1130 (1), 17–30.

Bundgaard, C., et al., 2007. Pharmacokinetic modelling of blood-brain barrier transport of escitalopram in rats. Biopharm. Drug Dispos. 28 (7), 349–360.

Butt, A.M., Jones, H.C., Abbott, N.J., 1990. Electrical resistance across the blood-brain barrier in anaesthetized rats: a developmental study. J. Physiol. 47–62.

Calabria, A.R., et al., 2006. Puromycin-purified rat brain microvascular endothelial cell cultures exhibit improved barrier properties in response to glucocorticoid induction. J. Neurochem. 97 (4), 922–933.

Calabria, A.R., Shusta, E.V., 2008. A genomic comparison of in vivo and in vitro brain microvascular endothelial cells. J. Cereb. Blood Flow Metabol. 28 (1), 135–148.

Cannon, R.E., et al., 2012. Targeting blood-brain barrier sphingolipid signaling reduces basal P-glycoprotein activity and improves drug delivery to the brain. Proc. Natl. Acad. Sci. U. S. A. 109 (39), 15930–15935.

Cardoso, F.L., Brites, D., Brito, M.A., 2010. Looking at the blood-brain barrier: molecular anatomy and possible investigation approaches. Brain Res. Rev. 64 (2), 328–363.

Carl, S.M., et al., 2010. ABC and SLC transporter expression and proton oligopeptide transporter (POT) mediated permeation across the human blood-brain barrier cell line, hCMEC/D3 [corrected]. Mol. Pharm. 7 (4), 1057–1068.
Carlson, S.D., et al., 2000. Blood barriers of the insect. Annu. Rev. Entomol. 45, 151–174.
Cecchelli et al, 1999. In vitro model for evaluating drug transport across the blood-brain barrier. Adv. Drug Deliv. Rev. 36 (2–3), 165–178.
Chen, T., et al., 2017. Pluronic P85/F68 micelles of baicalein could interfere with mitochondria to overcome MRP2-mediated efflux and offer improved anti-Parkinsonian activity. Mol. Pharm.
Chen, Y., Liu, L., 2012. Modern methods for delivery of drugs across the blood-brain barrier. Adv. Drug Deliv. Rev. 64 (7), 640–665.
Choi, K.-D., et al., 2009. Hematopoietic and endothelial differentiation of human induced pluripotent stem cells. Stem Cell (Dayton, OH) 27 (3), 559–567.
Clark, D., 2003. In silico prediction of blood-brain barrier permeation. Drug Discov. Today 8 (20), 927–933.
Coisne, C., et al., 2005. Mouse syngenic in vitro blood-brain barrier model: a new tool to examine inflammatory events in cerebral endothelium. Lab. Investig. 85 (6), 734–746.
Colgan, O.C., et al., 2008. Influence of basolateral condition on the regulation of brain microvascular endothelial tight junction properties and barrier function. Brain Res. 1193, 84–92.
Coomber, B.L., Stewart, P.A., 1985. Morphometric analysis of CNS microvascular endothelium. Microvasc. Res. 30 (1), 99–115.
Cordon-Cardo, C., et al., 1989. Multidrug-resistance gene (P-glycoprotein) is expressed by endothelial cells at blood-brain barrier sites. Proc. Natl. Acad. Sci. U. S. A. 86 (2), 695–698.
Cox, D.S., et al., 2001. Influence of multidrug resistance (MDR) proteins at the blood-brain barrier on the transport and brain distribution of enaminone anticonvulsants. J. Pharm. Sci. 90 (10), 1540–1552.
Crone, C., Olesen, S.P., 1982. Electrical resistance of brain microvascular endothelium. Brain Res. 241 (1), 49–55.
Cucullo, L., et al., 2008. Immortalized human brain endothelial cells and flow-based vascular modeling: a marriage of convenience for rational neurovascular studies. J. Cereb. Blood Flow Metabol. 28 (2), 312–328.
Cucullo, L., et al., 2011. The role of shear stress in blood-brain barrier endothelial physiology. BMC Neurosci. 40.
Cucullo, L., et al., 2013. A new dynamic in vitro modular capillaries-venules modular system: cerebrovascular physiology in a box. BMC Neurosci. 14, 18.
Culot, M., et al., 2008. An in vitro blood-brain barrier model for high throughput (HTS) toxicological screening. Toxicol. In Vitro 22 (3), 799–811.
Cunha, V., et al., 2017. Effects of pharmaceuticals and personal care products (PPCPs) on multixenobiotic resistance (MXR) related efflux transporter activity in zebrafish (*Danio rerio*) embryos. Ecotoxicol. Environ. Saf. 136, 14–23.
Dagenais, C., et al., 2000. Development of an in situ mouse brain perfusion model and its application to mdr1a P-glycoprotein-deficient mice. J. Cereb. Blood Flow Metabol. 20 (2), 381–386.
Dagenais, C., et al., 2009. P-glycoprotein deficient mouse in situ blood-brain barrier permeability and its prediction using an in combo PAMPA model. Eur. J. Pharm. Sci. 38 (2), 121–137.
Dallas, S., Miller, D.S., Bendayan, R., 2006. Multidrug resistance-associated proteins: expression and function in the central nervous system. Pharmacol. Rev. 58 (2), 140–161.

Daneman, R., Zhou, L., Kebede, A., et al., 2010a. Pericytes are required for blood-brain barrier integrity during embryogenesis. Nature 468 (7323), 562–566.

Daneman, R., Zhou, L., Agalliu, D., et al., 2010b. The mouse blood-brain barrier transcriptome: a new resource for understanding the development and function of brain endothelial cells. PLoS One 5 (10), e13741.

Daneman, R., Prat, A., 2015a. The blood-brain barrier. Cold Spring Harb. Perspect. Biol. 7(1).

Daneman, R., Prat, A., 2015b. The blood-brain barrier. Cold Spring Harb. Perspect. Biol.

DeBault, L.E., Cancilla, P.A., 1980. gamma-Glutamyl transpeptidase in isolated brain endothelial cells: induction by glial cells in vitro. Science (New York, N.Y.) 207 (4431), 653–655.

Dehouck, B., et al., 1994. Upregulation of the low density lipoprotein receptor at the blood-brain barrier: intercommunications between brain capillary endothelial cells and astrocytes. J. Cell Biol. 126 (2), 465–473.

Dehouck, M.P., et al., 1990. An easier, reproducible, and mass-production method to study the blood-brain barrier in vitro. J. Neurochem. 54 (5), 1798–1801.

Deli, M.A., et al., 2005. Permeability studies on in vitro blood-brain barrier models: physiology, pathology, and pharmacology. Cell. Mol. Neurobiol. 59–127.

Demeuse, P., et al., 2002. Compartmentalized coculture of rat brain endothelial cells and astrocytes: a syngenic model to study the blood-brain barrier. J. Neurosci. Methods 121 (1), 21–31.

Devaskar, S., et al., 1991. Developmental regulation of the distribution of rat brain insulin-insensitive (Glut 1) glucose transporter. Endocrinology 129 (3), 1530–1540.

Di, L., et al., 2008a. Applications of high throughput microsomal stability assay in drug discovery. Comb. Chem. High Throughput Screen. 11 (6), 469–476.

Di, L., et al., 2009. Comparison of blood-brain barrier permeability assays: in situ brain perfusion, MDR1-MDCKII and PAMPA-BBB. J. Pharm. Sci. 98 (6), 1980–1991.

Di, L., Kerns, E.H., Carter, G.T., 2008b. Strategies to assess blood-brain barrier penetration. Expert Opin. Drug Discov. 3 (6), 677–687.

Dieu, L.-H., et al., 2014. Polymersomes conjugated to 83-14 monoclonal antibodies: in vitro targeting of brain capillary endothelial cells. Eur. J. Pharm. Biopharm. 88 (2), 316–324.

Diotel, N., et al., 2011. Activity and expression of steroidogenic enzymes in the brain of adult zebrafish. Eur. J. Neurosci. 34 (1), 45–56.

Dishino, D.D., et al., 1983. Relationship between lipophilicity and brain extraction of C-11-labeled radiopharmaceuticals. J. Nucl. Med. 24 (11), 1030–1038.

Dohgu, S., et al., 2005. Brain pericytes contribute to the induction and up-regulation of blood-brain barrier functions through transforming growth factor-beta production. Brain Res. 1038 (2), 208–215.

Dohgu, S., et al., 2007. Adverse effect of cyclosporin A on barrier functions of cerebral microvascular endothelial cells after hypoxia-reoxygenation damage in vitro. Cell. Mol. Neurobiol. 27 (7), 889–899.

Dong, S., et al., 2014. Synthesis and cellular uptake of folic acid-conjugated cellulose nanocrystals for cancer targeting. Biomacromolecules 15 (5), 1560–1567.

Dutheil, F., et al., 2010. ABC transporters and cytochromes P450 in the human central nervous system: influence on brain pharmacokinetics and contribution to neurodegenerative disorders. Expert Opin. Drug Metab. Toxicol. 6 (10), 1161–1174.

Edwards, J.S., Swales, L.S., Bate, M., 1993. The differentiation between neuroglia and connective tissue sheath in insect ganglia revisited: the neural lamella and perineurial sheath cells are absent in a mesodermless mutant of Drosophila. J. Comp. Neurol. 333 (2), 301–308.

Eliceiri, B.P., Gonzalez, A.M., Baird, A., 2011. Zebrafish model of the blood-brain barrier: morphological and permeability studies. Methods Mol. Biol. (Clifton, NJ) 686, 371–378.

Etame, A.B., et al., 2012. Enhanced delivery of gold nanoparticles with therapeutic potential into the brain using MRI-guided focused ultrasound. Nanomedicine 8 (7), 1133–1142.

Fan, C.-H., et al., 2014. Submicron-bubble-enhanced focused ultrasound for blood-brain barrier disruption and improved CNS drug delivery. PLoS One 9 (5), e96327.

Farkas, A., et al., 2005. Hyperosmotic mannitol induces Src kinase-dependent phosphorylation of beta-catenin in cerebral endothelial cells. J. Neurosci. Res. 80 (6), 855–861.

Farrell, C.L., Pardridge, W.M., 1991. Blood-brain barrier glucose transporter is asymmetrically distributed on brain capillary endothelial lumenal and ablumenal membranes: an electron microscopic immunogold study. Proc. Natl. Acad. Sci. U. S. A. 88 (13), 5779–5783.

Fenart, L., et al., 1998. Inhibition of P-glycoprotein: rapid assessment of its implication in blood-brain barrier integrity and drug transport to the brain by an in vitro model of the blood-brain barrier. Pharm. Res. 15 (7), 993–1000.

Feng, L., et al., 2017. TiO_2-nanowired delivery of DL-3-*n*-butylphthalide (DL-NBP) attenuates blood-brain barrier disruption, brain edema formation, and neuronal damages following concussive head injury. Mol. Neurobiol.

Fischer, S., et al., 1999. Hypoxia induces permeability in brain microvessel endothelial cells via VEGF and NO. Am. J. Physiol. 276 (4 Pt 1), C812–20.

Fischer, S., et al., 2000. Effect of astroglial cells on hypoxia-induced permeability in PBMEC cells. Am. J. Physiol. Cell Physiol. 279 (4), C935–44.

Fischer, S., et al., 2013. Abcb4 acts as multixenobiotic transporter and active barrier against chemical uptake in zebrafish (*Danio rerio*) embryos. BMC Biol. 11, 69.

Fleming, A., Diekmann, H., Goldsmith, P., 2013. Functional characterisation of the maturation of the blood-brain barrier in larval zebrafish. PLoS One 8 (10), e77548.

Forster, C., et al., 2008. Differential effects of hydrocortisone and TNFalpha on tight junction proteins in an in vitro model of the human blood-brain barrier. J. Physiol. 586 (7), 1937–1949.

Furuse, M., et al., 2001. Conversion of zonulae occludentes from tight to leaky strand type by introducing claudin-2 into Madin-Darby canine kidney I cells. J. Cell Biol. 153 (2), 263–272.

Furuse, M., 2010. Molecular basis of the core structure of tight junctions. Cold Spring Harb. Perspect. Biol. 2 (1), a002907.

Furuse, M., Sasaki, H., Tsukita, S., 1999. Manner of interaction of heterogeneous claudin species within and between tight junction strands. J. Cell Biol. 147 (4), 891–903.

Gaber, M.W., et al., 2004. An intravital microscopy study of radiation-induced changes in permeability and leukocyte-endothelial cell interactions in the microvessels of the rat pia mater and cremaster muscle. Brain Res. Protocol. 13 (1), 1–10.

Gaillard, P.J., et al., 2001. Establishment and functional characterization of an in vitro model of the blood-brain barrier, comprising a co-culture of brain capillary endothelial cells and astrocytes. Eur. J. Pharm. Sci. 12 (3), 215–222.

Garberg, P., et al., 2005. In vitro models for the blood-brain barrier. Toxicol. In Vitro 19 (3), 299–334.

Geldenhuys, W.J., Allen, D.D., Bloomquist, J.R., 2012. Novel models for assessing blood-brain barrier drug permeation. Expert Opin. Drug Metab. Toxicol. 8 (6), 647–653.

Ghosh, A., et al., 2014. Assessment of blood-brain barrier function and the neuro-inflammatory response in the rat brain by using cerebral open flow microperfusion (cOFM). PLoS One. 9(5).

Ghosh, C., et al., 2010. Pattern of P450 expression at the human blood-brain barrier: roles of epileptic condition and laminar flow. Epilepsia 51 (8), 1408–1417.

Ghosh, C., et al., 2011. Blood-brain barrier P450 enzymes and multidrug transporters in drug resistance: a synergistic role in neurological diseases. Curr. Drug Metab. 12 (8), 742–749.

Giaginis, C., Tsantili-Kakoulidou, A., 2008. Alternative measures of lipophilicity: from octanol-water partitioning to IAM retention. J. Pharm. Sci. 97 (8), 2984–3004.

Gregoire, N., et al., 1983. Autoradiographic method for quantitative evaluation of the blood-brain barrier effects of contrast media. AJNR Am. J. Neuroradiol. 4 (3), 323–325.

Griep, L.M., et al., 2013. BBB on chip: microfluidic platform to mechanically and biochemically modulate blood-brain barrier function. Biomed. Microdevices 15 (1), 145–150.

Gumbleton, M., Audus, K.L., 2001. Progress and limitations in the use of in vitro cell cultures to serve as a permeability screen for the blood-brain barrier. J. Pharm. Sci. 90 (11), 1681–1698.

Gynther, M., et al., 2016. Systemic and brain pharmacokinetics of perforin inhibitor prodrugs. Mol. Pharm. 13 (7), 2484–2491.

Hall, C.N., et al., 2014. Capillary pericytes regulate cerebral blood flow in health and disease. Nature 508 (7494), 55–60.

Hammarlund-Udenaes, M. (2000) The use of microdialysis in CNS drug delivery studies. Pharmacokinetic perspectives and results with analgesics and antiepileptics. Adv. Drug Deliv. Rev., 45(2–3), pp. 283–294.

Hara, T., et al., 1988. Measurement of human blood brain barrier integrity using 11C-inulin and positron emission tomography. Eur. J. Nucl. Med. 14 (4), 173–176.

Harvilchuck, J.A., et al., 2013. In vivo acetylcholinesterase reactivation in male guinea pigs and rhesus macaques following cyclosarin exposure and treatment with 1,1′-methylenebis {4-[(hydroxyimino)methyl] pyridinium} dimethanesulfonate. Int. J. Toxicol. 32 (4 Suppl), 99S–107S.

Hatherell, K., et al., 2011. Development of a three-dimensional, all-human in vitro model of the blood-brain barrier using mono-, co-, and tri-cultivation transwell models. J. Neurosci. Methods 199 (2), 223–229.

Hawkins, B.T., Davis, T.P., 2005. The blood-brain barrier/neurovascular unit in health and disease. Pharmacol. Rev. 57 (2), 173–185.

Hawkins, R.A., et al., 2006. Structure of the blood-brain barrier and its role in the transport of amino acids. J. Nutr. 136 (1 Suppl) 218S-26S.

Hawkins, R.A., Mokashi, A., Simpson, I.A., 2005. An active transport system in the blood-brain barrier may reduce levodopa availability. Exp. Neurol. 195 (1), 267–271.

Hayashi, K., et al., 2004. Effects of hypoxia on endothelial/pericytic co-culture model of the blood-brain barrier. Regul. Pept. 123 (1–3 SPEC. ISS), 77–83.

He, Y., et al., 2014. Cell-culture models of the blood-brain barrier. Stroke 45 (8), 2514–2526.

Helms, H.C., et al., 2014. An electrically tight in vitro blood-brain barrier model displays net brain-to-blood efflux of substrates for the ABC transporters, P-gp, Bcrp and Mrp-1. AAPS J. 16 (5), 1046–1055.

Helms, H.C., et al., 2016. In vitro models of the blood-brain barrier: an overview of commonly used brain endothelial cell culture models and guidelines for their use. J. Cereb. Blood Flow Metab. 36 (5), 862–890.

Hersom, M., et al., 2016. Transferrin receptor expression and role in transendothelial transport of transferrin in cultured brain endothelial monolayers. Mol. Cell. Neurosci. 76, 59–67.

Hindle, S.J., Bainton, R.J., 2014. Barrier mechanisms in the Drosophila blood-brain barrier. Front. Neurosci. 8, 414.

Hoffmann, A., et al., 2011a. High and low molecular weight fluorescein isothiocyanate (FITC)-dextrans to assess blood-brain barrier disruption: technical considerations. Transl. Stroke Res. 2 (1), 106–111.
Hoffmann, A., et al., 2011b. Validation of in vivo magnetic resonance imaging blood-brain barrier permeability measurements by comparison with gold standard histology. Stroke 42 (7), 2054–2060.
Hori, S., et al., 2004. A pericyte-derived angiopoietin-1 multimeric complex induces occludin gene expression in brain capillary endothelial cells through Tie-2 activation in vitro. J. Neurochem. 89 (2), 503–513.
Huque, F.T.T., et al., 2004. Permeability through DOPC/dodecane membranes: measurement and LFER modelling. Eur. J. Pharm. Sci. 23 (3), 223–232.
Imaizumi, S., et al., 1996. The influence of oxygen free radicals on the permeability of the monolayer of cultured brain endothelial cells. Neurochem. Int. 29 (2), 205–211.
Van Itallie, C.M., Anderson, J.M., 2013. Claudin interactions in and out of the tight junction. Tissue Barriers 1 (3), e25247.
James, D., et al., 2010. Expansion and maintenance of human embryonic stem cell-derived endothelial cells by TGFbeta inhibition is Id1 dependent. Nat. Biotechnol. 28 (2), 161–166.
Jampilek, J., et al., 2015. Preparation of silica nanoparticles loaded with nootropics and their in vivo permeation through blood-brain barrier. Biomed. Res. Int. 812673.
Janzer, R.C., Raff, M.C., 1987. Astrocytes induce blood-brain barrier properties in endothelial cells. Nature 325 (6101), 253–257.
Jeong, J.-Y.Y., et al., 2008. Functional and developmental analysis of the blood-brain barrier in zebrafish. Brain Res. Bull. 75 (5), 619–628.
Jim, K.K., et al., 2016. Infection of zebrafish embryos with live fluorescent *Streptococcus pneumoniae* as a real-time pneumococcal meningitis model. J. Neuroinflammat. 13 (1), 188.
Johnson-Leger, C.A., et al., 2002. Junctional adhesion molecule-2 (JAM-2) promotes lymphocyte transendothelial migration. Blood 100 (7), 2479–2486.
Josserand, V., et al., 2006. Evaluation of drug penetration into the brain: a double study by in vivo imaging with positron emission tomography and using an in vitro model of the human blood-brain barrier. J. Pharmacol. Exp. Ther. 316 (1), 79–86.
Kalaria, R.N., 1992. The blood-brain barrier and cerebral microcirculation in Alzheimer disease. Cerebrovasc. Brain Metab. Rev. 4 (3), 226–260.
Kalvass, J.C., Maurer, T.S., 2002. Influence of nonspecific brain and plasma binding on CNS exposure: implications for rational drug discovery. Biopharm. Drug Dispos. 23 (8), 327–338.
Kamalinia, G., et al., 2015. Cationic albumin-conjugated chelating agent as a novel brain drug delivery system in neurodegeneration. Chem. Biol. Drug Des. 86 (5), 1203–1214.
Kang, E., Shin, J.W., 2016. Pericyte-targeting drug delivery and tissue engineering. Int. J. Nanomed. 2397–2406.
Kang, Y.-S., et al., 2016. Use of PEGylated immunoliposomes to deliver dopamine across the blood-brain barrier in a rat model of Parkinson's disease. CNS Neurosci. Therap. 22 (10), 817–823.
Kangwantas, K., Pinteaux, E., Penny, J., 2016. The extracellular matrix protein laminin-10 promotes blood-brain barrier repair after hypoxia and inflammation in vitro. J. Neuroinflammat. 13, 25.
Kendrick, K.M., 1990. Microdialysis measurement of in vivo neuropeptide release. J. Neurosci. Methods 34 (1–3), 35–46.
Kiener, J.L., Cho, E., Saba, T.M., 1986. Factor XIII as a modulator of plasma fibronectin alterations during experimental bacteremia. J. Trauma 26 (11), 1013–1023.

Kim, D.W., et al., 2011. Blood-brain barrier disruption is involved in seizure and hemianopsia in nonketotic hyperglycemia. Neurologist 17 (3), 164–166.

Kniesel, U., Wolburg, H., 2000. Tight junctions of the blood-brain barrier. Cell. Mol. Neurobiol. 20 (1), 57–76.

Knight, R.A., et al., 2009. Estimating blood and brain concentrations and blood-to-brain influx by magnetic resonance imaging with step-down infusion of Gd-DTPA in focal transient cerebral ischemia and confirmation by quantitative autoradiography with Gd-[(14)C] DTPA. J. Cereb. Blood Flow Metabol. 29 (5), 1048–1058.

Kusuhara, H., Sugiyama, Y., 2005. Active efflux across the blood-brain barrier: role of the solute carrier family. NeuroRx J. Am. Soc. Exp. NeuroTherap. 2 (1), 73–85.

Laksitorini, M.D., et al., 2015. Modulation of intercellular junctions by cyclic-ADT peptides as a method to reversibly increase blood-brain barrier permeability. J. Pharm. Sci. 104 (3), 1065–1075.

Larsen, J.M., Martin, D.R., Byrne, M.E., 2014. Recent advances in delivery through the blood-brain barrier. Curr. Top. Med. Chem. 14 (9), 1148–1160.

Lauenstein, L., et al., 1987. Uptake kinetics of 14C L-leucine and 14C L- and 14C D-methionine in rat brain and incorporation into protein. Neurosurg. Rev. 10 (2), 147–150.

League-Pascual, J.C., et al., 2017. Plasma and cerebrospinal fluid pharmacokinetics of select chemotherapeutic agents following intranasal delivery in a non-human primate model. J. Neuro-Oncol. 132 (3), 401–407.

Lee, S., et al., 2007. Autocrine VEGF signaling is required for vascular homeostasis. Cell 130 (4), 691–703.

Li, J.Y., Boado, R.J., Pardridge, W.M., 2001. Blood-brain barrier genomics. J. Cereb. Blood Flow Metabol. 21 (1), 61–68.

Li, Y., et al., 2017. Zebrafish: a promising in vivo model for assessing the delivery of natural products, fluorescence dyes and drugs across the blood-brain barrier. Pharmacol. Res. 125 (Pt B), 246–257.

Lippmann, E.S., et al., 2012. Derivation of blood-brain barrier endothelial cells from human pluripotent stem cells. Nat. Biotechnol. 30 (8), 783–791.

Lippmann, E.S., et al., 2014. A retinoic acid-enhanced, multicellular human blood-brain barrier model derived from stem cell sources. Sci. Rep. 4, 4160.

Liu, R., et al., 2011. Targeting the neurovascular unit: development of a new model and consideration for novel strategy for Alzheimer's disease. Brain Res. Bull. 86 (1–2), 13–21.

Liu, X., et al., 2004. Development of a computational approach to predict blood-brain barrier permeability. Drug Metab. Dispos. 32 (1), 132–139.

Liu, X., Chen, C., Smith, B.J., 2008. Progress in brain penetration evaluation in drug discovery and development. J. Pharmacol. Exp. Ther. 325 (2), 349–356.

Loscher, W., et al., 2005. Role of drug efflux transporters in the brain for drug disposition and treatment of brain diseases. Prog. Neurobiol. 76 (1), 22–76.

Loscher, W., Potschka, H., 2005. Blood-brain barrier active efflux transporters: ATP-binding cassette gene family. NeuroRx J. Am. Soc. Exp. NeuroTherap. 2 (1), 86–98.

Lowrence, R.C., et al., 2016. Dithiazole thione derivative as competitive NorA efflux pump inhibitor to curtail multi drug resistant clinical isolate of MRSA in a zebrafish infection model. Appl. Microbiol. Biotechnol. 100 (21), 9265–9281.

Ludwig, R.J., et al., 2005. Junctional adhesion molecules (JAM)-B and -C contribute to leukocyte extravasation to the skin and mediate cutaneous inflammation. J. Investig. Dermatol. 125 (5), 969–976.

Lundquist, S., et al., 2002. Prediction of drug transport through the blood-brain barrier in vivo: a comparison between two in vitro cell models. Pharm. Res. 19 (7), 976–981.

Lundquist, S., Renftel, M., 2002. The use of in vitro cell culture models for mechanistic studies and as permeability screens for the blood-brain barrier in the pharmaceutical industry—background and current status in the drug discovery process. Vasc. Pharmacol. 38 (6), 355–364.

Ma, S., et al., 2014. Transport of ginkgolides with different lipophilicities based on an hCMEC/D3 cell monolayer as a blood-brain barrier cell model. Life Sci. 114 (2), 93–101.

Machado, S.P., et al., 2014. Histopathological lesions, P-glycoprotein and PCNA expression in zebrafish (*Danio rerio*) liver after a single exposure to diethylnitrosamine. Environ. Toxicol. Pharmacol. 38 (3), 720–732.

Mann, G.E., Yudilevich, D.L., Sobrevia, L., 2003. Regulation of amino acid and glucose transporters in endothelial and smooth muscle cells. Physiol. Rev. 83 (1), 183–252.

Markoutsa, E., et al., 2011. Uptake and permeability studies of BBB-targeting immunoliposomes using the hCMEC/D3 cell line. Eur. J. Pharm. Biopharm. 77 (2), 265–274.

Martin-Padura, I., et al., 1998. Junctional adhesion molecule, a novel member of the immunoglobulin superfamily that distributes at intercellular junctions and modulates monocyte transmigration. J. Cell Biol. 142 (1), 117–127.

Marty, B., et al., 2012. Dynamic study of blood-brain barrier closure after its disruption using ultrasound: a quantitative analysis. J. Cereb. Blood Flow Metabol. 32 (10), 1948–1958.

Mayer, F., et al., 2009. Evolutionary conservation of vertebrate blood-brain barrier chemoprotective mechanisms in Drosophila. J. Neurosci. 29 (11), 3538–3550.

Mazur, C.S., et al., 2012. Human and rat ABC transporter efflux of bisphenol a and bisphenol a glucuronide: interspecies comparison and implications for pharmacokinetic assessment. Toxicol. Sci. 128 (2), 317–325.

McAllister, M.S., et al., 2001. Mechanisms of glucose transport at the blood-brain barrier: an in vitro study. Brain Res. 904 (1), 20–30.

Megard, I., et al., 2002. A co-culture-based model of human blood-brain barrier: application to active transport of indinavir and in vivo-in vitro correlation. Brain Res. 927 (2), 153–167.

Mena, I., Cotzias, G.C., 1975. Protein intake and treatment of Parkinson's disease with levodopa. N. Engl. J. Med. 292 (4), 181–184.

Mensch, J., et al., 2009. In vivo, in vitro and in silico methods for small molecule transfer across the BBB. J. Pharm. Sci. 98 (12), 4429–4468.

Mensch, J. et al. (2010) Application of PAMPA-models to predict BBB permeability including efflux ratio, plasma protein binding and physicochemical parameters. Int. J. Pharm., 395 (1–2), pp. 182–197.

Miletich, R.S., et al., 1993. 6-[18F]fluoro-L-dihydroxyphenylalanine metabolism and positron emission tomography after catechol-O-methyltransferase inhibition in normal and hemiparkinsonian monkeys. Brain Res. 626 (1–2), 1–13.

Mittapalli, R.K., et al., 2010. Exploiting nutrient transporters at the blood-brain barrier to improve brain distribution of small molecules. Ther. Deliv. 1 (6), 775–784.

Morita, K., et al., 1999. Endothelial claudin: claudin-5/TMVCF constitutes tight junction strands in endothelial cells. J. Cell Biol. 147 (1), 185–194.

Muruganandam, A., et al., 1997. Development of immortalized human cerebromicrovascular endothelial cell line as an in vitro model of the human blood-brain barrier. FASEB J. 11 (13), 1187–1197.

Naik, P., Cucullo, L., 2012. In vitro blood-brain barrier models: current and perspective technologies. J. Pharm. Sci. 101 (4), 1337–1354.

Nakagawa, S., et al., 2007. Pericytes from brain microvessels strengthen the barrier integrity in primary cultures of rat brain endothelial cells. Cell. Mol. Neurobiol. 27 (6), 687–694.

Nakagawa, S., et al., 2009. A new blood-brain barrier model using primary rat brain endothelial cells, pericytes and astrocytes. Neurochem. Int. 54 (3–4), 253–263.

Neuhaus, W., et al., 2006. A novel flow based hollow-fiber blood-brain barrier in vitro model with immortalised cell line PBMEC/C1-2. J. Biotechnol. 125 (1), 127–141.

Newton, H.B., 2006. Advances in strategies to improve drug delivery to brain tumors. Expert. Rev. Neurother. 6 (10), 1495–1509.

Nicolazzo, J.A., Charman, S.A., Charman, W.N., 2006. Methods to assess drug permeability across the blood-brain barrier. J. Pharm. Pharmacol. 58 (3), 281–293.

Nielsen, P.A., et al., 2011. Models for predicting blood-brain barrier permeation. Drug Discov. Today 16 (11–12), 472–475.

Niewoehner, J., et al., 2014. Increased brain penetration and potency of a therapeutic antibody using a monovalent molecular shuttle. Neuron 81 (1), 49–60.

Nitta, T., et al., 2003. Size-selective loosening of the blood-brain barrier in claudin-5-deficient mice. J. Cell Biol. 161 (3), 653–660.

O'Keeffe, E., Campbell, M., 2016. Modulating the paracellular pathway at the blood-brain barrier: current and future approaches for drug delivery to the CNS. Drug Discov. Today Technol. 35–39.

Ogunshola, O.O., 2011. In vitro modeling of the blood-brain barrier: simplicity versus complexity. Curr. Pharm. Des. 17 (26), 2755–2761.

Ohno, K., Pettigrew, K.D., Rapoport, S.I., 1978. Lower limits of cerebrovascular permeability to nonelectrolytes in the conscious rat. Am. J. Physiol. 235 (3), H299–307.

Ohtsuki, S., et al., 2014. Quantitative targeted proteomics for understanding the blood-brain barrier: towards pharmacoproteomics. Expert Rev. Proteomics 11 (3), 303–313.

Oldendorf, W.H., 1970. Measurement of brain uptake of radiolabeled substances using a tritiated water internal standard. Brain Res. 24 (2), 372–376.

Oldendorf, W.H., Cornford, M.E., Brown, W.J., 1977. The large apparent work capability of the blood-brain barrier: a study of the mitochondrial content of capillary endothelial cells in brain and other tissues of the rat. Ann. Neurol. 1 (5), 409–417.

Omidi, Y. et al. (2003) Evaluation of the immortalised mouse brain capillary endothelial cell line, b.End3, as an in vitro blood-brain barrier model for drug uptake and transport studies. Brain Res., 990(1–2), pp. 95–112.

On, N., et al., 2013. Examination of blood-brain barrier (BBB) integrity in a mouse brain tumor model. J. Neuro-Oncol. 133–143.

Ong, S., et al., 1995. Membrane partition coefficients chromatographically measured using immobilized artificial membrane surfaces. Anal. Chem. 67 (4), 755–762.

Ong, S., Liu, H., Pidgeon, C., 1996. Immobilized-artificial-membrane chromatography: measurements of membrane partition coefficient and predicting drug membrane permeability. J. Chromatogr. A 728 (1–2), 113–128.

Orunoglu, M., et al., 2017. Effects of curcumin-loaded PLGA nanoparticles on the RG2 rat glioma model. Mater. Sci. Eng. C Mater. Biol. Appl. 78, 32–38.

Pahuja, R., et al., 2015. Trans-blood brain barrier delivery of dopamine-loaded nanoparticles reverses functional deficits in parkinsonian rats. ACS Nano 9 (5), 4850–4871.

Palmer, A.M., Alavijeh, M.S., 2013. Overview of experimental models of the blood-brain barrier in CNS drug discovery. Curr. Protoc. Pharmacol. 1 (Suppl. 62), 1–30.

Palmiotti, C.A., et al., 2014. In vitro cerebrovascular modeling in the 21st century: current and prospective technologies. Pharm. Res. 31 (12), 3229–3250.

Pardridge, W., 1998. CNS drug design based on principles of blood-brain barrier transport. J. Neurochem. 70 (5), 1781–1792.

Pardridge, W.M., 2005. The blood-brain barrier and neurotherapeutics. NeuroRx J. Am. Soc. Exp. NeuroTherap. 1–2.
Pardridge, W.M., 2007. Blood-brain barrier delivery. Drug Discov. Today 54–61.
Pardridge, W.M., 2012. Drug transport across the blood-brain barrier. J. Cereb. Blood Flow Metabol. 32 (11), 1959–1972.
Pardridge, W. M. (2016). CSF, blood-brain barrier, and brain drug delivery, 5247 (March).
Passeleu-Le Bourdonnec, C., et al., 2013. Methodologies to assess drug permeation through the blood-brain barrier for pharmaceutical research. Pharm. Res. 2729–2756.
Patel, M.M., Patel, B.M., 2017. Crossing the blood-brain barrier: recent advances in drug delivery to the brain. CNS Drugs 31 (2), 109–133.
Patel, N.K., Gill, S.S., 2007. GDNF delivery for Parkinson's disease. Acta Neurochir. Suppl. 97 (Pt 2), 135–154.
Patel, R., Page, S., Al-Ahmad, A.J., 2017. Isogenic blood-brain barrier models based on patient-derived stem cells display inter-individual differences in cell maturation and functionality. J. Neurochem. 142 (1), 74–88.
Patnaik, R., et al., 2017. Histamine H3 inverse agonist BF 2649 or antagonist with partial H4 agonist activity clobenpropit reduces amyloid beta peptide-induced brain pathology in Alzheimer's disease. Mol. Neurobiol.
Peppiatt, C.M., et al., 2006. Bidirectional control of CNS capillary diameter by pericytes. Nature 443 (7112), 700–704.
Perel, P., et al., 2007. Comparison of treatment effects between animal experiments and clinical trials: systematic review. BMJ (Clin. Res. Ed.) 334 (7586), 197.
Perriere, N., et al., 2005. Puromycin-based purification of rat brain capillary endothelial cell cultures. Effect on the expression of blood-brain barrier-specific properties. J. Neurochem. 93 (2), 279–289.
Perriere, N., et al., 2007. A functional in vitro model of rat blood-brain barrier for molecular analysis of efflux transporters. Brain Res. 1150, 1–13.
Pidgeon, C., et al., 1995. IAM chromatography: an in vitro screen for predicting drug membrane permeability. J. Med. Chem. 38 (4), 590–594.
Poduslo, J.F., et al., 2001. Permeability of proteins at the blood-brain barrier in the normal adult mouse and double transgenic mouse model of Alzheimer's disease. Neurobiol. Dis. 8 (4), 555–567.
Poller, B., et al., 2008. The human brain endothelial cell line hCMEC/D3 as a human blood-brain barrier model for drug transport studies. J. Neurochem. 107 (5), 1358–1368.
Potschka, H., Luna-Munguia, H., 2014. CNS transporters and drug delivery in epilepsy. Curr. Pharm. Des. 20 (10), 1534–1542.
Prasad, S., et al., 2015. Impact of cigarette smoke extract and hyperglycemic conditions on blood-brain barrier endothelial cells. Fluids Barriers CNS 12, 18.
Prat, A., et al., 2001. Glial cell influence on the human blood-brain barrier. Glia 36 (2), 145–155.
Qosa, H., et al., 2016. High-throughput screening for identification of blood-brain barrier integrity enhancers: a drug repurposing opportunity to rectify vascular amyloid toxicity. J. Alzheimer's Dis. 1499–1516.
Rao, J., Dragulescu-Andrasi, A., Yao, H., 2007. Fluorescence imaging in vivo: recent advances. Curr. Opin. Biotechnol. 18 (1), 17–25.
Rascher, G., et al., 2002. Extracellular matrix and the blood-brain barrier in glioblastoma multiforme: spatial segregation of tenascin and agrin. Acta Neuropathol. 104 (1), 85–91.
Reichel, A., Begley, D.J., 1998. Potential of immobilized artificial membranes for predicting drug penetration across the blood-brain barrier. Pharm. Res. 15 (8), 1270–1274.

Roberts, L.M., et al., 2008. Subcellular localization of transporters along the rat blood-brain barrier and blood-cerebral-spinal fluid barrier by in vivo biotinylation. Neuroscience 155 (2), 423–438.

Roelcke, U., et al., 1995. Alteration of blood-brain barrier in human brain tumors: comparison of [18F]fluorodeoxyglucose, [11C]methionine and rubidium-82 using PET. J. Neurol. Sci. 132 (1), 20–27.

Rosenberg, Y.J., et al., 2017. Post-exposure treatment with the oxime RS194B rapidly reverses early and advanced symptoms in macaques exposed to sarin vapor. Chem. Biol. Interact. 274, 50–57.

Rubin, L.L., et al., 1991. A cell culture model of the blood-brain barrier. J. Cell Biol. 115 (6), 1725–1735.

Russo, G., et al., 2017. Determination of in vitro and in silico indexes for the modeling of blood-brain barrier partitioning of drugs via micellar and immobilized artificial membrane liquid chromatography. J. Med. Chem. 60 (9), 3739–3754.

Sahagun, G., Moore, S.A., Hart, M.N., 1990. Permeability of neutral vs. anionic dextrans in cultured brain microvascular endothelium. Am J. Physiol. 259 (1 Pt 2), 162–166.

Saitou, M., et al., 2000. Complex phenotype of mice lacking occludin, a component of tight junction strands. Mol. Biol. Cell 11 (12), 4131–4142.

Sajja, R.K., Prasad, S., Cucullo, L., 2014. Impact of altered glycaemia on blood-brain barrier endothelium: an in vitro study using the hCMEC/D3 cell line. Fluids Barriers CNS 11 (1), 8.

Sakurada, O., et al., 1978. Measurement of local cerebral blood flow with iodo [14C] antipyrine. Am J. Physiol. 234 (1), H59–66.

Salminen, T., Pulli, A., Taskinen, J., 1997. Relationship between immobilised artificial membrane chromatographic retention and the brain penetration of structurally diverse drugs. J. Pharm. Biomed. Anal. 15 (4), 469–477.

Samiotaki, G., et al., 2015. Enhanced delivery and bioactivity of the neurturin neurotrophic factor through focused ultrasound-mediated blood-brain barrier opening in vivo. J. Cereb. Blood Flow Metabol. 35 (4), 611–622.

Sarkar, G., et al., 2014. Peptide carrier-mediated non-covalent delivery of unmodified cisplatin, methotrexate and other agents via intravenous route to the brain. PLoS One 9 (5), e97655.

Saunders, N.R., et al., 2015. Markers for blood-brain barrier integrity: how appropriate is Evans blue in the twenty-first century and what are the alternatives? Front. Neurosci.

Scherrmann, J.-M., 2002. Drug delivery to brain via the blood-brain barrier. Vasc. Pharmacol. 38 (6), 349–354.

Schiera, G., et al., 2005. Permeability properties of a three-cell type in vitro model of blood-brain barrier. J. Cell. Mol. Med. 9 (2), 373–379.

Schinkel, A.H., et al., 1996. P-glycoprotein in the blood-brain barrier of mice influences the brain penetration and pharmacological activity of many drugs. J. Clin. Invest. 97 (11), 2517–2524.

Schmidt, K.C., Turkheimer, F.E., 2002. Kinetic modeling in positron emission tomography. Quart. J. Nucl. Med. 46 (1), 70–85.

Schoknecht, K., et al., 2014. Monitoring stroke progression: in vivo imaging of cortical perfusion, blood-brain barrier permeability and cellular damage in the rat photothrombosis model. J. Cereb. Blood Flow Metabol. 34 (11), 1791–1801.

Schulze, C., et al., 1997. Lysophosphatidic acid increases tight junction permeability in cultured brain endothelial cells. J. Neurochem. 68 (3), 991–1000.

Serlin, Y., et al., 2015. Anatomy and physiology of the blood-brain barrier. Semin. Cell Dev. Biol. 38, 2–6.

Sharom, F.J., 2011. The P-glycoprotein multidrug transporter. Essays Biochem. 50 (1), 161–178.

Shen, F., et al., 2011. Coexpression of angiopoietin-1 with VEGF increases the structural integrity of the blood-brain barrier and reduces atrophy volume. J. Cereb. Blood Flow Metabol. 31 (12), 2343–2351.

Shen, S., Zhang, W., 2010. ABC transporters and drug efflux at the blood-brain barrier. Rev. Neurosci. 21 (1), 29–53.

Shepro, D., Morel, N.M., 1993. Pericyte physiology. FASEB J. 7 (11), 1031–1038.

Shityakov, S., et al., 2016. Characterization, in vivo evaluation, and molecular modeling of different propofol-cyclodextrin complexes to assess their drug delivery potential at the blood-brain barrier level. J. Chem. Inf. Model. 56 (10), 1914–1922.

Simard, M., et al., 2003. Signaling at the gliovascular interface. J. Neurosci. 23 (27), 9254–9262.

Sims, D.E., 1986. The pericyte—a review. Tissue Cell 18 (2), 153–174.

Sinkó, B., et al., 2009. A PAMPA study of the permeability-enhancing effect of new ceramide analogues. In: Chemistry and Biodiversity.pp. 1867–1874.

Smith, M., Omidi, Y., Gumbleton, M., 2007. Primary porcine brain microvascular endothelial cells: biochemical and functional characterisation as a model for drug transport and targeting. J. Drug Target. 15 (4), 253–268.

Smith, Q.R., 1996. Brain perfusion systems for studies of drug uptake and metabolism in the central nervous system. Pharm. Biotechnol. 8, 285–307.

Sokoloff, L., et al., 1977. The [14C]deoxyglucose method for the measurement of local cerebral glucose utilization: theory, procedure, and normal values in the conscious and anesthetized albino rat. J. Neurochem. 28 (5), 897–916.

Sopasakis, V.R., et al., 2004. High local concentrations and effects on differentiation implicate interleukin-6 as a paracrine regulator. Obes. Res. 12 (3), 454–460.

Stanimirovic, D.B., et al., 2015. Blood-brain barrier models: in vitro to in vivo translation in preclinical development of CNS-targeting biotherapeutics. Expert Opin. Drug Discov. 10 (2), 141–155.

Stemmer, N., et al., 2012. Noninvasive fluorescence imaging in animal models of stroke. Curr. Med. Chem. 19 (28), 4786–4793.

Stewart, P.A., Wiley, M.J., 1981. Developing nervous tissue induces formation of blood-brain barrier characteristics in invading endothelial cells: a study using quail-chick transplantation chimeras. Dev. Biol. 84 (1), 183–192.

Stork, T., et al., 2008. Organization and function of the blood-brain barrier in Drosophila. J. Neurosci. 28 (3), 587–597.

Straus, W., 1959. Rapid cytochemical identification of phagosomes in various tissues of the rat and their differentiation from mitochondria by the peroxidase method. J. Biophys. Biochem. Cytol. 5 (2), 193–204.

Sugano, K., Hamada, H., Machida, M., Ushio, H., 2001a. High throughput prediction of oral absorption: improvement of the composition of the lipid solution used in parallel artificial membrane permeation assay. J. Biomol. Screen. 6 (3), 189–196.

Sugano, K., Hamada, H., Machida, M., Ushio, H., et al., 2001b. Optimized conditions of biomimetic artificial membrane permeation assay. Int. J. Pharm. 228 (1–2), 181–188.

Sugano, K., et al., 2003. Prediction of human intestinal permeability using artificial membrane permeability. Int. J. Pharm. 257 (1–2), 245–251.

Syvanen, S., et al., 2009. Species differences in blood-brain barrier transport of three positron emission tomography radioligands with emphasis on P-glycoprotein transport. Drug Metab. Disposit. 37 (3), 635–643.

Tajes, M., et al., 2014. The blood-brain barrier: structure, function and therapeutic approaches to cross it. Mol. Membr. Biol. 31 (5), 152–167.

Takasato, Y., Rapoport, S.I., Smith, Q.R., 1984. An in situ brain perfusion technique to study cerebrovascular transport in the rat. Am J. Physiol. 247 (3 Pt 2), 484–493.

Takata, F., et al., 2015. Elevated permeability of the blood-brain barrier in mice intratracheally administered porcine pancreatic elastase. J. Pharmacol. Sci. 129 (1), 78–81.

Takeshita, Y., et al., 2014. An in vitro Blood-brain barrier model combining shear stress and endothelial cell/astrocyte co-culture. J. Neurosci. Methods 30 (232), 165–172.

Tam, S.J., et al., 2012. Death receptors DR6 and TROY regulate brain vascular development. Dev. Cell 22 (2), 403–417.

Tamai, I., Tsuji, A., 2000. Transporter-mediated permeation of drugs across the blood-brain barrier. J. Pharm. Sci. 89 (11), 1371–1388.

Tan, S.F., et al., 2017. Characterisation, in vitro and in vivo evaluation of valproic acid-loaded nanoemulsion for improved brain bioavailability. J. Pharm. Pharmacol. 1–11.

Tepass, U., Hartenstein, V., 1994. The development of cellular junctions in the Drosophila embryo. Dev. Biol. 161 (2), 563–596.

Thiebaut, F., et al., 1989. Immunohistochemical localization in normal tissues of different epitopes in the multidrug transport protein P170: evidence for localization in brain capillaries and crossreactivity of one antibody with a muscle protein. J. Histochem. Cytochem. 37 (2), 159–164.

Thomsen, L.B., Thomsen, M.S., Moos, T., 2015. Targeted drug delivery to the brain using magnetic nanoparticles. Ther. Deliv. 6 (10), 1145–1155.

Thorne, R.G., et al., 2008. Delivery of interferon-beta to the monkey nervous system following intranasal administration. Neuroscience 152 (3), 785–797.

Tian, X., et al., 2012. In vitro and in vivo studies on gelatin-siloxane nanoparticles conjugated with SynB peptide to increase drug delivery to the brain. Int. J. Nanomed. 7, 1031–1041.

Tomkins, O., et al., 2008. Blood-brain barrier disruption in post-traumatic epilepsy. J. Neurol. Neurosurg. Psychiatry 79 (7), 774–777.

Tong, H.-I., et al., 2016. Monocyte trafficking, engraftment, and delivery of nanoparticles and an exogenous gene into the acutely inflamed brain tissue—evaluations on monocyte-based delivery system for the central nervous system. PLoS One. 11(4).

Turner, M.H., Ullmann, J.F.P., Kay, A.R., 2012. A method for detecting molecular transport within the cerebral ventricles of live zebrafish (*Danio rerio*) larvae. J. Physiol. 590 (10), 2233–2240.

Ujiie, M., et al., 2003. Blood-brain barrier permeability precedes senile plaque formation in an Alzheimer disease model. Microcirculation (New York, NY: 1994) 10 (6), 463–470.

Ulapane, K.R., et al., 2017. Improving brain delivery of biomolecules via BBB modulation in mouse and rat: detection using MRI, NIRF, and mass spectrometry. Nanotheranostics 1 (2), 217–231.

Umans, R.A., Taylor, M.R., 2012a. Zebrafish as a model to study drug transporters at the blood-brain barrier. Clin. Pharmacol. Ther. 92 (5), 567–570.

Umans, R.A., Taylor, M.R., 2012b. Zebrafish as a model to study drug transporters at the blood-brain barrier. Clin. Pharmacol. Therap. 92 (5), 567–570.

Unno, K., et al., 2017. Blood-brain barrier permeability of green tea catechin metabolites and their neuritogenic activity in human neuroblastoma SH-SY5Y cells. Mol. Nutr. Food Res.

Van Rooy, I., et al., 2011. In vivo methods to study uptake of nanoparticles into the brain. Pharm. Res. 28 (3), 456–471.

Vazana, U., et al., 2016. Glutamate-mediated blood-brain barrier opening: implications for neuroprotection and drug delivery. J. Neurosci. 36 (29), 7727–7739.

Verwilst, P., et al., 2017. Rational design of in vivo tau tangle-selective near-infrared fluorophores: expanding the BODIPY universe. J. Am. Chem. Soc. 139 (38), 13393–13403.

Vizseralek, G., et al., 2014. PAMPA study of the temperature effect on permeability. Eur. J. Pharm. Sci. 53, 45–49.

Wang, T., Agarwal, S., Elmquist, W.F., 2012. Brain distribution of cediranib is limited by active efflux at the blood-brain barrier. J. Pharmacol. Exp. Ther. 341 (2), 386–395.

Wang, W., Dentler, W.L., Borchardt, R.T., 2001. VEGF increases BMEC monolayer permeability by affecting occludin expression and tight junction assembly. Am. J. Physiol. Heart Circ. Physiol. 280 (1), 434–440.

Watson, P.M.D., et al., 2013. Modelling the endothelial blood-CNS barriers: a method for the production of robust in vitro models of the rat blood-brain barrier and blood-spinal cord barrier. BMC Neurosci. 59.

Weksler, B.B., et al., 2005. Blood-brain barrier-specific properties of a human adult brain endothelial cell line. FASEB J. 19 (13), 1872–1874.

Westerfield et al, 1997. An on-line database for zebrafish development and genetics research. Semin. Cell Dev. Biol. 8 (5), 477–488.

Wilhelm, I., Fazakas, C., Krizbai, I.A., 2011. In vitro models of the blood-brain barrier. Acta Neurobiol. Exp. (Wars) 71 (1), 113–128.

Wilhelm, I., Krizbai, I.A., 2014. In vitro models of the blood-brain barrier for the study of drug delivery to the brain. Mol. Pharm. 11 (7), 1949–1963.

Wisniewski, N., et al., 2001. Decreased analyte transport through implanted membranes: differentiation of biofouling from tissue effects. J. Biomed. Mater. Res. 57 (4), 513–521.

Wolburg, H., Lippoldt, A., 2002. Tight junctions of the blood-brain barrier: development, composition and regulation. Vasc. Pharmacol. 38 (6), 323–337.

Wolff, A., et al., 2015. In vitro blood-brain barrier models—an overview of established models and new microfluidic approaches. J. Pharm. Sci. 2727–2746.

Wu, V.M., Beitel, G.J., 2004. A junctional problem of apical proportions: epithelial tube-size control by septate junctions in the Drosophila tracheal system. Curr. Opin. Cell Biol. 16 (5), 493–499.

Xie, Y.-T.T., et al., 2012. Brain-targeting study of stearic acid-grafted chitosan micelle drug-delivery system. Int. J. Nanomed. 7, 3235–3244.

Yamagata, K., et al., 2003. Polyunsaturated fatty acids induce tight junctions to form in brain capillary endothelial cells. Neuroscience 116 (3), 649–656.

Yamamoto, M., et al., 1997. Increased expression of low density lipoprotein receptor-related protein/alpha2-macroglobulin receptor in human malignant astrocytomas. Cancer Res. 57 (13), 2799–2805.

Yamamoto, Y., et al., 2017. Predicting drug concentration-time profiles in multiple CNS compartments using a comprehensive physiologically-based pharmacokinetic model. In: CPT: Pharmacometrics & Systems Pharmacology.

Yang, F.-Y., et al., 2014. Pharmacokinetic analysis and uptake of 18F-FBPA-Fr after ultrasound-induced blood-brain barrier disruption for potential enhancement of boron delivery for neutron capture therapy. J. Nucl. Med. 55 (4), 616–621.

Yang, T., et al., 2015. Exosome delivered anticancer drugs across the blood-brain barrier for brain cancer therapy in *Danio rerio*. Pharm. Res. 32 (6), 2003–2014.

Yao, Y., Tsirka, S.E., 2011. Truncation of monocyte chemoattractant protein 1 by plasmin promotes blood-brain barrier disruption. J. Cell Sci. 124 (Pt 9), 1486–1495.

Yi, T., et al., 2017. Enhancing both oral bioavailability and brain penetration of puerarin using borneol in combination with preparation technologies. Drug Deliv. 24 (1), 422–429.

Yoon, C.H., et al., 2006. Rapid screening of blood-brain barrier penetration of drugs using the immobilized artificial membrane phosphatidylcholine column chromatography. J. Biomol. Screen. 11 (1), 13–20.
Yu, Y.J., et al., 2011. Boosting brain uptake of a therapeutic antibody by reducing its affinity for a transcytosis target. Sci. Transl. Med. 3, 84. 84ra44.
Zenker, D., et al., 2003. Human blood-derived macrophages enhance barrier function of cultured primary bovine and human brain capillary endothelial cells. J. Physiol. 551 (Pt 3), 1023–1032.
Zhang, J., et al., 2012. Involvement of claudins in zebrafish brain ventricle morphogenesis. Ann. N. Y. Acad. Sci. 1257, 193–198.
Zhang, L., Lu, J., Qiu, L., 2016. Synergistic effects of A-B-C-type amphiphilic copolymer on reversal of drug resistance in MCF-7/ADR breast carcinoma. Int. J. Nanomed. 11, 5205–5220.
Zheng, P.-P., et al., 2010. Glut1/SLC2A1 is crucial for the development of the blood-brain barrier in vivo. Ann. Neurol. 68 (6), 835–844.
Zhou, Q.-H., et al., 2011. Delivery of a peptide radiopharmaceutical to brain with an IgG-avidin fusion protein. Bioconjug. Chem. 22 (8), 1611–1618.

Further reading

Ghoroghchian, P.P., Therien, M.J., Hammer, D.a., 2009. In vivo fluorescence imaging: a personal perspective. Wiley Interdiscip. Rev. Nanomed. Nanobiotechnol. 1 (2), 156–167.
Ramalingam, P., Ko, Y.T., 2016. Validated LC-MS/MS method for simultaneous quantification of resveratrol levels in mouse plasma and brain and its application to pharmacokinetic and brain distribution studies. J. Pharm. Biomed. Anal. 119, 71–75.
Steuer, A.E., Poetzsch, M., Kraemer, T., 2016. MALDI-MS drug analysis in biological samples: opportunities and challenges. Bioanalysis 8 (17), 1859–1878.

Part II

Nanoparticles-based brain targeting delivery strategies

Receptor-mediated transportation through BBB

5

*Zui Zhang**, *Changyou Zhan**,†
*School of Basic Medical Sciences & State Key Laboratory of Molecular Engineering of Polymers, Fudan University, Shanghai, P.R. China, †Key Laboratory of Smart Drug Delivery (Fudan University), Ministry of Education, Shanghai, P.R. China

1 Introduction

The blood-brain barrier (BBB) is mainly composed of brain endothelial cells and tight junction proteins (Abbott et al., 2006; Armulik et al., 2010; Abbott et al., 2010). BBB is a physical and biochemical barrier that prevents toxic compounds from reaching the brain, but allows the transport of gas and trophic molecules (Hawkins and Davis, 2005; Pardridge, 2005b). BBB plays pivotal roles in remaining brain homeostasis; however, it also presents an obstacle to the delivery of most of drugs into the brain, severely restricting the development of therapeutics for many brain diseases (Abbott, 2013; Pardridge, 2005a).

A variety of endogenous peptides or proteins that are necessary for normal brain functions traverse the BBB via receptor-mediated transcytosis (RMT), which is one of the most promising approaches to circumvent BBB and facilitate the delivery of biomacromolecules and nanocarriers (Jones and Shusta, 2007). RMT has been found in the process of brain influx of nutrients like insulin, leptin, transferrin, among many others. These receptors expressed on the brain capillary endothelial cells bind the endogenous ligands or ligand-modified prodrug/drug delivery systems; then, mediate the endocytosis and transport to the brain parenchyma. The receptor-mediated transcytosis occurs at least in four steps: (1) recognition and binding of ligand at the luminal side; (2) receptor-mediated endocytosis at the luminal side of the brain capillary endothelium (Donahue et al., 2006); (3) recycling of receptor to the luminal side of brain capillary endothelial cells; and (4) exocytosis of ligand at the abluminal side of the brain capillary endothelium and transport into the brain (Lajoie and Shusta, 2015) (Fig. 1).

There are various receptors involved in the RMT process, including insulin receptor (IR), transferrin receptor (TfR), low-density lipoprotein receptor (LDLR) and LDLR-related protein-1 (LRP-1), scavenger receptor class B type 1 (SR-B1), leptin receptor, lactoferrin receptor, nicotinic acetylcholine receptors (nAChRs), diphtheria toxin receptor, and single domain llama antibody (sdAb) receptor (Wang et al., 2009). In this chapter, we discuss the mechanisms of receptor-mediated transcytosis, as well as their applications in developing brain-targeted drug delivery systems.

Brain Targeted Drug Delivery Systems. https://doi.org/10.1016/B978-0-12-814001-7.00005-6

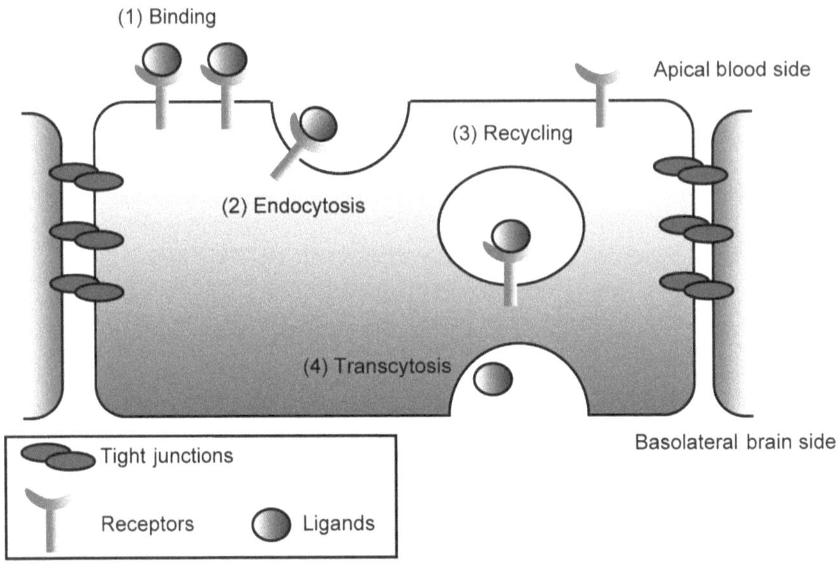

Fig. 1 Schematic diagram of the process of receptor-mediated transcytosis.

2 Insulin receptor

The insulin receptor (IR) on blood vessels throughout the central nervous system (CNS) was first found to rapidly and specifically bind plasma insulin in 1979 (Jacobs et al., 1979). Later in 1981, William Pardridge demonstrated the existence of IR in isolated brain capillaries by radioimmunoassay for the first time (Frank and Pardridge, 1981). From then on, the role of IR in crossing BBB has been extensively studied. IR can mediate the transport of endogenous insulin to the brain parenchyma. IR is composed of four subunits (two α and two β subunits) that are linked by disulfide bonds, among which the two α-subunits form an insulin-binding pocket. Once insulin is recognized and binds to the pocket, the tyrosine phosphorylation increases in β subunits of IR, resulting in conformational change of the IR to switch on a channel and allowing the insulin or engineered vector to cross the cell membrane (Becker and Roth, 1990). However, the use of insulin as a ligand to trigger brain transport of nanocarriers is limited by its undesirable hypoglycemic effect. To solve the problem, two murine monoclonal antibodies (MAb83-7 and MAb83-14) have been produced to bind α-subunit of human IR. Both antibodies can strongly associate with capillary endothelium in vitro immunocytochemical analysis of brain section. These antibodies also showed efficient transcytosis through the BBB of rhesus monkeys in vivo. At 3 h after a single intravenous injection, 3.8% of the injected MAb83-14 was found in per 100 g brain of rhesus monkey, while no brain uptake was found of the negative control antibody (the mouse IgG2a isotype control antibody) (Pardridge et al., 1995). In 2013, Kuo and Huang modified solid lipid nanoparticles with MAb83-14 to load carmustine (BCNU, a dialkylating agent mainly used for chemotherapy) and found that MAb83-14 stimulated endocytosis of nanoparticles by human brain-microvascular endothelial cells, resulting in enhanced permeability of BCNU across the BBB (Kuo and Shih-Huang, 2013). At early of 2011, Kreurer and coworkers have already conjugated another anti-IR monoclonal antibody (29B4) to human serum albumin nanoparticles (HSA-NP) and found that the loaded loperamide could cross the brain to induce significant antinociceptive effects after intravenous injection (Ulbrich et al., 2011). These results encouraged scientists to modify anti-IR antibodies to other formulations such as PDMS-b-PMOXA-based polymersome and solid lipid nanoparticles for enhanced brain transport of therapeutics (Dieu et al., 2014).

For drug delivery in humans, genetically engineered forms of the human insulin receptor monoclonal antibody (HIRMAb) were subsequently produced. A chimeric HIRMAb could bind to the IR on human brain capillaries with the comparable affinity to the murine HIRMAb, and the uptake of the chimeric HIRMAb by the rhesus monkey brain in vivo was similar to that of the murine HIRMAb (Coloma et al., 2000). To further enhance the immunocompatibility of HIRMAbs in humans, they were humanized by grafting the complementarity determining region of human IgG onto the framework regions. Although the affinity of the humanized HIRMAb for the HIR was decreased to 27% of that of the murine HIRMAb, the 125-iodine radiolabeled humanized HIRMAb could rapidly transport into all parts of the primate brain after intravenous administration in rhesus monkey (Boado et al., 2007).

In addition, biologic drugs, including therapeutic enzymes, neurotrophic factors, decoy receptors, monoclonal antibodies, and avidin, have been fused with the HIRMAb for efficient brain-targeted delivery. The challenge of design of HIRMAb fusion proteins lies in retaining the bioactivity of both segments. For example, β-glucuronidase (GUSB), a lysosomal enzyme mutated in mucopolysaccharidosis type VII (Miller et al., 1990), could be fused to either the amino terminus or the carboxyl terminus of either the heavy chain (HC) or the light chain (Palchetti et al., 2016) of the HIRMAb. Unexpectedly, GUSB lost more than 95% activity when fused to the carboxyl terminus of the HC while the high binding affinity for the HIR was retained. In contrast, when the GUSB was fused to the amino terminus of the HC of HIRMAb, GUSB enzymatic activity was retained, but most of HIR-binding activity got lost (Boado and Pardridge, 2010). A successful example has been achieved by fusing α-L-Iduronidase (IDUA), a lysosomal enzyme mutated in Hurler's syndrome, to HIRMAb (Scott et al., 1991). Lu et al. fused human IDUA to the carboxyl terminus of the HC of HIRMAb and found that the resultant fusion protein retained both the IDUA enzymatic activity and binding affinity to HIR (Lu et al., 2010). Moreover, 1% of the injected HIRMAb-IDUA fusion protein was able to cross the BBB and distributed in the brain of rhesus monkey (Boado et al., 2008c). Other examples include: (1) HIRMAb-GDNF (glial cell-derived neurotrophic factor) fusion protein. Intracerebral injection of HIRMAb-GDNF in rat resulted in 90% reduction of stroke volume in a middle cerebral artery occlusion (MCAO) model. The CHO-derived HIRMAb-GDNF fusion protein could transport into primate brain in vivo, resulting in pharmacologic elevation of brain GDNF, while no brain transport of GDNF itself was found after intravenous injection (Boado et al., 2008a). (2) The HIRMAb-TNFR (tumor necrosis factor-alpha receptor) fusion protein, in which human TNFR extracellular domain was fused with the HIRMAb. HIRMAb-TNFR bound both the HIR and human TNFα. As expected, the HIRMAb-TNFR fusion protein suppressed the cytotoxic effects of the TNFα in a human bioassay (Boado et al., 2010b). Other biomacromolecules like erythropoietin (EPO) (Thomas Tayra et al., 2013; Boado et al., 2010a) and paraoxonase-1 (Boado et al., 2008b) have also been transported into the brain by taking advantage of fusion protein technique.

3 Transferrin receptor

Transferrin (Tf), encoded by the TF gene, belongs to the family of iron-binding plasma glycoproteins that control the free iron (Fe) level in biological fluid (Ponka et al., 1998). It is a ~80kDa protein, containing two specific high-affinity Fe(III) binding pockets. The binding affinity of Fe(III) to Tf is highly pH-dependent, progressively decreasing at acidic pH values (Dautry-Varsat et al., 1983). The Tf receptor (TfR), a transmembrane glycoprotein, consists of two identical 90-kDa monomers linked by intermolecular disulfide bonds (Huebers and Finch, 1987). TfR has been found highly expressed on the brain capillary endothelial cells (BCECs) (Jefferies et al., 1984) and is capable of mediating brain transport of iron in vivo.

Tf is biodegradable, nontoxic, and nonimmunogenic. Several studies have showed that Tf enhanced brain delivery of nanoparticles (NPs) in vitro and/or in vivo. For example, DiI (derivatives of indocarbocyanine iodide)-PLGA NPs were modified with Tf and incubated with BCECs. The cellular uptake of Tf-NPs was about 20-fold higher than that of plain NPs (without Tf modification) and two folds greater than that of BSA-NPs within 1h in 37°C (Chang et al., 2009). In vivo, DiI accumulation in cortex in Tf-NPs group was two folds higher than that in BSA-NPs group (Chang et al., 2012). Tf has also been used to modify other nanocarriers like micelle and polymersome. The BCECs uptake of Tf-micelle loaded with c(RGDfK)-paclitaxel conjugates (cRGDfK is a cyclic peptide that specifically binds to integrins) increased significantly in comparison to that of unadorned micelle. In vivo, Tf-micelle loaded with c[RGDfK]-paclitaxel conjugates could significantly prolong the mean survival time of nude mice bearing intracranial U87 MG glioma (42.8 days) compared with free paclitaxel (33.6 days) (Zhang et al., 2012). When Tf was anchored on the surface of biodegradable polymersome (Tf-PO), Tf-PO showed 2.3 folds of the ID % per gram of brain higher than did the undecorated polymersome. Fluorescent microscopy of brain coronal sections showed higher accumulation of Tf-PO in the cerebral cortex, periventricular region of the lateral ventricle, and the third ventricle than that of plain PO (without surface modification) (Pang et al., 2011). To discern the precise mechanism of the Tf-mediated transcytosis, Chang et al. studied the endocytosis of Tf-PLGA-NPs (<90nm) in an in vitro BBB model (BCECs coculture with astrocytes). Tf-labeled NPs were taken up in an energy-dependent manner and entered the cells via the caveolae-dependent pathway (Chang et al., 2009). However, Tf-PO (around 100 nm) were taken up via a clathrin-mediated, energy-dependent pathway in bEnd.3 cells (Pang et al., 2011). The results suggested that Tf-modified nonocarriers might transport BBB through different pathways depending on the materials and/or size of the vehicles.

Tf-modified polypropylenimine dendrimer has been used to transport the plasmid DNA to the brain. After 2 h coculture with Tf-modified dendrimer, the uptake of DNA by bEnd.3 cells increased 1.4 folds compared with that of unmodified dendrimer. In vivo, gene expression got enhanced by two folds after Tf modification (Somani et al., 2014).

The Tf-IDUA fusion protein was engineered by Osborn et al., of which the N-terminal Tf motif maintained preferential specificity for the TfR and the C-terminal IDUA retained enzymatic activity and substrate specificity. The Tf-IDUA fusion protein entered the cytoplasm of cerebellar Purkinje cells of the brain to reduce cerebellar GAG storage in adult MPS 1 (Mucopolysaccharidosis 1) mice (Osborn et al., 2008).

However, the in vivo application of Tf is limited by its high endogenous concentration in plasma, for $<0.1\%$ of endogenous Tf can bind to the BBB TfR (Ulbrich et al., 2009). The administered Tf-vectors have to compete with the excess amount of endogenous Tf for binding to the TfR. The use of monoclonal antibody against TfR (TfRmAbs) can tackle this dilemma, because the binding site of the TfRmAb on the TfR is different from that of endogenous Tf. The TfRmAbs bind to the receptor on the surface of endothelial cells and allow the conjugated therapeutics across the BBB via receptor-mediated transcytosis (Pardridge, 2015).

Boado et al. engineered a chimeric TfRMAb, subsequently conjugated it with a single chain Fv (ScFv) antibody. In the fusion protein, the affinity for murine TfR was retained. The brain uptake of the chimeric TfRMAb-ScFv fusion protein in mouse reached as high as 3.5% of ID/g brain (Boado et al., 2009). OX26, a rat anti-TfR IgG2a, which was prepared by William Pardridge's group in 1991, has been widely used for brain-targeted drug delivery afterwards. At 5 h after the injection of the OX26 antibody into the rats, the distribution of brain volume of OX26 was 18 folds higher than that of the control IgG2a (Pardridge et al., 1991). OX26 has been used to modify nanocarrier to increase brain uptake, including nanoparticle, liposome, and polymersome (Ulbrich et al., 2009). Z-DEVD-FMK, a caspase-3 inhibitor, is a neuronal protective peptide unable to cross the BBB and diffuse into the brain. Chitosan (CS) nanospheres conjugated with PEG bearing the OX26 (CS-PEG-OX26) was produced to transport Z-DEVD-FMK into brain. Fluorescently labeled CS-PEG-OX26 nanoparticles were intravenously injected into mice in order to elevate their efficacy for brain translocation, showing that positive fluorescent signal scattered all over the hemispheres, while free NPs were undetectable (Aktas et al., 2005). OX26-modified α-cobrotoxin (an analgesic peptide) PEG-PLA NPs also showed transport across BBB after intranasal administration in rats (Liu et al., 2013a). For the delivery of genetic materials, the OX26-modified PEGylated liposome coupled with chlorotoxin (CTX) could transport hTERTC27 (plasmid of a 27 kDa C-terminal peptide of human telomerase reverse transcriptase) into brain and treat brain glioma via inhibiting tumor cell growth (Yue et al., 2014).

Researchers also engineered 8D3 antibody (for mouse TfR) to the β-Galactosidase (a candidate for enzyme replacement therapy of lysosomal storage disorder) to facilitate brain transport. After intravenous injection, the β-galactosidase-8D3 conjugate showed 10-fold increase in mice brain than β-galactosidase by measuring enzyme activity. The results of capillary depletion assay demonstrated that more than 90% of the β-galactosidase-8D3 conjugate that entered into the endothelial compartment of brain circumvented the BBB and was transported into brain parenchyma (Zhang and Pardridge, 2005). 8D3 antibody was also used to engineer fusion protein like cTfRmAb-EPO carrying erythropoietin (a neuroprotective drug) across the BBB (Zhou et al., 2010). Vilaplana and colleagues coated gold nanoparticles (AuNPs) with 8D3, and intravenously administered to mice. The transcytosis mechanism was analyzed by a transmission electron microscope. Two individual trafficking routes occurred at the same time, including a TfR-mediated and a clathrin-dependent internalization pathways (Cabezon et al., 2015). TfR-mediated transcytosis is complicated and multiple intracellular pathways may be involved in the process. Other TfRMAbs like R17217 also can cross the BBB via TfR-mediated transcytosis in vitro and in vivo (Ulbrich et al., 2009; Lee et al., 2000).

The biomedical application of large proteins still suffers from drawbacks including high synthesis cost, instability, and immunological response; instead of TfR antibodies, peptides targeting TfR have been explored through phage display technology. In 2000, a B6 peptide with affinity for TfR was identified as a substitute for transferrin (Xia et al., 2000). It demonstrated potential as a ligand for brain-targeted drug delivery. B6-modified PEG-PLA NPs exhibited significant cellular uptake into the mouse BCECs via lipid raft-mediated and clathrin-mediated endocytosis. In addition, biodistribution studies revealed that fluorescently labeled B6-NPs exhibited much higher brain accumulation than did plain NPs (without peptide modification) (Liu et al., 2013b). In an Alzheimer's mouse model, B6-NPs could facilitate the delivery of a functional neuroprotective peptide NAPVSIPQ (NAP) across the BBB, ameliorating in behavior impairments and pathological index even at low doses (Gregori et al., 2015). In another study, a 9-mer peptide targeting TfR named CRT peptide (CRTIGPSVC) was developed. CRT peptide accumulated in the brain after i.v. administration to mice. Furthermore, CRT peptide facilitated brain transport in a glioblastoma mouse model, resulting in a significant decrease in tumor size (Staquicini et al., 2011).

TfR-mediated transport across BBB has been successful in various cases and is widely used in brain drug delivery; however, the expression of TfR is unspecific in BBB, and it widely distributes in peripheral organs. Thus, off-target effect may restrict the application of Tf or TfRMAb-modified cargo for brain-targeted drug delivery to some extent. In addition, low iron concentration in plasma induces the increase of TfR expression. Administration of high-affinity TfRAb may induce the down-regulation of TfR expression, which would interrupt the physiological iron homeostasis. TfR degeneration would decrease the transcytosis efficiency and disrupt the iron uptake in brain.

4 Low-density lipoprotein receptor and low-density lipoprotein receptor-related proteins

The low-density lipoprotein receptor (LDLR), encoded by the LDLR gene, is a cell-surface receptor that mediates the endocytosis of cholesterol-rich low-density lipoprotein (LDL) (Goldstein et al., 1985). The LDL such as cholesterol, tocopherol, and apolipoproteins (Lanthier et al., 2002) bind to the LDLR, which locates in the caveolae membrane fraction and mediates the transport of LDL into the brain (Meresse et al., 1989; Candela et al., 2008). Therefore, it is a promising method to make use of LDLR for brain-targeted delivery (Spencer and Verma, 2007).

In 1989, Meresse et al. isolated brain capillaries and identified a high-affinity binding site for LDL (Meresse et al., 1989). It demonstrated the LDLR-mediated transcytosis of nanocarriers in vivo. Apolipoproteins (Lanthier et al., 2002) have been conjugated to many nanomaterials to increase the brain transport. For example, poly(butyl cyanoacrylate) nanoparticles (PBCA NPs) modified with ApoB or ApoE and loaded with antinociceptive medicine (hexapeptide dalargin or loperamide) were able to cross the BBB. The analgesic effect could be enhanced by precoating hexapeptide dalargin or loperamide-loaded PBCA NPs with polysorbate 80 (PS80) before apolipoprotein modification (Kreuter et al., 2002). The mechanism of PS80 increasing brain transport is that PS80 promotes the plasma ApoB and/or ApoE absorption on the surface of the NPs; therefore, PS80-NPs surrounded by Apo were recognized by the LDLR and transcytosed by the brain capillary endothelial cells (Alyaudtin et al., 2001; Luck et al., 1997). Another supportive evidence is that the ApoE-3-modified PS80-coated PBCA-NPs were transported across the porcine BCECs 1.8 folds more than the PS80-coated PBCA-NPs (Kim et al., 1996). As the PBCA-NPs have low drug loading capacity and low biodegradation, the biodegradable and biocompatible solid lipid nanoparticles (Kaur et al., 2008) have been produced as a drug carrier alternatively (Kaur et al., 2008). The transcytosis efficiency of ApoE-SLNs was evaluated in hCMEC/D3 cell monolayers, and the results showed a 1.8-fold increase of cellular uptake for SLN-Palmitate-ApoE and 1.9-fold for SLN-DSPE-ApoE than that for the plain SLNs (without functionalization) (Neves et al., 2015). In 2014, Song and coworkers prepared a biomimetic nanostructure ApoE3-reconstituted high-density lipoprotein (ApoE3-rHDL), which presents high binding affinity to Aβ, and demonstrated that ApoE3-rHDL has 0.4% ID/g of access to the brain 1 h after intravenous administration in Alzheimer's Disease (AD) animal model. In addition, a 4-week treatment of ApoE3-rHDL to AD animal model decreased Aβ deposition, attenuated microgliosis, ameliorated neurologic changes, and rescued memory deficits (Song et al., 2014). Later in 2016, the same group loaded the ApoE-reconstituted high-density lipoprotein nanocarrier (ANC) with α-Mangostin (α-M) (ANC-α-M), a polyphenolic drug that can inhibit the Aβ oligomers and fibrils formation and accelerate Aβ cellular degradation. The data showed that ANC-α-M exhibited the highest efficiency in decreasing amyloid deposition, attenuating microgliosis, and rescuing memory defect compared with liposome or ANC treatment in AD mouse model (Song et al., 2016). Except for the protein ligands, a peptide ligand of LDLR, termed peptide-22, has been identified using phage display technique. Peptide-22 was modified on the surface of paclitaxel-loaded NPs, which could be taken up by BCECs and rat glioma C6 cells. Intravenous injection of peptide-22-modified paclitaxel-loaded NPs significantly prolonged the survival time of mice bearing intracranial glioma mice (Zhang et al., 2013a).

Low-density lipoprotein receptor-related proteins (LRPs) are endocytic receptors that mediate the transport of ligands into endothelial cells, including receptor-associated protein (Staquicini et al., 2011), melanotransferrin (P97), and angiopep-2 (Pan et al., 2004; Rahmanto et al., 2012). One of the LRPs identified on BBB is class A scavenger receptor, but following studies demonstrated that SR do not undergo trancytosis across the BBB (Husemann and Silverstein, 2001). Another two members of LRPs are LRP1 (known as alpha-2-macroglobulin receptor, apolipoprotein E receptor, or cluster of differentiation 91) and LRP2 (Megalin), which are expressed on the cerebral vascular epithelial cells.

Angiopep-2, a 19-mer peptide ligand of LRP1, belongs to the Kunitz domain-derived peptides family (Demeule et al., 2008). Angiopep-2 has been widely applied for brain-targeted drug delivery via LPR1-mediated tanscytosis. Cy5.5-labeled Angiopep-2 could rapidly transport into the brain parenchyma, as measured by in vivo imaging followed by fluorescence analysis of brain slices (Yan et al., 2011). Thomas et al. conjugated Angiopep-2 with paclitaxel (ANG1005) to design new therapeutics for the treatment of brain cancers. By radiolabelling method, they verified that the BBB transfer efficiency (Kin) of ANG1005 ($7.3 \pm 0.2 \times 10^{-3}$ mL/s/g) was 86-fold higher than that of paclitaxel ($8.5 \pm 0.5 \times 10^{-5}$ mL/s/g). In addition, the brain uptake of ANG1005 was more than 10-fold higher than that of free PTX in mice bearing brain metastases of breast cancer (Thomas et al., 2009). Although the brain uptake of ANG1005 by mouse brain following intravenous injection was unexpectedly as low as 0.34% ID/g, ANG1005 showed significantly improved delivery to brain and brain metastases of breast cancer in comparison to free paclitaxel, indicating that therapeutic dose of ANG1005 was delivered to the intracranial tumor.

Angiopep-2 has also been applied to modify nanocarriers such as NPs, micelle, and carbon nanotube for brain-targeted drug delivery. The angiopep-2-modified Au-PEG-NPs could deliver doxorubicin across the BBB to treat the intracranial glioma, resulting in 2.89-fold longer median survival time than that of the control group (Ruan et al., 2015). Angiopep-2 was also used to modify polymeric micelles loading AmB (amphotericin B, a hydrophobic antibiotic) by Shao and colleagues. The data showed that angiopep-2-functionalized group could effectively deliver AmB into the brain to achieve the highest AmB level among all treated groups (Shao et al., 2012). A recent study has explored a retro-inverso isomer of traditional angiopep-2, named D-angiopep-2. Since more than 85% of L-angiopep-2 degraded within 2h in rat blood serum, D-angiopep-2 could escape from the proteolysis. Although the binding affinity with the LRP1 of D-angiopep-2 is lower than angiopep-2, the stability in serum helps it to be a promising alternative for brain targeting delivery (Wei et al., 2014).

P97 (melanotransferrin), a glycosylated protein that reversibly binds iron, is another ligand of LRP1, which is closely related to Tf and lactoferrin (Tartaglia et al., 1995; Rahmanto et al., 2012). Compared to transferrin, P97 has 5.7 folds higher efficiency of brain transport 1 h after i.v. injection (Demeule et al., 2002). In addition, the results of in vitro BCEC monolayer experiment demonstrated that the transcytosis efficiency of P97 was 14-fold higher than that of transferrin (Beliveau, 2003). P97 was also used to form conjugates with drugs or to modify nanocarriers to enhance the brain transport. For example, adriamycin (ADR, a classic antitumor drug) was conjugated with P97 and intravenously injected into mice, and the brain uptake of P97-ADR was 10 folds higher than that of bovine serum albumin or Lf-modified conjugates 1 h after injection. In vivo, P97-ADR treatment could induce 20.8% and 44% increase of median survival time of mice bearing intracranial ZR-75-1 mammary tumors and C6 gliomas, respectively (Karkan et al., 2008). For the delivery of genetic materials, P97 was also used to form conjugates with the extracellular domain of the coxsackie-adenovirus receptor (CAR), and the adaptor protein was validated to redirect the Ad5 (adenovirus serotype 5, a gene delivery vector) to significant transport across the BBB in vitro, with an efficiency of 40–50 folds higher than the control (Tang et al., 2007). P97-modified etoposide-entrapped SLNs were recently found to cross the BBB for efficient brain tumor therapy (Kuo and Wang, 2016).

5 Nicotinic acetylcholine receptors

The nicotinic acetylcholine receptors (nAchRs) have been reported in previous studies to mediate the transport of the rabies virus glycoprotein (RVG, 505 amino acids) into the neuron cells. Thus, scientists developed a 29-mer peptide named RVG29 from RVG, expecting to drive drugs or genetic materials into brain via nAchRs-mediated transcytosis. The RVG29-derived peptide is likely to traverse the BBB via binding to the nicotinic acetylcholine receptor α-subunit as implicated in its internalization into cultured neurons. For gene delivery, a nona-arginine (R9) sequence was conjugated to RVG29 peptide to enable electrostatic interaction with siRNA cargo, and RVG29 peptide facilitated efficient delivery of siRNA to the mouse brain parenchyma as well as primary mouse neurons.

RVG29 has also been modified on polyamidoamine dendrimers (PAMAM) through a PEG spacer and coupled with DNA to obtain PAMAM-PEG-RVG29/DNA nanoparticles. The conjugated NPs loading DNA showed higher brain transport efficiency than unconjugated NPs in vitro and in vivo. The report gene expression of the PAMAM-PEG-RVG29/DNA NPs-treated group was detected significantly higher than unmodified NPs (Liu et al., 2009). The recombinant RVG29-9R-6His was successfully expressed and purified from *Escherichia coli* and validated to bind plasmid DNA and deliver it into the Neuro 2a cells effectively (Yang et al., 2014). RVG29 was also conjugated to the itraconazole (ITZ)-loaded albumin NPs via biotin and streptavidin crosslinkage, producing RVG29-ITZ-NPs. Flow cytometry data showed that cellular uptake of RVG29-ITZ-NPs was significantly enhanced in comparison to unmodified NPs. There was more ITZ accumulation in the brain of RVG29-ITZ-NPs-treated group than ITZ-NPs in vivo (Chen et al., 2011). In addition, RVG29 has also been employed to facilitate the brain transport of exosomes. Dendritic cells-secreted exosomes expressing Lamp2b (exosomal membrane protein) were produced from engineered self-derived dendritic cells, fused with neuron-specific RVG29 and loaded GAPDH siRNA. Systemic injection of RVG-targeted exosome loading GAPDH siRNA induced specific gene knockdown in neurons, microglia, and oligodendrocytes. RVG29-modified exosome was then used to deliver BACE1 siRNA for treatment of Alzheimer disease, and it exhibited strong knockdown of target mRNA (60%) and protein (62%) in wild-type mice (Alvarez-Erviti et al., 2011).

Snake neurotoxins are well-known for their high binding affinities and specificities to nAChRs. In our group, loop 2 fragment of *Ophiophagus hannah* toxin b (KC2S, aa 25–44) was developed as another nAChRs ligand for brain targeting drug delivery. KC2S competitively inhibited the interaction between ^{125}I-α-bungarotoxin (a natural antagonist of nAChRs) and hippocampus nAChRs (Zhan et al., 2010). KS2S could be specifically taken up by BCECs in vitro (Lentz, 1991). KC2S was further conjugated on the surface of PEG–PLA micelles to facilitate brain transport of payloads. Of note, nude mice bearing intracranial glioma were administered KC2S-micelles loading paclitaxel and showed a significant longer survival time (Zhan et al., 2010; Lentz, 1991).

Since the disulfide bond of KC2S that essentially enhances receptor binding is instable during blood circulation, a short peptide without disulfide bond is expected to enhance in vivo brain targeting. The loop 2 region of candoxin (CDX, aa 27–42) was derived from candoxin from the Malayan krait *Bungarus candidus* (Nirthanan et al., 2002). Receptor-binding affinity of CDX to α7 nAChRs was experimentally validated as sub-micromolar. In vitro, CDX could efficiently enter the primary rat brain capillary endothelial cells. CDX-modified PEG-PLA micelles loading paclitaxel (CDX-PEG-PLA-PTX) substantially improved the therapeutic efficacy and significantly prolonged the survival time of nude mice bearing intracranial glioma (Zhan et al., 2011). In another study, paclitaxel and a plasmid encoding tumor necrosis factor-related apoptosis-inducing ligand were co-delivered through CDX-modified micelles and glioma homing gene carrier for the treatment of intracranial glioma (Zhan et al., 2012). The prolonged survival after programmed therapies that aim to overcome the BBB and blood-brain tumor barrier further verified the brain targeting ability of the CDX peptide.

However, CDX peptide displayed extremely rapid degradation in lysosomal homogenates, in which almost 100% of intact peptide was disappeared within 15 min. The result suggested that BBB might act as an enzymatic barrier to the CDX peptide. The retro-inverso isomer of CDX (^{D}CDX), a ligand of nAChRs that is fully resistant to proteolysis, was developed to enhance brain targeting efficiency by overcoming intracellular degradation. ^{D}CDX displayed fivefold stronger binding affinity to the neuronal nAChRs than did CDX. Moreover, ^{D}CDX demonstrated exceptional stability in the fresh rat serum and lysosomal homogenate. ^{D}CDX facilitated significantly brain-targeted delivery of liposomes in vitro and in vivo when modified on liposomal surface. As a result, brain-targeted delivery of ^{D}CDX-modified liposomes enhanced therapeutic efficiency of encapsulated doxorubicin for glioma. After receiving four doses of doxorubicin-loaded ^{D}CDX-liposomes, nude mice bearing intracranial glioma exhibited a median survival of 33.5 days, which was 5.5 days longer than that of mice receiving doxorubicin-loaded CDX-liposomes with the same therapeutic regimen (Wei et al., 2015) (Fig. 2).

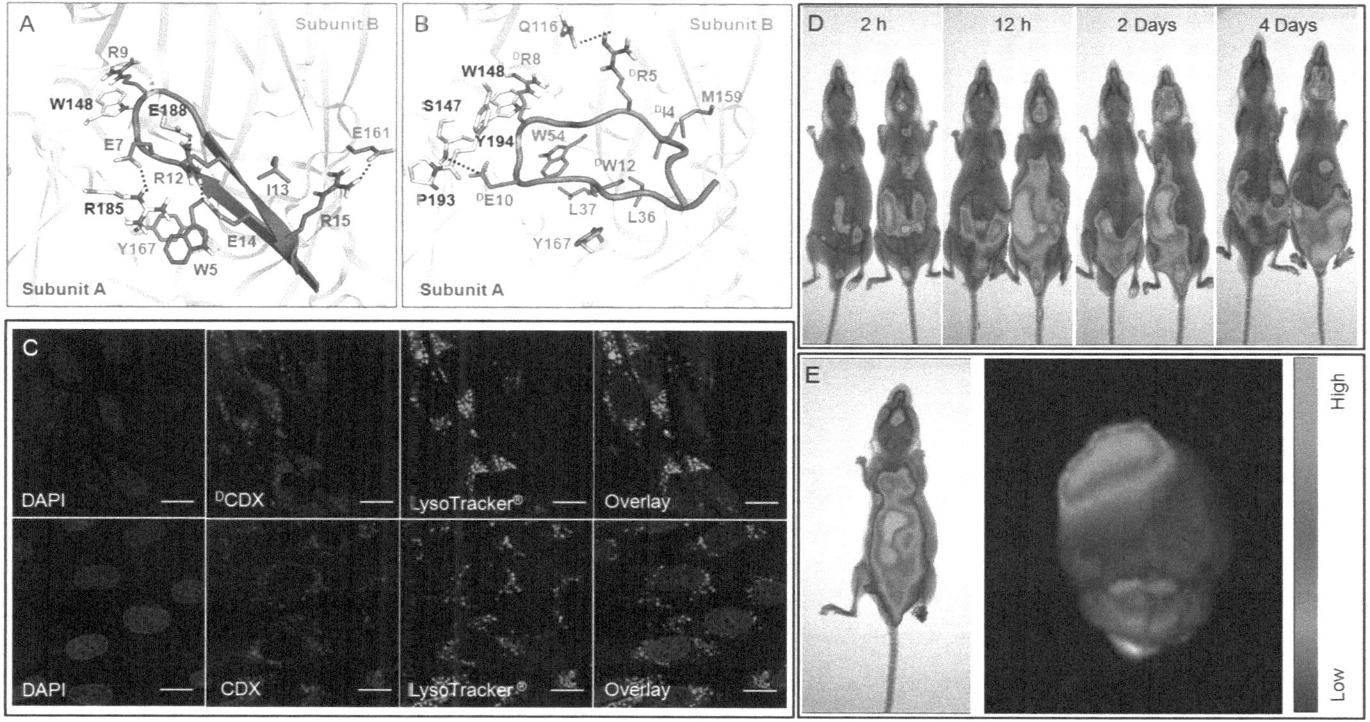

Fig. 2 Binding modes of CDX (A, *green*) and ^{D}CDX (B, *aqua*) with α7 nAChRs. Subunits A and B are respectively shown in white and yellow. (C) Intracellular colocalization of CDX and ^{L}CDX (in *green*) in the BBB monolayer after 2h incubation (lysosomes are shown in *red*). Near-infrared optical images of DiR-encapsulated micelles injected in the caudal vein of intracranial glioma-bearing nude mice 5 days (D) and 15 days (E) post-tumor implantation. The mouse on the left-hand side in four pairwise comparisons in panel (D) was injected with DiR-encapsulated mPEG-PLA micelles, and that on the right-hand side was injected with CDX-PEG-PLA micelles loaded with the same dose of DiR. The mouse in panel (E) was sacrificed 12h after injection of DiR-encapsulated CDX-PEG-PLA micelles, and the brain was dissected for imaging. Represent with permission from reference Zhan, C., Li, C., Wei, X., Lu, W., Lu, W. 2015. Toxins and derivatives in molecular pharmaceutics: drug delivery and targeted therapy. Adv. Drug Deliv. Rev. 90, 101–118.

6 Lactoferrin receptor

Lactoferrin (Tartaglia et al., 1995), known as lactotransferrin (LTf), is an iron-binding cationic glycoprotein with a molecular mass of about 80 kDa. It belongs to the trans ferrin family and is widely distributed in various secretory fluids such as milk, saliva, tears, and nasal secretions (Lonnerdal and Iyer, 1995). Lf crosses the BBB via receptor-mediated transcytosis. Lactoferrin receptor, with a molecular mass of 105 kDa, has been identified in many cells, including monocytes, lymphocytes, liver cells, and mammary epithelial cells (Suzuki and Lonnerdal, 2002). The Lf receptor has also been identified on the BCECs and is composed of two types of binding sites, including a high-affinity site (Kd = 6.77 nM) and a low-affinity site (Kd = 4815 nM) (Fillebeen et al., 1999). The brain uptake of Lf is much higher than that of Tf and TfRMAb OX26 in vivo 1 h after intravenous injection (Ji et al., 2006). Unexpectedly, in many previous reports Lf-modified nanocarriers did not show higher brain transport efficiency. For example, Lf-polymersome exhibited much less uptake by bEnd.3 cells compared to Tf-polymersome (Gao et al., 2010). Lf-liposome loading senktide (a selective NK3 receptor agonist) showed less brain uptake than did OX26-liposome (De Luca et al., 2015). However, the Lf-modified NPs loading gene had 2.3 folds of transport efficiency higher than that of Tf-NPs (Huang et al., 2008). Lf and folic acid were modified on the surface of PLGA-NPs loading etoposide, and the results showed the permeability coefficient across the BBB of LF/FA PLGA-NPs group was twofold of that of unmodified PLGA-NPs (Kuo and Chen, 2015). Lf-conjugated LDL-mimic nanostructured lipid carriers (NLC) have been explored to transport curcumin to the AD brain. The BCECs uptake of LfH-mNLC was 1.39-fold higher than that of NLC, and the in vivo imaging results revealed that the level of Lf-mNLC was 2.78 times greater than that of NLC (Meng et al., 2015).

7 Scavenger receptor class B type 1

Scavenger receptor class B type 1 (SR-B1), a plasma membrane glycoprotein, is a receptor for high-density lipoprotein (HDL) (Goti et al., 2001). SR-B1 is located in caveolae of apical membrane of brain capillary endothelial cells, mediating cholesterol transfer to and from HDL (Acton et al., 1996). Apo A-I (apolipoprotein A-I), which belongs to the HDL family, is a plasma ligand for SR-B1. Balazs and coworkers' study suggested that part of cerebral apolipoprotein A-I and HDL-associated α-TocH across the BBB were facilitated by SR-B1 (Balazs et al., 2004). Doxorubicin (DOX)-loaded PBCA NPs coated with PS80 demonstrated to have high efficiency to deliver DOX to mouse brain, and the investigation of plasma protein adsorption on the surface of the drug-loaded nanoparticles revealed that it absorbed considerable amount of Apo A-I, which may interact with the scavenger receptor class B type I located at the blood-brain barrier to facilitate brain transport (Petri et al., 2007). Apo A-I was also directly modified on the surface of nanocarriers for brain-targeted drug delivery. Apo A-I was modified on protamine-oligonucleotide nanoparticles, and the cellular uptake and transcytosis in primary porcine BCECs were assessed. The results of radiolabelling experiment showed that particles coated with Apo A-I exhibited significantly increased uptake and transcytosis when compared to uncoated particles. Moreover, the enhancement could be reversed by blocking SR-B1, indicating that the Apo A-I and SR-BI pathway played a key role in the transcytosis process (Kratzer et al., 2007). Apo A-I was covalently attached to human serum albumin nanoparticles via the NHS-PEG-Mal 3400 linker by Jörg Kreuter et al., and an antinociceptive drug Loperamide was loaded. Drug-loaded Apo A-I-HSA-NPs showed considerable antinociceptive effect (Kreuter et al., 2007).

8 Leptin receptor

Leptin receptor, also known as LEP-R or OB-R, is a single transmembrane protein belonging to the cytokine receptor family. There are two isoforms of OB-R, the short one OB-Ra and the long one OB-Rb. OB-Ra has been identified on the brain capillary endothelium and is the major receptor for leptin (Tartaglia et al., 1995). Leptin is an appetite regulatory hormone with a molecular mass of 16-kDa. It is secreted into the blood circulation by adipose tissues and functions in the central nerve system (i.e., hypothalamus) after crossing the BBB. The mechanism of leptin transport across the BBB is considered as OB-R-mediated transcytosis (Golden et al., 1997). Lep70–89, a peptide derived from leptin, exhibited significantly higher cellular uptake by mouse brain-derived endothelial cells (MBEC4) than unmodified liposomes. Lep70–89-modified PEGylated liposomes were taken up via macropinocytosis and subject to nonclassical intracellular trafficking, resulting in the circumvention of lysosomal degradation in endothelial cells. Another leptin-derived peptide is a 30-mer peptide (leptin-30), which has been modified on dendrigraft poly-L-lysine (DGL) to deliver DNA plasmid into brain. Luciferase activity data showed that leptin-30 vector could increase the transfection efficiency by four folds compared to unmodified vector (Tamaru et al., 2010). Therefore, leptin and its derivatives have the potential to facilitate the BBB transport of drug delivery systems.

9 Diphtheria toxin receptor

CRM197, a nontoxic mutation of diphtheria toxin (DT), can be taken up by BCECs via binding the receptor of the precursor of heparin-binding epidermal growth factor-like growth factor (HB-EGF), also known as the diphtheria toxin receptor (DTR) (Naglich et al., 1992). DTR is expressed on the BCECs, neurons, and glial cells. CRM197, coupled with PLGA NPs, could cross the BBB and accumulate in CNS cells, such as glial cells, astrocytes. In addition, CRM197-grafted PBCA NPs could carry the zidovudine (AZT) across the BBB. The results showed that the permeability coefficient of AZT and loading efficiency increased when the size of the AZT-loaded CRM197-PBCA NPs decreased (Kuo and Chung, 2012). In another study, CRM197 was conjugated with horse radish peroxidase (HRP) and tested in an in vitro model of the BBB (cocultured bovine brain capillary endothelial cells with newborn rat astrocytes) (Wang et al., 2010). The results showed that CRM197-HRP successfully crossed the BBB model. A previous research provided supportive evidence that a fraction of intravenously administered CRM197-HRP was found in the brain parenchyma in guinea pigs. Using this vector, Gaillard et al. developed a product for the treatment of Japanese encephalitis virus (JEV) (Gaillard and De Boer, 2006; Gaillard et al., 2005). All of these indicated that the CRM197 is a promising ligand to effectively deliver drug into the brain. However, the use of CRM197 is problematic as it has been used for vaccination against diphtheria, and the presence of antibodies may hinder the efficacy of this vector. In addition, it has been recently reported that CRM197 has a weak toxicity and specific care has to be taken in the use of CRM197 at high dose, although the toxicity of CRM197 is about 100 times less than that of the wild-type diphtheria.

10 Single domain llama antibody receptor

Phage display technique has been used to screen single domain llama antibodies (sdAbs). The average molecular mass of these sdAbs is 14 kDa, approximately half of the size of a scFv and 10-fold smaller than that of IgG. They consist of a heavy chain variable domains (VHHs) of the llama antibodies and a substantial number of typical conventional antibody heavy chain variable sequences (VHs) (Tanha et al., 2002). In 2002, two BBB-specific sdAbs, FC5 and FC44, were selected from llama sdAb phage display library by Arumugam and colleagues. FC5 and FC44 could selectively bind cerebral microvascular endothelial cells and transport across the human BBB model (Muruganandam et al., 2002).

Some studies showed that FC5 interacts with luminal α(2,3)-sialoglycoprotein receptor to trigger lathrin-mediated endocytosis (Abulrob et al., 2005). The FC5 and FC44 demonstrated high brain uptake efficiency, and the accumulation in mouse brain of FC5 and FC44 was $4.5 \pm 2.7\%$ and $2.9 \pm 1.7\%$ of injecting dose/g of brain, respectively (Muruganandam et al., 2002). Recently, a highly sensitive SRM-ILIS (selected reaction monitoring isotopically labeled internal standard) method has been employed to evaluate brain delivery of FC5 and FC44. The results showed the efficiency of FC5 and FC44 across the BBB model was 50–100 folds higher than that of the control groups. In addition, the level of both FC5 and FC44 was significantly higher (10–25 folds) than that of the control as analyzed by the multiplexed SRM-ILIS method (Haqqani et al., 2013).

11 Concluding remarks

Over the decades, receptor-mediated transcytosis has been verified as a promising method to achieve brain-targeted drug delivery. A variety of ligands, including peptides, protein, and antibodies, have been employed to mediate brain transport (Table 1). Those protein or antibody ligands normally have to be functionalized after the preparation of formulations, which is due to the incompatibility to the organic

Table 1 General comparison of peptide and protein/antibody ligands for brain-targeted drug delivery

	Peptide	Protein/antibody
Size	Small	Large
Potency	High	Very high
Selectivity	High	Very high
High-throughput screening	Yes	Yes
Cost	Low	High
Stability in storage	High	Low
Stability in vivo	Very low	Low
Immunogenicity	Low	High
Functionalization	Easy	Difficult

solvents or unfavorable pH used in the preparation process. Peptide-based ligands identified using structure-based design (Demeule et al., 2008) and phage display (Zhang et al., 2013b; Li et al., 2011) are capable of targeting the corresponding receptors with high affinity and specificity. In addition, peptide-based ligands have been widely used to facilitate brain-targeted drug delivery for the ease of functionalization. In comparison to protein and antibody ligands, peptide ligands are always less costly and more stable in storage. In most cases, peptide ligands are non-immunogenic to avoid unwanted immune responses (Oller-Salvia et al., 2016a). However, peptide ligands are subject to proteolysis in vivo, severely restricting the clinical application for targeted drug delivery in vivo. Even though stable peptides have been developed to achieve long-term targeting (Oller-Salvia et al., 2016b; Liu et al., 2016; Prades et al., 2015), insightful studies need to be conducted to better understand the interaction of those stable peptide ligands with plasma proteins, immune cells, and also target organs. Short peptides are thought to be non-immunogenic; however, it remains elusive if the conjugated-form of peptide ligands (with nanocarriers) produces immune response.

The binding affinity of ligand to receptor is one of the important factors that affect the efficiency of BBB penetration. Yu and coworkers designed antibodies with different affinities to TfR and found that the optimal antibody with highest brain transport efficiency was neither the high-affinity nor the low-affinity one. The reason is that high-affinity binding to TfR results in a rapid clearance of antibody and TfR degradation, limiting sustained brain exposure to antibody. On the other hand, although low-affinity binding to TfR results in a reduced target-mediated clearance and thus substantially better antibody exposure, the brain uptake is also limited by the low affinity of antibody for TfR (Yu et al., 2014).

Moreover, the intracellular pathway of receptor-mediated transcytosis process remains elusive. The receptor of the BBB might participate in more than one substance transport. Some of the ligands might be competitively inhibited by each other if they share the same binding site. They can also affect other agents across the BBB and disrupt the homeostasis in the brain. The majority of receptors are expressed not only on the BBB, but also in other peripheral organs. Therefore, the content of ligand in the brain might be much lower than other tissues. For example, brain uptake of 8D3 antibody in the liver and kidney reached $16.9 \pm 6.1\%$ID/g and $4.9 \pm 0.1\%$ID/g, respectively, significantly higher than brain ($3.1 \pm 0.4\%$ID/g) after intravenous injection in mice (Lee et al., 2000).

Lastly, maybe the most important point is the formed protein corona when the nonocarriers enter into the body. Those brain-targeted drug delivery systems interact with blood plasma, peritoneal fluid, cerebrospinal fluid, or nasal fluid which differs from the route of administration (Guan et al., 2017). For example, intravenously injected NPs interact with more than 2000 kinds of plasma proteins and a bunch of them are absorbed on the surface of the NPs. It is unknown if peptide or antibody conjugated with the vector retains the affinity with the cognate receptor on BBB when surrounded by various absorbed proteins. It was reported that transferrin lost the binding ability with TfR after incubation with plasma, in which the protein corona may block the binding domain for receptor.

References

Abbott, N.J., 2013. Blood-brain barrier structure and function and the challenges for CNS drug delivery. J. Inherit. Metab. Dis. 36, 437–449.

Abbott, N.J., Ronnback, L., Hansson, E., 2006. Astrocyte-endothelial interactions at the blood-brain barrier. Nat. Rev. Neurosci. 7, 41–53.

Abbott, N.J., Patabendige, A.A., Dolman, D.E., Yusof, S.R., Begley, D.J., 2010. Structure and function of the blood-brain barrier. Neurobiol. Dis. 37, 13–25.

Abulrob, A., Sprong, H., Henegouwen, P.V.B.E., Stanimirovic, D., 2005. The blood-brain barrier transmigrating single domain antibody: mechanisms of transport and antigenic epitopes in human brain endothelial cells. J. Neurochem. 95, 1201–1214.

Acton, S., Rigotti, A., Landschulz, K.T., Xu, S.Z., Hobbs, H.H., Krieger, M., 1996. Identification of scavenger receptor SR-BI as a high density lipoprotein receptor. Science 271, 518–520.

Aktas, Y., Yemisci, M., Andrieux, K., Gursoy, R.N., Alonso, M.J., Fernandez-Megia, E., Novoa-Carballal, R., Quinoa, E., Riguera, R., Sargon, M.F., Celik, H.H., Demir, A.S., Hincal, A.A., Dalkara, T., Capan, Y., Couvreur, P., 2005. Development and brain delivery of chitosan-PEG nanoparticles functionalized with the monoclonal antibody OX26. Bioconjug. Chem. 16, 1503–1511.

Alvarez-Erviti, L., Seow, Y.Q., Yin, H.F., Betts, C., Lakhal, S., Wood, M.J.A., 2011. Delivery of siRNA to the mouse brain by systemic injection of targeted exosomes. Nat. Biotechnol. 29, 341-U179.

Alyaudtin, R.N., Reichel, A., Lobenberg, R., Ramge, P., Kreuter, J., Begley, D.J., 2001. Interaction of poly(butylcyanoacrylate) nanoparticles with the blood-brain barrier in vivo and in vitro. J. Drug Target. 9, 209.

Armulik, A., Genove, G., Mae, M., Nisancioglu, M.H., Wallgard, E., Niaudet, C., He, L., Norlin, J., Lindblom, P., Strittmatter, K., Johansson, B.R., Betsholtz, C., 2010. Pericytes regulate the blood-brain barrier. Nature 468, 557–561.

Balazs, Z., Panzenboeck, U., Hammer, A., Sovic, A., Quehenberger, O., Malle, E., Sattler, W., 2004. Uptake and transport of high-density lipoprotein (HDL) and HDL-associated alpha-tocopherol by an in vitro blood-brain barrier model. J. Neurochem. 89, 939–950.

Becker, A.B., Roth, R.A., 1990. Insulin receptor structure and function in normal and pathological conditions. Annu. Rev. Med. 41, 99–115.

Beliveau, R., 2003. Vectorization of proteins across the blood-brain barrier: high transcytosis of melanotransferrin (P97). J. Neurochem. 85, 7.

Boado, R.J., Pardridge, W.M., 2010. Genetic engineering of IgG-glucuronidase fusion proteins. J. Drug Target 18, 205–211.

Boado, R.J., Zhang, Y., Zhang, Y., Pardridge, W.M., 2007. Humanization of anti-human insulin receptor antibody for drug targeting across the human blood-brain barrier. Biotechnol. Bioeng. 96, 381–391.

Boado, R.J., Zhang, Y., Zhang, Y., Wang, Y., Pardridge, W.M., 2008a. GDNF fusion protein for targeted-drug delivery across the human blood-brain barrier. Biotechnol. Bioeng. 100, 387–396.

Boado, R.J., Zhang, Y., Zhang, Y., Wang, Y., Pardridge, W.M., 2008b. IgG-paraoxonase-1 fusion protein for targeted drug delivery across the human blood-brain barrier. Mol. Pharm. 5, 1037–1043.

Boado, R.J., Zhang, Y., Zhang, Y., Xia, C.F., Wang, Y., Pardridge, W.M., 2008c. Genetic engineering of a lysosomal enzyme fusion protein for targeted delivery across the human blood-brain barrier. Biotechnol. Bioeng. 99, 475–484.

Boado, R.J., Zhang, Y., Wang, Y., Pardridge, W.M., 2009. Engineering and expression of a chimeric transferrin receptor monoclonal antibody for blood-brain barrier delivery in the mouse. Biotechnol. Bioeng. 102, 1251–1258.

Boado, R.J., Hui, E.K., Lu, J.Z., Pardridge, W.M., 2010a. Drug targeting of erythropoietin across the primate blood-brain barrier with an IgG molecular Trojan horse. J. Pharmacol. Exp. Ther. 333, 961–969.

Boado, R.J., Hui, E.K., Lu, J.Z., Zhou, Q.H., Pardridge, W.M., 2010b. Selective targeting of a TNFR decoy receptor pharmaceutical to the primate brain as a receptor-specific IgG fusion protein. J. Biotechnol. 146, 84–91.

Cabezon, I., Manich, G., Martin-Venegas, R., Camins, A., Pelegri, C., Vilaplana, J., 2015. Trafficking of gold nanoparticles coated with the 8D3 anti-transferrin receptor antibody at the mouse blood-brain barrier. Mol. Pharm. 12, 4137–4145.

Candela, P., Gosselet, F., Miller, F., Buee-Scherrer, V., Torpier, G., Cecchelli, R., Fenart, L., 2008. Physiological pathway for low-density lipoproteins across the blood-brain barrier: transcytosis through brain capillary endothelial cells in vitro. Endothelium 15, 254–264.

Chang, J., Jallouli, Y., Kroubi, M., Yuan, X.B., Feng, W., Kang, C.S., Pu, P.Y., Betbeder, D., 2009. Characterization of endocytosis of transferrin-coated PLGA nanoparticles by the blood-brain barrier. Int. J. Pharm. 379, 285–292.

Chang, J., Paillard, A., Passirani, C., Morille, M., Benoit, J.P., Betbeder, D., Garcion, E., 2012. Transferrin adsorption onto PLGA nanoparticles governs their interaction with biological systems from blood circulation to brain cancer cells. Pharm. Res. 29, 1495–1505.

Chen, W., Zhan, C.Y., Gu, B., Meng, Q.G., Wang, H., Lu, W.Y., Hou, H.M., 2011. Targeted brain delivery of itraconazole via RVG29 anchored nanoparticles. J. Drug Target. 19, 228–234.

Coloma, M.J., Lee, H.J., Kurihara, A., Landaw, E.M., Boado, R.J., Morrison, S.L., Pardridge, W.M., 2000. Transport across the primate blood-brain barrier of a genetically engineered chimeric monoclonal antibody to the human insulin receptor. Pharm. Res. 17, 266–274.

Dautry-Varsat, A., Ciechanover, A., Lodish, H.F., 1983. pH and the recycling of transferrin during receptor-mediated endocytosis. Proc. Natl. Acad. Sci. U. S. A. 80, 2258–2262.

De Luca, M.A., Lai, F., Corrias, F., Caboni, P., Bimpisidis, Z., Maccioni, E., Fadda, A.M., Di Chiara, G., 2015. Lactoferrin- and antitransferrin-modified liposomes for brain targeting of the NK3 receptor agonist senktide: Preparation and in vivo evaluation. Int. J. Pharm. 479, 129–137.

Demeule, M., Poirier, J., Jodoin, J., Bertrand, Y., Desrosiers, R.R., Dagenais, C., Nguyen, T., Lanthier, J., Gabathuler, R., Kennard, M., Jefferies, W.A., Karkan, D., Tsai, S., Fenart, L., Cecchelli, R., Beliveau, R., 2002. High transcytosis of melanotransferrin (P97) across the blood brain barrier. J. Neurochem. 83, 924–933.

Demeule, M., Currie, J.C., Bertrand, Y., Che, C., Nguyen, T., Regina, A., Gabathuler, R., Castaigne, J.P., Beliveau, R., 2008. Involvement of the low-density lipoprotein receptor-related protein in the transcytosis of the brain delivery vector Angiopep-2. J. Neurochem. 106, 1534–1544.

Dieu, L.H., Wu, D., Palivan, C.G., Balasubramanian, V., Huwyler, J., 2014. Polymersomes conjugated to 83-14 monoclonal antibodies: in vitro targeting of brain capillary endothelial cells. Eur. J. Pharm. Biopharm. 88, 316–324.

Donahue, J.E., Flaherty, S.L., Johanson, C.E., Duncan 3rd, J.A., Silverberg, G.D., Miller, M.C., Tavares, R., Yang, W., Wu, Q., Sabo, E., Hovanesian, V., Stopa, E.G., 2006. RAGE, LRP-1, and amyloid-beta protein in Alzheimer's disease. Acta Neuropathol. 112, 405–415.

Fillebeen, C., Descamps, L., Dehouck, M.P., Fenart, L., Benaissa, M., Spik, G., Cecchelli, R., Pierce, A., 1999. Receptor-mediated transcytosis of lactoferrin through the blood-brain barrier. J. Biol. Chem. 274, 7011–7017.

Frank, H.J., Pardridge, W.M., 1981. A direct in vitro demonstration of insulin binding to isolated brain microvessels. Diabetes 30, 757–761.

Gaillard, P.J., De Boer, A.G., 2006. A novel opportunity for targeted drug delivery to the brain. J. Control. Release. 116, e60-2.

Gaillard, P.J., Visser, C.C., De Boer, A.G., 2005. Targeted delivery across the blood-brain barrier. Expert Opin. Drug Deliv. 2, 299–309.

Gao, H.L., Pang, Z.Q., Fan, L., Hu, K.L., Wu, B.X., Jiang, X.G., 2010. Effect of lactoferrin- and transferrin-conjugated polymersomes in brain targeting: in vitro and in vivo evaluations. Acta Pharmacol. Sin. 31, 237–243.

Golden, P.L., Maccagnan, T.J., Pardridge, W.M., 1997. Human blood-brain barrier leptin receptor—binding and endocytosis in isolated human brain microvessels. J. Clin. Invest. 99, 14–18.

Goldstein, J.L., Brown, M.S., Anderson, R.G.W., Russell, D.W., Schneider, W.J., 1985. Receptor-mediated endocytosis—concepts emerging from the Ldl receptor system. Annu. Rev. Cell Biol. 1, 1–39.

Goti, D., Hrzenjak, A., Levak-Frank, S., Frank, S., Van Der Westhuyzen, D.R., Malle, E., Sattler, W., 2001. Scavenger receptor class B, type I is expressed in porcine brain capillary endothelial cells and contributes to selective uptake of HDL-associated vitamin E. J. Neurochem. 76, 498–508.

Gregori, M., Masserini, M., Mancini, S., 2015. Nanomedicine for the treatment of Alzheimer's disease. Nanomedicine 10, 1203–1218.

Guan, J., Zhang, Z., Hu, X., Yang, Y., Chai, Z., Liu, X., Liu, J., Gao, B., Lu, W., Qian, J., Zhan, C., 2017. Cholera toxin subunit B enabled multifunctional glioma-targeted drug delivery. Adv. Healthc. Mater. 6, 201700709.

Haqqani, A.S., Caram-Salas, N., Ding, W., Brunette, E., Delaney, C.E., Baumann, E., Boileau, E., Stanimirovic, D., 2013. Multiplexed evaluation of serum and CSF pharmacokinetics of brain-targeting single-domain antibodies using a NanoLC-SRM-ILIS method. Mol. Pharm. 10, 1542–1556.

Hawkins, B.T., Davis, T.P., 2005. The blood-brain barrier/neurovascular unit in health and disease. Pharmacol. Rev. 57, 173–185.
Huang, R.Q., Ke, W.L., Liu, Y., Jiang, C., Pei, Y.Y., 2008. The use of lactoferrin as a ligand for targeting the polyamidoamine-based gene delivery system to the brain. Biomaterials 29, 238–246.
Huebers, H.A., Finch, C.A., 1987. The physiology of transferrin and transferrin receptors. Physiol. Rev. 67, 520–582.
Husemann, J., Silverstein, S.C., 2001. Expression of scavenger receptor class B, type I, by astrocytes and vascular smooth muscle cells in normal adult mouse and human brain and in Alzheimer's disease brain. Am. J. Pathol. 158, 825–832.
Jacobs, S., Hazum, E., Shechter, Y., Cuatrecasas, P., 1979. Insulin receptor: covalent labeling and identification of subunits. Proc. Natl. Acad. Sci. U. S. A. 76, 4918–4921.
Jefferies, W.A., Brandon, M.R., Hunt, S.V., Williams, A.F., Gatter, K.C., Mason, D.Y., 1984. Transferrin receptor on endothelium of brain capillaries. Nature 312, 162–163.
Ji, B., Maeda, A., Higuchi, M., Inoue, K., Akita, H., Harashima, H., Suhara, T., 2006. Pharmacokinetics and brain uptake of lactoferrin in rats. Life Sci. 78, 851–855.
Jones, A.R., Shusta, E.V., 2007. Blood-brain barrier transport of therapeutics via receptor-mediation. Pharm. Res. 24, 1759–1771.
Karkan, D., Pfeifer, C., Vitalis, T.Z., Arthur, G., Ujiie, M., Chen, Q.Q., Tsai, S., Koliatis, G., Gabathuler, R., Jefferies, W.A., 2008. A unique carrier for delivery of therapeutic compounds beyond the blood-brain barrier. PLoS One. 3.
Kaur, I.P., Bhandari, R., Bhandari, S., Kakkar, V., 2008. Potential of solid lipid nanoparticles in brain targeting. J. Control. Release 127, 97–109.
Kim, D.H., Iijima, H., Goto, K., Sakai, J., Ishii, H., Kim, H.J., Suzuki, H., Kondo, H., Saeki, S., Yamamoto, T., 1996. Human apolipoprotein E receptor 2—a novel lipoprotein receptor of the low density lipoprotein receptor family predominantly expressed in brain. J. Biol. Chem. 271, 8373–8380.
Kratzer, I., Wernig, K., Panzenboeck, U., Bernhart, E., Reicher, H., Wronski, R., Windisch, M., Hammer, A., Malle, E., Zimmer, A., Sattler, W., 2007. Apolipoprotein A-I coating of protamine-oligonucleotide nanoparticles increases particle uptake and transcytosis in an in vitro model of the blood-brain barrier. J. Control. Release 117, 301–311.
Kreuter, J., Shamenkov, D., Petrov, V., Ramge, P., Cychutek, K., Koch-Brandt, C., Alyautdin, R., 2002. Apolipoprotein-mediated transport of nanoparticle-bound drugs across the blood-brain barrier. J. Drug Target. 10, 317–325.
Kreuter, J., Hekmatara, T., Dreis, S., Vogel, T., Gelperina, S., Langer, K., 2007. Covalent attachment of apolipoprotein A-I and apolipoprotein B-100 to albumin nanoparticles enables drug transport into the brain. J. Control. Release 118, 54–58.
Kuo, Y.C., Chen, Y.C., 2015. Targeting delivery of etoposide to inhibit the growth of human glioblastoma multiforme using lactoferrin- and folic acid-grafted poly(lactide-co-glycolide) nanoparticles. Int. J. Pharm. 479, 138–149.
Kuo, Y.C., Chung, C.Y., 2012. Transcytosis of CRM197-grafted polybutylcyanoacrylate nanoparticles for delivering zidovudine across human brain-microvascular endothelial cells. Colloids Surf. B Biointerfaces 91, 242–249.
Kuo, Y.C., Shih-Huang, C.Y., 2013. Solid lipid nanoparticles carrying chemotherapeutic drug across the blood-brain barrier through insulin receptor-mediated pathway. J. Drug Target. 21 (8), 730.
Kuo, Y.C., Wang, I.H., 2016. Enhanced delivery of etoposide across the blood-brain barrier to restrain brain tumor growth using melanotransferrin antibody-and tamoxifen-conjugated solid lipid nanoparticles. J. Drug Target. 24, 645–654.

Lajoie, J.M., Shusta, E.V., 2015. Targeting receptor-mediated transport for delivery of biologics across the blood-brain barrier. Annu. Rev. Pharmacol. Toxicol. 55, 613–631.

Lanthier, J., Bouthillier, A., Lapointe, M., Demeule, M., Beliveau, R., Desrosiers, R.R., 2002. Down-regulation of protein L-isoaspartyl methyltransferase in human epileptic hippocampus contributes to generation of damaged tubulin. J. Neurochem. 83, 581–591.

Lee, H.J., Engelhardt, B., Lesley, J., Bickel, U., Pardridge, W.M., 2000. Targeting rat antimouse transferrin receptor monoclonal antibodies through blood-brain barrier in mouse. J. Pharmacol. Exp. Ther. 292, 1048–1052.

Lentz, T.L., 1991. Structure-function-relationships of curaremimetic neurotoxin loop-2 and of a structurally similar segment of rabies virus glycoprotein in their interaction with the nicotinic acetylcholine-receptor. Biochemistry 30, 10949–10957.

Li, J., Feng, L., Fan, L., Zha, Y., Guo, L., Zhang, Q., Chen, J., Pang, Z., Wang, Y., Jiang, X., Yang, V.C., Wen, L., 2011. Targeting the brain with PEG-PLGA nanoparticles modified with phage-displayed peptides. Biomaterials 32, 4943–4950.

Liu, Y., Huang, R.Q., Han, L., Ke, W.L., Shao, K., Ye, L.Y., Lou, J.N., Jiang, C., 2009. Brain-targeting gene delivery and cellular internalization mechanisms for modified rabies virus glycoprotein RVG29 nanoparticles. Biomaterials 30, 4195–4202.

Liu, L., Zhang, X.Y., Li, W.C., Sun, H.Z., Lou, Y., Zhang, X.G., Li, F.Z., 2013a. Transferrin receptor antibody-modified alpha-cobrotoxin-loaded nanoparticles enable drug delivery across the blood-brain barrier by intranasal administration. J. Nanopart. Res. 15.

Liu, Z.Y., Gao, X.L., Kang, T., Jiang, M.Y., Miao, D.Y., Gu, G.Z., Hu, Q.Y., Song, Q.X., Yao, L., Tu, Y.F., Chen, H.Z., Jiang, X.G., Chen, J., 2013b. B6 peptide-modified PEG-PLA nanoparticles for enhanced brain delivery of neuroprotective peptide. Bioconjug. Chem. 24, 997–1007.

Liu, M., Li, X., Xie, Z., Xie, C., Zhan, C., Hu, X., Shen, Q., Wei, X., Su, B., Wang, J., Lu, W., 2016. D-peptides as recognition molecules and therapeutic agents. Chem. Rec. 16, 1772–1786.

Lonnerdal, B., Iyer, S., 1995. Lactoferrin—molecular-structure and biological function. Annu. Rev. Nutr. 15, 93–110.

Lu, J.Z., Hui, E.K., Boado, R.J., Pardridge, W.M., 2010. Genetic engineering of a bifunctional IgG fusion protein with iduronate-2-sulfatase. Bioconjug. Chem. 21, 151–156.

Luck, M., Schroder, W., Harnisch, S., Thode, K., Blunk, T., Paulke, B.R., Kresse, M., Muller, R.H., 1997. Identification of plasma proteins facilitated by enrichment on particulate surfaces: analysis by two-dimensional electrophoresis and N-terminal microsequencing. Electrophoresis 18, 2961–2967.

Meng, F.F., Asghar, S., Gao, S.Y., Su, Z.G., Song, J., Huo, M.R., Meng, W.D., Ping, Q.N., Xiao, Y.Y., 2015. A novel LDL-mimic nanocarrier for the targeted delivery of curcumin into the brain to treat Alzheimer's disease. Colloids Surf. B Biointerfaces 134, 88–97.

Meresse, S., Delbart, C., Fruchart, J.C., Cecchelli, R., 1989. Low-density lipoprotein receptor on endothelium of brain capillaries. J. Neurochem. 53, 340–345.

Miller, R.D., Hoffmann, J.W., Powell, P.P., Kyle, J.W., Shipley, J.M., Bachinsky, D.R., Sly, W.S., 1990. Cloning and characterization of the human beta-glucuronidase gene. Genomics 7, 280–283.

Muruganandam, A., Tanha, J., Narang, S., Stanimirovic, D., 2002. Selection of phage-displayed llama single-domain antibodies that transmigrate across human blood-brain barrier endothelium. FASEB J. 16 (2), 240.

Naglich, J.G., Metherall, J.E., Russell, D.W., Eidels, L., 1992. Expression cloning of a diphtheria toxin receptor: Identity with a heparin-binding EGF-like growth factor precursor. Cell 69, 1051–1061.

Neves, A.R., Queiroz, J.F., Weksler, B., Romero, I.A., Couraud, P.O., Reis, S., 2015. Solid lipid nanoparticles as a vehicle for brain-targeted drug delivery: two new strategies of functionalization with apolipoprotein E. Nanotechnology 26, 495103.

Nirthanan, S., Charpantier, E., Gopalakrishnakone, P., Gwee, M.C.E., Khoo, H.E., Cheah, L.S., Bertrand, D., Kini, R.M., 2002. Candoxin, a novel toxin from Bungarus candidus, is a reversible antagonist of muscle (alpha beta gamma delta) but a poorly reversible antagonist of neuronal alpha 7 nicotinic acetylcholine receptors. J. Biol. Chem. 277, 17811–17820.

Oller-Salvia, B., Sanchez-Navarro, M., Ciudad, S., Guiu, M., Arranz-Gibert, P., Garcia, C., Gomis, R.R., Cecchelli, R., Garcia, J., Giralt, E., Teixido, M., 2016a. MiniAp-4: a Venom-inspired peptidomimetic for brain delivery. Angew. Chem. Int. Ed. Engl. 55, 572–575.

Oller-Salvia, B., Sanchez-Navarro, M., Giralt, E., Teixido, M., 2016b. Blood-brain barrier shuttle peptides: an emerging paradigm for brain delivery. Chem. Soc. Rev. 45, 4690–4707.

Osborn, M.J., Mcelmurry, R.T., Peacock, B., Tolar, J., Blazar, B.R., 2008. Targeting of the CNS in MPS-IH using a nonviral transferrin-alpha-L-iduronidase fusion gene product. Mol. Ther. 16, 1459–1466.

Palchetti, S., Colapicchioni, V., Digiacomo, L., Caracciolo, G., Pozzi, D., Capriotti, A.L., La Barbera, G., Lagana, A., 2016. The protein corona of circulating PEGylated liposomes. Biochim. Biophys. Acta 1858, 189–196.

Pan, W.H., Kastin, A.J., Zankel, T.C., Van Kerkhof, P., Terasaki, T., Bu, G.J., 2004. Efficient transfer of receptor-associated protein (RAP) across the blood-brain barrier. J. Cell Sci. 117, 5071–5078.

Pang, Z., Gao, H., Yu, Y., Chen, J., Guo, L., Ren, J., Wen, Z., Su, J., Jiang, X., 2011. Brain delivery and cellular internalization mechanisms for transferrin conjugated biodegradable polymersomes. Int. J. Pharm. 415, 284–292.

Pardridge, W.M., 2005a. The blood-brain barrier: bottleneck in brain drug development. NeuroRx 2, 3–14.

Pardridge, W.M., 2005b. Molecular biology of the blood-brain barrier. Mol. Biotechnol. 30, 57–70.

Pardridge, W.M., 2015. Blood-brain barrier drug delivery of IgG fusion proteins with a transferrin receptor monoclonal antibody. Expert Opin. Drug Deliv. 12, 207–222.

Pardridge, W.M., Buciak, J.L., Friden, P.M., 1991. Selective transport of an anti-transferrin receptor antibody through the blood-brain barrier in vivo. J. Pharmacol. Exp. Ther. 259, 66–70.

Pardridge, W.M., Kang, Y.S., Buciak, J.L., Yang, J., 1995. Human insulin receptor monoclonal antibody undergoes high affinity binding to human brain capillaries in vitro and rapid transcytosis through the blood-brain barrier in vivo in the primate. Pharm. Res. 12, 807–816.

Petri, B., Bootz, A., Khalansky, A., Hekmatara, T., Muller, R., Uhl, R., Kreuter, J., Gelperina, S., 2007. Chemotherapy of brain tumour using doxorubicin bound to surfactant-coated poly(butyl cyanoacrylate) nanoparticles: revisiting the role of surfactants. J. Control. Release 117, 51–58.

Ponka, P., Beaumont, C., Richardson, D.R., 1998. Function and regulation of transferrin and ferritin. Semin. Hematol. 35, 35–54.

Prades, R., Oller-Salvia, B., Schwarzmaier, S.M., Selva, J., Moros, M., Balbi, M., Grazu, V., De La Fuente, J.M., Egea, G., Plesnila, N., Teixido, M., Giralt, E., 2015. Applying the retro-enantio approach to obtain a peptide capable of overcoming the blood-brain barrier. Angew. Chem. Int. Ed. Engl. 54, 3967–3972.

Rahmanto, Y.S., Bal, S., Loh, K.H., Yu, Y., Richardson, D.R., 2012. Melanotransferrin: search for a function. BBA-Gen. Subjects 1820, 237–243.

Ruan, S.B., Yuan, M.Q., Zhang, L., Hu, G.L., Chen, J.T., Cun, X.L., Zhang, Q.Y., Yang, Y.T., He, Q., Gao, H.L., 2015. Tumor microenvironment sensitive doxorubicin delivery and release to glioma using angiopep-2 decorated gold nanoparticles. Biomaterials 37, 425–435.

Scott, H.S., Nelson, P.V., Hopwood, J.J., Morris, C.P., 1991. PCR of a KpnI RFLP in the alpha-L-iduronidase (IDUA) gene. Nucleic Acids Res. 19, 5796.

Shao, K., Wu, J.Q., Chen, Z.Q., Huang, S.X., Li, J.F., Ye, L.Y., Lou, J.N., Zhu, L.P., Jiang, C., 2012. A brain-vectored angiopep-2 based polymeric micelles for the treatment of intracranial fungal infection. Biomaterials 33, 6898–6907.

Somani, S., Blatchford, D.R., Millington, O., Stevenson, M.L., Dufes, C., 2014. Transferrin-bearing polypropylenimine dendrimer for targeted gene delivery to the brain. J. Control. Release 188, 78–86.

Song, Q., Huang, M., Yao, L., Wang, X., Gu, X., Chen, J., Chen, J., Huang, J., Hu, Q., Kang, T., Rong, Z., Qi, H., Zheng, G., Chen, H., Gao, X., 2014. Lipoprotein-based nanoparticles rescue the memory loss of mice with Alzheimer's disease by accelerating the clearance of amyloid-beta. ACS Nano 8, 2345–2359.

Song, Q., Song, H., Xu, J., Huang, J., Hu, M., Gu, X., Chen, J., Zheng, G., Chen, H., Gao, X., 2016. Biomimetic ApoE-reconstituted high density lipoprotein Nanocarrier for blood-brain barrier penetration and amyloid Beta-targeting drug delivery. Mol. Pharm. 13, 3976–3987.

Spencer, B.J., Verma, I.M., 2007. Targeted delivery of proteins across the blood-brain barrier. Proc. Natl. Acad. Sci. U. S. A. 104, 7594–7599.

Staquicini, F.I., Ozawa, M.G., Moya, C.A., Driessen, W.H.P., Barbu, E.M., Nishimori, H., Soghomonyan, S., Flores, L.G., Liang, X.W., Paolillo, V., Alauddin, M.M., Basilion, J.P., Furnari, F.B., Bogler, O., Lang, F.F., Aldape, K.D., Fuller, G.N., Hook, M., Gelovani, J.G., Sidman, R.L., Cavenee, W.K., Pasqualini, R., Arap, W., 2011. Systemic combinatorial peptide selection yields a non-canonical iron-mimicry mechanism for targeting tumors in a mouse model of human glioblastoma. J. Clin. Investig. 121, 161–173.

Suzuki, Y.A., Lonnerdal, B., 2002. Characterization of mammalian receptors for lactoferrin. Biochem. Cell Biol. 80, 75–80.

Tamaru, M., Akita, H., Fujiwara, T., Kajimoto, K., Harashima, H., 2010. Leptin-derived peptide, a targeting ligand for mouse brain-derived endothelial cells via macropinocytosis. Biochem. Biophys. Res. Commun. 394, 587–592.

Tang, Y., Han, T., Everts, M., Zhu, Z.B., Gillespie, G.Y., Curiel, D.T., Wu, H., 2007. Directing adenovirus across the blood-brain barrier via melanotransferrin (P97) transcytosis pathway in an in vitro model. Gene Ther. 14, 523–532.

Tanha, J., Dubuc, G., Hirama, T., Narang, S.A., Mackenzie, C.R., 2002. Selection by phage display of llama conventional V(H) fragments with heavy chain antibody V(H)H properties. J. Immunol. Methods 263, 97–109.

Tartaglia, L.A., Dembski, M., Weng, X., Deng, N.H., Culpepper, J., Devos, R., Richards, G.J., Campfield, L.A., Clark, F.T., Deeds, J., Muir, C., Sanker, S., Moriarty, A., Moore, K.J., Smutko, J.S., Mays, G.G., Woolf, E.A., Monroe, C.A., Tepper, R.I., 1995. Identification and expression cloning of a leptin receptor, OB-R. Cell 83, 1263–1271.

Thomas Tayra, J., Kameda, M., Yasuhara, T., Agari, T., Kadota, T., Wang, F., Kikuchi, Y., Liang, H., Shinko, A., Wakamori, T., Vcelar, B., Weik, R., Date, I., 2013. The neuroprotective and neurorescue effects of carbamylated erythropoietin Fc fusion protein (CEPO-Fc) in a rat model of Parkinson's disease. Brain Res. 1502, 55–70.

Thomas, F.C., Taskar, K., Rudraraju, V., Goda, S., Thorsheim, H.R., Gaasch, J.A., Mittapalli, R.K., Palmieri, D., Steeg, P.S., Lockman, P.R., Smith, Q.R., 2009. Uptake of ANG1005, a novel paclitaxel derivative, through the blood-brain barrier into brain and experimental brain metastases of breast Cancer. Pharm. Res. 26, 2486–2494.

Ulbrich, K., Hekmatara, T., Herbert, E., Kreuter, J., 2009. Transferrin- and transferrin-receptor-antibody-modified nanoparticles enable drug delivery across the blood-brain barrier (BBB). Eur. J. Pharm. Biopharm. 71, 251–256.

Ulbrich, K., Knobloch, T., Kreuter, J., 2011. Targeting the insulin receptor: nanoparticles for drug delivery across the blood-brain barrier (BBB). J. Drug Target. 19, 125–132.

Wang, Y.Y., Lui, P.C., Li, J.Y., 2009. Receptor-mediated therapeutic transport across the blood-brain barrier. Immunotherapy 1, 983–993.

Wang, P., Xue, Y., Shang, X., Liu, Y., 2010. Diphtheria toxin mutant CRM197-mediated transcytosis across blood-brain barrier in vitro. Cell. Mol. Neurobiol. 30, 717–725.

Wei, X.L., Zhan, C.Y., Chen, X.S., Hou, J.P., Xie, C., Lu, W.Y., 2014. Retro-inverso isomer of Angiopep-2: a stable D-peptide ligand inspires brain-targeted drug delivery. Mol. Pharm. 11, 3261–3268.

Wei, X.L., Zhan, C.Y., Shen, Q., Fu, W., Xie, C., Gao, J., Peng, C.M., Zheng, P., Lu, W.Y., 2015. A D-peptide ligand of nicotine acetylcholine receptors for brain-targeted drug delivery. Angew. Chem. Int. Ed. 54, 3023–3027.

Xia, H.B., Anderson, B., Mao, Q.W., Davidson, B.L., 2000. Recombinant human adenovirus: targeting to the human transferrin receptor improves gene transfer to brain microcapillary endothelium. J. Virol. 74, 11359–11366.

Yan, H.H., Wang, J.Y., Yi, P.W., Lei, H., Zhan, C.Y., Xie, C., Feng, L.L., Qian, J., Zhu, J.H., Lu, W.Y., Li, C., 2011. Imaging brain tumor by dendrimer-based optical/paramagnetic nanoprobe across the blood-brain barrier. Chem. Commun. 47, 8130–8132.

Yang, Y.J., Zhao, P.S., Wu, H.X., Wang, H.L., Zhao, L.L., Xue, X.H., Gai, W.W., Gao, Y.W., Yang, S.T., Xia, X.Z., 2014. Production and characterization of a fusion peptide derived from the rabies virus glycoprotein (RVG29). Protein Expr. Purif. 104, 7–13.

Yu, Y.J., Atwal, J.K., Zhang, Y., Tong, R.K., Wildsmith, K.R., Tan, C., Bien-Ly, N., Hersom, M., Maloney, J.A., Meilandt, W.J., Bumbaca, D., Gadkar, K., Hoyte, K., Luk, W., Lu, Y., Ernst, J.A., Scearce-Levie, K., Couch, J.A., Dennis, M.S., Watts, R.J., 2014. Therapeutic bispecific antibodies cross the blood-brain barrier in nonhuman primates. Sci. Transl. Med. 6261ra154.

Yue, P.J., He, L., Qiu, S.W., Li, Y., Liao, Y.J., Li, X.P., Xie, D., Peng, Y., 2014. OX26/CTX-conjugated PEGylated liposome as a dual-targeting gene delivery system for brain glioma. Mol. Cancer. 13.

Zhan, C.Y., Yan, Z.Q., Xie, C., Lu, W.Y., 2010. Loop 2 of Ophiophagus hannah toxin b binds with neuronal nicotinic acetylcholine receptors and enhances intracranial drug delivery. Mol. Pharm. 7, 1940–1947.

Zhan, C.Y., Li, B., Hu, L.J., Wei, X.L., Feng, L.Y., Fu, W., Lu, W.Y., 2011. Micelle-based brain-targeted drug delivery enabled by a nicotine acetylcholine receptor ligand. Angew. Chem. Int. Ed. 50, 5482–5485.

Zhan, C.Y., Wei, X.L., Qian, J., Feng, L.L., Zhu, J.H., Lu, W.Y., 2012. Co-delivery of TRAIL gene enhances the anti-glioblastoma effect of paclitaxel in vitro and in vivo. J. Control. Release 160, 630–636.

Zhang, Y., Pardridge, W.M., 2005. Delivery of beta-galactosidase to mouse brain via the blood-brain barrier transferrin receptor. J. Pharmacol. Exp. Ther. 313, 1075–1081.

Zhang, P., Hu, L., Yin, Q., Feng, L., Li, Y., 2012. Transferrin-modified c[RGDfK]-paclitaxel loaded hybrid micelle for sequential blood-brain barrier penetration and glioma targeting therapy. Mol. Pharm. 9, 1590–1598.

Zhang, B., Sun, X.Y., Mei, H., Wang, Y., Liao, Z.W., Chen, J., Zhang, Q.Z., Hu, Y., Pang, Z.Q., Jiang, X.G., 2013a. LDLR-mediated peptide-22-conjugated nanoparticles for dual-targeting therapy of brain glioma. Biomaterials 34, 9171–9182.

Zhang, X., Liu, L., Chai, G., Zhang, X., Li, F., 2013b. Brain pharmacokinetics of neurotoxin-loaded PLA nanoparticles modified with chitosan after intranasal administration in awake rats. Drug Dev. Ind. Pharm. 39, 1618–1624.

Zhou, Q.H., Boado, R.J., Lu, J.Z., Hui, E.K.W., Pardridge, W.M., 2010. Re-engineering erythropoietin as an IgG fusion protein that penetrates the blood-brain barrier in the mouse. Mol. Pharm. 7, 2148–2155.

Further reading

Zhan, C., Li, C., Wei, X., Lu, W., Lu, W., 2015. Toxins and derivatives in molecular pharmaceutics: drug delivery and targeted therapy. Adv. Drug Deliv. Rev. 90, 101–118.

Carrier-mediated transportation through BBB

6

Naveed Ullah Khan, Tongtong Miao, Xiufeng Ju, Qian Guo, Liang Han
Department of Pharmaceutics, College of Pharmaceutical Sciences, Soochow University, Suzhou, People's Republic of China

1 Introduction

The brain is the most energy-consuming organ in the body. About 20% of the total energy produced by the body is consumed by the brain for its proper functioning (Kou et al., 2017a). Blood-brain barrier (BBB) plays the lion's share in providing the energy and energy-related water-soluble nutrients like sugars, amino acids, peptides, and vitamins to the brain (Krizbai et al., 2016). However, the tight junctions between brain capillary endothelial cells at the BBB confine paracellular transfer of these small nutrient molecules and then limit the transportation of various molecules from the periphery to the brain (Abbott et al., 2010; Agrawal et al., 2017). BBB is considered to be a dynamic interface which has physiological functions of specific and selective membrane transport from blood to brain and active efflux from brain to blood for various compounds (Tsuji and Tamai, 1999a,b). The various transporters expressed at the BBB have been considered to play a critical role in supplying the brain with many essential nutrients (Mittapalli et al., 2010; Geldenhuys et al., 2015b; Pardridge, 2015). A large number of solute-like carrier (SLC) transporters use either facilitative transport or secondary active transport for transferring the energy and energy-related nutrients (Krizbai et al., 2016). In other words, the BBB possesses a carrier role, mediated mainly by SLC transporters. These transporters are responsible for the nutrient and energy supply of the central nervous system (CNS) (i.e., uptake of glucose and amino acids from the blood to the brain). Thus, transporters for various nutrients are expressed at high levels at the BBB (Mittapalli et al., 2010; Bhutia et al., 2014).

Current drug treatments for many CNS diseases remain mostly ineffective because it is very hard for drug delivery to reach therapeutic concentration in brain parenchyma for effective treatment. The underlying mechanisms are likely to include the limited drug permeability across the BBB, the presence of degrading enzyme inside brain capillary endothelial cells, and the efflux pumps of the BBB. Among these factors, the major challenge for effective drug delivery to brain is the efficient cross of the BBB and entry of therapeutic drugs into the brain parenchyma (Pardridge, 1999). BBB prevents the entry of all toxic molecules as well as most drug molecules to protect the brain thereof (Pardridge, 1999; Cardoso et al., 2010). In fact, BBB is only permeable to some small molecules with strictly specified structure (Pardridge, 1999).

Brain Targeted Drug Delivery Systems. https://doi.org/10.1016/B978-0-12-814001-7.00006-8

Nanotechnology has been widely and is being extensively applied in drug delivery field to construct nano drug delivery systems by formulating all kinds of therapeutic agents into biocompatible nanostructures or nanocomposites such as conjugates, liposomes, nanoparticles, nanocapsules, and micellar systems (Singh et al., 2015). Over the past few decades, nano drug delivery systems have made great contributions in increasing delivery efficiency, bioavailability, and in vivo drug stability (Wang et al., 2017; Shi et al., 2016). In recent years, nano drug delivery systems have been examined and are being developed to overcome the hurdle of the BBB (Petri et al., 2007).

The rich SLC transporters at the BBB imply the promising important role of the carrier-mediated transportation (CMT) in brain-targeted drug delivery (Geier et al., 2013). The high expression of these SLC transporters at the BBB makes them ideal targets for nano drug delivery systems to cross the BBB. Many related specific substrates have been already used to functionalize nano drug delivery systems to enhance brain-targeted drug delivery (Mittapalli et al., 2010; Bhutia et al., 2014). The combination of CMT systems and nano drug delivery systems may lead to the development of efficient approaches for the BBB penetration and systemic brain targeting drug delivery. An attempt has been made in this chapter to comprehensively summarize the understanding about CMT transporters and the related application for designing brain-targeted nano drug delivery systems.

2 CMT systems at the BBB

CMT transcytosis is one major mechanism for substance transport across the BBB and the portal for brain uptake of energy and nutrients. As shown in Fig. 1, most nutrients are transported from blood to brain by the BBB selective transporters, such as hexose, amino acid, or monocarboxylate transporters, overexpressed on the brain capillary endothelial cells (Agrawal et al., 2017). The turnover number is the approximation of number of substrate molecules that one specific transporter can transport per second. The turnover number for these transporters at the BBB has been estimated to be

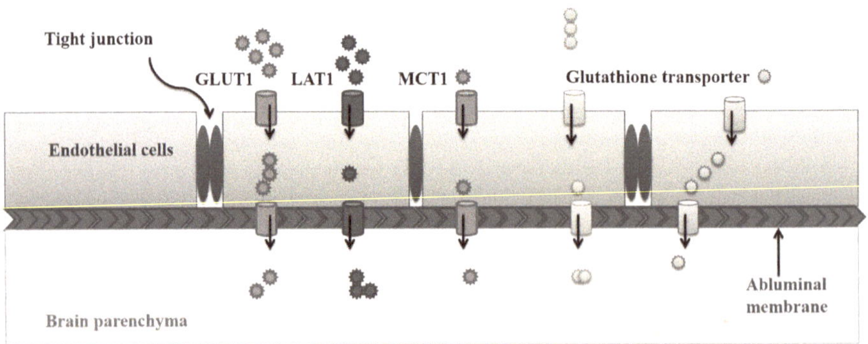

Fig. 1 CMT systems at the BBB for supplying nutrients to brain parenchyma.

270–3000 molecules/s. For example, the turnover number for sucrose transporter is 500 molecules/s (Schulz et al., 2011). It should be also noted that the electrochemical sodium ion gradient, the so-called sodium-motive force, is the main driving force for the active/facilitated transportations of a variety of biomolecules such as amino acids and carbohydrates in most of living cells (Barar et al., 2016).

These plasma membrane nutrient transporters at the BBB have attracted increasing interest in recent years as they can be used as promising portals for brain-targeted drug delivery. These transporters at the BBB belong to the SLC superfamily. And they are comprised of two functional groups that include the mediation of solute influx or efflux from the brain capillary endothelial cells (Barar et al., 2016). The SLC transporters involved in influx at the BBB may be divided into different groups (Fig. 2) and are listed as follows:

(a) Hexose transport system for glucose and mannose such as glucose transporters (Mantych et al., 1993; Pardridge et al., 1990).

(b) Amino acid transporters including neutral amino acid transporters, cationic amino acid transporters, anionic amino acid transporters, and β-amino acid transporters. Neutral amino acid transport system is for transportation of neutral amino acids and can be divided into large and small neutral amino acid transporters (Kido et al., 2001b; Kageyama et al., 2000; Rautio et al., 2013). Cationic amino acid transport system is for transportation of L-lysine, L-arginine, and L-ornithine (O'Kane et al., 2006; Stoll et al., 1993). Anionic amino acid transport system is for transportation of aspartate and glutamate (Sakaeda et al., 2000; O'Kane et al., 1999; Benrabh and Lefauconnier, 1996). β-Amino acid transport system is for transportation of β-alanine and taurine (Benrabh et al., 1995; Tamai et al., 1995; Komura et al., 1997).

(c) Peptide transport system for transportation of peptides, including (i) oligopeptide transporters such as glutathione transporter, PepT1, and PepT2; and (ii) polypeptide transporters such as OATP2, OAT-K1, and OATP (Tsuji, 1999; Tsuji and Tamai, 1999a,b).

(d) Monocarboxylic acid transport system is for transportation of lactate, short-chain fatty acids, biotin, salicylic acid, valproic acid, phenylbutyrate, and 3,5,3′-triiodo-L-thyronine

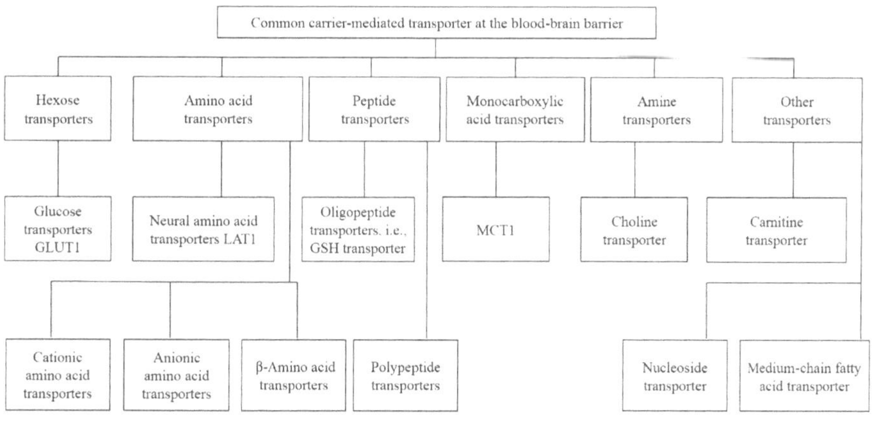

Fig. 2 Common CMT transporters at the BBB. The transporters at the second row have already been used for mediating the brain targeting of nano drug delivery system.

(Halestrap, 2013; Miller and Oldendorf, 1986; Oldendorf, 1973; Conn et al., 1983; Ceballos et al., 2009).

(e) Choline transport system may belong to amine transport system and is for transportation of choline and thiamine (Murakami et al., 2000; Kang et al., 1990a; Karlsson et al., 1984; Li et al., 2013a).

(f) Other transport systems including carnitine transporter, nucleoside transport system (Masereeuw et al., 1994), medium-chain fatty acid transporter (Adkison and Shen, 1996), and so on.

The current increased understanding and frontier research of the biology of the BBB have identified many specific transporters expressed at the BBB endothelial cells (Mittapalli et al., 2010; Agarwal et al., 2011). In addition to the above mentioned transport systems, other transport systems such as organic anion transporters are also present at the BBB. The BBB is rich in SLC transporters implying an important role of CMT in drug delivery (Geier et al., 2013).

Among these SLC transporters at the BBB, the most important and widely used transporters for mediating the transport of nano drug delivery systems to brain include the glucose transporter, neutral amino acids transporter, glutathione transporter, monocarboxylic acid transporter, choline transporter, and carnitine transporter. In the following, discussions are provided on the application of these transporters for designing CMT-based brain-targeted nano drug delivery systems.

3 Nano drug delivery systems

There are many types of nano drug delivery systems that have been developed over the past few decades, such as nanoparticles, liposomes, and micelles. In general, nano drug delivery systems possess many advantages for drug delivery: prolonged blood circulation, enhanced drug stability, increased drug bioavailability, and passively targeted therapeutic effect with decreased side effects and toxicity. Nano drug delivery systems found renowned attention in tumor-targeted drug delivery field because of the efficiently passive targeting effect to various types of tumor (Singh et al., 2014). However, nano drug delivery systems without subtle design and functionalization can't provide satisfactory permeation across the BBB (Zhan and Lu, 2012). This non-specific nature restricts their role as potential brain targeting drug delivery systems (Allen and Cullis, 2004).

So the important factor to be taken into account, for designing systemic brain targeting nano drug delivery systems, is the development of functionalization of nano drug delivery systems to assist their translocation across the BBB. Among many different types of nano drug delivery systems, nanoparticles and liposomes hold an additional advantage since they can be easily modified or functionalized to efficiently target a particular site of interest (e.g., BBB). So the most widely developed types of nano drug delivery systems, for application of brain targeting, are nanoparticles and liposomes (Gaillard et al., 2014b; Alexander et al., 2012, 2013, 2014, 2016; Sahu et al., 2013; Ajazuddin et al., 2012; Vyas et al., 2010; Dashora et al., 2006).

Nanoparticles are able to incorporate diverse targeting moieties for enhancing the penetration across the BBB (i.e., CMT). In other words, nanoparticles can be easily modified to enhance the BBB crossing efficiency, making this nano drug delivery system advantageous for brain targeting delivery (Petros and DeSimone, 2010). Hence, functionalized nanoparticles are highly efficient drug vehicles interacting with brain capillary endothelial cells and able to overcome the barrier and release drug molecules encapsulated within, or adsorbed or bound on the surface. There are some differences for liposomes. Unmodified liposomes can enhance drug delivery to brain because liposome's unique phospholipid bilayer structure makes it more compatible with the lipoidal layer of the BBB and helps the drug to enter the brain. However, liposome itself does not allow to cross the BBB. Hence, various modifications have been made to enable the penetration of liposomal carrier across the BBB (Spuch and Navarro, 2011; Vieira and Gamarra, 2016).

Targeted therapy is an advanced approach for the administration of drugs to be delivered to specific regions and has received growing attention, not only for the enhancement of therapeutic efficacy, but also for the reduction in systemic side effects (Liu et al., 2006). Advanced nano drug delivery systems, which are capable of overcoming the BBB after functionalized modification, have great future perspectives for the drug management of many diseases of the CNS (Kou et al., 2017a). Advanced brain-targeted nano drug delivery systems represent a constantly developing field in the last few years. Various kinds of modification methods on nano drug delivery systems have been developed to improve the efficiency of drug delivery to brain in recent years. These methods include the encapsulation of the BBB modulators and specific P-glycoprotein inhibitors, and conjugation with targeting or penetration ligands (Han et al., 2016). Among all the methods, a key strategy is to functionalize the surface of nano drug delivery systems with specific ligands, such as peptides and antibodies, which can specifically bind to highly expressed targets at the BBB (Liu and Lu, 2012). Many specific transporters at the brain capillary endothelial cells (mentioned in the above section) can be the targets of the nano drug delivery systems to achieve enhanced drug delivery to the CNS (Fig. 3).

4 CMT of nano drug delivery systems across the BBB

Using the method of functionalizing the surface of nano drug delivery systems with specific ligands, the advantages of CMT have been grafted onto the nano drug delivery systems (Fig. 3). Nutrients like glucose and glutathione, as substrates of the SLC transporters at the BBB, have already been utilized to modify liposome to facilitate the translocation of liposome to brain (Noble et al., 2014; Vieira and Gamarra, 2016). For example: (i) many glucose-modified liposomes have been developed to specifically bind to glucose transporter proteins (GLUTs) at the BBB to enhance the transcytosis and the brain penetration (Du et al., 2014; Xie et al., 2012; Qu et al., 2014). (ii) Another case is the so-called G-Technology® which applies the strategy of modification with glutathione to target the highly expressed glutathione transporter at the BBB to effectively deliver drugs to brain (Salem et al., 2015; Lindqvist et al., 2016;

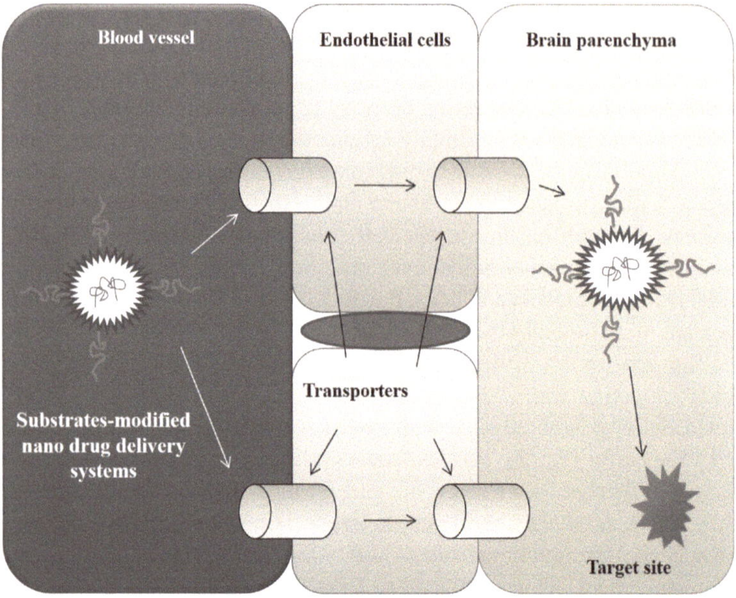

Fig. 3 CMT-based brain targeting nano drug delivery.

Markoutsa et al., 2014; Maussang et al., 2016). For nanoparticle-based drug delivery systems, substrates of many transporters including GLUT1, LAT1, and choline transporter have also been examined for mediating brain drug delivery by modifying nanoparticle surface (Li et al., 2013a; Shao et al., 2014; Jiang et al., 2014; Salmaso et al., 2009; Lin et al., 2016b).

This functionalization combines advantages of nano drug delivery systems with high BBB crossing efficiency of CMT and improves permeation across the BBB by targeting the transporters that are expressed at endothelial cells that form the BBB. These CMT-based nano drug delivery systems are considered to enable improved brain penetration efficacy (Mittapalli et al., 2010; Agarwal et al., 2011) and have great future perspectives for the diagnosis and treatment of brain-located diseases. The same logic could be used for drug delivery into tumor cells like glioma cells because these nutrient transporters may be also upregulated in tumor cells to support their rapid growth. It has been reported that the nutrient transporters GLUT1, LAT1, and choline transporters show significant promise for the delivery of drugs in the form of nanoparticles for glioma therapy (Lin et al., 2016b; Salmaso et al., 2009; Jiang et al., 2014; Shao et al., 2014; Li et al., 2013a).

4.1 Hexose transport system

The transport of hexoses including glucose into most mammalian cells is mediated by 13 transporters, GLUTs 1-12, and the myo-inositol transporter HMIT (Simpson et al., 2007). Except ubiquitously expressed GLUT1, other transporters have fairly distinct tissue- and cell-specific patterns of expression. The functional expression of glucose transporters was initially identified in the brain microvessels of rat and pig (Dick et al., 1984). Later on, the GLUT1 isoform was shown to be expressed at the BBB in bovine brain cortex. All glucose transporter-binding sites at the BBB can be attributed to the GLUT1 isoform (Pardridge et al., 1990). It is important to note that many of the transporters present in mammalian brain are either unable to transport glucose (GLUTs 5, 6, 11, & HMIT have very low affinity for glucose) or have very limited localization and concentrations (GLUT 2 & 4), while for others their location, ability, and/or capacity to transport glucose have yet to be assessed (GLUTs 8 &10). Thus, with all of the above exclusions, the predominant transporters in mammalian brain involved in cerebral glucose utilization are GLUTs 1 and 3, which are expressed throughout the brain and whose localization and kinetic characteristics are well-established.

From pharmacological perspective, GLUT1 may be the most promising target transporter because of the high and selective expression in the microvascular endothelial cells of the BBB and glia (Patching, 2017; Qin et al., 2010; Simpson et al., 2007). However, GLUT3 in brain has been localized almost exclusively to neurons (Simpson et al., 2007). The GLUT1 are present on both the luminal side and the abluminal side of the BBB (Béduneau et al., 2007; Tsuji, 2005). In human and monkey brain, the GLUT1 expression was found in the gray matter and white matter endothelial cells, astrocyte foot processes surrounding gray matter blood vessels, and astrocytes adjacent to synaptic contacts. While the immunoblots of adult human frontal cortex were reported to have two forms of GLUT1 (45 and 52 kDa), the immunoblots of vessel-depleted frontal lobe showed the 45 kDa form solely in gray matter fractions. Such findings confirmed linkage to GLUT1 in both astrocyte and astrocyte-associated neuronal energy metabolism (Morgello et al., 1995).

GLUT1 has been demonstrated as robust CMT pathway for systemic drug delivery to brain by efficiently crossing the BBB. Glucose is able to traverse the BBB by binding to GLUT1 (Béduneau et al., 2007; Tsuji, 2005). Conjugating glucose to a drug molecule can significantly increase the ability of the drug to enter the brain through the GLUT1. In this respect, the D-glucose ester of 7-chlorokynurenic acid, but not the unconjugated form, was protective against seizures in mice (Battaglia et al., 2000). D-Glucose esters of dopamine or L-DOPA showed promising central effects (Bonina et al., 2003). Now, brain-targeted drug delivery utilizing GLUT1-based CMT pathway has expanded to nano drug delivery systems from prodrug strategy.

4.1.1 GLUT1-targeted nanoparticles for brain-targeted drug delivery

Various nanoparticles have been covalently decorated with glucose for ensuring selective brain accumulation of the loaded drug. For instance, Jiang et al. prepared 2-deoxy-D-glucose-modified poly(ethylene glycol)-co-poly(trimethylene carbonate) nanoparticles for targeting drug delivery to brain tumor. The overall survivability of orthotopically established rat glioblastoma bearing nude mice was enhanced up to 48 days, while the control mouse group survived only 34 days (Jiang et al., 2014).

Comprehensive understanding of the specific binding of glucose analogs to GLUT1 can give more detailed information on using such molecules for mediating brain targeting drug delivery. Not only glucose itself, but mannose or mannose analogs can also be used for targeting GLUT1 (Du et al., 2014; Singh et al., 2015; Kuo and Lee, 2015). Compared with glucose or other glucose analogs, mannose and mannose analogs can be better recognized by the GLUT1 transporter (Umezawa and Eto, 1988). p-Aminophenyl-a-D-mannopyranoside, a mannose analog, was found to have high affinity for the GLUT1 transporter present at the BBB (Singh et al., 2015). Singh et al. prepared p-aminophenyl-a-D-mannopyranoside-modified docetaxel-loaded solid lipidic nanoparticles for targeting docetaxel delivery to brain and proved increased drug concentration in brain, revealing the prospective of p-Aminophenyl-a-D-mannopyranoside-conjugated lipidic nanoparticles as an efficient vehicle for drug delivery to brain (Singh et al., 2015).

4.1.2 GLUT1-targeted liposomes for brain-targeted drug delivery

Fulan et al. worked on the GLUT1 strategy by preparing glucose-modified drug-loaded liposome. The liposome was modified by glucose through polyethylene glycol (PEG) with varying chain length. PEG was also used to stabilize the formulation and reduce the phagocytosis effect of the reticuloendothelial system as well as liposome accumulation in spleen and liver (Xie et al., 2012; Cruz et al., 2011). The liposome size was small (<200 nm) so that glucose-modified liposome can make good use of the CMT to easily cross the BBB (Kaur et al., 2008). The results showed that glucose-modified liposome was stable enough and able to easily cross the BBB through the GLUT1 transporter. Glucose-modified liposome with a medium-chain PEG displayed a higher concentration in the brain, while less in peripheral organs (Xie et al., 2012). In contrast, the liposome prepared with shorter chain PEG showed greater concentration in the periphery than brain because strong stereospecific blockade effect from shorter chain length PEG made liposome unable to cross the BBB through the GLUT1 transporter. Likewise, longer chain PEG with strong flexibility and folding ability may cover the glucose and also reduces the ability of liposome to cross the BBB. (Xie et al., 2012). Zhang et al. developed a functional targeting epirubicin-loaded liposomes modified with aminophenyl glucose for transferring epirubicin across the BBB. 4-Aminophenyl β-D-glucopyranoside, a glucose derivative that can be transported across the BBB through the GLUT1 transporter, was used as a targeting ligand for guiding the transport of epirubicin-loaded liposome vesicles across the BBB (Pardridge, 2007). The results showed that the constructed liposomes were able to be transported across the BBB. The action mechanisms of functional targeting epirubicin liposomes correlated with the following features: the long circulation in the blood system and the ability to be transported across the BBB via the GLUT1 transporter. In conclusion, functional targeting epirubicin liposomes could be used as a potential therapy for treating brain diseases (Zhang et al., 2015).

In addition, Ying et al. conjugated p-aminophenyl-a-D-mannopyranoside on daunorubicin-loaded liposomes for transporting daunorubicin across the BBB and evaluating the BBB crossing efficiency of p-aminophenyl-a-D-mannopyranoside

(Ying et al., 2010). Hao et al. prepared p-aminophenyl-a-D-mannopyranoside-modified liposomes to target various functional regions of the brain and demonstrated the potential of CMT by p-aminophenyl-a-D-mannopyranoside (Hao et al., 2013).

4.2 Amino acid transporters

Many kinds of amino acid transport systems function at the BBB to maintain brain homeostasis by transferring amino acids (Barar et al., 2016). Of these, the glycoprotein-associated amino acid transport systems play the important role in amino acid homeostasis in brain parenchyma. Based upon the discrepant binding affinity of a particular transporter to different amino acids, along with its dependency on sodium ion, amino acid transporters can be classified into different groups such as system L, y +L, Xc^- (consisting of xCT and 4F2hc), asc, and b0,+. However, along with the gradual development of research, these different groups of amino acid transporters have been found with some commonalities and differences in terms of binding affinity to different amino acid substrates. System L and other groups share somewhat commonalities in terms of amino acid identity (around 40%–89%). For example, alanine can be transported into the brain through systems L and/or asc, which is an overlapped function between these transporters. Furthermore, some of these transporters act as obligatory exchangers. For example, xCT/4F2hc functions as the exchanger of L-cysteine and L-glutamic acid (Hosoya et al., 2002). A number of studies have also shown that the subunits of system L act as an obligatory exchanger, so that the inward transportation of one amino acid may associate with the outward transportation of other amino acid (Meier et al., 2002). Such exchange functionality, which may be indirectly related to ATP-dependent transporters activities, seems to provide the driving force for the sodium ion-independent amino acid transport systems including system L. Nevertheless, the molecular mechanism(s) of this process is yet to be fully understood.

4.2.1 Neutral amino acid transporters

System L plays a key role upon traverse of the neutral amino acids in and out of the brain, maintaining desired concentrations of neutral amino acids in brain. More precisely, the system L functions as a sodium ion-independent bidirectional transporter that is responsible for both branched and aromatic neutral amino acids in almost all types of cells with different affinity to a range of large and small neutral amino acids (Kido et al., 2001b; Kageyama et al., 2000; Matsuo et al., 2000; Nii et al., 2001). Depending on the site of the biological membrane studied, luminal and abluminal transportation of amino acids show different pattern. Since system L functions bi-directionally, the inward and outward traverses of amino acids appear to differ one another, significantly. For example, the outward trafficking of L-phenylalanine seems to be greater than L-leucine whose inward transportation happens to be markedly high. As a member of glycoprotein-associated amino acid transporter family, system L comprises of light (LAT) and heavy (4F2hc) chains and two types of

LAT1/4F2hc and LAT2/4F2hc (Kido et al., 2001b). Affinity of LAT1/4F2hc and LAT2/4F2hc transporters vary for different amino acids. The apparent affinity constants or the Michaelis-Menten constant, K_m, equals the substrate concentration at half maximal reaction rate. In this case, K_m is a good approximation for the dissociation constant and thus describes the affinity of the substrate for the enzyme. The lower the K_m value, the higher the binding affinity. LAT1 is a ubiquitous transporter with a high affinity for large neutral amino acids and with K_m values in the μM range, whereas LAT2 shows a lower affinity to large neutral amino acids and higher affinity to small neutral amino acids and possessing a K_m value in the mM range for neutral amino acids (Kageyama et al., 2000; Matsuo et al., 2000; Kim et al., 2002; Kanai and Endou, 2003). So LAT1 is supposed to have a higher transport efficiency than LAT2 for large neutral amino acids. In the absence of 4F2hc, the LAT1 is found in the intracellular compartments. Upon complexation with 4F2hc, it can reach to the plasma membrane, while the 4F2hc itself reaches the plasma membrane independently. The surface conformation of 4F2hc seems to be altered in the presence of LAT1, confining it to cell-cell adhesion sites. The 4F2hc comprises 529 amino acids (94 kDa, glycosylated; 72 kDa unglycosylated). The LAT1 protein consists of 507 amino acids with a molecular mass of 55 kDa, whose association with 4F2hc (LAT1/4F2hc heterodimeric complex) induces transportation of large neutral amino acids into the brain (Boado et al., 1999; Kageyama et al., 2000). The light chain LAT1 is widely expressed in nonepithelial cells including brain, spleen, thymus, testis, skin, liver, placenta, skeletal muscle, and stomach. In brain, LAT1 expression is found predominantly in capillary endothelial cells that form the BBB. LAT1 transports a wide range of substrates including large amino acids (e.g., L-tyrosine) and thyroid hormones across the BBB (Kanai et al., 1998). There are also a few neurotherapeutics which can be transported into the brain by LAT1. They are: L-3,4-dihydroxyphenylalanine (L-DOPA, a BBB permeable dopamine precursor used in Parkinson's disease), gabapentin (a cyclic amino acid used as antiepileptic drug), and melphalan (an alkylating agent used to treat brain cancers) (Pardridge, 2012).

Abundant and selective expression on both luminal and abluminal membrane sides of the BBB combined with markedly enhanced substrate affinity (by ~1000 times compared to that on peripheral tissues) makes LAT1-mediated drug delivery to brain an attractive therapeutic strategy (Boado et al., 1999; Peura et al., 2011; Killian et al., 2007). LAT1-mediated drug delivery to brain has begun (Lin et al., 2016b; Kharya et al., 2013). Many prodrugs have been developed by conjugating the substrates to the drug molecules or preparing a fusion molecule mimicking the substrates of LAT1. These prodrugs generally possess both the negatively charged alpha-carboxyl and the positively charged alpha-amino groups (Rautio et al., 2014). Ylikangas et al. developed tryptophan-conjugated prodrugs and demonstrated that tryptophan can be used as the promoiety for designing LAT1-specific prodrugs with high affinity (Ylikangas et al., 2014). In another study, Peura et al. designed phenylalanine derivatives of valproic acid by introducing the meta-substituted phenylalanine analogue promoiety as the LAT1-specific ligand and demonstrated the high efficiency of the LAT1-mediated brain targeting (Peura et al., 2011). Likewise in another study, L-cysteine was covalently attached to either

6-mercaptopurine or 2-methyl-1-propanethiol via a disulfide bond to synthesize the LAT1-specific prodrugs. And these prodrug conjugates showed high affinity to LAT1 expressed by cerebral vessels (Killian et al., 2007). From these above studies, it can be seen that LAT1-mediated drug delivery holds great perspective for significant brain accumulation (Lin et al., 2016b; Kharya et al., 2013).

Furthermore, LAT1 is overexpressed in many types of cancer cells including glioblastoma (Lin et al., 2016b; Kobayashi et al., 2008; Kaira et al., 2008a,b; Sakata et al., 2009). Thus, high expression level of LAT1 on brain capillary endothelial cells and glioma cells makes it a "dual target" for antiglioma therapy. Wu et al. developed a LAT1-mediated chemotherapeutic agent aspartate-conjugated doxorubicin. The aspartate-conjugated doxorubicin showed high affinity to LAT1 and could substantially inhibit the LAT1 overexpressing cancer cells. Such findings were further confirmed by pharmacokinetic data. The significant accumulation of aspartate-conjugated doxorubicin within the tumor tissue was most likely through LAT1 uptake. Upon all results, the aspartate-conjugated doxorubicin was proposed as a new treatment strategy for the LAT1 overexpressing cancer cells including glioblastoma (Wu et al., 2015).

Nano drug delivery systems are being studied to be fabricated with specific ligands of LAT1 transporters on their exosurface for enhanced brain accumulation via CMT. Vyas et al. explored facilitated transport of an anti-HIV agent efavirenz (a nonnucleoside reverse transcriptase inhibitor) across the BBB into the brain using phenylalanine-anchored solid lipid nanoparticles. The amino acid micronutrient phenylalanine was used as the ligand to facilitate CMT via LAT1 to traverse the BBB. Nanoparticles were around 150 nm and possessed good entrapment efficiency (around 70%). in vivo studies showed 2–3 folds and 7–8 folds accumulation of phenylalanine-anchored solid lipid nanoparticles in brain as compared to unmodified nanoparticles and free drug, respectively. Transcytosis studies confirmed about 10-fold higher BBB crossing efficiency compared to free drug. Phenylalanine-anchored solid lipid nanoparticles improved the drug bioavailability and maintained therapeutic levels in the brain for an extended period of time that can result in significant eradication of the viral load therein (Vyas et al., 2015). In another study, tryptophan derivate-functionalized Pluronic micelles encapsulating an antiepilectic drug were successfully used for drug delivery to the hippocampus in brain (Liu et al., 2016). In addition, Li et al. reported the design of LAT1-mediated PEGylated liposomal system containing glutamate functionality (large amino acid) in its exosurface region for selective delivery of docetaxel to glioma tissue and showed significant brain accumulations (Lin et al., 2016b). L-DOPA, a well-known drug to treat Parkinson's disease, is previously reported to cross the BBB via LAT1 (Kageyama et al., 2000). More recently, Bhunia et al. reported on the development of a nanometric (100–135 nm) promising LAT1 selective liposomal drug carrier prepared from L-DOPA-functionalized amphiphile for efficient targeting of potent chemotherapeutics to orthotopically established mouse glioblastoma. in vitro studies revealed LAT1-mediated cellular uptake. Intravenously administered liposomes of Amphi-DOPA showed preferential accumulation in brain tissue (Bhunia et al., 2017). These studies demonstrated that LAT1-mediated drug targeting could bring forth advances in biocompatible and biodegradable drug delivery systems and also the feasibility of LAT1-mediated systemic chemotherapy of brain diseases.

Recently, antibody against CD98hc (the heavy chain 4F2hc of system L) showed robust accumulation in brain after systemic dosing and a significant pharmacodynamic response as measured by brain Aβ reduction. Anti-CD98hc antibodies showed even better accumulation in the brain than anti-transferrin receptor antibodies without altering CD98hc expression or amino acid transport. Anti-CD98hc/β-secretase bispecific antibodies reduced brain amyloid levels in mice (Zuchero et al., 2016). The study of antibody against CD98hc expands the current approaches available for enhancing brain uptake of therapeutic antibodies.

4.2.2 Cationic amino acid transporters

Transportation of cationic amino acids is mediated through two transporter families (Barar et al., 2016). The first transporter family is system y+ so-called cationic amino acid transporter, and the second one is broad-scope amino acid transporters consisting of systems b0,+, B0,+, and y+L (Barar et al., 2016). However, the functional expression and distribution of these two transporter families by brain capillary endothelial cells have not been fully addressed (Barar et al., 2016). It has been reported that the cationic amino acid transporter was found to be the only cationic amino acid transporter present, mostly on the abluminal membrane of bovine brain microvessels (Barar et al., 2016). The cationic amino acid transporter showed voltage dependency and K_m values at μM range for amino acids such as L-lysine, L-arginine, and L-ornithine. The inhibitor constant, K_i, is an indication of how potent an inhibitor is; it is the concentration required to produce half maximum inhibition. The cationic amino acid transporter, in the presence of sodium ion, was inhibited by several essential neutral amino acids with K_i values of 3–10 times greater than the plasma concentrations (Barar et al., 2016). However, some small nonessential amino acids (i.e., serine, glutamine, alanine, and glycine) were able to inhibit the cationic amino acid transporter with K_i values similar to their plasma concentrations, implying that the cationic amino acid transporter might be involved in the BBB traverse of these amino acids (Barar et al., 2016). Further, the cationic amino acid transporter could be a key transporter in traverse of arginine that is necessary for the synthesis of nitric oxide in cerebral endothelial cells (O'Kane et al., 2006). Taken all, it seems that this system is the only cationic amino acid transport machinery at the BBB (O'Kane et al., 2006; Stoll et al., 1993). Hawkins et al. reported that cationic amino acid transporter or system y+ is the only transporter at the BBB that transports the cationic amino acids into the CNS (O'Kane et al., 2006).

It is possible to deliver drug across the BBB to brain via cationic amino acid transporter by drug substrate conjugate or cationic amino acid transporter-specific drug delivery system (Stoll et al., 1993). Cationic amino acid transporter has affinity for some neurotrophic viruses. [3H]-L-ornithine is structurally a substrate for cationic amino acid transporter. Sharma et al. prepared poly-L-arginine and transferrin co-modified liposomes for specific gene delivery to brain. The brain accumulation or uptake of co-modified liposomes was significantly much higher than transferrin-bound liposomes. Besides being cell penetrating peptide, the poly-L-arginine may be also a substrate for cationic amino acid transporter, which can mediate the CMT to cross the BBB. The study suggested an efficient and safe brain-targeted gene delivery system (Sharma et al., 2013).

4.2.3 Efflux amino acid transporters

The system Xc^- is critical in amino acid exchanger function in various cell types such as brain capillary endothelial cells (Barar et al., 2016). The system Xc^- is critical in glutamate-glutamine cycle (Barar et al., 2016). At the BBB, the system Xc^- pumps the glutamine molecules out of the extracellular fluid of the CNS into the endothelial cells and then to the blood. Further, the brain capillary endothelial cells are also able to hydrolyze glutamine and use it for production of glutathione (Barar et al., 2016). So as an ABC transporter, the system Xc^- has not been exploited for designing brain drug delivery via CMT.

4.3 Peptide transporters

The uptake of many small peptides such as dipeptides and tripeptides in brain capillary endothelial cells can be saturable. These small peptides cross the BBB and enter brain mainly through the peptide transporters (Barar et al., 2016). Peptide transporters were found as an integral part of the plasma membrane proteins. Many oligopeptide transporters have been found to be expressed in brain such as glutathione transporter, PepT1, PepT2, and HPT (Tsuji and Tamai, 1999a,b). It has not been clarified yet whether PepT1, PepT2, and HPT exist at the BBB or not. But it has been reported that the expression of PepT1 and PepT2 was found at the choroid plexus of the human brain (Berger and Hediger, 1999; Novotny et al., 2000). Peptide transporters including PepT1, PepT2, and HPT neither recognize nor transport glutathione. The usefulness of glutathione transporters at the BBB for the specific brain delivery of small peptides or peptide-mimetic drugs remains to be fully investigated.

For the active/facilitated transportations of amino acids and carbohydrates in most of living cells as well as the mammalian cells, the electrochemical sodium ion gradient was thought to be the main driving force (Barar et al., 2016). The peptide transport process, nevertheless, seems to be an evolutionary shift in the coupling ion and favors hydrogen ion, through which a proton-motive force energizes active traverse of peptides through cell membrane. Peptide transporters function as proton-coupled oligopeptide symporters with the uptake of small peptides coupled to the efflux of a proton.

PepT1 is also highly expressed in the intestine (Tsuji and Tamai, 1999a,b). PepT1 seems to be a key transporter in the intestine for overall amino acids/peptide absorption only after high dietary protein intake (Nässl et al., 2011). PepT2 is highly expressed in kidney and also expressed in liver (Tsuji and Tamai, 1999a,b). Importantly, in the renal proximal tubule, PepT2 is responsible for conserving the peptide-bound amino nitrogen, otherwise it can be excreted through the urine. Both transporters PepT1 and PepT2 deliver orally effective β-lactam antibiotics, angiotensin-converting enzyme inhibitors, bestatin, and the other peptide-mimetic drugs (Tsuji and Tamai, 1996). Another oligopeptide transporter, HPT, is responsible for transport of histidine oligopeptides and histidine itself. These transporters including PepT1, PepT2, and HPT also mediate the trafficking of peptide-mimetic drugs. PepT1 can be used for peptidomimetic oral drug delivery through intestine (Tsuji, 1999). The bioavailability of prodrugs specific to PepT1 was shown to be higher than those of the corresponding parent compounds, mainly because of the improved transportation. Such phenomenon has emerged as a new field of peptide transporter-mediated targeted therapy, so-called PepT1-targeted prodrugs (Zhang et al., 2013). Valganciclovir, a valyl ester of ganciclovir, was clinically shown to possess markedly higher bioavailability than ganciclovir when taken orally by patients with cytomegalovirus infection, in large part for being substrate of both PepT1 and PepT2 (Sugawara et al., 2000). A number of drugs seem to be substrate to these transporters, including amoxicillin, benazepril, captopril, cefixime, cephalexin, enalapril, levodopa, oxacillin, Ramipril, tolbutamide, and valaciclovir. PepT1 and PepT2 are relatively stereoselective, while showing greater affinity to the peptides formed from L isomer amino acids than those that possess D isomer amino acids. Kinetically, depending upon the substrate, PepT1 is considered as a low-affinity and high-capacity system which yields K_m ranging from 0.2 to 10 mM. However, PepT2 is considered as a high-affinity and low-capacity transport system showing K_m values of 5–500 μM.

Although not completely characterized, glutathione transporter is present on brain capillary endothelial cells (Peterson et al., 2013). Glutathione is an endogenous tripeptide with important antioxidant properties and is able to cross the BBB through the specific glutathione transporter (Gaillard et al., 2014a; Kannan et al., 2000; Rip et al., 2014; Koshkaryev et al., 2013; Markoutsa et al., 2011). The consideration of glutathione-coated brain-targeted nano drug delivery systems can be rationalized since large number of glutathione transporters are present at the BBB (Wang et al., 2014; Liang et al., 2010; Gaillard, 2010b). The prodrug approach via conjugation of glutathione can obtain drug delivery to brain via CMT. Glutathione ligand should bind to the BBB glutathione transporter, subsequently increasing the number of prodrugs or nano drug delivery systems at the BBB interface. G-Technology®, based on glutathione, is a well-established, patented, FDA-approved technology proved to enhance the brain targeting of drug molecules. Various attempts made using this approach to target the BBB have been reported. Based on the G-Technology®, Rip et al. prepared glutathione-modified PEGylated liposomes and studied the pharmacokinetic behavior, brain endothelial cellular uptake, and brain distribution ability (Rip et al., 2014). The results demonstrated approximately 1.8-folds higher cell uptake by the endothelial cells for glutathione-modified PEGylated liposomes and a temperature-dependent uptake of the liposome that decreases with decreasing temperature. The microdialysis was performed to study the drug concentration in brain and it showed a significant increase in drug concentration with glutathione-modified PEGylated liposome than the PEGylated liposome. It can be concluded that glutathione modification of PEGylated liposomal system (G-Technology®) offers a promising approach to target the drug molecule to the brain and protect the drug as well by providing a safe and stable homing/carrier system (Rip et al., 2014). The approach of using glutathione-modified liposomal doxorubicin has already reached phase 2 clinical trial (Rip et al., 2014). Lin et al. prepared gefitinib-loaded liposomes, which were further modified with glutathione to enhance gefitinib trafficking across the BBB. Like earlier reports, surface glutathione successfully enhanced the drug delivery across the BBB (Lin et al., 2016a). Glutathione-conjugated ribavirin-loaded liposomes were found to have dose-dependent ability of brain penetration. The accumulated extents of liposomes in brain were dependent upon the extent of glutathione used for liposomes conjugation (Maussang et al., 2016). Marteen et al. prepared glutathione-targeted PEGylated liposome for brain delivery of amyloid β antibody to facilitate the entry into brain. Glutathione PEGylated liposome increases the drug retention time and reduces the rapid clearance of antibody, thereby enhancing the drug efficacy, while the glutathione ligand ensures drug targeting into brain. Hence, the study proves that G-Technology® offers an effective carrier for drug delivery into the brain (Rotman et al., 2015). Glutathione conjugation facilitates the drug transport across the BBB, while PEGylation prolongs the liposomal retention time in the blood and at the same time offers a biocompatible carrier system (Kannan et al., 2000, 1990; Zlokovic et al., 1994). Lindqvist et al. prepared glutathione-conjugated PEGylated liposomes for improved brain targeting of an opioid peptide DAMGO, to study the effectiveness of glutathione-conjugated drug carrier in efficient brain delivery and the pharmacokinetic and pharmacodynamic behavior of DAMGO in animal model (Lindqvist et al., 2013; Gaillard, 2010a; Gaillard et al., 2012; Hammarlund-Udenaes et al., 2008; Gupta et al., 2006). However, in contrast with the other work in G-Technology®, the present study suggests that ligand-mediated brain targeting does not inevitably need increased brain uptake of drug substances.

The glutathione transporter pathway has been also exploited in the construction of other types of nano drug delivery systems, including glutathione-modified PLGA nanoparticles loaded with paclitaxel (Geldenhuys et al., 2011) or docetaxel (Grover et al., 2014). The glutathione-coated nanoparticles will give enhanced drug transport via brain by either a facilitated transport or increased passive diffusion due to an increased concentration gradient at the BBB interface (Geldenhuys et al., 2011). Geldenhuys et al. developed glutathione-coated PLGA-PEG nanoparticles loaded with doxorubicin for the treatment of brain tumor. In this study, glutathione was used as ligand to enable CMT of nanoparticles across the BBB. Doxorubicin was potentially delivered into tumor cells, spreading light on the possible future applications of glutathione-modified nanocarriers for brain tumor targeting (Geldenhuys et al., 2015a).

4.4 Monocarboxylic acid transport systems

The monocarboxylic acid transport systems (MCTs) can transport lactate, pyruvate, short-chain monocarboxylic acids such as acetic acid, and ketone bodies such as β-hydroxybutyric acid and acetoacetate, which are essential for brain metabolism (Pardridge, 1995). Salicylic acid and valproic acid showed significant competitive inhibitory effects on the transport of acetic acid on both in vitro and in vivo levels. However, dicarboxylic acids and tricarboxylic acids were not inhibitory (Terasaki et al., 1991; Kang et al., 1990b; Tamai and Tsuji, 1996). These results suggest that acidic drugs bearing a monocarboxylic acid moiety may cross the BBB via the MCTs (Tsuji and Tamai, 1999a,b). Simvastatin acid, lovastatin acid, and pravastatin, all of which contain a carboxylic acid moiety, have been shown to be transported by MCTs at the BBB (Tsuji et al., 1993; Saheki et al., 1994).

The MCTs have 14 members (Halestrap and Meredith, 2004). Of these 14 family members, only MCT1 to 4 are found in brain and have been definitively shown to transport metabolically relevant monocarboxylic acids. However, MCT2 protein expression was definitively localized to neurons in intact brain. MCT3 expression is limited to choroid plexus and the pigment epithelial cells of the retina where it is abundant. While MCT4 is widely distributed in rodent brain and yet appears to be localized exclusively to astrocytes (Halestrap and Meredith, 2004), expression in human brain is not mentioned. In addition, MCT4 has the affinity for both lactate (K_m 28 mM) and pyruvate (K_m 150 mM) significantly low than that of MCT1 to 3.

MCT1 has been identified at the BBB as well as in various tissues (Takanaga et al., 1995). Recently, MCT1 was found on both the luminal and abluminal membranes of brain capillary endothelial cells (Gerhart et al., 1997). MCT1 at the BBB functions for the bi-directional transport of lactic acid and other monocarboxylate compounds. Since a Na^+/H^+ exchanger exists at the luminal membrane of the brain capillary endothelial cells (Ennis et al., 1996), protons are expected to provide the driving force to MCT1 for the enhanced transport of monocarboxylates across the BBB from blood to brain extracellular fluid. The abundance of MCT1 in cerebral microvessels of suckling rats suggests an important role of the transporter in the delivery of energy substrates to the neonatal brain (Gerhart et al., 1997). Under normal physiological conditions in adult rats, however, this MCT1 presumably facilitates efflux of lactate, which is produced from glucose in the brain, from the brain into blood.

Another monocarboxylate valproic acid is known to inhibit the BBB transport of lactate, pyruvate, and short-chain fatty acids such as acetate; the uptake of valproic acid at the BBB into the brain was demonstrated to be mediated via a medium-chain fatty acid transporter (Adkison and Shen, 1996). The apparent Michaelis constant for the saturable process ranged from 10 mM in the cortical regions to 23 mM in the thalamus (Tsuji and Tamai, 1999a,b). The uptake of valproic acid was not inhibited by short-chain (less than C_4) fatty acids, but was significantly inhibited by medium-chain (C_6–C_{12}) fatty acids, suggesting that the short-chain monocarboxylate transporter at the BBB is not involved in the luminal uptake of valproic acid. *Para*-amino-hippuric acid inhibited the uptake of valproic acid (Adkison and Shen, 1996). These observations indicate that the putative valproic acid transporter at the BBB may be an anion exchanger that operates in a manner similar to that reported for the *Para*-amino-hippuric acid transporter, OAT1, expressed at the basolateral membrane of the renal tubular epithelium (Sekine et al., 1997). Although OAT is exclusively expressed in the kidney, an OAT family member may exist at the BBB.

The limitation for CMT via MCT1 across the BBB from blood to brain is that the molecular weight of the monocarboxylate moiety should be less than 200 kDa. Substrates including nicotinic acid, salicylic acid, benzoic acid, and butyrate satisfy this requirement and may be transported by MCT1 across the BBB (Kang et al., 1990b).

Aromatic short-chain fatty acid, 4-phenylbutyrate, is a small molecule drug. The investigation of 4-phenylbutyrate transportation across the BBB demonstrated that CMT via MCT1 may be an efficient penetration pathway for brain penetration. This finding has clinical significance in designing targeted drug delivery to brain (Lee and Kang, 2016). Similar results were found as to aluminum citrate and γ-hydroxy butyrate.

In fact, nano drug delivery systems have been developed to be modified with MCT1-related substrates for transportation across the BBB. Venishetty et al. explored β-hydroxybutyric acid grafted solid lipid nanoparticles and demonstrated that the transportation of this nano drug delivery system relied on the transport of the ligand β-hydroxybutyric acid by MCT1. Increased and saturable uptake was revealed for β-hydroxybutyric acid grafted solid lipid nanoparticles in brain endothelial cells and in brain tissue. β-Hydroxybutyric acid present on the surface of solid lipid nanoparticles caused the nanoparticles to be taken up by MCT1 transporter as normal β-hydroxybutyric acid and improved the brain uptake of loaded drug compared with unmodified solid lipid nanoparticles (Venishetty et al., 2013). Devi et al. developed lactic acid-conjugated solid lipid nanoparticles bearing both albendazole and prednisolone for effective management of neurocysticercosis. Transendothelial transport study depicted selective brain uptake of lactic acid-conjugated solid lipid nanoparticles compared to solid lipid nanoparticles attributed to CMT via MCT transporter. Organ distribution studies reflected high accumulation of drugs in the brain in case of lactic acid-conjugated solid lipid nanoparticles as compared to plain drugs solution (Devi et al., 2015). So substrates of MCT1 can play important roles in the brain transportation of drug or drug delivery systems.

4.5 Amine transport systems

The transport mechanisms for amine drugs have not yet been well-elucidated. CMT may participate in the influx of several amine drugs (Tsuji and Tamai, 1999a, b). An endogenous hydrophilic amine, choline, is taken up by amine transport systems, more accurately, choline transporter. Uptake of choline was inhibited by amine compounds such as eperisone, scopolamine, thiamine, isoproterenol, and hemicholinium-3, whereas zwitterionic or anionic compounds were not inhibitory (Kang et al., 1990a). For the BBB transport of amine compounds, there are at least two different CMT mechanisms specific to choline and amine drugs (Tsuji and Tamai, 1999a,b). Nevertheless, the molecular mechanism(s) of the process still needs to be fully investigated.

Acetylcholine is an endogenous hydrophilic amine. However, brain cannot synthesize acetylcholine by itself. Choline is a biochemical precursor of the neurotransmitter acetylcholine and other essential components of cell membrane phospholipids such as phosphatidylcholine. So choline transporter is expressed at the BBB to mediate the transport of acetylcholine. Besides the expression in the brain endothelial cells, the choline transporter is expressed at choroid plexus as well. Choline influx via choline transporter at the BBB regulates the formation of acetylcholine in the CNS. The uptake of choline to brain has been found to be saturable, with high-affinity K_m at

0.22 mM. The high choline concentration in the brain demonstrates the amazing ability of the BBB choline transporter to transport choline across the BBB (Zeisel, 2004; Allen and Smith, 2001). Furthermore, the low physiologic plasma concentration of choline (approximately 25% of the K_m for the binding of choline with choline transporter) makes the BBB choline transporter free to transport choline derivates without interrupting the supply of choline to the CNS (Allen and Lockman, 2003). Therefore, the BBB choline transporter is considered a potential target for active drug delivery into the CNS.

As a very effective approach, a choline derivate with high choline transporter affinity had been coupled to polymeric nanoparticles for preparing a BBB targeting vector (Li et al., 2013a). Li et al. conjugated choline to the surface of nanoparticles with co-delivery of doxorubicin and therapeutic gene and found great BBB penetration and high cellular uptake (Li et al., 2013a). In another research, Li et al. used choline derivatives as ligands for mediating gene delivery into brain and proved choline transporter-mediated significant high accumulation of nanoparticles in brain (Li et al., 2011). Glioma is the very common type of the CNS cancer in adults and lethal in children. Gadolium chelate contrast-enhanced magnetic resonance imaging is the most preferred technique to diagnose glioma. Choline derivatives were also used to modify dendrimer-based magnetic resonance imaging nano contrast agents for enhanced penetration of the BBB and glioma diagnosis. In this work, choline transporter was used for the CMT of modified nanoprobes to facilitate the glioma detection (Li et al., 2013b). From the above results, it can be seen that the utilization of choline derivatives as targeting ligands can build up efficient nano drug delivery systems and could make a promising strategy for drug delivery to treat the CNS manifestations.

4.6 Carnitine transporter

In brain capillary endothelial cells, there exists a saturable L-carnitine transport system OCTN2 (Tsuji and Tamai, 1999a,b). OCTN2 is highly expressed in brain capillary endothelial cells of the BBB (Kido et al., 2001a; Miecz et al., 2008; Berezowski et al., 2004; Inano et al., 2003). OCTN2 takes up L-carnitine in a Na^+-dependent manner. Luminal uptake of L-carnitine through the saturable system can be inhibited by butyrobetaine, whereas the abluminal uptake of L-carnitine was diminished by phenylalanine, leucine, and L-system inhibitors. It seems that L-carnitine enters the brain through the luminal membrane of the BBB via OCTN2 and effluxes through the abluminal membrane of the BBB via amino acid transport systems (Mroczkowska et al., 1997). OCTN2 also exists abundantly in kidney, skeletal muscle, heart, and placenta (Tamai et al., 1998).

L-Carnitine is a small molecule absolutely obligatory for β-oxidation of long-chain fatty acids in mitochondria (Wu et al., 1998; Tamai et al., 1998). Even though brain cells do not utilize β-oxidation of fatty acids to any significant extent to generate energy, acetyl-L-carnitine plays a critical role in brain function and energy status (Inano et al., 2003; Virmani and Binienda, 2004). OCTN2 at the BBB facilitates the transfer of this important metabolite from systemic circulation to brain across the BBB. Pharmacological treatment of patients with Alzheimer's disease is becoming more important and acyl-L-carnitines are one group of candidate drugs. Cerebrospinal fluid levels of acetyl-L-carnitine achieved under treatment were significantly higher than those at baseline, reflecting a good penetration through the BBB (Tsuji and Tamai, 1999a,b).

L-Carnitine-conjugated prodrugs have been studied to overcome the BBB and enhance drug accumulation in brain using OCTN2-mediated pathway (Napolitano et al., 2009). OCTN2 is also highly expressed in glioblastoma multiforme. As such, OCTN2 could be exploited as a portal for designing nano drug delivery systems to facilitate drug permeation across the BBB and also to selectively target glioma cells (Kou et al., 2017a). Kou et al. prepared L-carnitine-modified PLGA nanoparticles and demonstrated that L-carnitine-mediated recognition and internalization into the BBB endothelial cells via OCTN2 significantly facilitated the transcytosis of nanoparticles across the BBB. L-Carnitine-modified nanoparticles mainly employed caveolin- and clathrin-co-dependent endocytosis, and macropinocytosis, strongly implicating that OCTN2-mediated endocytosis are involved in the cellular uptake (Kou et al., 2017a,b, 2013). The accumulation of loaded paclitaxel in brain was significantly increased by L-carnitine, indicating that OCTN2 was an effective target for nano drug delivery systems for enhancing the BBB permeation. These results indicated that L-carnitine-modified PLGA nanoparticles were able to significantly improve brain drug delivery efficacy by targeting OCTN2, providing a promising strategy for brain disease therapy (Kou et al., 2017a,b, 2013).

5 Conclusion and perspective

The transportation of therapeutics across the BBB has been one of the most challenging parts while designing brain-targeted drug delivery systems for treating the CNS diseases. A great deal of previous work on drug delivery to the brain has been directed to the strategies of, (i) adding lipophilicity to candidate drugs, on the assumption that transport of drugs across the lipoidal membrane barrier of brain capillary endothelial cells that form the BBB is diffusion-limited. From the viewpoint of drug delivery, designing drugs (including peptides) with greater lipophilicity to enhance their BBB permeation seems to be an easy approach. However, such a strategy would not only increase the permeation into tissues other than brain, but also decrease the bioavailability due to the hepatic first-pass metabolism in the case of oral administration; (ii) conjugating substrates of highly expressed receptors at the BBB onto drug delivery systems or to macromolecule drugs to mediate the BBB crossing via receptor-mediated transcytosis. These efforts have been made to try to overcome the BBB. Indeed, some designs or strategies have been demonstrated successfully for the transportation of therapeutic agents across the BBB. However, the BBB crossing efficiency is still not therapeutically enough for treating the CNS diseases and deeper and more comprehensive investigations are eagerly needed to develop efficient brain-targeted drug delivery systems.

A detailed understanding of the uptake and efflux mechanisms at the BBB would be very helpful for targeting drugs to the brain to provide the expected CNS pharmacological effect. Accordingly, for the development of brain-specific drug delivery systems for neuroactive drugs, it may be effective to utilize the specific transport mechanisms at the BBB. The main strategy is to conjugate substrates of highly expressed transporters at the BBB to synthesize prodrugs or onto drug delivery systems to mediate the BBB crossing via CMT. Prodrug approach and nano drug delivery systems modified with substrates of related transporters (e.g., GLUT1, LAT1) have been extensively investigated for drug delivery to the CNS. Various methods using CMT for the BBB crossing and brain penetration of small molecules and nano drug delivery systems have been reviewed in this chapter. This review presented here provide strong support to the idea that plasma membrane transporters represent ideal portals for targeting nano drug delivery system for enhanced BBB crossing and brain penetration.

In should be also noted that there exist some limitations or controversies for CMT of nano drug delivery system across the BBB: (i) the exposure of various other organs to the drugs encapsulated in transporter-targeted drug delivery systems because of the expression of the transporters in other tissues as well. Additional more subtle designs are needed to prevent the off-target exposure of the drugs; (ii) CMT transporters can only transport molecules with similar structure and size to their natural substrates. Since CMT systems are typically small, stereospecific pores, they are not particularly suitable to the transport of large-molecule therapeutics (Pottiez et al., 2009). For example, the molecular weight of the monocarboxylate moiety should be less than 200 kDa, to be successfully transported across the BBB via MCT1; (iii) the transporter targeting may interrupt the supply of the CNS; (iv) some substrates of the CMT transporters have serious adverse effects if administered into human blood circulation (e.g., cocaine, nicotine, valporic acid); and (v) conjugation of ligands (substrates) to nano drug delivery system may result in low affinity for targeted transporters as compared to the free substrates.

References

Abbott, N.J., Patabendige, A.A., Dolman, D.E., Yusof, S.R., Begley, D.J., 2010. Structure and function of the blood-brain barrier. Neurobiol. Dis. 37, 13–25.

Adkison, K.D., Shen, D.D., 1996. Uptake of valproic acid into rat brain is mediated by a medium-chain fatty acid transporter. J. Pharmacol. Exp. Ther. 276, 1189–1200.

Agarwal, S., Sane, R., Oberoi, R., Ohlfest, J.R., Elmquist, W.F., 2011. Delivery of molecularly targeted therapy to malignant glioma, a disease of the whole brain. Expert Rev. Mol. Med. 13, e17. https://doi.org/10.1017/S1462399411001888.

Agrawal, M., Ajazuddin, Tripathi, D. K., Saraf, S., Saraf, S., Antimisiaris, S. G., et al., 2017. Recent advancements in liposomes targeting strategies to cross blood-brain barrier (BBB) for the treatment of Alzheimer's disease. J. Control. Release 260, 61-77.

Ajazuddin, Alexander, A., Khan, J., Giri, T. K., Tripathi, D. K., Saraf, S., et al., 2012. Advancement in stimuli triggered in situ gelling delivery for local and systemic route. Expert Opin. Drug Deliv. 9, 1573-1592.

Alexander, A., Dwivedi, S., Ajazuddin, Giri, T.K., Saraf, S., Saraf, S., et al., 2012. Approaches for breaking the barriers of drug permeation through transdermal drug delivery. J. Control. Release 164, 26–40.

Alexander, A., Ajazuddin, Khan, J., Saraf, S., Saraf, S., 2013. Poly(ethylene glycol)-poly(lactic-co-glycolic acid) based thermosensitive injectable hydrogels for biomedical applications. J. Control. Release 172, 715–729.
Alexander, A., Ajazuddin, Khan, J., Saraf, S., Saraf, S., 2014. Polyethylene glycol (PEG)-poly (N-isopropylacrylamide) (PNIPAAm) based thermosensitive injectable hydrogels for biomedical applications. Eur. J. Pharm. Biopharm. 88, 575–585.
Alexander, A., Ajazuddin, Patel, R.J., Saraf, S., Saraf, S., 2016. Recent expansion of pharmaceutical nanotechnologies and targeting strategies in the field of phytopharmaceuticals for the delivery of herbal extracts and bioactives. J. Control. Release 241, 110–124.
Allen, D.D., Smith, Q.R., 2001. Characterization of the blood-brain barrier choline transporter using the in situ rat brain perfusion technique. J. Neurochem. 76, 1032–1041.
Allen, D.D., Lockman, P.R., 2003. The blood-brain barrier choline transporter as a brain drug delivery vector. Life Sci. 73, 1609–1615.
Allen, T.M., Cullis, P.R., 2004. Drug delivery systems: entering the mainstream. Science 303, 1818–1822.
Béduneau, A., Saulnier, P., Benoit, J.P., 2007. Active targeting of brain tumors using nanocarriers. Biomaterials 28, 4947–4967.
Barar, J., Rafi, M.A., Pourseif, M.M., Omidi, Y., 2016. Blood-brain barrier transport machineries and targeted therapy of brain diseases. Bioimpacts 6, 225–248.
Berezowski, V., Miecz, D., Marszałek, M., Bröer, A., Bröer, S., Cecchelli, R., et al., 2004. Involvement of OCTN2 and B0,+ in the transport of carnitine through an in vitro model of the blood-brain barrier. J. Neurochem. 91, 860–872.
Battaglia, G., La Russa, M., Bruno, V., Arenare, L., Ippolito, R., Copani, A., et al., 2000. Systemically administered D-glucose conjugates of 7-chlorokynurenic acid are centrally available and exert anticonvulsant activity in rodents. Brain Res. 860, 149–156.
Benrabh, H., Bourre, J.M., Lefauconnier, J.M., 1995. Taurine transport at the blood-brain barrier: an in vivo brain perfusion study. Brain Res. 692, 57–65.
Benrabh, H., Lefauconnier, J.M., 1996. Glutamate is transported across the rat blood-brain barrier by a sodium-independent system. Neurosci. Lett. 210, 9–12.
Berger, U.V., Hediger, M.A., 1999. Distribution of peptide transporter PEPT2 mRNA in the rat nervous system. Anat. Embryol. 199, 439–449.
Bhunia, S., Vangala, V., Bhattacharya, D., Ravuri, H.G., Kuncha, M., Chakravarty, S., et al., 2017. Large amino acid transporter 1 selective liposomes of L-DOPA functionalized amphiphile for combating glioblastoma. Mol. Pharm. 14, 3834–3847.
Bhutia, Y.D., Babu, E., Prasad, P.D., Ganapathy, V., 2014. The amino acid transporter SLC6A14 in cancer and its potential use in chemotherapy. Asian J. Pharm. Sci. 9, 293–303.
Boado, R.J., Li, J.Y., Nagaya, M., Zhang, C., Pardridge, W.M., 1999. Selective expression of the large neutral amino acid transporter at the blood-brain barrier. Proc. Nat. Acad. Sci. U. S. A. 96, 12079–12084.
Cardoso, F.L., Brites, D., Brito, M.A., 2010. Looking at the blood-brain barrier: molecular anatomy and possible investigation approaches. Brain Res. Rev. 64, 328–363.
Ceballos, A., Belinchon, M.M., Sanchez-Mendoza, E., Grijota-Martinez, C., Dumitrescu, A.M., Refetoff, S., et al., 2009. Importance of monocarboxylate transporter 8 for the blood-brain barrier-dependent availability of 3,5,3′-triiodo-L-thyronine. Endocrinology 150, 2491–2496.
Conn, A.R., Fell, D.I., Steele, R.D., 1983. Characterization of alpha-keto acid transport across blood-brain barrier in rats. Am. J. Physiol. 245, E253–260.
Dashora, K., Saraf, S., Saraf, S., 2006. In vitro studies of tizanidine controlled-release microcapsular matrices. Pak. J. Pharm. Sci. 19, 177–181.

Devi, R., Jain, A., Hurkat, P., Jain, S.K., 2015. Dual drug delivery using lactic acid conjugated SLN for effective management of neurocysticercosis. Pharm. Res. 32, 3137–3148.
Dick, A.P., Harik, S.I., Klip, A., Walker, D.M., 1984. Identification and characterization of the glucose transporter of the blood-brain barrier by cytochalasin B binding and immunological reactivity. Proc. Nat. Acad. Sci. U. S. A. 81, 7233–7237.
Du, D., Chang, N., Sun, S., Li, M., Yu, H., Liu, M., et al., 2014. The role of glucose transporters in the distribution of p-aminophenyl-α-D-mannopyranoside modified liposomes within mice brain. J. Control. Release 182, 99–110.
Ennis, S.R., Ren, X.D., Betz, A.L., 1996. Mechanisms of sodium transport at the blood-brain barrier studied with in situ perfusion of rat brain. J. Neurochem. 66, 756–763.
Bonina, F., Puglia, C., Rimoli, M.G., Melisi, D., Boatto, G., Nieddu, M., et al., 2003. Glycosyl derivatives of dopamine and L-DOPA as anti-Parkinson prodrugs: synthesis, pharmacological activity and in vitro stability studies. J. Drug Target. 11, 25–36.
Gaillard, P.J., 2010a. Crossing barriers from blood-to-brain and academia-to-industry. Ther. Deliv. 1, 495–500.
Gaillard, P. J., 2010b. Glutathione-based drug delivery system. PCT Int. Appl. 52pp. CODEN: PIXXD2 WO 2010095940 A2 20100826.
Gaillard, P.J., Visser, C.C., Appeldoorn, C.C.M., Rip, J., 2012. Enhanced brain drug delivery: safely crossing the blood-brain barrier. Drug Discov. Today Technol. 9, e155–e160.
Gaillard, P.J., Appeldoorn, C.C., Dorland, R., van Kregten, J., Manca, F., Vugts, D.J., et al., 2014a. Pharmacokinetics, brain delivery, and efficacy in brain tumor-bearing mice of glutathione pegylated liposomal doxorubicin (2B3-101). PLoS One. 9, e82331. https://doi.org/10.1371/journal.pone.0082331.
Gaillard, P. J., Visser, C. C., Boer, M. D., Appeldoorn, C. C. M., Rip, J., 2014b. Blood-to-Brain Drug Delivery Using Nanocarriers. Springer, New York.
Geier, E.G., Chen, E.C., Webb, A., Papp, A.C., Yee, S.W., Sadee, W., et al., 2013. Profiling solute carrier transporters in the human blood-brain barrier. Clin. Pharmacol. Therap. 94, 636–639.
Geldenhuys, W., Mbimba, T., Bui, T., Harrison, K., Sutariya, V., 2011. Brain-targeted delivery of paclitaxel using glutathione-coated nanoparticles for brain cancers. J. Drug Target. 19, 837–845.
Geldenhuys, W., Wehrung, D., Groshev, A., Hirani, A., Sutariya, V., 2015a. Brain-targeted delivery of doxorubicin using glutathione-coated nanoparticles for brain cancers. Pharm. Dev. Technol. 20, 497–506.
Geldenhuys, W.J., Mohammad, A.S., Adkins, C.E., Lockman, P.R., 2015b. Molecular determinants of blood-brain barrier permeation. Ther. Deliv. 6, 961–971.
Gerhart, D.Z., Enerson, B.E., Zhdankina, O.Y., Leino, R.L., Drewes, L.R., 1997. Expression of monocarboxylate transporter MCT1 by brain endothelium and glia in adult and suckling rats. Am. J. Physiol. 273, E207–213.
Grover, A., Hirani, A., Pathak, Y., Sutariya, V., 2014. Brain-targeted delivery of docetaxel by glutathione-coated nanoparticles for brain cancer. AAPS PharmSciTech 15, 1562–1568.
Gupta, A., Chatelain, P., Massingham, R., Jonsson, E.N., Hammarlund-Udenaes, M., 2006. Brain distribution of cetirizine enantiomers: comparison of three different tissue-to-plasma partition coefficients: K(p), K(p,u), and K(p,uu). Drug Metab. Dispos. 34, 318–323.
Halestrap, A.P., Meredith, D., 2004. The SLC16 gene family-from monocarboxylate transporters (MCTs) to aromatic amino acid transporters and beyond. Pflügers Arch. 447, 619–628.
Halestrap, A.P., 2013. Monocarboxylic acid transport. Compr. Physiol. 3, 1611–1643.

Hammarlund-Udenaes, M., Fridén, M., Syvänen, S., Gupta, A., 2008. On the rate and extent of drug delivery to the brain. Pharm. Res. 25, 1737–1750.

Han, L., Kong, D.K., Zheng, M.Q., Murikinati, S., Ma, C., Yuan, P., et al., 2016. Increased nanoparticle delivery to brain tumors by autocatalytic priming for improved treatment and imaging. ACS Nano 10, 4209–4218.

Hao, Z.F., Cui, Y.X., Li, M.H., Du, D., Liu, M.F., Tao, H.Q., et al., 2013. Liposomes modified with P-aminophenyl-α-D-mannopyranoside: a carrier for targeting cerebral functional regions in mice. Eur. J. Pharm. Biopharm. 84, 505–516.

Hosoya, K., Tomi, M., Ohtsuki, S., Takanaga, H., Saeki, S., Kanai, Y., et al., 2002. Enhancement of L-cystine transport activity and its relation to xCT gene induction at the blood-brain barrier by diethyl maleate treatment. J. Pharmacol. Exp. Ther. 302, 225–231.

Inano, A., Sai, Y., Nikaido, H., Hasimoto, N., Asano, M., Tsuji, A., et al., 2003. Acetyl-L-carnitine permeability across the blood-brain barrier and involvement of carnitine transporter OCTN2. Biopharm. Drug Dispos. 24, 357–365.

Jiang, X., Xin, H., Ren, Q., Gu, J., Zhu, L., Du, F., et al., 2014. Nanoparticles of 2-deoxy-D-glucose functionalized poly(ethylene glycol)-co-poly(trimethylene carbonate) for dual-targeted drug delivery in glioma treatment. Biomaterials 35, 518–529.

Kageyama, T., Nakamura, M., Matsuo, A., Yamasaki, Y., Takakura, Y., Hashida, M., et al., 2000. The 4F2hc/LAT1 complex transports L-DOPA across the blood-brain barrier. Brain Res. 879, 115–121.

Kaira, K., Oriuchi, N., Imai, H., Shimizu, K., Yanagitani, N., Sunaga, N., et al., 2008a. L-type amino acid transporter 1 and CD98 expression in primary and metastatic sites of human neoplasms. Cancer Sci. 99, 2380–2386.

Kaira, K., Oriuchi, N., Imai, H., Shimizu, K., Yanagitani, N., Sunaga, N., et al., 2008b. Prognostic significance of L-type amino acid transporter 1 expression in resectable stage I–III nonsmall cell lung cancer. Br. J. Cancer 98, 742–748.

Kanai, Y., Segawa, H., Miyamoto, K., Uchino, H., Takeda, E., Endou, H., 1998. Expression cloning and characterization of a transporter for large neutral amino acids activated by the heavy chain of 4F2 antigen (CD98). J. Biol. Chem. 273, 23629–23632.

Kanai, Y., Endou, H., 2003. Functional properties of multispecific amino acid transporters and their implications to transporter-mediated toxicity. J. Toxicol. Sci. 28, 1–17.

Kang, Y.S., Terasaki, T., Ohnishi, T., Tsuji, A., 1990a. In vivo and in vitro evidence for a common carrier mediated transport of choline and basic drugs through the blood-brain barrier. J. Pharmacobiodyn. 13, 353–360.

Kang, Y.S., Terasaki, T., Tsuji, A., 1990b. Acidic drug transport in vivo through the blood-brain barrier. A role of the transport carrier for monocarboxylic acids. J. Pharmacobiodyn. 13, 158–163.

Kannan, R., Kuhlenkamp, J.F., Jeandidier, E., Trinh, H., Ookhtens, M., Kaplowitz, N., 1990. Evidence for carrier-mediated transport of glutathione across the blood-brain barrier in the rat. J. Clin. Invest. 85, 2009–2013.

Kannan, R., Chakrabarti, R., Tang, D., Kim, K.J., Kaplowitz, N., 2000. GSH transport in human cerebrovascular endothelial cells and human astrocytes: evidence for luminal localization of Na^+-dependent GSH transport in HCEC. Brain Res. 852, 374–382.

Karlsson, C., Mäepea, O., Alm, A., 1984. Choline transport through the blood-retinal and the blood-brain barrier in vivo. Acta Ophthalmol. 62, 763–766.

Kaur, I.P., Bhandari, R., Bhandari, S., Kakkar, V., 2008. Potential of solid lipid nanoparticles in brain targeting. J. Control. Release 127, 97–109.

Kharya, P., Jain, A., Gulbake, A., Shilpi, S., Jain, A., Hurkat, P., et al., 2013. Phenylalanine-coupled solid lipid nanoparticles for brain tumor targeting. J. Nanopart. Res. 15, 1228–1230.

Kido, Y., Tamai, I., Ohnari, A., Sai, Y., Kagami, T., Nezu, J., et al., 2001a. Functional relevance of carnitine transporter OCTN2 to brain distribution of L-carnitine and acetyl-L-carnitine across the blood-brain barrier. J. Neurochem. 79, 959–969.

Kido, Y., Tamai, I., Uchino, H., Suzuki, F., Sai, Y., Tsuji, A., 2001b. Molecular and functional identification of large neutral amino acid transporters LAT1 and LAT2 and their pharmacological relevance at the blood-brain barrier. J. Pharm. Pharmacol. 53, 497–503.

Killian, D.M., Hermeling, S., Chikhale, P.J., 2007. Targeting the cerebrovascular large neutral amino acid transporter (LAT1) isoform using a novel disulfide-based brain drug delivery system. Drug Deliv. 14, 25–31.

Kim, D.K., Kanai, Y., Choi, H.W., Tangtrongsup, S., Chairoungdua, A., Babu, E., et al., 2002. Characterization of the system L-amino acid transporter in T24 human bladder carcinoma cells. Biochim. Biophys. Acta 1565, 112–121.

Kobayashi, K., Ohnishi, A., Promsuk, J., Shimizu, S., Kanai, Y., Shiokawa, Y., et al., 2008. Enhanced tumor growth elicited by L-type amino acid transporter 1 in human malignant glioma cells. Neurosurgery 62, 493–503.

Komura, J., Tamai, I., Senmaru, M., Terasaki, T., Sai, Y., Tsuji, A., 1997. Brain-to-blood active transport of β-alanine across the blood-brain barrier. FEBS Lett. 400, 131–135.

Koshkaryev, A., Sawant, R., Deshpande, M., Torchilin, V., 2013. Immunoconjugates and long circulating systems: origins, current state of the art and future directions. Adv. Drug Deliv. Rev. 65, 24–35.

Kou, L., Sun, J., Zhai, Y., He, Z., 2013. The endocytosis and intracellular fate of nanomedicines: implication for rational design. Asian J. Pharm. Sci. 8, 1–10.

Kou, L., Hou, Y., Yao, Q., Guo, W., Wang, G., Wang, M., et al., 2017a. L-Carnitine-conjugated nanoparticles to promote permeation across blood-brain barrier and to target glioma cells for drug delivery via the novel organic cation/carnitine transporter OCTN2. Artif. Cells Nanomed. Biotechnol. 1–12. https://doi.org/10.1080/21691401.2017.1384385.

Kou, L., Yao, Q., Sun, M., Wu, C., Wang, J., Luo, Q., et al., 2017b. Cotransporting ion is a trigger for cellular endocytosis of transporter-targeting nanoparticles: a case study of high-efficiency SLC22A5 (OCTN2)-mediated carnitine-conjugated nanoparticles for oral delivery of therapeutic drugs. Adv. Healthc. Mater. 6(17). https://doi.org/10.1002/adhm.201700165.

Krizbai, I.A., Nyúltóth, Á., Bauer, H.C., Farkas, A.E., Traweger, A., Haskó, J., et al., 2016. Pharmaceutical targeting of the brain. Curr. Pharm. Des. 22, 5442–5462.

Kuo, Y.C., Lee, C.H., 2015. Inhibition against growth of glioblastoma multiforme in vitro using etoposide-loaded solid lipid nanoparticles with p-aminophenyl-α-D-manno-pyranoside and folic acid. J. Pharm. Sci. 104, 1804–1814.

Lee, N.Y., Kang, Y.S., 2016. In vivo and in vitro evidence for brain uptake of 4-phenylbutyrate by the monocarboxylate transporter 1 (MCT1). Pharm. Res. 33, 1711–1722.

Li, J., Zhou, L., Ye, D., Huang, S., Shao, K., Huang, R., et al., 2011. Choline-derivate-modified nanoparticles for brain-targeting gene delivery. Adv. Mater. 23, 4516–4520.

Li, J., Guo, Y., Kuang, Y., An, S., Ma, H., Jiang, C., 2013a. Choline transporter-targeting and co-delivery system for glioma therapy. Biomaterials 34, 9142–9148.

Li, J., Huang, S., Shao, K., Liu, Y., An, S., Kuang, Y., et al., 2013b. A choline derivate-modified nanoprobe for glioma diagnosis using MRI. Sci. Rep. 31623. https://doi.org/10.1038/srep01623.

Liang, H. F., Chen, Y. C., Yang, T. F., Chang, L. W., Wang, A. J., Lu, J. M., et al., 2010. Glutathione-based delivery system. U.S. Pat. Appl. Publ. 18pp., Cont.-in-part of U.S. Ser. No. 303,934.

Lin, K.H., Hong, S.T., Wang, H.T., Lo, Y.L., Lin, A.M., Yang, J.C., 2016a. Enhancing anticancer effect of gefitinib across the blood-brain barrier model using liposomes modified with one α-helical cell-penetrating peptide or glutathione and Tween 80. Int. J. Mol. Sci. 17, E1998. https://doi.org/10.3390/ijms17121998.

Lin, L., Di, X., Zhang, S., Kan, Q., Hao, L., Lu, T., et al., 2016b. Large amino acid transporter 1 mediated glutamate modified docetaxel-loaded liposomes for glioma targeting. Colloids Surf. B Biointerfaces 141, 260–267.

Lindqvist, A., Rip, J., Gaillard, P.J., Björkman, S., Hammarlundudenaes, M., 2013. Enhanced brain delivery of the opioid peptide DAMGO in glutathione pegylated liposomes: a microdialysis study. Mol. Pharm. 10, 1533–1541.

Lindqvist, A., Rip, J., van Kregten, J., Gaillard, P.J., Hammarlund-Udenaes, M., 2016. In vivo functional evaluation of increased brain delivery of the opioid peptide DAMGO by glutathione-PEGylated liposomes. Pharm. Res. 33, 177–185.

Liu, C.C., Shen, Z., Kung, H.F., Lin, M.C., 2006. Cancer gene therapy targeting angiogenesis: an updated review. World J. Gastroenterol. 12, 6941–6948.

Liu, J., He, Y., Zhang, J., Li, J., Yu, X., Cao, Z., et al., 2016. Functionalized nanocarrier combined seizure-specific vector with P-glycoprotein modulation property for antiepileptic drug delivery. Biomaterials 74, 64–76.

Liu, Y., Lu, W., 2012. Recent advances in brain tumor-targeted nano-drug delivery systems. Expert Opin. Drug Deliv. 9, 671–686.

Cruz, L.J., Tacken, P.J., Fokkink, R., Figdor, C.G., 2011. The influence of PEG chain length and targeting moiety on antibody-mediated delivery of nanoparticle vaccines to human dendritic cells. Biomaterials 32, 6791–6803.

Mantych, G.J., James, D.E., Devaskar, S.U., 1993. Jejunal/kidney glucose transporter isoform (Glut-5) is expressed in the human blood-brain barrier. Endocrinology 132, 35–40.

Markoutsa, E., Pampalakis, G., Niarakis, A., Romero, I.A., Weksler, B., Couraud, P.O., et al., 2011. Uptake and permeability studies of BBB-targeting immunoliposomes using the hCMEC/D3 cell line. Eur. J. Pharm. Biopharm. 77, 265–274.

Markoutsa, E., Papadia, K., Giannou, A.D., Spella, M., Cagnotto, A., Salmona, M., et al., 2014. Mono and dually decorated nanoliposomes for brain targeting, in vitro and in vivo studies. Pharm. Res. 31, 1275–1289.

Masereeuw, R., Jaehde, U., Langemeijer, M. W., de Boer, A. G., Breimer, D. D., 1994. in vitro and in vivo transport of zidovudine (AZT) across the blood-brain barrier and the effect of transport inhibitors. Pharm. Res. 11, 324-330.

Matsuo, H., Tsukada, S., Nakata, T., Chairoungdua, A., Kim, D.K., Cha, S.H., et al., 2000. Expression of a system L neutral amino acid transporter at the blood-brain barrier. Neuroreport 11, 3507–3511.

Maussang, D., Rip, J., van Kregten, J., van den Heuvel, A., van der Pol, S., van der Boom, B., et al., 2016. Glutathione conjugation dose-dependently increases brain-specific liposomal drug delivery in vitro and in vivo. Drug Discov. Today Technol. 20, 59–69.

Meier, C., Ristic, Z., Klauser, S., Verrey, F., 2002. Activation of system L heterodimeric amino acid exchangers by intracellular substrates. EMBO J. 21, 580–589.

Miecz, D., Januszewicz, E., Czeredys, M., Hinton, B.T., Berezowski, V., Cecchelli, R., et al., 2008. Localization of organic cation/carnitine transporter (OCTN2) in cells forming the blood-brain barrier. J. Neurochem. 104, 113–123.

Miller, L.P., Oldendorf, W.H., 1986. Regional kinetic constants for blood-brain barrier pyruvic acid transport in conscious rats by the monocarboxylic acid carrier. J. Neurochem. 46, 1412–1416.

Mittapalli, R.K., Manda, V.K., Adkins, C.E., Geldenhuys, W.J., Lockman, P.R., 2010. Exploiting nutrient transporters at the blood-brain barrier to improve brain distribution of small molecules. Ther. Deliv. 1, 775–784.

Morgello, S., Uson, R.R., Schwartz, E.J., Haber, R.S., 1995. The human blood-brain barrier glucose transporter (GLUT1) is a glucose transporter of gray matter astrocytes. Glia 14, 43–54.

Mroczkowska, J.E., Galla, H.J., Nalecz, M.J., Nalecz, K.A., 1997. Evidence for an asymmetrical uptake of L-carnitine in the blood-brain barrier in vitro. Biochem. Biophys. Res. Commun. 241, 127–131.

Murakami, H., Sawada, N., Koyabu, N., Ohtani, H., Sawada, Y., 2000. Characteristics of choline transport across the blood-brain barrier in mice: correlation with in vitro data. Pharm. Res. 17, 1526–1530.

Napolitano, C., Scaglianti, M., Scalambra, E., Manfredini, S., Ferraro, L., Beggiato, S., et al., 2009. Carnitine conjugate of nipecotic acid: a new example of dual prodrug. Molecules 14, 3268–3274.

Nässl, A.M., Rubio-Aliaga, I., Fenselau, H., Marth, M.K., Kottra, G., Daniel, H., 2011. Amino acid absorption and homeostasis in mice lacking the intestinal peptide transporter PEPT1. Am. J. Physiol. Gastrointest. Liver Physiol. 301, G128–137.

Nii, T., Segawa, H., Taketani, Y., Tani, Y., Ohkido, M., Kishida, S., et al., 2001. Molecular events involved in up-regulating human Na^+-independent neutral amino acid transporter LAT1 during T-cell activation. Biochem. J. 358, 693–704.

Noble, G.T., Stefanick, J.F., Ashley, J.D., Kiziltepe, T., Bilgicer, B., 2014. Ligand-targeted liposome design: challenges and fundamental considerations. Trends Biotechnol. 32, 32–45.

Novotny, A., Xiang, J., Stummer, W., Teuscher, N.S., Smith, D.E., Keep, R.F., 2000. Mechanisms of 5-aminolevulinic acid uptake at the choroid plexus. J. Neurochem. 75, 321–328.

O'Kane, R.L., Martínez-López, I., Dejoseph, M.R., Viña, J.R., Hawkins, R.A., 1999. Na(+)-dependent glutamate transporters (EAAT1, EAAT2, and EAAT3) of the blood-brain barrier. A mechanism for glutamate removal. J. Biol. Chem. 274, 31891–31895.

O'Kane, R.L., Viña, J.R., Simpson, I., Zaragozá, R., Mokashi, A., Hawkins, R.A., 2006. Cationic amino acid transport across the blood-brain barrier is mediated exclusively by system y+. Am. J. Physiol. Endocrinol. Metab. 291, E412–419.

Oldendorf, W.H., 1973. Carrier-mediated blood-brain barrier transport of short-chain monocarboxylic organic acids. Am. J. Physiol. 224, 1450–1453.

Pardridge, W.M., Boado, R.J., Farrell, C.R., 1990. Brain-type glucose transporter (GLUT-1) is selectively localized to the blood-brain barrier. Studies with quantitative western blotting and in situ hybridization. J. Biol. Chem. 265, 18035–18040.

Pardridge, W.M., 1995. Transport of small molecules through the blood-brain barrier: biology and methodology. Adv. Drug Deliv. Rev. 15, 5–36.

Pardridge, W.M., 1999. Blood-brain barrier biology and methodology. J. Neurovirol. 5, 556–569.

Pardridge, W.M., 2007. Blood-brain barrier delivery. Drug Discov. Today 12, 54–61.

Pardridge, W.M., 2012. Drug transport across the blood-brain barrier. J. Cereb. Blood Flow Metab. 32, 1959–1972.

Pardridge, W.M., 2015. Blood-brain barrier endogenous transporters as therapeutic targets: a new model for small molecule CNS drug discovery. Expert Opin. Ther. Targets 19, 1059–1072.

Patching, S.G., 2017. Glucose transporters at the blood-brain barrier: function, regulation and gateways for drug delivery. Mol. Neurobiol. 54, 1046–1077.

Peterson, D.R., Sukowski, E.J., Zikos, D., 2013. Blood-brain barrier transport pathways for cytoprotective thiols. Am. J. Ther. 20, 469–479.

Petri, B., Bootz, A., Khalansky, A., Hekmatara, T., Muller, R., Uhl, R., et al., 2007. Chemotherapy of brain turnour using doxorubicin bound to surfactant-coated poly(butyl cyanoacrylate) nanoparticles: revisiting the role of surfactants. J. Control. Release 117, 51–58.

Petros, R.A., DeSimone, J.M., 2010. Strategies in the design of nanoparticles for therapeutic applications. Nat. Rev. Drug Discovery 9, 615–627.

Peura, L., Malmioja, K., Laine, K., Leppänen, J., Gynther, M., Isotalo, A., et al., 2011. Large amino acid transporter 1 (LAT1) prodrugs of valproic acid: new prodrug design ideas for central nervous system delivery. Mol. Pharm. 8, 1857–1866.

Pottiez, G., Flahaut, C., Cecchelli, R., Karamanos, Y., 2009. Understanding the blood-brain barrier using gene and protein expression profiling technologies. Brain Res. Rev. 62, 83–98.

Qin, Y., Fan, W., Chen, H., Yao, N., Tang, W., Tang, J., et al., 2010. In vitro and in vivo investigation of glucose-mediated brain-targeting liposomes. J. Drug Target. 18, 536–549.

Qu, B., Li, X., Guan, M., Li, X., Hai, L., Wu, Y., 2014. Design, synthesis and biological evaluation of multivalent glucosides with high affinity as ligands for brain targeting liposomes. Eur. J. Med. Chem. 72, 110–118.

Rautio, J., Gynther, M., Laine, K., 2013. LAT1-mediated prodrug uptake: a way to breach the blood-brain barrier? Ther. Deliv. 4, 281–284.

Rautio, J., Kärkkäinen, J., Huttunen, K.M., Gynther, M., 2014. Amino acid ester prodrugs conjugated to the α-carboxylic acid group do not display affinity for the L-type amino acid transporter 1 (LAT1). Eur. J. Pharm. Sci. 66, 36–40.

Rip, J., Chen, L., Hartman, R., van den Heuvel, A., Reijerkerk, A., van Kregten, J., et al., 2014. Glutathione PEGylated liposomes: pharmacokinetics and delivery of cargo across the blood-brain barrier in rats. J. Drug Target. 22, 460–467.

Rotman, M., Welling, M.M., Bunschoten, A., de Backer, M.E., Rip, J., Nabuurs, R.J., et al., 2015. Enhanced glutathione PEGylated liposomal brain delivery of an anti-amyloid single domain antibody fragment in a mouse model for Alzheimer's disease. J. Control. Release 203, 40–50.

Saheki, A., Terasaki, T., Tamai, I., Tsuji, A., 1994. In vivo and in vitro blood-brain barrier transport of 3-hydroxy-3-methylglutaryl coenzyme A (HMG-CoA) reductase inhibitors. Pharm. Res. 11, 305–311.

Sahu, S., Saraf, S., Kaur, C.D., Saraf, S., 2013. Biocompatible nanoparticles for sustained topical delivery of anticancer phytoconstituent quercetin. Pak. J. Biol. Sci. 16, 601–609.

Sakaeda, T., Siahaan, T.J., Audus, K.L., Stella, V.J., 2000. Enhancement of transport of D-melphalan analogue by conjugation with L-glutamate across bovine brain microvessel endothelial cell monolayers. J. Drug Target. 8, 195–204.

Sakata, T., Ferdous, G., Tsuruta, T., Satoh, T., Baba, S., Muto, T., et al., 2009. L-type amino-acid transporter 1 as a novel biomarker for high-grade malignancy in prostate cancer. Pathol. Int. 59, 7–18.

Salem, H.F., Ahmed, S.M., Hassaballah, A.E., Omar, M.M., 2015. Targeting brain cells with glutathione-modulated nanoliposomes: in vitro and in vivo study. Drug Des. Devel. Ther. 9, 3705–3727.

Salmaso, S., Pappalardo, J.S., Sawant, R.R., Musacchio, T., Rockwell, K., Caliceti, P., et al., 2009. Targeting glioma cells in vitro with ascorbate-conjugated pharmaceutical nanocarriers. Bioconjug. Chem. 20, 2348–2355.

Schulz, A., Beyhl, D., Marten, I., Wormit, A., Neuhaus, E., Poschet, G., et al., 2011. Proton-driven sucrose symport and antiport are provided by the vacuolar transporters SUC4 and TMT1/2. Plant J. 68, 129–136.

Sekine, T., Watanabe, N., Hosoyamada, M., Kanai, Y., Endou, H., 1997. Expression cloning and characterization of a novel multispecific organic anion transporter. J. Biol. Chem. 272, 18526–18529.
Shao, K., Ding, N., Huang, S., Ren, S., Zhang, Y., Kuang, Y., et al., 2014. Smart nanodevice combined tumor-specific vector with cellular microenvironment-triggered property for highly effective antiglioma therapy. ACS Nano 8, 1191–1203.
Sharma, G., Modgil, A., Layek, B., Arora, K., Sun, C., Law, B., et al., 2013. Cell penetrating peptide tethered bi-ligand liposomes for delivery to brain in vivo: Biodistribution and transfection. J. Control. Release 167, 1–10.
Shi, J., Zhang, H., Chen, Z., Xu, L., Zhang, Z., 2016. A multi-functional nanoplatform for efficacy tumor theranostic applications. Asian J. Pharm. Sci. 12, 235–249.
Simpson, I.A., Carruthers, A., Vannucci, S.J., 2007. Supply and demand in cerebral energy metabolism: the role of nutrient transporters. J. Cereb. Blood Flow Metab. 27, 1766–1791.
Singh, I., Swami, R., Jeengar, M.K., Khan, W., Sistla, R., 2015. p-Aminophenyl-α-D-mannopyranoside engineered lipidic nanoparticles for effective delivery of docetaxel to brain. Chem. Phys. Lipids 188, 1–9.
Singh, I., Swami, R., Khan, W., Sistla, R., 2014. Lymphatic system: a prospective area for advanced targeting of particulate drug carriers. Expert Opin. Drug Deliv. 11, 211–229.
Spuch, C., Navarro, C., 2011. Liposomes for targeted delivery of active agents against neurodegenerative diseases (Alzheimer's disease and Parkinson's disease). J. Drug Deliv. 2011, 469679. https://doi.org/10.1155/2011/469679.
Stoll, J., Wadhwani, K.C., Smith, Q.R., 1993. Identification of the cationic amino acid transporter (System y+) of the rat blood-brain barrier. J. Neurochem. 60, 1956–1959.
Sugawara, M., Huang, W., Fei, Y.J., Leibach, F.H., Ganapathy, V., Ganapathy, M.E., 2000. Transport of valganciclovir, a ganciclovir prodrug, via peptide transporters PEPT1 and PEPT2. J. Pharm. Sci. 89, 781–789.
Takanaga, H., Tamai, I., Inaba, S., Sai, Y., Higashida, H., Yamamoto, H., et al., 1995. cDNA cloning and functional characterization of rat intestinal monocarboxylate transporter. Biochem. Biophys. Res. Commun. 217, 370–377.
Tamai, I., Senmaru, M., Terasaki, T., Tsuji, A., 1995. Na(+)- and Cl(−)-dependent transport of taurine at the blood-brain barrier. Biochem. Pharmacol. 50, 1783–1793.
Tamai, I., Tsuji, A., 1996. Drug delivery through the blood-brain barrier. Adv. Drug Deliv. Rev. 19, 401–424.
Tamai, I., Ohashi, R., Nezu, J., Yabuuchi, H., Oku, A., Shimane, M., et al., 1998. Molecular and functional identification of sodium ion-dependent, high affinity human carnitine transporter OCTN2. J. Biol. Chem. 273, 20378–20382.
Terasaki, T., Takakuwa, S., Moritani, S., Tsuji, A., 1991. Transport of monocarboxylic acids at the blood-brain barrier: studies with monolayers of primary cultured bovine brain capillary endothelial cells. J. Pharmacol. Exp. Ther. 258, 932–937.
Tsuji, A., Saheki, A., Tamai, I., Terasaki, T., 1993. Transport mechanism of 3-hydroxy-3-methylglutaryl coenzyme A reductase inhibitors at the blood-brain barrier. J. Pharmacol. Exp. Ther. 267, 1085–1090.
Tsuji, A., Tamai, I., 1996. Carrier-mediated intestinal transport of drugs. Pharm. Res. 13, 963–977.
Tsuji, A., 1999. Tissue selective drug delivery utilizing carrier-mediated transport systems. J. Control. Release 62, 239–244.
Tsuji, A., Tamai, I., 1999a. Carrier-mediated or specialized transport of drugs across the blood-brain barrier. Adv. Drug Deliv. Rev. 36, 277–290.
Tsuji, A., Tamai, I., 1999b. Organic anion transporters. Pharm. Biotechnol. 12, 471–491.

Tsuji, A., 2005. Small molecular drug transfer across the blood-brain barrier via carrier-mediated transport systems. NeuroRx 2, 54–62.
Umezawa, F., Eto, Y., 1988. Liposome targeting to mouse brain: mannose as a recognition marker. Biochem. Biophys. Res. Commun. 153, 1038–1044.
Venishetty, V.K., Samala, R., Komuravelli, R., Kuncha, M., Sistla, R., Diwan, P.V., 2013. β-Hydroxybutyric acid grafted solid lipid nanoparticles: a novel strategy to improve drug delivery to brain. Nanomedicine 9, 388–397.
Vieira, D.B., Gamarra, L.F., 2016. Getting into the brain: liposome-based strategies for effective drug delivery across the blood-brain barrier. Int. J. Nanomed. 11, 5381–5414.
Virmani, A., Binienda, Z., 2004. Role of carnitine esters in brain neuropathology. Mol. Aspects Med. 25, 533–549.
Vyas, A., Jain, A., Hurkat, P., Jain, A., Jain, S.K., 2015. Targeting of AIDS related encephalopathy using phenylalanine anchored lipidic nanocarrier. Colloids Surf. B Biointerfaces 131, 155–161.
Vyas, A., Saraf, S., Saraf, S., 2010. Encapsulation of cyclodextrin complexed simvastatin in chitosan nanocarriers: a novel technique for oral delivery. J. Incl. Phenom. Macro. 66, 251–259.
Wang, A. J., Jian, C. H., Li, S. D., Lin, Y. F., Liu, S. J., 2014. Glutathione-based delivery system. U.S. Pat. Appl. Publ. 13pp. CODEN: USXXCO US 2007141133 A1 20070621 CAN 147:102147 AN 2007:672399.
Wang, Z., Guo, W., Kuang, X., Hou, S., Liu, H., 2017. Nanopreparations for mitochondria targeting drug delivery system: current strategies and future prospective. Asian J. Pharm. Sci. 12, 498–508.
Wu, W., Dong, Y., Gao, J., Gong, M., Zhang, X., Kong, W., et al., 2015. Aspartate-modified doxorubicin on its N-terminal increases drug accumulation in LAT1-overexpressing tumors. Cancer Sci. 106, 747–756.
Wu, X., Prasad, P.D., Leibach, F.H., Ganapathy, V., 1998. cDNA sequence, transport function, and genomic organization of human OCTN2, a new member of the organic cation transporter family. Biochem. Biophys. Res. Commun. 246, 589–595.
Xie, F., Yao, N., Qin, Y., Zhang, Q., Chen, H., Yuan, M., et al., 2012. Investigation of glucose-modified liposomes using polyethylene glycols with different chain lengths as the linkers for brain targeting. Int. J. Nanomed. 7, 163–175.
Ying, X., Wen, H., Lu, W.L., Du, J., Guo, J., Tian, W., et al., 2010. Dual-targeting daunorubicin liposomes improve the therapeutic efficacy of brain glioma in animals. J. Control. Release 141, 183–192.
Ylikangas, H., Malmioja, K., Peura, L., Gynther, M., Nwachukwu, E.O., Leppänen, J., et al., 2014. Quantitative insight into the design of compounds recognized by the L-type amino acid transporter 1 (LAT1). ChemMedChem 9, 2699–2707.
Zeisel, S.H., 2004. Nutritional importance of choline for brain development. J. Am. Coll. Nutr. 23, 621S–626S.
Zhan, C., Lu, W., 2012. The blood-brain/tumor barriers: challenges and chances for malignant gliomas targeted drug delivery. Curr. Pharm. Biotechnol. 13, 2380–2387.
Zhang, C.X., Zhao, W.Y., Liu, L., Ju, R.J., Mu, L.M., Zhao, Y., et al., 2015. A nanostructure of functional targeting epirubicin liposomes dually modified with aminophenyl glucose and cyclic pentapeptide used for brain glioblastoma treatment. Oncotarget 6, 32681–32700.
Zhang, Y., Sun, J., Sun, Y., Wang, Y., He, Z., 2013. Prodrug design targeting intestinal PepT1 for improved oral absorption: design and performance. Curr. Drug Metab. 14, 675–687.

Zlokovic, B.V., Mackic, J.B., McComb, J.G., Weiss, M.H., Kaplowitz, N., Kannan, R., 1994. Evidence for transcapillary transport of reduced glutathione in vascular perfused guinea-pig brain. Biochem. Biophys. Res. Commun. 201, 402–408.

Zuchero, Y.J., Chen, X., Bien-Ly, N., Bumbaca, D., Tong, R.K., Gao, X., et al., 2016. Discovery of novel blood-brain barrier targets to enhance brain uptake of therapeutic antibodies. Neuron 89, 70–82.

Brain drug delivery by adsorption-mediated transcytosis

7

Xiaowen Zhu, Kai Jin, Yilan Huang, Zhiqing Pang
School of Pharmacy, Fudan University, Key Laboratory of Smart Drug Delivery, Ministry of Education, Shanghai, PR China

1 Introduction

The unique property of the blood-brain barrier (BBB) characterized by its endothelial tight junction and a complete absence of pinocytic activity restricts >98% drugs to enter the central nervous system (CNS) from systemic circulation. For small-molecule drugs, they can be transported into brain by lipidation, chemical delivery system, or transporter-mediated way. In contrast, it is very difficult to transport large molecular drugs such as proteins and gene drugs into brain because of their hydrophilicities, protein-bound properties, and large molecular weights, although they have the potential to be curative therapeutics for brain disorders.

The BBB drug targeting technology based on receptor-mediated transcytosis (RMT) and adsorptive-mediated transcytosis (AMT) brings hope to these large molecules (Lu et al., 2005b; Pang et al., 2008). RMT, which is initiated by the interaction between the ligands and their endogenous receptors on the BBB, can effectively increase brain drug delivery, especially macromolecular drug delivery (Agrawal et al., 2017). Similar to RMT, AMT may involve transcytosis initiated by the binding of polycationic substances to negative components on the plasma membrane and helps deliver drugs into brain (Gonatas et al., 1984). The surface of brain capillary endothelial cells (BCECs) composing the BBB is negative under physiological pH conditions, and anions are polarized on the luminal side and abluminal side of BCECs (Vorbrodt, 1989). The anionic components on membranous side are beneficial for cationic substances to absorb and can mediate endocytosis of cells. The transcellular transport of cationic substances across the BBB is mainly clathrin-mediated and caveolae-mediated. However, the pathway of endocytosis and transcellular transport of cationic substances is not clear. The process of AMT lasts a few minutes, which is far slower than the velocity of transporter-mediated nutrient transport. Unlike specific RMT, adsorptive-mediated binding is nonspecific. The binding affinity of AMT is low, but its binding capacity is high. It is not easy to cause saturation-inhibition which happens to RMT. In general, the efficiency of AMT to transport through the BBB is similar to that of RMT (Bickel et al., 2001).

Brain Targeted Drug Delivery Systems. https://doi.org/10.1016/B978-0-12-814001-7.00007-X

A variety of proteins or peptides can transport through BBB into the brain via AMT, such as cationic proteins, basic polypeptides, and cell-penetrating peptides (CPPs). Cationic proteins can be prepared by the reaction between carboxylic groups of proteins (such as the C-terminal end of the protein chain and the side chain carboxylic acid of glutamic acid and aspartic acid) and cationic amine reagents (such as two amines and polyamines). For example, natural bovine serum albumin (BSA) is negative-charged under neutral physiological conditions, and the protein chain contains more acidic amino acid residues than basic amino acid residues. When BSA is coupled up with cationic reagents, such as hexamethylenediamine, under appropriate catalysts, the isoelectric point (p*I*) increases from 4 to 8–9, or even >10 (Lu et al., 2005b). Carotid artery perfusion and cerebrovascular removal experiments showed that the brain transport of this cationic bovine serum albumin (CBSA) is obviously better than that of BSA. Basic polypeptides and proteins are positive-charged under physiological conditions and can transport through the BBB via AMT. For instance, Ebiratide, a polypeptide whose structure is similar to adreno cortico tropic hormone (ACTH), can bind BCECs (Shimura et al., 1992) and be transported into the brain via AMT (Shimura et al., 1991). CPPs refer to the amino acid sequence with cell-penetrating function, which generally come from different protein families. The length of CPPs is 10–27 amino acids. Most of CPPs are positive-charged, such as TAT peptide, Syn-B peptide, and poly-arginine (Arg9). The transport of CPPs across the BBB is not clear, but recent studies have shown that its entry into cells is probably or partly via AMT.

Since most drugs do not have cationic properties themselves, they cannot be transported directly into the brain by AMT. Coupling drugs or drug delivery systems with these cationic proteins, basic peptides, or CPPs, adsorptive-mediated brain targeting delivery systems are constructed, which will be helpful for transporting drugs including small molecules and large molecules into brain. In this chapter, we will discuss these adsorptive-mediated brain targeting delivery systems in detail and try to provide an in-depth look at the design of these brain drug delivery systems to maximize their benefits for brain disease treatment.

2 Mechanism of AMT

As is known to all, the BBB is a nonfenestrated endothelium with narrow tight junctions between BCECs and prevents water-soluble and polar substances from blood to brain. Generally, the diffusion of a substance across the BBB via passive transport depends on its lipid solubility, molecular mass, and charge. Large molecules such as proteins and genes are generally excluded from passive diffusion due to their hydrophilicity and high molecular mass. AMT has attracted much attention because of its potential in large-molecule drug delivery to brain. Understanding the mechanism of AMT is very important for designing brain targeting drug delivery systems.

AMT is initiated by the binding of polycationic substances to negative components on the plasma membrane of BCECs and helps deliver drugs into brain (Gonatas et al., 1984). Generally, the anion components are asymmetrically distributed on the luminal side and abluminal side of BCECs (Vorbrodt, 1989). As illustrated in Fig. 1, the main anion components on luminal side are carboxylic acid groups of sialoglycoproteins

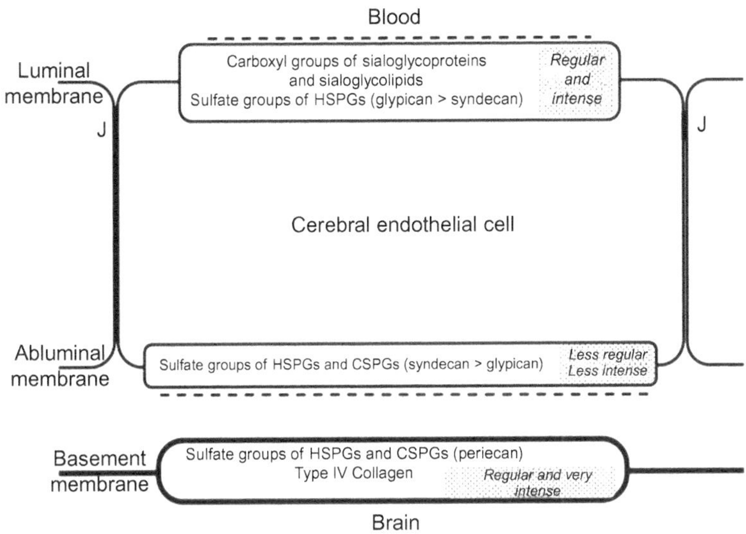

Fig. 1 Brain endothelial cell-surface and basement membrane components with negative charges. Abbreviations: *HSPGs*, heparan sulfate proteoglycans; *CSPGs*, chondroitin sulfate proteoglycans; *J*, tight junction.
Reproduced with permission from Hervé, F., Ghinea, N., Scherrmann, J.-M., 2008. CNS delivery via adsorptive transcytosis. AAPS J. 10, 455–472 and by copyright holder, Françoise Hervé.

and sialoglycolipids and, to a lesser degree, sulfate groups of heparan sulfate proteoglycans. However, the basolateral anion compositions are mainly heparan sulfates of heparan sulfate proteoglycans (HSPGs) and chondroitin sulfate proteoglycans (CSPGs). The dominating cell-surface heparan sulfate proteoglycans (HSPGs) at the endothelial cell surface are the syndecans and glypicans. Cell-surface HSPGs play a critical role in cellular internalization of basic peptides, regulation of growth factor or cytokine signaling, and coagulation factor activity, which may be associated with protein brain delivery (Belting, 2003). The basement membrane adjacent to the bas olateral side of BCECs is also a negatively charged barrier due to its chondroitin sulfates and heparan sulfates. The anionic components on luminal side are beneficial for cationic substances to absorb and can mediate endocytosis of cells, while anionic components on basal lamina are beneficial for the exocytosis of cationic substances to transport into the gap of brain parenchyma cells. All these three successive electronegative barriers create an environment to selectively bind cationic substances and transport them through BBB.

Generally, the transcellular transport of BCECs is mainly clathrin-mediated and caveolae-mediated. There are two kinds of vesicles on BCECs, caveolae vesicles and clathrin-coated pits/vesicles, which are found at both luminal and abluminal plasma membranes of BCECs. Both caveolae and clathrin-coated vesicles are much more abundant at the luminal side than at the abluminal side. This indicates that these two pathways may mainly function from blood to brain (Hervé et al., 2008). Caveolae and clathrin-coated vesicles mediate the transcytosis of different kinds of molecules across BBB. Caveolae may bud to form free, apparently intact vesicles and then internalize specific ligands and fuse apparently intact with large spherical vesicular structures for direct transendothelial transport (Schnitzer, 2001). Once the clathrin-coated vesicles have formed, they lose their clathrin coat. The uncoated vesicles may fuse with a transcytotic endosome (Hervé et al., 2008). Therefore, the internalized receptors and ligands can cross cell membrane and be delivered to the opposite membrane. This process is called transcytosis. However, there is another situation where the molecules internalized by clathrin-coated vesicles or caveolae vesicles can converge with each another within downstream endosomes and eventually lysosomes (Schnitzer, 2001).

The vesicular route used for AMT of cationic substances through BBB is still not clear. It is believed that specific plasma membrane receptors may not involve in AMT. Endocytosis is initiated through electrostatic interaction between cationic substances and negative charges on the surface of BCECs. For example, the clathrin-coated pits along the luminal surface of BCECs are negatively charged, which are capable of binding positively charged substances, such as protamine, histone, and CBSA. A few studies have suggested that caveolae participates in the endocytosis of cationic substances, such as cationic $F(ab')_2$ fragment (Girod et al., 1999). It was reported that AMT was energy-, time-, and concentration-dependent (Bickel et al., 2001).

Although the processes following endocytosis are similar in AMT and RMT, the main difference lies in the affinity and capacity of these two pathways (Bickel et al., 2001).Generally, RMT is characterized by high affinity (K_d values in the low nanomolar range) and low capacity (maximum binding capacities of <1 pmol/mg membrane protein). For instance, the isolated human brain microvessels avidly bind insulin with a high affinity dissociation constant (K_d) of 1.2 ± 0.5 nM (Pardridge et al., 1985). The binding of holotransferrin with isolated human brain capillaries has a K_d value of 5.6 ± 1.4 nM and a maximal binding constant of 8.0 ± 1.5 ng/mg proteins (Pardridge et al., 1987a). In contrast, AMT is characterized by micromolar half-saturation constants and maximum binding capacities of several nmol/mg membrane proteins. Take CBSA ($pI > 8$) as an example; isolated bovine brain capillaries rapidly bind CBSA with a maximal binding capacity of 5.5 ± 0.7 micrograms/mg proteins, and a half-saturation constant of 0.8 ± 0.1 mM (Kumagai et al., 1987). In general, occupancy of the binding sites depends on both affinity and capacity, and the efficiency of AMT to transport through BBB is similar to that of RMT (Bickel et al., 2001).

3 Adsorptive-mediated brain drug delivery systems

3.1 Cationic albumin-mediated brain drug delivery system

3.1.1 Brain delivery of cationic albumin

When BSA, rat serum albumin (RSA), immunoglobulin (IgG), and monoclonal antibody are cationized, the brain transport capacity of these proteins is enhanced significantly, which can be used in the diagnosis and treatment of brain diseases (Bickel et al., 2001). Although protein cationization, to some extent, improves the brain uptake ability, it also improves the liver and kidney uptake and plasma clearance rate, which is not conducive to brain tissue uptake. The plasma half-life of RSA is about 4.8 h, while that of cationic RSA (CRSA) is about 2.5 h, when p*I* is 8–9. When p*I* is 10, the clearance curves of CRSA in plasma are double exponential, and the initial elimination half-life is <1 min (Bickel et al., 2001). Therefore, how to choose the suitable cationic degree is critical for brain delivery. We generally recommend that the p*I* of proteins is 8–9 after cationization (Bickel et al., 2001; Thole et al., 2002; Lu et al., 2005b; Xu et al., 2009). It is demonstrated that molecular weight of CBSA remained unaltered at this cationization in comparison with that of BSA, i.e., approximately 66 kDa, and only a minimal dimerization of CBSA was generated (Lu et al., 2005b; Agarwal et al., 2011). Binding of CBSA to the luminal side of rat brain capillaries in vivo was found using the carotid injection technique in adult male SD rats. The brain uptake of CBSA (p*I* 8.5–9) was 1.58-fold greater than that of native albumin (Kumagai et al., 1987).

Among cationic proteins, CBSA appeared to have favorable pharmacokinetic profiles with a longer circulation in blood and a greater degree of selectivity to brain tissue as compared to other organs (liver, heart, lung) (Bickel et al., 2001). Furthermore, compared with cationic antibodies and immunoglobulin, CBSA was easier to prepare. With these traits, CBSA was found to be a promising brain targeting moiety designed to couple with drugs and drug delivery systems. The following part will introduce recent advances in CBSA-drug conjugates and CBSA-conjugated nanoparticle delivery systems for brain drug delivery.

3.1.2 Brain delivery of cationic albumin-drug conjugates

Coupling drugs with CBSA results in brain delivery of drugs through AMT. For instance, β-endorphin is an endogenous opioid neuropeptide which mainly exists in hypothalamus and pituitary gland. Function of β-endorphin has been known as exerting an analgesic effect by involving in the regulation of information, such as modulation of pain perception. β-endorphin was coupled with CBSA using N-succinimidyl-3-(2-pyridyldithio)propionate (SPDP) to deliver the peptide through the BBB (Kumagai et al., 1987). It was shown that conjugation of CBSA to β-endorphin led to significant increase in binding rate with isolated brain capillary, which was many times greater than that of the unconjugated group. The binding exhibited to be temperature-dependent, while over 50% was inhibited by incubation at cold temperature. In addition, approximately 70% of the chimeric peptide was resistant to mild acid wash due to their entry into a microvessel space (Kumagai et al., 1987). The in vivo uptake of β-endorphin-CBSA chimeric peptide was measured in Sprague-Dawley rats with the carotid injection technique. It was demonstrated that the brain uptake of β-endorphin-CBSA peptide was 7-fold that of native β-endorphin, indicating that cationic albumin provided a viable approach to enhance delivery of therapeutic peptide through the BBB (Pardridge et al., 1987b).

3.1.3 Brain delivery of CBSA-conjugated nanoparticle delivery systems

For CBSA-drug conjugates, the technique is complicated for their chemical modifications and suffers for their lower drug carrying capacity, slow drug releasing, and short half-life in blood. Coupling CBSA with nanoparticle drug delivery systems is proved to be successful in brain drug delivery. Compared with CBSA-drug conjugates technique, its advantages were the large drug loading capacity, disguise of limiting characteristics of drugs with physical nature of nanoparticles, controllable drug release, and reduction of drug degradation in vivo. Moreover, the surface modification of PEG enabled nanoparticles to escape the arrest of mononuclear phagocytic system (MPS) so as to prolong its half-life in blood and increase the possibility to transport across the BBB.

Different kinds of nanoparticle drug delivery systems have been explored to couple with CBSA to develop adsorptive-mediated brain drug delivery systems. Liposome is a kind of artificial membrane. It has a vesicular structure with an aqueous core surrounded by a hydrophobic membrane bilayer composed of phospholipids, whose hydrophobic tail is inserted into the bilayer and hydrophilic head extends into the water (Torchilin, 2005). CBSA-conjugated PEGylated liposomes were taken up into brain endothelium via an AMT pathway and proved to be a suitable carrier for brain drug delivery under the confocal laser scanning fluorescence microscopy (Thole et al., 2002).

Polymersomes are self-assembled polymeric vesicles which are made of various amphiphilic block copolymers. These vesicles have numerous advantages including stealthiness, high stability, a large drug loading capacity, biodegradability, and sustained drug release. They were also proven to be more robust and less water-permeable compared with liposomes (Discher et al., 1999). Finally, polymersomes can easily be functionalized, making them good candidates for medical application, especially brain drug delivery (Discher et al., 2007; Georgieva et al., 2012). In our group, biodegradable polymersomes conjugated with CBSA (CBSA-PO) were exploited for brain drug delivery (Pang et al., 2012). Biodegradable polymersomes were made by using a blend of MPEG-PCL and maleimide-PEG-PCL via nanoprecipitation method. Subsequently, polymersomes were conjugated with thiolated CBSA with a thiol group to maleimide group molar ratio of 1:3 and the resulting CBSA-PO was purified through passing a Sepharose CL-4B column. Compared with unconjugated polymersomes, the size of CBSA-PO increased slightly, which had an average value of around 101 nm. A dramatic increase in zeta potential was observed for CBSA-PO, from −20 mV to around 9 mV, which was attributed to surface CBSA on polymersomes. The uptake of CBSA-PO by bEnd.3 cells, an immortalized brain endothelial cell line which was isolated from mice and showed specific endothelial properties and blood-brain barrier characteristics (Brown et al., 2007; Hu et al., 2009), was significantly higher than that of unconjugated polymersomes, but was inhibited by low temperature, free CBSA, and poly-L-lysine, indicating that endocytosis was energy-driven and adsorption-mediated. Pharmacokinetics results revealed that CBSA-PO had long circulation times, and CBSA conjugation on the polymersomes significantly increased the BBB permeability surface area product by 3.6-fold and the percentage of injected dose per gram brain (% ID/g brain) by 2.1-fold. Further capillary depletion experiments demonstrated that CBSA-PO was distributed into the brain parenchyma in a time-dependent manner, while few polymersomes were detected in the brain parenchyma. These results indicated that CBSA conjugation with polymersomes significantly improved their transcytosis across the BBB through AMT.

Polymer nanoparticles refer to solid particles composed of macromolecular polymers, with particle size ranging from 10 nm to 1000 nm. Low toxicity, good biocompatibility, and biodegradation at specific sites are the main advantages of polymer nanoparticles as drug carriers (Feng et al., 2013). We first reported the brain delivery property of CBSA-conjugated nanoparticles (CBSA-NP) (Lu et al., 2005b). The copolymers of methoxy-PEG-PLA and maleimide-PEG-PLA were applied to prepare PEGylated nanoparticles by double emulsion and solvent evaporation method. CBSA was thiolated and conjugated to nanoparticles through the maleimide function located at the distal end of PEG surrounding the nanoparticle's surface. In vitro cellular uptake of CBSA-NP showed that BCECs took in much more CBSA-NP than BSA-NP at 37°C, with different concentrations and incubation time. Uptake process was demonstrated to be dependent on the concentration of CBSA-NP, incubation time, and energy (Xu et al., 2009). In an in vitro BBB model constructed by coculture of primary BCECs and astrocytes, the permeability of CBSA-NP was about 7.76 times higher than that of BSA-NP, while it was inhibited in the excess of free CBSA (Lu et al., 2005a). In addition, CBSA-NP had a good safety profile on BCECs and did not impact the integrity of BBB endothelial tight junctions. Further fluorescent microscopy of brain coronal sections demonstrated CBSA-NP accumulated significantly more in the lateral ventricle, third ventricle, and periventricular region than BSA-NP (Lu et al., 2005b). It was concluded that CBSA-NP was a promising brain drug delivery platform with low toxicity. By using CBSA-NP platform, chemotherapeutics, peptides, and genes were delivered to brain for brain disease treatment (Lu et al., 2006, 2007; Xu et al., 2009). NC-1900 is a synthetic fragment analog of arginine vasopression (AVP_{4-9}) and has been proved to have facilitative effects on the spatial memory impairments and improve memory deficits in passive avoidance test. However, the i.c.v. administration was hard for patients to accept although a thimble of NC-1900 was needed, while a relatively high dose was required for p.o. administration due to its low bioavailability and low permeability to the BBB. Thus, NC-1900 was incorporated into CBSA-NP (CBSA-NP-NC) to improve its performance on memory impairments (Xie et al., 2006). It was shown NC-1900 was released from CBSA-NP-NC in a sustained release manner and the half-life of NC-1900 loaded in CBSA-NP in plasma was 4-fold longer than that of free NC-1900. The active avoidance behavioral results in scopolamine-induced memory deficits mouse models revealed that NC-1900 didn't produce any positive effects by i.v. administration, but CBSA-NP-NC greatly improved memory impairments to a normal level (Xie et al., 2006). Tanshinone IIA (TIIA) is one of the most abundant constituents of the root of *Salvia miltiorrhiza*, which has been widely used in clinics for the treatment of cerebrovascular disease (Han et al., 2008). However, the delivery of TIIA to central nervous system (CNS) has been ineffective due to its poor solubility, short half-life in circulation, and limited brain penetration through the BBB (Du et al., 2008). Thus, CBSA-NP was developed to enhance the brain-specific delivery of TIIA (Liu et al., 2013). TIIA was encapsulated CBSA-NP (CBSA-NP-TIIA) with a high encapsulation efficiency. Pharmacokinetic experiments demonstrated that the MRT for CBSA-NP-TIIA and TIIA were 7.96 ± 0.68 and 3.36 ± 0.21 h, respectively. The MRT and $AUC_{0\text{-}inf}$ of CBSA-NP-TIIA were 2.37 and 3.40 times that of TIIA, respectively. The neuroprotective effects of CBSA-NP-TIIA on ischemic stroke were evaluated by infarct volume, neurological deficiencies, neutrophils infiltration, microglia activation, and pro-inflammatory cytokines. Compared with TIIA solution group, CBSA-NP-TIIA showed a remarkable reduction of cerebral infarct volume and ameliorated neurological deficit which was induced by ischemia reperfusion. There was also obvious superiority in suppressing neutrophil infiltration compared with TIIA solution, which might be one of protective mechanisms of CBSA-NP-TIIA. In addition, CBSA-NP-TIIA could significantly downregulate microglia activation and levels of pro-inflammatory cytokines TNF-α and IL-8 in brain tissue. All these results suggested CBSA-NP-TIIA was promising for the treatment of stroke (Liu et al., 2013). Aclarubicin (ACL), one of the anthracyclines, exerted a great antitumor activity by acting as a catalytic inhibitor of topoisomerase II and as a topoisomerase I poison. However, as the substrate of P-glycoprotein, ACL was speculated to be inaccessible to brain tumor because of the presence of P-glycoprotein at the neoplastic cells and the BBB. Therefore, incorporating ACL into CBSA-NP (CBSA-NP-ACL) played a key role in enhancing glioma chemotherapy of ACL. The therapeutic potential of CBSA-NP-ACL was investigated in C6 glioma-bearing rats. When the tumor rat model was subjected to 4 cycles of CBSA-NP-ACL treatment, a significant increase of median survival time was found compared with other groups. Terminal deoxynucleotidyl transferase-mediated dUTP nick-end-labeling (TUNEL) results further showed that CBSA-NP-ACL could induce more tumor cell apoptosis than other treatments (Lu et al., 2007). To investigate the potential of CBSA-NP as a nonviral vector for gene therapy of brain disease, hTRAIL-encoding plasmid (pORF-hTRAIL) was selected as a model therapeutic gene for malignant glioma (Lu et al., 2006). It was shown that hTRAIL mRNA and protein were detected in normal brain and tumors 24 and 48 h post i.v. injection of CBSA-NP-hTRAIL, respectively. Antiglioma tests revealed that repeated i.v. injections of CBSA-NP-hTRAIL induced tumor cell apoptosis in vivo and significantly delayed tumor growth, indicating CBSA-NP-hTRAIL is promising for noninvasive gene therapy of malignant glioma.

Solid lipid nanoparticles (SLN) refer to nanoparticles mainly made of biocompatible high-melting-point lipids (Mukherjee et al., 2009). Since solid lipid nanoparticles are solid at room temperature, they have the advantages of polymer nanoparticles, such as high physical stability, less drug leakage, slow releasing, passive targeting, and ease to be sterilized. At the same time, solid lipid nanoparticles also have some characteristics of liposomes, such as low toxicity and being apt for large-scale production (Thukral et al., 2014). SLN coupling with CBSA (CBSA-SLN) could also enhance brain drug delivery. Agarwal et al. investigated the potential of CBSA-SLN for the treatment of brain tumor using Doxorubicin (DOX) as a model drug (Agarwal et al., 2011). BCECs and astrocytes were cocultured to establish a simple

BBB model to study the transcytosis ability of free DOX, SLN-DOX, and CBSA-SLN-DOX in vitro. Their permeability coefficient (Pe) were 0.8×10^{-6}cm/s, 1.9×10^{-6}cm/s, 2.5×10^{-5}cm/s, and 1.1×10^{-6}cm/s, respectively, suggesting that maximum transendothial transport was obtained in case of CBSA-DOX-SLN. Pharmacokinetics studies demonstrated that compared with the free DOX, the $t_{1/2}$ of SLN-DOX and CBSA-SLN-DOX were prolonged from 1.48 h to 4.65 h and 5.29 h, respectively. Biodistribution results revealed that CBSA-SLN-DOX exhibited a significant increase of drug accumulation in brain compared with the unmodified counterparts.

3.2 Basic proteins-mediated brain drug delivery systems

3.2.1 Brain delivery of basic proteins

Basic polypeptides and proteins are positive-charged under physiological conditions. It has been confirmed that a variety of basic peptides and proteins can be transported into the brain via adsorptive-mediated transcytosis, such as ebiratide, 001-C8, E-2078, TAPA, histone, avidin, wheat germ agglutinin (WGA), *Ricinus communis* agglutinin I (RCA I), protamine, and human basic fibroblast growth factor (Pardridge et al., 1989, 1993; Raub and Audus, 1990; Pardridge and Boado, 1991; Shimura et al., 1991; Terasaki et al., 1991; Villegas and Broadwell, 1993; Tamai et al., 1997; Deguchi et al., 2000, 2003). Histones, basic proteins with low molecular weight, can combine with separate bovine BCECs. The binding degree is closely related to temperature and time and the process of binding can be inhibited by basic proteins such as protamine and poly-lysine. Avidin is a kind of basic proteins with high molecular weight and can also be transported into the brain via adsorptive-mediated transcytosis (Pardridge and Boado, 1991). Like histones, avidin is easy to be cleared in plasma, which weakens its application in drug delivery in the brain. Protamine is a 7-kD arginine-rich, basic protein that is produced in sperm cells. It possesses high arginine content and mediate cellular transport of attached cargos. Protamine enhances the permeability of brain endothelial wall and penetrates BBB (Pardridge et al., 1993). Basic polypeptides and proteins are similar to cationic proteins. The p*I* of basic polypeptides and proteins has great influence on its transport ability and in vivo pharmacokinetics. Too high p*I* speeds up the liver and kidney uptake and plasma clearance rate, which is not conducive to brain tissue uptake. It is generally considered that the suitable p*I* of basic polypeptide and protein is for 8–9.

The mechanism of transport through the BBB of basic proteins and polypeptides is not clear. Only parts of studies show that caveolae mediates the transcellular transport of basic proteins and polypeptides. For example, the endocytosis and exocytosis in primary microvascular endothelial cells of RCAI are ATP-dependent. Caveolae mediates the endocytosis of RCAI, and trans-Golgi network mediates the intracellular transport of RCAI (Villegas and Broadwell, 1993). A hypothesis concludes the transcellular transport of WGA-HRP is by a variety of pathways: endosomes, lysosomes, and Golgi complexes are involved in the transcellular transport of WGA-HRP (Broadwell et al., 1988).

3.2.2 Brain delivery of basic protein-drug conjugates

Linking basic peptides or proteins to drugs helps to transport drugs into the brain via adsorptive-mediated transcytosis, such as the connection of protamine and albumin, which can significantly increase albumin delivery in the brain (Pardridge et al., 1993). Because of the short in vivo half-life of basic polypeptide or protein, when basic polypeptide or protein is linked to drug, the plasma clearance of drug will be accelerated, which is not conducive to drug transport.

3.2.3 Brain delivery of basic protein-conjugated nanoparticle drug delivery system

Using basic polypeptide or protein as a targeting molecule, when drug is loaded in basic protein-modified nanoparticles with long circulation function, the brain delivery ability of basic protein can be greatly improved. For instance, cisplatin can induce apoptosis in glioblastoma cells, but it does not cross BBB efficiently. To enhance the brain uptake of cisplatin, it was encapsulated in protamine sulphate-modified poly(lactide-*co*-glycolide) nanoparticles (Pr-NP-Cis) for the treatment of glioblastoma (Dhami et al., 2014). In vitro bovine BCEC assay was used to examine the ability of cisplatin, NP-Cis, and Pr-NP-Cis to cross BBB. This assay demonstrated that Pr-NP-Cis have significantly greater uptake than cisplatin. The cytotoxicity of Pr-NP-Cis against U87 glioblastoma cells was higher than NP-Cis and cisplatin, which might be due to the greater uptake of Pr-NP-Cis via adsorptive-mediated transcytosis. Cellular uptake of Pr-NP-Cis against U87 glioblastoma cells showed that Pr-NP-Cis had greater uptake through adsorptive-mediated transcytosis because of the negative charge on the surface of tumor cells.

3.3 CPPs-mediated brain drug delivery system

3.3.1 Brain delivery of CPPs

Cell-penetrating peptides (CPPs) are short peptides that facilitate cellular intake and uptake of linked "cargo". CPPs typically have an amino acid composition that either contains a high relative abundance of positively charged amino acids such as lysine or arginine or has sequences that contain an alternating pattern of polar/charged amino acids and nonpolar, hydrophobic amino acids. Compared with the majority of delivery systems that suffer from various limitations when applied in clinical situations for the transport of therapeutic molecules into the CNS, CPP-based delivery systems exhibit a great ability in carrying macromolecules across cellular membranes with high efficiency but low cellular toxicity (Derossi et al., 1994). Considering their smaller size (up to 30 amino acids in length), cationic and/or amphipathic CPPs have a greater potential to penetrate the BBB than other transport systems, enabling them to be used as very promising tools for therapeutic purposes in CNS-related diseases (Mae and Langel, 2006).

CPPs can be classified by whether they are naturally derived or artificially synthesized. The first CPP, trans-activator of transcription (TAT), derived from human immunodeficiency virus-1 (HIV-1), can be efficiently taken up from the surrounding media (Derossi et al., 1994; Mae and Langel, 2006). Another penetratin, also known as Antp, derived from the third helix of the antennapedia transcription factor of *Drosophila melanogaster* (Vives et al., 1997), together with TAT, is regarded to be the first group of CPPs derived from natural proteins. Since then, the number of CPPs with effective transduction properties has greatly expanded. The second group of CPPs consists of chimeric molecules, such as transportan (TP), which consists of 12 amino acids derived from the neuropeptide galanin fused with a 14 amino acid peptide from the wasp venom mastoparan (Pooga et al., 1998). The third group of CPPs consists of the synthetic peptide family, of which Poly-L-arginine are the best studied (Rothbard et al., 2000; El-Andaloussi et al., 2005). Poly-L-arginine is a synthetic cationic peptide consisting of eight or more arginine residues and has been used to facilitate the intracellular translocation of a wide variety of molecular cargos (Sharma et al., 2012, 2013).

Much attention has been put into figuring out the mechanisms facilitating membrane permeation of the CPPs, but the puzzle is still not fully understood (El-Andaloussi et al., 2005). Nevertheless, it is today generally accepted that both endocytosis and direct translocation contribute to membrane translocation of CPPs, though it was previously believed that only direct translocation was involved. However, since protocols involving the use of fixatives were shown to cause artifacts in membrane permeability (Richard et al., 2003), several studies have demonstrated endocytosis to be a mechanism of cellular uptake of CPPs (Fittipaldi et al., 2003; Nakase et al., 2004; Pujals et al., 2006). It is important to note that whether CPPs exploit endocytosis or direct translocation across a membrane is dependent on multiple factors, such as the specific CPP sequence (Lundin et al., 2008), the CPP concentration (Jones and Sayers, 2012), the specific cell type (Trehin et al., 2004), and the state of cellular differentiation (Foerg et al., 2007). Moreover, the cargo (Fischer et al., 2002; Tunnemann et al., 2006; Barany-Wallje et al., 2007) as well as the CPP-cargo formulation design being either covalent conjugation or physical complexation (Kristensen et al., 2015), and the conjugation of a label for detection (Fischer et al., 2002; Hirose et al., 2012), may be decisive for the mode of membrane permeation. Additionally, it is likely that multiple mechanisms are active simultaneously, depending on the above mentioned factors, thereby further complicating the search for common conclusions on the mechanism responsible for cellular internalization of the CPPs and their cargos.

Direct penetration of CPPs occurs via an energy-independent cellular process and it is believed that the translocation across biological membranes can progress at 4°C and most likely involves a direct electrostatic interaction with negatively charged phospholipids (Luo and Saltzman, 2000). Lowering the incubation temperature to 4°C or depletion of cellular ATP did not inhibit the rapid transduction of TAT into cells, suggesting that TAT-mediated protein transduction is endocytosis-independent (Vives et al., 1997; Futaki et al., 2001; Mai et al., 2002). Other arguments in favor of an energy-independent mechanism include the absence of effect of metabolic or endocytosis inhibitors on CPPs internalization and the failure of radiolabeled CPPs to label endocytotic vesicles (Suzuki et al., 2002). Moreover, structure activity studies indicate that the internalization is equally effective whether CPPs were in inverse or retro forms, which implies receptor-independent recognition (Derossi et al., 1996).

A direct penetration mechanism is thus proposed which emphasizes the positive charges on most CPPs including TAT and Antp. It is suggested that the unfolded fusion protein interacts with the membrane through electrostatic interactions between the basic amino acids on CPPs and the negatively charged cell membrane polysaccharides or phospholipids, and then nucleates a pore, which enables protein translocation across the membrane (Derossi et al., 1996; Prochiantz, 2000; Deshayes et al., 2004; Herce and Garcia, 2007). According to this theory, once inside the cell, the fusion protein is refolded into its active form with the help of the endogenous chaperone system. Different modes by which CPPs directly translocate across the plasma membrane have been proposed: the carpet and the barrel-stave models (Clayton et al., 2006), the inverted micelle model (Derossi et al., 1996), the electroporation-like model (Binder and Lindblom, 2003), and the counterion model (Sakai et al., 2005). In some studies, penetratin has been demonstrated to translocate across membranes via mechanisms explained by the carpet and the barrel-stave models, which both involve pore formation, but differ according to the orientation of CPPs relative to the membrane lipids (Clayton et al., 2006). With the inverted micelle model, electrostatic interactions between CPPs and negatively charged membrane phospholipids facilitate insertion into the membrane, after which interaction between hydrophobic CPP residues and the membrane core leads to changes in membrane curvature, resulting in the formation of vesicles in which CPPs are taken up. This mechanism was first demonstrated for penetratin in 1996 (Derossi et al., 1996). However, later studies have demonstrated the involvement of energy-independent vesicular CPPs uptake differing from endocytosis by the smaller size of the formed vesicles, as well as by the fact that this mechanism is active at 4°C (Alves et al., 2008; Joanne et al., 2009). The electroporation-like model and the counterion model involve either local charge neutralization or the formation of a transient electrical field, respectively. The former mode of translocation has been used to explain uptake of penetratin into cells (Binder and Lindblom, 2003), whereas the latter is found relevant for the guanidinium-rich polyarginines (Sakai et al., 2005).

However, several studies have challenged the energy- and receptor-independent CPP translocation theory. It has been argued that uptake of CPPs arises following fixation procedures used for fluorescence microscopy. In addition, CPPs such as TAT or penetratin strongly bind to the plasma membrane and cannot be removed by the standard washing protocol used in FACS analysis. These membrane-bound peptides might be mistaken by FACS as internalized peptides, leading to questionable conclusions with respect to direct CPP penetration (Richard et al., 2003). The application of procedures avoiding these experimental artifacts yielded an alternative internalization mechanism favoring endocytosis-mediated entry.

Endocytosis-mediated entry is the process of cellular ingestion, where the plasma membrane folds inward to bring substances into the cell. During this process, cells absorb substances from outside of the cell by imbibing it with their cell membrane. Phagocytosis and pinocytosis are two overall endocytic mechanisms, which involve energy-dependent formation of vesicles with various sizes. Phagocytosis, also referred to as "cell eating", takes place in specialized scavenger cells, such as the macrophages, and is responsible for the engulfment of cell debris, bacteria, and other large particulate matter (Doherty and Mcmahon, 2009). On the other hand, pinocytosis, or "cell drinking", contributes to the control of cellular homeostasis and takes place in all cell types (Conner and Schmid, 2003). Pinocytosis is further segregated into the pathways macropinocytosis, clathrin-mediated endocytosis, caveolin-mediated endocytosis, or clathrin- and caveolin-independent endocytosis, all of which differ by the mechanism of vesicle formation as well as the resulting size of these vesicles (Conner and Schmid, 2003).

Various studies have demonstrated cellular uptake of arginine-rich CPPs, such as TAT and polyarginines, by macropinocytosis for which membrane ruffling plays an important role (Khalil et al., 2006). Studies on TAT internalization with chemical inhibition of specific endocytotic pathways point to the involvement of multiple mechanisms. In support of lipid raft-mediated endocytosis involving caveolae, Fittipaldi et al. showed that the internalization of TAT-EGFP endosomes was resistant to non-ionic detergents and co-localized with caveolae markers. Moreover, both the disruption of lipid rafts and the disturbance of caveolar trafficking impaired the internalization of TAT-GFP (Fittipaldi et al., 2003). They also showed that conjugated TAT was not internalized in clathrin-coated endosomes. In contrast, using unconjugated TAT, Richard and colleagues showed that specific inhibitors of clathrin-dependent endocytosis partially inhibit TAT peptide uptake, while inhibitors of raft/caveolin-dependent pathway or genetic deficient of caveolin-1 expression could not inhibit the internalization of TAT (Richard et al., 2005). Taken together, these results suggest that unconjugated TAT peptide might follow a clathrin-mediated endocytic pathway, whereas conjugated TAT follows a caveolae-mediated endocytic pathway. Furthermore, lipid raft-dependent macropinocytosis, yet another form of endocytosis that is independent of either caveloe or clathrin, was also implicated in the endocytosis of large TAT-fusion proteins above 30 kDa (Wadia et al., 2004) as well as unconjugated TAT (Kaplan et al., 2005). Dose-dependent inhibition of TAT uptake was observed when cells were pretreated with amiloride, an inhibitor of the Na^+/K^+ exchanger required for macropinocytosis, and when cholesterol was removed from the cell membrane (Wadia et al., 2004; Kaplan et al., 2005). In addition, uptake of a TAT-conjugated protein was shown to exploit caveolae-mediated endocytosis (Fittipaldi et al., 2003), whereas a TAT-conjugated fluorophore was demonstrated to be taken up via clathrin-mediated endocytosis (Richard et al., 2005), thereby underlining that the physicochemical properties of the cargo are highly relevant for the main mechanism exploited for the CPP-mediated cellular uptake. Indeed, the coexistence of different routes of endocytosis is not unique for TAT, but true for many other CPPs such as homoarginine peptide (Nakase et al., 2004; Khalil et al., 2006) and penetratin (Saalik et al., 2004; Alves et al., 2010).

Suitable methodologies to demonstrate endocytic uptake include the use of microscopy to localize fluorescently tagged CPPs in the cytosol or in vesicular structures (Fretz et al., 2007; Amand et al., 2008), and the specific active endocytic mechanism may be identified by the use of chemical inhibitors (Duchardt et al., 2007) or by the more recently developed methodology employing siRNA inhibition of individual endocytic mechanisms (Al Soraj et al., 2012). If an endocytic mechanism is hijacked by a CPP for intracellular delivery of its cargo, a successful outcome relates to the potential for endosomal escape before being directed to lysosomes for degradation or recycling of endosomes for transport back to the plasma membrane and subsequent extracellular release. A study demonstrated that cyclic CPPs facilitate membrane destabilization at the low pH (approximately 5.5) in endosomes and are thus a strategy for enhancing endosomal escape (Qian et al., 2014). If transepithelial or transendothelial CPP-mediated transport of a cargo drug is intended, the prominent criterion for efficient drug delivery relates to whether transcytosis follows the endocytic uptake. Transcytosis is exploited by various toxins subsequent to oral ingestion in order to transverse the epithelium for gaining access to the systemic circulation (Ahsan et al., 2005; Lukyanenko et al., 2011), but may also be the mechanism by which peptide and protein drugs are translocated across epithelia and endothelia when CPPs are employed as delivery vectors.

3.3.2 Brain delivery of CPPs-drug conjugates

A number of CPPs including TAT, penetratin, TP, rabies virus glycoprotein (RVG), prion peptide, and SynB have already shown great ability in improving therapeutic molecule delivery across the BBB to treat CNS diseases (Snyder and Dowdy, 2005). Recently, Wei et al. designed a special CPP called CB5005 that can target and inhibit intracellular NF-κB activation. In vitro cellular evaluation confirmed that CB5005 was effectively taken up by brain capillary endothelial cell bEnd.3 and glioma cells U87. The intracellular localization analysis further demonstrated that CB5005 could not only penetrate into the cells, but also enter into their nuclei. More interestingly, CB5005 permeated deeply into the tumor spheroids of U87 cell in vitro and distributed itself into the brain after intravenous injection when coupled with a fluorescence dye, showing promising potential in brain drug delivery (Zhang et al., 2016).

Considering the high expression of activating transcription factor 5 (ATF5) in glioma and its expression and function during the onset of glioma, Cates et al. designed a novel deliverable truncated-dominant-negative (d/n) form of ATF5 fused to a cell-penetrating domain (Pen-d/n-ATF5) that can be intraperitoneally or subcutaneously administered to mice harboring malignant gliomas. In vitro tests showed that Pen-d/n-ATF5-RP entered into glioma cells and triggered massive cell apoptosis. Moreover, subcutaneously administered Pen-d/n-ATF5-RP transported the BBB and entered into normal brain and tumor cells, causing rapid and selective tumor cell death (Cates et al., 2016).

Notch pathway was found to be activated in most glioblastomas, underlining the importance of Notch in the formation and recurrence of glioblastomas. A Notch inhibitory peptide, dominant negative MAML (dnMAML), was conjugated to elastin-like polypeptide (ELP) for tumor-targeted delivery. ELP is a thermally responsive polypeptide that can be actively and passively targeted to the tumor site by localized application of hyperthermia. This complex was further modified with SynB1 (SynB1-ELP-dnMAML) for improved cellular uptake and BBB penetration. SynB1-ELP-dnMAML inhibited the growth of D54 and U251 cells in vitro by inducing apoptosis and cell cycle arrest, especially in the presence of hyperthermia. Hyperthermia increased overall uptake of the polypeptide by the cells and enhanced the resulting pharmacological effects of dnMAML (Opacak-Bernardi et al., 2017).

CPPs are not only explored for brain peptide delivery by a hybrid of CPPs sequence and therapeutic peptide sequence as described above, but also can be exploited for brain protein delivery. Lim et al. identified a cell-permeable peptide, dNP2, which efficiently delivered proteins into T cells and into brain tissues as well (Lim et al., 2015). This peptide showed prospect in multiple sclerosis treatment, since multiple sclerosis is a human autoimmune disease caused by the induction of inflammation in the central nervous system by myelin-specific T cells that cross the protective environment of the BBB. Their results demonstrated that the intracellular delivery mechanism of dNP2 was partly identical to the mechanism of other CPPs, which also utilized multiple pathways depending on the cargos it carried, including lipid raft-mediated endocytosis following heparan sulphate interaction. They then conjugated dNP2 with cytoplasmic domain of cytotoxic T-lymphocyte antigen 4 (dNP2-ctCTLA-4) which negatively regulates activated T cells and showed inhibitory effects on experimental autoimmune encephalomyelitis in both preventive and therapeutic mouse models, resulting in the reduction of demyelination and CNS-infiltrating T helper 1 and T helper 17 cells (Lim et al., 2015).

3.3.3 Brain delivery of CPPs-conjugated nanoparticle drug delivery system

Similar to cationic proteins and basic proteins, CPP has long been used to improve the BBB-penetrating capability of nanoparticle drug delivery systems. As shown in Table 1, different CPPs are conjugated to nanoparticle drug delivery systems for brain disease treatment. For instance, albumin nanoparticles (BSA-NP) can be used for glioma treatment with the help of low molecular weight protamine (LMWP) (Lin et al., 2016). Due to rapid growth, the metabolically active tumors are hungry for nutrients. As a result, albumin intake into tumor tissues is greatly increased for use as a source of amino acids and energy for cancer cells. Albumin-binding proteins, such as SPARC (secreted protein acidic and rich in cysteine) and glycoprotein 60 (gp60), are the major mechanisms responsible for albumin uptake by tumors, a process including transcytosis across endothelium and endocytosis in tumor cells. It has been reported that SPARC and gp60 are overexpressed in brain tumors, serving as promoters to glioma progression and invasion, suggesting its potential therapeutic value. The albumin nanoparticles can penetrate the BBB by the help of LMWP and target glioma cells via the mechanisms of SPARC- and gp60-mediated biomimetic transport. In an in vitro BBB-tumor cell model, the uptake of LMWP-modified albumin nanoparticles (L-BSA-NP) by U87 cells was 2.5-fold higher than that of BSA-NP, demonstrating the ability of LMWP for enhancing permeation of the NPs through the bEnd.3 monolayer and uptake by the U87 cells. Lin et al. further investigated the therapeutic effect of

Table 1 Summary of representative CPPs-conjugated nanoparticle drug delivery system for treatment of brain diseases

CPPs	Nanoparticles	Drugs	Target and brain disease	Reference
Tandem peptide R8-c(RGD)	Liposome	Paclitaxel	Vasculogenic mimicry and cancer stem cells in malignant glioma	Liu et al. (2015)
LMWP	Albumin nanoparticle	Paclitaxel and fenretinide	Glioma cells	Lin et al. (2016)
NFL-TBS.40-63	Lipid nanocapsule	Paclitaxel	Glioblastoma cells	Balzeau et al. (2013)
RGD-R8	Liposome	Paclitaxel	Glioma cells	Liu et al. (2014)
Nucleolar translocation signal sequence of the LIM Kinase 2 protein	Dendrigraft poly-L-lysines nanoparticle	Plasmid DNA-encoding inhibitor of growth 4	Gene therapy of glioma	Yao et al. (2015)
Bi-ligand (transferrin-poly-L-arginine)	Liposome	Beta-galactosidase(beta-gal) plasmid	Brain penetration and transfection	Sharma et al. (2013)
Tandem peptide R8-dGR (RRRRRRRRdGR)	Liposome	Paclitaxel	Antiglioma therapy including antitumor cells, antivasculogenic mimicry, and antibrain cancer stem cells	Liu et al. (2016)

L-BSA-NP loaded with paclitaxel and fenretinide on the orthotopic glioma (Luc-U87) model (Lin et al., 2016). The size of the intracranial glioma was monitored using the IVIS imaging system by giving the luciferase substrate luciferin. The L-BSA-NP group displayed clearly weaker bioluminescence intensity than other groups, with a smaller bioluminescence area at the same time (Fig. 2). The survival rate also demonstrated the improved treatment outcomes by applying the L-BSA-NP; the median survival time was 24, 29, 31, 33, and 37 days for PBS, PTX, 4-HPR/PTX, BSA-NP, and L-BSA-NP group, respectively. The L-BSA-NP group displayed the longest survival time among all of the groups, with statistical significance compared with other groups, and sustained less body weight loss than the BSA-NP group (Fig. 2) (Lin et al., 2016).

Chemotherapeutic agents like paclitaxel can be delivered toward brain, while gene therapeutics can also be carried by CPPs-modified nanoparticles. Yao et al. developed a new gene vector connecting PEGylated dendrigraft poly-L-lysines (DGL) nanoparticles with a cell-penetrating peptide; the nucleolar translocation signal (NoLS) sequence of the LIM Kinase 2 (LIMK2) protein (LIMK2-NP) using plasmid DNA-encoding inhibitor of growth 4 as the therapeutic gene for the treatment of glioma. Anti-glioma results demonstrated that LIMK2-NP produced the strongest and most intensive apoptosis on the tumor site and the longest median survival time of glioma-bearing mice among all treatment groups (Yao et al., 2015).

4 Conclusion and perspectives

In the past, a lot of strategies have been developed to deliver drugs to CNS to treat brain diseases. Most of drugs are macromolecules, such as proteins, polypeptides, and genes, which increase the difficulty in transport from blood to brain. AMT gives us a new method to transport drugs to brain. The positively charged proteins or peptides can produce an electrostatic interaction with negatively charged brain endothelial cells and create a vesicle to endocytosis. However, the mechanism of adsorptive-mediated transcytosis is still not clear and the mechanism study of AMT needs to be continued. Although adsorptive-mediated nanoparticle targeting delivery systems can increase drug delivery to brain, from the data available, the percentage of injected drug dose found in brain after administration is <1% (Costantino and Boraschi, 2012). Here comes the question: How to increase the brain drug delivery efficiency? Combining AMT with advanced nanotechnology may pave the way for brain drug delivery, but there still has a long way to find the answer.

Acknowledgments

This work was supported by the National Natural Science Foundation of China (81773283, 81472757, 81361140344).

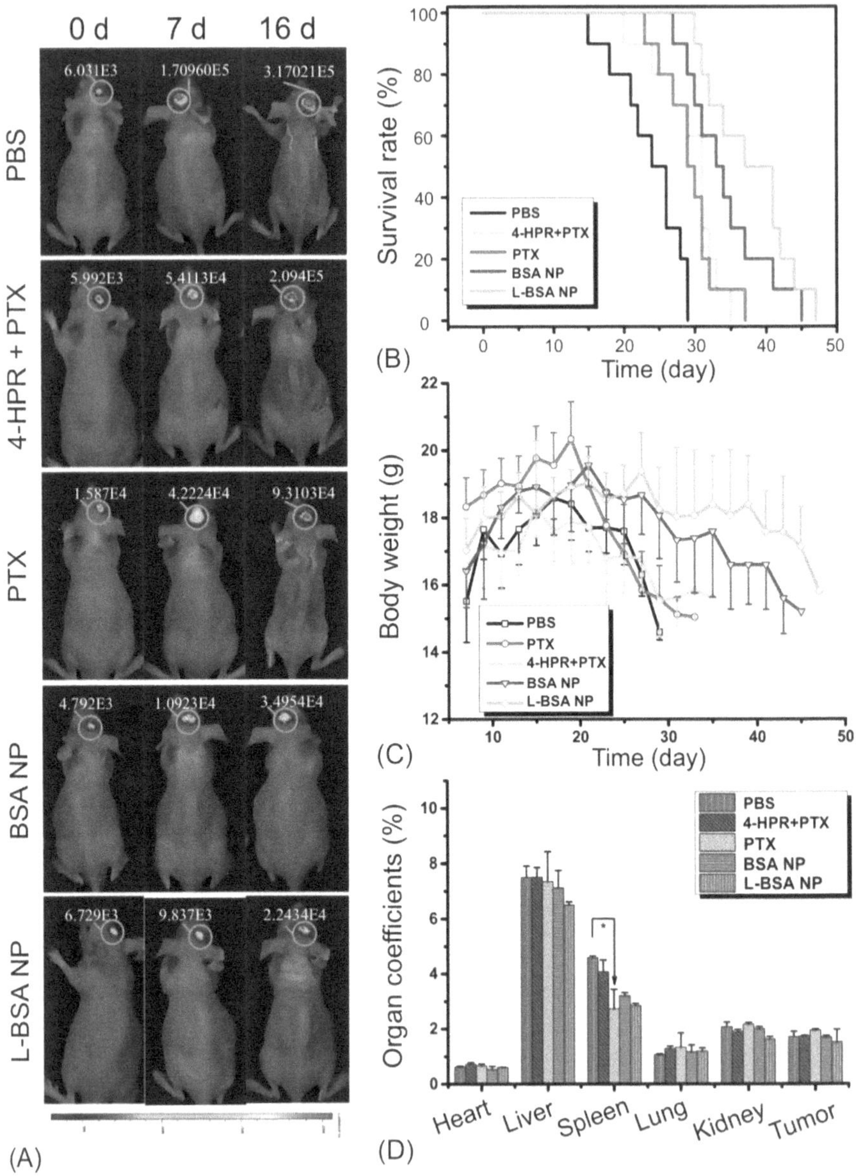

Fig. 2 Antiglioma efficacy of LMWP-BSA-NP loaded with paclitaxel and fenretinide. (A) Glioma growth inhibition monitored by using in vivo bioluminescence images. (B) Survival curve of different groups after different treatments. (C) Body weight variations of different groups in the treatment course. (D) Organ coefficients.

Reproduced with permission from Lin, T., Zhao, P., Jiang, Y., Tang, Y., Jin, H., Pan, Z., He, H., Yang, V.C., Huang, Y., 2016. Blood-brain-barrier-penetrating albumin nanoparticles for biomimetic drug delivery via albumin-binding protein pathways for antiglioma therapy. ACS Nano, 10, 9999–10012. Copyright (2016) American Chemical Society.

References

Agarwal, A., Agrawal, H., Tiwari, S., Jain, S., Agrawal, G.P., 2011. Cationic ligand appended nanoconstructs: a prospective strategy for brain targeting. Int. J. Pharm. 421, 189–201.

Agrawal, M., Ajazuddin, Tripathi, D.K., Saraf, S., Antimisiaris, S.G., Mourtas, S., Hammarlund-Udenaes, M., Alexander, A., 2017. Recent advancements in liposomes targeting strategies to cross blood-brain barrier (BBB) for the treatment of Alzheimer's disease. J. Control. Release 260, 61–77.

Ahsan, C.R., Hajnoczky, G., Maksymowych, A.B., Simpson, L.L., 2005. Visualization of binding and transcytosis of botulinum toxin by human intestinal epithelial cells. J. Pharmacol. Exp. Ther. 315, 1028–1035.

Al Soraj, M., He, L., Peynshaert, K., Cousaert, J., Vercauteren, D., Braeckmans, K., De Smedt, S.C., Jones, A.T., 2012. siRNA and pharmacological inhibition of endocytic pathways to characterize the differential role of macropinocytosis and the actin cytoskeleton on cellular uptake of dextran and cationic cell penetrating peptides octaarginine (R8) and HIV-Tat. J. Control. Release 161, 132–141.

Alves, I.D., Goasdoue, N., Correia, I., Aubry, S., Galanth, C., Sagan, S., Lavielle, S., Chassaing, G., 2008. Membrane interaction and perturbation mechanisms induced by two cationic cell penetrating peptides with distinct charge distribution. Biochim. Biophys. Acta 1780, 948–959.

Alves, I.D., Jiao, C.Y., Aubry, S., Aussedat, B., Burlina, F., Chassaing, G., Sagan, S., 2010. Cell biology meets biophysics to unveil the different mechanisms of penetratin internalization in cells. Biochim. Biophys. Acta 1798, 2231–2239.

Amand, H.L., Fant, K., Norden, B., Esbjorner, E.K., 2008. Stimulated endocytosis in penetratin uptake: effect of arginine and lysine. Biochem. Biophys. Res. Commun. 371, 621–625.

Balzeau, J., Pinier, M., Berges, R., Saulnier, P., Benoit, J.P., Eyer, J., 2013. The effect of functionalizing lipid nanocapsules with NFL-TBS.40-63 peptide on their uptake by glioblastoma cells. Biomaterials 34, 3381–3389.

Barany-Wallje, E., Gaur, J., Lundberg, P., Langel, U., Graslund, A., 2007. Differential membrane perturbation caused by the cell penetrating peptide Tp10 depending on attached cargo. FEBS Lett. 581, 2389–2393.

Belting, M., 2003. Heparan sulfate proteoglycan as a plasma membrane carrier. Trends Biochem. Sci. 28, 145–151.

Bickel, U., Yoshikawa, T., Pardridge, W.M., 2001. Delivery of peptides and proteins through the blood–brain barrier. Adv. Drug Deliv. Rev. 46, 247–279.

Binder, H., Lindblom, G., 2003. Charge-dependent translocation of the Trojan peptide penetratin across lipid membranes. Biophys. J. 85, 982–995.

Broadwell, R.D., Balin, B.J., Salcman, M., 1988. Transcytotic pathway for blood-borne protein through the blood-brain barrier. Proc. Natl. Acad. Sci. 85, 632–636.

Brown, R.C., Morris, A.P., O'neil, R.G., 2007. Tight junction protein expression and barrier properties of immortalized mouse brain microvessel endothelial cells. Brain Res. 1130, 17–30.

Cates, C.C., Arias, A.D., Nakayama Wong, L.S., Lame, M.W., Sidorov, M., Cayanan, G., Rowland, D.J., Fung, J., Karpel-Massler, G., Siegelin, M.D., Greene, L.A., Angelastro, J.M., 2016. Regression/eradication of gliomas in mice by a systemically-deliverable ATF5 dominant-negative peptide. Oncotarget 7, 12718–12730.

Clayton, A.H., Atcliffe, B.W., Howlett, G.J., Sawyer, W.H., 2006. Conformation and orientation of penetratin in phospholipid membranes. J. Pept. Sci. 12, 233–238.

Conner, S.D., Schmid, S.L., 2003. Regulated portals of entry into the cell. Nature 422, 37–44.
Costantino, L., Boraschi, D., 2012. Is there a clinical future for polymeric nanoparticles as brain-targeting drug delivery agents? Drug Discov. Today 17, 367–378.
Deguchi, Y., Miyakawa, Y., Sakurada, S., Naito, Y., Morimoto, K., Ohtsuki, S., Hosoya, K.I., Terasaki, T., 2003. Blood-brain barrier transport of a novel μ1-specific opioid peptide, H-Tyr-d-Arg-Phe-β-Ala-OH (TAPA). J. Neurochem. 84, 1154–1161.
Deguchi, Y., Naito, T., Yuge, T., 2000. Blood-brain barrier transport of 125I-labeled basic fibroblast growth factor. Pharm. Res. 17, 63–69.
Derossi, D., Calvet, S., Trembleau, A., Brunissen, A., Chassaing, G., Prochiantz, A., 1996. Cell internalization of the third helix of the Antennapedia homeodomain is receptor-independent. J. Biol. Chem. 271, 18188–18193.
Derossi, D., Joliot, A.H., Chassaing, G., Prochiantz, A., 1994. The third helix of the Antennapedia homeodomain translocates through biological membranes. J. Biol. Chem. 269, 10444–10450.
Deshayes, S., Gerbal-Chaloin, S., Morris, M.C., Aldrian-Herrada, G., Charnet, P., Divita, G., Heitz, F., 2004. On the mechanism of non-endosomial peptide-mediated cellular delivery of nucleic acids. Biochim. Biophys. Acta 1667, 141–147.
Dhami, N.K., Pandey, R.S., Jain, U.K., Chandra, R., Madan, J., 2014. Non-aggregated protamine-coated poly (lactide-co-glycolide) nanoparticles of cisplatin crossed blood–brain barrier, enhanced drug delivery and improved therapeutic index in glioblastoma cells: in vitro studies. J. Microencapsul. 31, 685–693.
Discher, B.M., Won, Y.Y., Ege, D.S., Lee, J.C., Bates, F.S., Discher, D.E., Hammer, D.A., 1999. Polymersomes: tough vesicles made from diblock copolymers. Science 284, 1143–1146.
Discher, D.E., Ortiz, V., Srinivas, G., Klein, M.L., Kim, Y., Christian, D., Cai, S., Photos, P., Ahmed, F., 2007. Emerging applications of polymersomes in delivery: from molecular dynamics to shrinkage of tumors. Prog. Polym. Sci. 32, 838–857.
Doherty, G.J., Mcmahon, H.T., 2009. Mechanisms of endocytosis. Annu. Rev. Biochem. 78, 857–902.
Du, W., Wei, Y., Zhao, G., Qin, H.Y., Wu, X.A., 2008. Simultaneous determination of four Tanshinones in rat plasma by high performance liquid chromatography and its application to pharmacokinetic studies. Chin. Pharm. J. 43, 786–789.
Duchardt, F., Fotin-Mleczek, M., Schwarz, H., Fischer, R., Brock, R., 2007. A comprehensive model for the cellular uptake of cationic cell-penetrating peptides. Traffic 8, 848–866.
El-Andaloussi, S., Holm, T., Langel, U., 2005. Cell-penetrating peptides: mechanisms and applications. Curr. Pharm. Des. 11, 3597–3611.
Feng, L., Zhu, C., Yuan, H., Liu, L., Lv, F., Wang, S., 2013. Conjugated polymer nanoparticles: preparation, properties, functionalization and biological applications. Chem. Soc. Rev. 42, 6620–6633.
Fischer, R., Waizenegger, T., Kohler, K., Brock, R., 2002. A quantitative validation of fluorophore-labelled cell-permeable peptide conjugates: fluorophore and cargo dependence of import. Biochim. Biophys. Acta 1564, 365–374.
Fittipaldi, A., Ferrari, A., Zoppe, M., Arcangeli, C., Pellegrini, V., Beltram, F., Giacca, M., 2003. Cell membrane lipid rafts mediate caveolar endocytosis of HIV-1 Tat fusion proteins. J. Biol. Chem. 278, 34141–34149.
Foerg, C., Ziegler, U., Fernandez-Carneado, J., Giralt, E., Merkle, H.P., 2007. Differentiation restricted endocytosis of cell penetrating peptides in MDCK cells corresponds with activities of Rho-GTPases. Pharm. Res. 24, 628–642.

Fretz, M.M., Penning, N.A., Al-Taei, S., Futaki, S., Takeuchi, T., Nakase, I., Storm, G., Jones, A.T., 2007. Temperature-, concentration- and cholesterol-dependent translocation of L- and D-octa-arginine across the plasma and nuclear membrane of CD34+ leukaemia cells. Biochem. J. 403, 335–342.

Futaki, S., Suzuki, T., Ohashi, W., Yagami, T., Tanaka, S., Ueda, K., Sugiura, Y., 2001. Arginine-rich peptides. An abundant source of membrane-permeable peptides having potential as carriers for intracellular protein delivery. J. Biol. Chem. 276, 5836–5840.

Georgieva, J.V., Brinkhuis, R.P., Stojanov, K., Weijers, C.A., Zuilhof, H., Rutjes, F.P., Hoekstra, D., Van Hest, J.C., Zuhorn, I.S., 2012. Peptide-mediated blood-brain barrier transport of polymersomes. Angew. Chem. Int. Ed. Engl. 51, 8339–8342.

Girod, J., Fenart, L., Régina, A., Dehouck, M.-P., Hong, G., Scherrmann, J.-M., Cecchelli, R., Roux, F., 1999. Transport of cationized anti-tetanus Fab'2 fragments across an in vitro blood-brain barrier model: involvement of the transcytosis pathway. J. Neurochem. 73, 2002–2008.

Gonatas, N.K., Stieber, A., Hickey, W.F., Herbert, S.H., Gonatas, J.O., 1984. Endosomes and golgi vesicles in adsorptive and fluid phase endocytosis. J. Cell Biol. 99, 1379–1390.

Han, J.Y., Fan, J.Y., Horie, Y., Miura, S., Cui, D.H., Ishii, H., Hibi, T., Tsuneki, H., Kimura, I., 2008. Ameliorating effects of compounds derived from *Salvia miltiorrhiza* root extract on microcirculatory disturbance and target organ injury by ischemia and reperfusion. Pharmacol. Ther. 117, 280–295.

Herce, H.D., Garcia, A.E., 2007. Molecular dynamics simulations suggest a mechanism for translocation of the HIV-1 TAT peptide across lipid membranes. Proc. Natl. Acad. Sci. USA 104, 20805–20810.

Hervé, F., Ghinea, N., Scherrmann, J.-M., 2008. CNS delivery via adsorptive transcytosis. AAPS J. 10, 455–472.

Hirose, H., Takeuchi, T., Osakada, H., Pujals, S., Katayama, S., Nakase, I., Kobayashi, S., Haraguchi, T., Futaki, S., 2012. Transient focal membrane deformation induced by arginine-rich peptides leads to their direct penetration into cells. Mol. Ther. 20, 984–993.

Hu, K., Li, J., Shen, Y., Lu, W., Gao, X., Zhang, Q., Jiang, X., 2009. Lactoferrin-conjugated PEG-PLA nanoparticles with improved brain delivery: in vitro and in vivo evaluations. J. Control. Release 134, 55–61.

Joanne, P., Galanth, C., Goasdoue, N., Nicolas, P., Sagan, S., Lavielle, S., Chassaing, G., El Amri, C., Alves, I.D., 2009. Lipid reorganization induced by membrane-active peptides probed using differential scanning calorimetry. Biochim. Biophys. Acta 1788, 1772–1781.

Jones, A.T., Sayers, E.J., 2012. Cell entry of cell penetrating peptides: tales of tails wagging dogs. J. Control. Release 161, 582–591.

Kaplan, I.M., Wadia, J.S., Dowdy, S.F., 2005. Cationic TAT peptide transduction domain enters cells by macropinocytosis. J. Control. Release 102, 247–253.

Khalil, I.A., Kogure, K., Futaki, S., Harashima, H., 2006. High density of octaarginine stimulates macropinocytosis leading to efficient intracellular trafficking for gene expression. J. Biol. Chem. 281, 3544–3551.

Kristensen, M., De Groot, A.M., Berthelsen, J., Franzyk, H., Sijts, A., Nielsen, H.M., 2015. Conjugation of cell-penetrating peptides to parathyroid hormone affects its structure, potency, and transepithelial permeation. Bioconjug. Chem. 26, 477–488.

Kumagai, A.K., Eisenberg, J.B., Pardridge, W.M., 1987. Absorptive-mediated endocytosis of cationized albumin and a beta-endorphin-cationized albumin chimeric peptide by isolated brain capillaries. Model system of blood-brain barrier transport. J. Biol. Chem. 262, 15214–15219.

Lim, S., Kim, W.J., Kim, Y.H., Lee, S., Koo, J.H., Lee, J.A., Yoon, H., Kim, D.H., Park, H.J., Kim, H.M., Lee, H.G., Yun Kim, J., Lee, J.U., Hun Shin, J., Kyun Kim, L., Doh, J., Kim, H., Lee, S.K., Bothwell, A.L., Suh, M., Choi, J.M., 2015. dNP2 is a blood-brain barrier-permeable peptide enabling ctCTLA-4 protein delivery to ameliorate experimental autoimmune encephalomyelitis. Nat. Commun. 6, 8244.

Lin, T., Zhao, P., Jiang, Y., Tang, Y., Jin, H., Pan, Z., He, H., Yang, V.C., Huang, Y., 2016. Blood-brain-barrier-penetrating albumin nanoparticles for biomimetic drug delivery via albumin-binding protein pathways for antiglioma therapy. ACS Nano 10, 9999–10012.

Liu, X., Ye, M., An, C., Pan, L., Ji, L., 2013. The effect of cationic albumin-conjugated PEGylated tanshinone IIA nanoparticles on neuronal signal pathways and neuroprotection in cerebral ischemia. Biomaterials 34, 6893–6905.

Liu, Y., Mei, L., Xu, C., Yu, Q., Shi, K., Zhang, L., Wang, Y., Zhang, Q., Gao, H., Zhang, Z., He, Q., 2016. Dual receptor recognizing cell penetrating peptide for selective targeting, efficient intratumoral diffusion and synthesized anti-glioma therapy. Theranostics 6, 177–191.

Liu, Y., Mei, L., Yu, Q., Xu, C., Qiu, Y., Yang, Y., Shi, K., Zhang, Q., Gao, H., Zhang, Z., He, Q., 2015. Multifunctional tandem peptide modified paclitaxel-loaded liposomes for the treatment of vasculogenic mimicry and cancer stem cells in malignant glioma. ACS Appl. Mater. Interfaces 7, 16792–16801.

Liu, Y., Ran, R., Chen, J., Kuang, Q., Tang, J., Mei, L., Zhang, Q., Gao, H., Zhang, Z., He, Q., 2014. Paclitaxel loaded liposomes decorated with a multifunctional tandem peptide for glioma targeting. Biomaterials 35, 4835–4847.

Lu, W., Sun, Q., Wan, J., She, Z., Jiang, X.G., 2006. Cationic albumin-conjugated pegylated nanoparticles allow gene delivery into brain tumors via intravenous administration. Cancer Res. 66, 11878–11887.

Lu, W., Tan, Y.Z., Hu, K.L., Jiang, X.G., 2005a. Cationic albumin conjugated pegylated nanoparticle with its transcytosis ability and little toxicity against blood-brain barrier. Int. J. Pharm. 295, 247–260.

Lu, W., Wan, J., Zhang, Q., She, Z., Jiang, X., 2007. Aclarubicin-loaded cationic albumin-conjugated pegylated nanoparticle for glioma chemotherapy in rats. Int. J. Cancer 120, 420–431.

Lu, W., Zhang, Y., Tan, Y.-Z., Hu, K.-L., Jiang, X.-G., Fu, S.-K., 2005b. Cationic albumin-conjugated pegylated nanoparticles as novel drug carrier for brain delivery. J. Control. Release 107, 428–448.

Lukyanenko, V., Malyukova, I., Hubbard, A., Delannoy, M., Boedeker, E., Zhu, C., Cebotaru, L., Kovbasnjuk, O., 2011. Enterohemorrhagic Escherichia coli infection stimulates Shiga toxin 1 macropinocytosis and transcytosis across intestinal epithelial cells. Am. J. Physiol. Cell Physiol. 301, C1140–9.

Lundin, P., Johansson, H., Guterstam, P., Holm, T., Hansen, M., Langel, U., El Andaloussi, S., 2008. Distinct uptake routes of cell-penetrating peptide conjugates. Bioconjug. Chem. 19, 2535–2542.

Luo, D., Saltzman, W.M., 2000. Synthetic DNA delivery systems. Nat. Biotechnol. 18, 33–37.

Mae, M., Langel, U., 2006. Cell-penetrating peptides as vectors for peptide, protein and oligonucleotide delivery. Curr. Opin. Pharmacol. 6, 509–514.

Mai, J.C., Shen, H., Watkins, S.C., Cheng, T., Robbins, P.D., 2002. Efficiency of protein transduction is cell type-dependent and is enhanced by dextran sulfate. J. Biol. Chem. 277, 30208–30218.

Mukherjee, S., Ray, S., Thakur, R.S., 2009. Solid lipid nanoparticles: a modern formulation approach in drug delivery system. Indian J. Pharm. Sci. 71, 349–358.

Nakase, I., Niwa, M., Takeuchi, T., Sonomura, K., Kawabata, N., Koike, Y., Takehashi, M., Tanaka, S., Ueda, K., Simpson, J.C., Jones, A.T., Sugiura, Y., Futaki, S., 2004. Cellular uptake of arginine-rich peptides: roles for macropinocytosis and actin rearrangement. Mol. Ther. 10, 1011–1022.

Opacak-Bernardi, T., Ryu, J.S., Raucher, D., 2017. Effects of cell penetrating Notch inhibitory peptide conjugated to elastin-like polypeptide on glioblastoma cells. J. Drug Target. 25, 523–531.

Pang, Z., Gao, H., Chen, J., Shen, S., Zhang, B., Ren, J., Guo, L., Qian, Y., Jiang, X., Mei, H., 2012. Intracellular delivery mechanism and brain delivery kinetics of biodegradable cationic bovine serum albumin-conjugated polymersomes. Int. J. Nanomed. 7, 3421–3432.

Pang, Z., Lu, W., Gao, H., Hu, K., Chen, J., Zhang, C., Gao, X., Jiang, X., Zhu, C., 2008. Preparation and brain delivery property of biodegradable polymersomes conjugated with OX26. J. Control. Release 128, 120–127.

Pardridge, W.M., Boado, R.J., 1991. Enhanced cellular uptake of biotinylated antisense oligonucleotide or peptide mediated by avidin, a cationic protein. FEBS Lett. 288, 30–32.

Pardridge, W.M., Buciak, J.L., Kang, Y.-S., Boado, R.J., 1993. Protamine-mediated transport of albumin into brain and other organs of the rat. Binding and endocytosis of protamine-albumin complex by microvascular endothelium. J. Clin. Investig. 92, 2224.

Pardridge, W.M., Eisenberg, J., Yang, J., 1985. Human blood-brain barrier insulin receptor. J. Neurochem. 44, 1771–1778.

Pardridge, W.M., Eisenberg, J., Yang, J., 1987a. Human blood-brain barrier transferrin receptor. Metabolism 36, 892–895.

Pardridge, W.M., Kumagai, A.K., Eisenberg, J.B., 1987b. Chimeric peptides as a vehicle for peptide pharmaceutical delivery through the blood-brain barrier. Biochem. Biophys. Res. Commun. 146, 307–313.

Pardridge, W.M., Triguero, D., Buciak, J., 1989. Transport of histone through the blood-brain barrier. J. Pharmacol. Exp. Ther. 251, 821–826.

Pooga, M., Hallbrink, M., Zorko, M., Langel, U., 1998. Cell penetration by transportan. FASEB J. 12, 67–77.

Prochiantz, A., 2000. Messenger proteins: homeoproteins, TAT and others. Curr. Opin. Cell Biol. 12, 400–406.

Pujals, S., Fernandez-Carneado, J., Lopez-Iglesias, C., Kogan, M.J., Giralt, E., 2006. Mechanistic aspects of CPP-mediated intracellular drug delivery: relevance of CPP self-assembly. Biochim. Biophys. Acta 1758, 264–279.

Qian, Z., Larochelle, J.R., Jiang, B., Lian, W., Hard, R.L., Selner, N.G., Luechapanichkul, R., Barrios, A.M., Pei, D., 2014. Early endosomal escape of a cyclic cell-penetrating peptide allows effective cytosolic cargo delivery. Biochemistry 53, 4034–4046.

Raub, T.J., Audus, K.L., 1990. Adsorptive endocytosis and membrane recycling by cultured primary bovine brain microvessel endothelial cell monolayers. J. Cell Sci. 97, 127–138.

Richard, J.P., Melikov, K., Brooks, H., Prevot, P., Lebleu, B., Chernomordik, L.V., 2005. Cellular uptake of unconjugated TAT peptide involves clathrin-dependent endocytosis and heparan sulfate receptors. J. Biol. Chem. 280, 15300–15306.

Richard, J.P., Melikov, K., Vives, E., Ramos, C., Verbeure, B., Gait, M.J., Chernomordik, L.V., Lebleu, B., 2003. Cell-penetrating peptides. A reevaluation of the mechanism of cellular uptake. J. Biol. Chem. 278, 585–590.

Rothbard, J.B., Garlington, S., Lin, Q., Kirschberg, T., Kreider, E., Mcgrane, P.L., Wender, P.A., Khavari, P.A., 2000. Conjugation of arginine oligomers to cyclosporin A facilitates topical delivery and inhibition of inflammation. Nat. Med. 6, 1253–1257.

Saalik, P., Elmquist, A., Hansen, M., Padari, K., Saar, K., Viht, K., Langel, U., Pooga, M., 2004. Protein cargo delivery properties of cell-penetrating peptides. A comparative study. Bioconjug. Chem. 15, 1246–1253.

Sakai, N., Takeuchi, T., Futaki, S., Matile, S., 2005. Direct observation of anion-mediated translocation of fluorescent oligoarginine carriers into and across bulk liquid and anionic bilayer membranes. ChemBioChem 6, 114–122.

Schnitzer, J.E., 2001. Caveolae: from basic trafficking mechanisms to targeting transcytosis for tissue-specific drug and gene delivery in vivo. Adv. Drug Deliv. Rev. 49, 265–280.

Sharma, G., Modgil, A., Layek, B., Arora, K., Sun, C., Law, B., Singh, J., 2013. Cell penetrating peptide tethered bi-ligand liposomes for delivery to brain in vivo: biodistribution and transfection. J. Control. Release 167, 1–10.

Sharma, G., Modgil, A., Sun, C., Singh, J., 2012. Grafting of cell-penetrating peptide to receptor-targeted liposomes improves their transfection efficiency and transport across blood-brain barrier model. J. Pharm. Sci. 101, 2468–2478.

Shimura, T., Tabata, S., Ohnishi, T., Terasaki, T., Tsuji, A., 1991. Transport mechanism of a new behaviorally highly potent adrenocorticotropic hormone (ACTH) analog, ebiratide, through the blood-brain barrier. J. Pharmacol. Exp. Ther. 258, 459–465.

Shimura, T., Tabata, S., Terasaki, T., Deguchi, Y., Tsuji, A., 1992. In-vivo blood-brain barrier transport of a novel adrenocorticotropic hormone analogue, ebiratide, demonstrated by brain microdialysis and capillary depletion methods. J. Pharm. Pharmacol. 44, 583–588.

Snyder, E.L., Dowdy, S.F., 2005. Recent advances in the use of protein transduction domains for the delivery of peptides, proteins and nucleic acids in vivo. Expert Opin. Drug Deliv. 2, 43–51.

Suzuki, T., Futaki, S., Niwa, M., Tanaka, S., Ueda, K., Sugiura, Y., 2002. Possible existence of common internalization mechanisms among arginine-rich peptides. J. Biol. Chem. 277, 2437–2443.

Tamai, I., Sai, Y., Kobayashi, H., Kamata, M., Wakamiya, T., Tsuji, A., 1997. Structure-internalization relationship for adsorptive-mediated endocytosis of basic peptides at the blood-brain barrier. J. Pharmacol. Exp. Ther. 280, 410–415.

Terasaki, T., Deguchi, Y., Sato, H., Hirai, K.-I., Tsuji, A., 1991. In vivo transport of a dynorphin-like analgesic peptide, E-2078, through the blood-brain barrier: an application of brain microdialysis. Pharm. Res. 8, 815–820.

Thole, M., Nobmann, S., Huwyler, J., Bartmann, A., Fricker, G., 2002. Uptake of cationzied albumin coupled liposomes by cultured porcine brain microvessel endothelial cells and intact brain capillaries. J. Drug Target 10, 337–344.

Thukral, D.K., Dumoga, S., Mishra, A.K., 2014. Solid lipid nanoparticles: promising therapeutic nanocarriers for drug delivery. Curr. Drug Deliv. 11, 771–791.

Torchilin, V.P., 2005. Recent advances with liposomes as pharmaceutical carriers. Nat. Rev. Drug Discov. 4, 145–160.

Trehin, R., Krauss, U., Beck-Sickinger, A.G., Merkle, H.P., Nielsen, H.M., 2004. Cellular uptake but low permeation of human calcitonin-derived cell penetrating peptides and Tat(47-57) through well-differentiated epithelial models. Pharm. Res. 21, 1248–1256.

Tunnemann, G., Martin, R.M., Haupt, S., Patsch, C., Edenhofer, F., Cardoso, M.C., 2006. Cargo-dependent mode of uptake and bioavailability of TAT-containing proteins and peptides in living cells. FASEB J. 20, 1775–1784.

Villegas, J., Broadwell, R., 1993. Transcytosis of protein through the mammalian cerebral epithelium and endothelium. II. Adsorptive transcytosis of WGA-HRP and the blood-brain and brain-blood barriers. J. Neurocytol. 22, 67–80.

Vives, E., Brodin, P., Lebleu, B., 1997. A truncated HIV-1 Tat protein basic domain rapidly translocates through the plasma membrane and accumulates in the cell nucleus. J. Biol. Chem. 272, 16010–16017.
Vorbrodt, A., 1989. Ultracytochemical characterization of anionic sites in the wall of brain capillaries. J. Neurocytol. 18, 359–368.
Wadia, J.S., Stan, R.V., Dowdy, S.F., 2004. Transducible TAT-HA fusogenic peptide enhances escape of TAT-fusion proteins after lipid raft macropinocytosis. Nat. Med. 10, 310–315.
Xie, Y.L., Lu, W., Jiang, X.G., 2006. Improvement of cationic albumin conjugated pegylated nanoparticles holding NC-1900, a vasopressin fragment analog, in memory deficits induced by scopolamine in mice. Behav. Brain Res. 173, 76–84.
Xu, F., Lu, W., Wu, H., Fan, L., Gao, X., Jiang, X., 2009. Brain delivery and systemic effect of cationic albumin conjugated PLGA nanoparticles. J. Drug Target 17, 423–434.
Yao, H., Wang, K., Wang, Y., Wang, S., Li, J., Lou, J., Ye, L., Yan, X., Lu, W., Huang, R., 2015. Enhanced blood-brain barrier penetration and glioma therapy mediated by a new peptide modified gene delivery system. Biomaterials 37, 345–352.
Zhang, L., Zhang, Y., Tai, L., Jiang, K., Xie, C., Li, Z., Lin, Y.Z., Wei, G., Lu, W., Pan, W., 2016. Functionalized cell nucleus-penetrating peptide combined with doxorubicin for synergistic treatment of glioma. Acta Biomater. 42, 90–101.

Efflux pump inhibition to enhance brain targeting delivery

8

Rujing Chen, Xiao Zhao, Kaili Hu
Institute of Interdisciplinary Integrative Medicine Research, Shanghai University of Traditional Chinese Medicine, Shanghai, China

1 Introduction

The blood-brain barrier (BBB) plays an important role by maintaining homeostasis and preventing macromolecules, infectious agents, and potential neurotoxins from entering the brain (Pardridge, 2005). However, the BBB also significantly limits the ability of therapeutic agents to reach their targets in the CNS at the same time. >98% of all small-molecule chemical agents and nearly 100% of all larger therapeutics are prevented from crossing the BBB (Pardridge, 2005). In addition, those few drugs that can cross the BBB may be actively transported back into the vasculature by efflux transporters, such as P-gp, a member of the ABC family (van Tellingen et al., 2015). These active efflux transporters can recognize a wide range of compounds (>60% of all marketed drugs) and contribute to drug resistance (Demeule et al., 2002). Several approaches have been used to decrease the activity of ABC efflux transporters. These strategies not only include the techniques to inhibit the transporters, but also to sidestep from them. Recent studies applied nanotechnology to overcome the drug resistance offered by drug efflux pumps(Kaur et al., 2014). The purpose of this chapter is to discuss the nanotechnological development in the inhibition of ABC efflux transporters (mainly P-gp) to enhance the brain delivery of therapeutics. Also, the ABC transporter inhibitors and the role of ABC transporters in inhibiting the entry of drug molecules are reviewed.

2 Efflux pump

ABC transporters, an example of ATP-powered pumps, are ubiquitous membrane-bound proteins, which use energy released by ATP hydrolysis to move substrates in or out of cells or into cellular vesicles, against their electrochemical gradient. In mammals, ABC transporters comprising one of the largest protein superfamilies are expressed mainly in the liver, intestine, BBB, blood-testis barrier, placenta, and kidney (Vasiliou et al., 2009). ABC transporters can transport a number of endogenous substrates, including inorganic anions, metal ions, peptides, amino acids, sugars, a large number of hydrophobic compounds, etc. (Vasiliou et al., 2009). In humans, ABC transporters are coded by 49 genes that are classified into seven subfamilies, on the basis of sequence homology and functional similarities (Moitra and Dean, 2011),

Brain Targeted Drug Delivery Systems. https://doi.org/10.1016/B978-0-12-814001-7.00008-1

designated from A to G, and they can broadly be categorized as importers or exporters, depending on the direction of transport relative to the cytoplasm (Dassa and Bouige, 2001). The three ABC subfamilies, B, C, and G, contain efflux transporters that extrude metabolic waste products, foreign chemicals (xenobiotics), and a large number of drugs from the brain into the blood (Hartz and Bauer, 2011). Therefore, ABC transporters are not only responsible for transport of nutrients from blood to brain, but also play an important role in maintaining the strength of the BBB. These efflux transporters (Qosa et al., 2015) limit CNS uptake of certain drugs and molecules to provide protection for the CNS from exposure to circulating chemicals, thus becoming major obstacles to CNS pharmacotherapy (Miller and Cannon, 2014). Among these subfamilies, ABCB1 (multidrug resistance proteins, MDR1 or P-gp), ABCC (multidrug resistance-associated protein, MRPs), and ABCG2 (breast cancer resistance protein, BCRP) are the utmost studied (Miller, 2015).

ABCB1 or P-gp is the 170-kDa glycoprotein product of the MDR1 gene which is highly expressed on the luminal membrane of the endothelial cells at the BBB and, to a much lesser extent, in brain parenchyma, neuronal, and glial cells (Sharom, 2008). Several studies have suggested that P-gp expression in brain parenchymal cells is nominal, although it may be significantly enhanced in pathologic conditions (Qosa et al., 2015). Strategic localization of P-gp at the luminal membrane of BBB endothelial cells and its wide substrate selectivity make it an effective defense against a wide spectrum of endogenous ligands, therapeutic drugs, and xenobiotics (Qosa et al., 2015). Therefore, P-gp plays a vital role in both neuroprotection and pharmacoresistance by efficiently restricting the entry of exogenous molecules into brain. However, it can limit the entry of therapeutics, particularly in certain conditions when its expression at the BBB is increased significantly contributing to the development of pharmacoresistance (Miller et al., 2008) (Fig. 1).

P-gp has numerous substrates, most of which are lipophilic, including antiepileptic drugs (phenobarbital, carbamazepine, phenytoin, and lamotrigine), antitumor drugs, immunosuppressants, adrenocortical hormone, analgesics, cytokines, histamines, calcium channel blockers, cardiac glycosides, antidepressant drugs, and antibiotics (Löscher and Potschka, 2005).

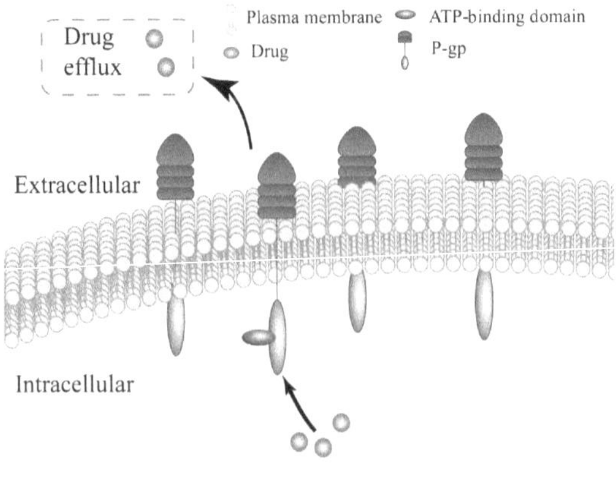

Fig. 1 Efflux of drugs by P-glycoprotein.

Dozens of P-gp inhibitors can be divided into several categories, which are calcium channel blockers, such as verapamil and nifedipine; calmodulin antagonists, such as trifluoperazine and chlorpromazine; cyclosporines, such as cyclosporine A; hormones and antihormone compounds, such as progesterone; isoquinolinetype alkaloids, such as berberine; and others (Xiong et al., 2015). The research of Futscher et al. suggests that verapamil inhibits P-gp activity by direct competition with P-gp substrates (Futscher et al., 1996). Shin et al. found that trifluoperazine induced the down-regulation of P-gp protein and mdr1b mRNA in a dose- and time-dependent manner in L1210/Adr cells (Shin et al., 2006). In the study of Sakata et al., it has been demonstrated that cyclosporine A competed with the substrates of P-gp to bind to the drug-binding site of P-gp, and learning from their study, a series of clinical trials on the combination of anticancer drugs that were MDR substrates and cyclosporine A have been originated (Sakata et al., 1994).

The family of multidrug resistance-associated proteins (MRPs or ABCC) has nine members involved in drug transport of humans (Dallas et al., 2006). Among them, MRP1, MRP2, and MRP4, which have definitive localization in brain capillaries, are the most studied (Miller, 2014). In the CNS, MRP1 localizes at the basolateral membrane of choroid plexus epithelial cells, and it is also detected at the luminal and abluminal membranes of capillary endothelium (Gazzin et al., 2011). MRP2 is expressed mainly on the apical side of capillary endothelium (Dallas et al., 2006). MRP4 seems to be expressed on both the luminal and abluminal membranes of the brain capillary endothelium (Qosa et al., 2015). The range of MRP-mediated efflux drug is relatively narrow. Antitumor drugs and some antiepileptic drugs are basically contained (Robey et al., 2010).

Inhibitors of MRP include probenecid, sulfinpyrazone, benzbromarone, dipyridamole, quinolines, and cyclosporines (Xiong et al., 2015). Wang et al. used probenecid as a MRP and organic anion transporter (OAT) inhibitor, to investigate the impact of MRPs and OATs on the distribution of fluconazole in the rat brain. The results showed that probenecid increased the penetration of fluconazole into the BBB, but did not alter the penetration of fluconazole into the blood-cerebrospinal fluid barrier of rats (Wang et al., 2017). Nagasaka et al. examined the in vitro inhibitory effect of aripiprazole and its active metabolite dehydroaripiprazole on the activities of human MDR1, BCRP, and MRP4. They found that the two compounds had relatively strong inhibition potencies against MDR1 and BCRP, while the two compounds showed almost no effects on MRP4 activity. In their study, it was also clarified that the potencies of aripiprazole and dehydroaripiprazole were stronger than those of risperidone, paliperidone, olanzapine, and ziprasidone (Nagasaka et al., 2012).

ABCG2 or BCRP is a 72-kDa half ABC transporter with only one nucleotide-binding domain and one membrane-spanning domain, predominantly expressed at the luminal membrane of the BBB cells and displaying substrate overlap with P-gp (Aronica et al., 2005). BCRP is thought to act in concert with P-gp to exert a synergistic effect in limiting BBB permeability.

BCRP has a wide range of substrates, such as antitumor medicines (e.g., mitoxantrone and topotecan), tyrosine kinase inhibitors (e.g., TKI, imatinib, and gefitinib), and some antibiotic and HMG-CoA inhibitors (Robey et al., 2010). The substrates overlap partly with those of P-gp and MRP2. Studies have shown that some antiviral drugs have inhibitory effects on BCRP. The potency of the inhibitory effects of these drugs on BCRP is in the following order: lopinavir > nelfinavir > efavirenz > saquinavir > atazanavir >amprenavir > abacavir (Weiss et al., 2007a, 2007b). Wang et al. investigated the effects of several antipsychotic drugs, including risperidone, 9-hydroxy-risperidone (paliperidone), olanzapine, quetiapine, clozapine, haloperidol, and chlorpromazine, and a positive control inhibitor Ko143 on functions of BCRP in MCF7 and BCRP overexpressing MCF7/MX100 cell lines using a BCRP prototypical substrate mitoxantrone. Their findings indicated that the tested antipsychotics rank order of potency of inhibition of BCRP according to concentrations required to reach 50% of maximum inhibition (IC_{50}) was as follows: Ko143 (0.07 μM) > risperidone (38.1 μM) > clozapine (42.0 μM) > paliperidone (51 μM) > chlorpromazine (52.2 μM) > quetiapine (66.1 μM) > olanzapine = haloperidol (>100.0 μM) (Wang et al., 2008).

ABC transporters can perform the functions of drug efflux pumps, which can reduce the effective drug concentration at lesions by reducing the permeability of the BBB to therapeutic drugs, thereby limiting their efficacy (Xiong et al., 2015). Several approaches have been used to decrease the activity of ABC efflux transporters (Qosa et al., 2015). These strategies not only include the techniques to inhibit the transporters, but also to sidestep from them. Firstly, various ABC efflux transporter substrates were given along with the competitive or noncompetitive ABC efflux transporter inhibitors. These specific inhibitors inhibit the ABC efflux transporters, thus allowing the drug molecules to enter inside the cell. However, the usages of these inhibitors were not explored so much as they have their own pharmacological actions and they are themselves toxics (Varma et al., 2003). Then, the researchers found that many pharmaceutical excipients also have ABC efflux transporter inhibitory activity, although they are inert in nature (Hugger et al., 2002). These excipients are commonly used in pharmaceutical formulations as they are reported to be safe, nontoxic, and are highly acceptable in formulations. After that, the arrival of nanotechnological techniques gives a new path to overcome the problem of efflux pumps. In this technique, ABC efflux transporter inhibitors can be encapsulated along with the therapeutics. And at the same time, the pharmaceutical excipients can also be used in these formulations. Some of the novel nanocarriers like liposomes and nanoparticles can bypass the efflux pumps (Huang et al., 2011; Huwyler et al., 2002). Other novel formulations such as polymeric micelles can inhibit the ABC efflux transporter activity (Kaur et al., 2014).

Nanotechnology has shown considerable applications in the drug delivery through various nanoformulations such as nanoparticles, liposomes, and micelles. Recent studies applied this technique to overcome the drug resistance offered by drug efflux pumps, mainly the P-gp efflux (Kaur et al., 2014). Nanocarrier systems including liposomes, solid lipid nanoparticles (SLNs), polymeric nanoparticles, and polymeric micelles have many advantages, such as protect drugs from premature degradation, enhance absorption of drugs in selected tissue, control of pharmacokinetic and tissue distribution profile, prevent premature interaction of drugs with biological environment, and improve intracellular penetration (Mahmoudzadeh et al., 2013).

3 Modulating the efflux pump by nanoparticles to improve brain delivery

3.1 Liposomes

Liposomes are vesicles made of phospholipid bilayer and an aqueous core, with vesicle size typically between 50 nm and 5 μm that was first reported by Alec Bangham, a British hematologist, who noticed its formation while staining dry phospholipids for evaluating an electron microscope (Bangham and Horne, 1964). As regard the variety of sizes and lamellar structures, liposomes can be loaded with hydrophobic, hydrophilic, or amphipathic drugs, using relatively simple techniques. Drugs can be encapsulated within or adsorbed on the lipid shell, depending on their hydrophobicity, and can be released from the same type of liposome with different kinetics, achieving superior therapeutic efficacy than free drugs (Pinzón-Daza et al., 2013). Liposome-encapsulated drugs have shown selective intratumor drug delivery, lower side effects, and particular efficacy against aggressive and chemoresistant tumors (Riganti et al., 2011). Liposome-encapsulated drugs have been proposed as vehicles that are able to cross the BBB and deliver their cargo into the CNS (Deeken and Löscher, 2007). It has been reported that liposomal drugs are less potent inducers of P-gp than free drugs (Zalipsky et al., 2007). Pinzón-Daza group reported that liposomal doxorubicin acts as an allosteric inhibitor of P-gp, reduces ATP hydrolysis, and competes with verapamil and colchicine for P-gp binding (Pinzón-Daza et al., 2013). Also, empty liposomes inhibit the activity of P-gp, because they alter the composition of phospholipids and fatty acids in membrane micro domains (i.e., lipid rafts) where P-gp operates (Riganti et al., 2011).

Inhibitory properties of liposomes on ABC transporters make liposomal drugs potentially useful not only against drug-resistant tumors, but also for drug delivery across the BBB (Pinzón-Daza et al., 2013). Patel et al. investigated the co-delivery of the P-gp inhibitor, tariquidar, and cytotoxic drug, paclitaxel, into tumor cells to reverse the MDR using long-circulating liposomes. They found that a simultaneous delivery of tariquidar and paclitaxel by long-circulating liposomes resulted in greater cytotoxicity in SKOV-3TR cells at a paclitaxel dose that was ineffective in the absence of tariquidar, demonstrating a significant reversal of the MDR towards paclitaxel (Patel et al., 2011). Du et al. assessed the potential of dual-targeting topotecan liposomes modified with tamoxifen (TAM) and wheat germ agglutinin (WGA); they found that the dual-targeting effects in vivo of topotecan liposomes modified with TAM and WGA could be related to an enhanced effect by TAM via inhibiting efflux of MDR proteins in the BBB and the brain tumor, and an enhanced effect by WGA via endocytosis in the BBB and in the brain tumor, which suggested that topotecan liposomes modified with TAM and WGA significantly improve topotecan transport across the BBB and the survival of brain tumor-bearing animals, showing dual-targeting effects (Du et al., 2009).

3.2 Solid lipid nanoparticles

SLNs are colloidal systems that consist of spherical solid lipid particles in the nanometer range, dispersed in water or in aqueous surfactant solution. They are generally made up of solid hydrophobic core having a monolayer of phospholipid coating. The solid core can contain the drug dissolved or dispersed in the solid high melting fat matrix with the hydrophobic end of the phospholipid chains embedded in the fat matrix. Thus, they have a potential to carry both lipophilic and hydrophilic drugs or diagnostics (Reddy and Venkateswarlu, 2004). SLN made from biodegradable or biocompatible solid lipids were developed in the beginning of the 1990s as an alternative colloidal carrier system for controlled drug delivery. SLNs as one of the promising drug delivery systems offer an attractive mean for drug delivery. They are with low toxicity potential like emulsions and liposomes and could produce sustained release due to their solid matrix, similar to polymeric nanoparticles (Kakkar et al., 2013). A number of studies have shown that SLN could increase the local drug concentration gradients and facilitate drug transport into the brain via endocytotic pathways and inhibiting the P-gp function (Kaur et al., 2008). Using MDA-MB-436 cells, Cavaco et al. found that SLNs efficiently blinded plasma membrane P-gp and coupling anti-CD44v6 promoted cancer CD44+ cells targeting, decreased the P-gp expression, and protected the drug against cell efflux events (Cavaco et al., 2017). Zhou et al. prepared and evaluated Venlafaxine (VLX) SLNs to investigate whether the efflux function and increased expression of P-gp could be reversed by utilizing SLNs. They found that, after i.v. injection of VLX formulations, the brain concentration of VLX from VLX-SLN and VLX-Verapamil was significantly higher than that obtained with the VLX solution ($P < 0.01$), respectively. Furthermore, there was no significant difference between VLX and VLX+empty SLN ($P > 0.05$). Their study results indicated that SLN could overcome P-gp and achieve brain target by intravenous administration (Zhou et al., 2015). Kumar et al. developed streptomycin sulfate (STRS)-loaded SLNs (STRS-SLNs) for noninvasive intranasal (IN) delivery. Biodistribution studies showed a 3.15 and 11.0 times higher concentrations in the brain and blood of mice, respectively, on IN administration of STRS-SLNs in comparison to free (F)-STRS. According to their study results, they concluded that lipophillic enclosure imparted to STRS, coupled with small particle size, and its purported ability to inhibit P-gp efflux due to the presence of tween 80 were considered to be responsible for a better bioavailability shown by STRS upon incorporation into SLNs (Kumar et al., 2014).

3.3 Polymeric nanoparticles

Polymer nanoparticle is a new type of drug carrier with small particle characteristics, which can pass through the barrier of biological membranes and reach specific parts of the human body that are inaccessible to the conventional drugs. The drug can be dissolved, entrapped, encapsulated, or attached to a nanoparticle matrix (Kaur et al., 2014). A number of therapeutic agents have been delivered to the brain using polymeric nanoparticles. For example, dalargin, kyotorphin, loperamide, tubocurarine, doxorubicin, clioquinol, D-penicillamine, paclitaxel, rivastigmine, dexamethasone, and 5-fluorouracil have been encapsulated in polymeric nanoparticles composed of dextran, chitosan, propylene glycol, polypropylene oxide, polyethylene glycol (PEG), poly(lactic-*co*-glycolic) acid (PLGA), a copolymer of poly(oxyethylene)-poly(oxypropylene), poly(butylcyanoacrylate), poly(N-isopropylacrylamide), or dendrimers (Alam et al., 2010). The variety of polymer carriers gives many new characteristics to drugs. Thus, biodegradable polymer-based nanoparticles have been widely administered as drug delivery systems for reversing MDR (Niazi et al., 2016). In the study of Geldenhuys et al., glutathione-coated poly-(lactide-*co*-glycolide) (PLGA) nanoparticles of paclitaxel were developed for treatment of brain cancers. The nanoparticles showed a sustained drug release behavior and were not substrates of P-gp and would not be effluxed by the P-gp pump across the BBB. Their results suggested that the proposed brain-targeted nanoparticle delivery of paclitaxel could be an effective treatment for brain cancers because glutathione-coated NP containing paclitaxel would target the brain and would provide the better cytotoxicity to the brain tumor. But they did not elucidate the exact interaction mechanism between the NPs and P-gp in this study (Geldenhuys et al., 2011). Chavanpatil et al. evaluated the drug delivery potential of Aerosol OT (AOT)-alginate nanoparticles in drug-resistant cells overexpressing the drug efflux transporter, P-gp. They found that an AOT-alginate nanoparticle system enhanced the cellular delivery and therapeutic efficacy of P-gp substrates in P-gp-overexpressing cells (Chavanpatil et al., 2007).

It is reported that small interfering RNA (siRNA)-mediated silencing of the P-gp gene is one possible strategy to improve the delivery of drugs to the brain (Niazi et al., 2016). By directly down-regulating efflux transporters expression and transport activity, siRNA could be the key for brain over protective issues (Malmo et al., 2013). Many researches proposed a nanosystem that will able to carry siRNA against P-gp to the BBB; in order to further silence this protein receptor, temporarily transform BBB in a more permeable membrane for P-gp substrates. Malmo et al. investigated the potential of siRNA-chitosan nanoparticles in silencing P-gp in a BBB model, and the results showed that P-gp silencing using chitosan siRNA nanoparticles resulted in improved delivery and efficacy of doxorubicin, indicating that this strategy could be suitable to improve the drug delivery into the CNS (Malmo et al., 2013). In the work of Gomes et al., they aimed to develop a nanosystem able to transport siRNA against P-gp towards the brain endothelial cells. In their study, polymeric PLGA nanoparticles were around 115 nm in size and had 50% of siRNA association efficiency. The nanoparticle surface was functionalized with a peptide binding to transferrin receptor (TfR), and their targeting ability against human brain endothelial cells was successfully demonstrated by fluorescence microscopy and flow cytometry. They found that the best system obtained through their experiments was polymeric nanoparticles (PLGA and PLGA:PLGA-PEG-NH2 (95:5)), which were effectively functionalized with TfR-peptides, and they concluded that the nanosystem, which was demonstrated to be safe for human brain endothelial cells, without significant cytotoxicity, bring new hope to the future of brain diseases therapies (Gomes et al., 2017).

3.4 Polymeric micelles

Micellar nanoparticles are composed of amphiphilic polymers which have a hydrophobic inner core in aqueous phase (Gill et al., 2015). The size of polymeric micelles usually varies from 10 to 100 nm (Sharma et al., 2016). The core of polymeric micelles is made of hydrophobic polymer blocks, mainly pluronic block copolymers that contain two hydrophilic PEG and one hydrophobic PPG blocks (PEG-PPG-PEG). The micelles can cross the membranes of cultured brain microvessel endothelial cells and inhibit P-gp (Batrakova and Kabanov, 2008). Thus, polymeric micelles can be used as efficient carriers for compounds, which alone exhibit poor solubility, undesired pharmacokinetics, and low stability in a physiological environment (Kabanov et al., 2002). Liu et al. prepared lamotrigine(LTG)-loaded Pluronic® P123 (P123) polymeric micelles (P123/LTG) by thin-film hydration to develop a nano-scale delivery system to improve the solubility and brain penetration of the antiepileptic drug lamotrigine. Their results indicated that P123 micelles have the potential to overcome the activity of P-gp expressed on the BBB and therefore showed potential for the targeted delivery of antiepileptic drugs (Liu et al., 2014). Liu et al. developed a tryptophan derivate (TD) functionalized Pluronic P123/F127 mixed micelles encapsulating LTG (TD-PF/LTG) to promote antiepileptic drugs delivery to epileptogenic focus. They found that the enhanced targeted delivery could be ascribed to the increased tryptophan uptake at epileptogenic focus as well as P-gp modulation property of the nanomaterial. Their study results suggested that TD-conjugated pluronic micelles showed promising potential as a nanoplatform for the delivery of antiepileptic drugs in refractory epilepsy (Liu et al., 2016).

4 Conclusion and perspectives

The strength of the BBB in offering protection to the CNS from exposure to circulating chemicals is maintained by tight junctions between endothelial cells and by a broad range of transporter proteins which regulate exchange between CNS and blood. The most important transporters that restrict the permeability of a large number of toxins as well as therapeutic agents are the ABC transporters (Qosa et al., 2015). Among them, P-gp is considered to play an important role in the permeation and absorption of P-gp substrates. Different generations of P-gp inhibitors are used to address the problem of efflux of drugs, but unfortunately, the selectivity and pharmacological actions of these inhibitors hinder their use. The exploration of novel drug delivery systems gives a new hope to solve this issue and to enhance the bioavailability of drugs. The co-formulation of P-gp inhibitors with P-gp substrate in a single nanocarrier system offers advantages to tackle the hindrance caused in the delivery of drugs due to the presence of P-gp efflux. These delivery systems basically work through two different mechanisms. They can either bypass the P-gp-mediated efflux or can inhibit the P-gp (Fig. 2). These delivery systems that have temporal co-localization of the drug as well as inhibiting agents prevent nonspecific distribution and the toxicity of inhibiting agents, playing a significant role in the delivery of

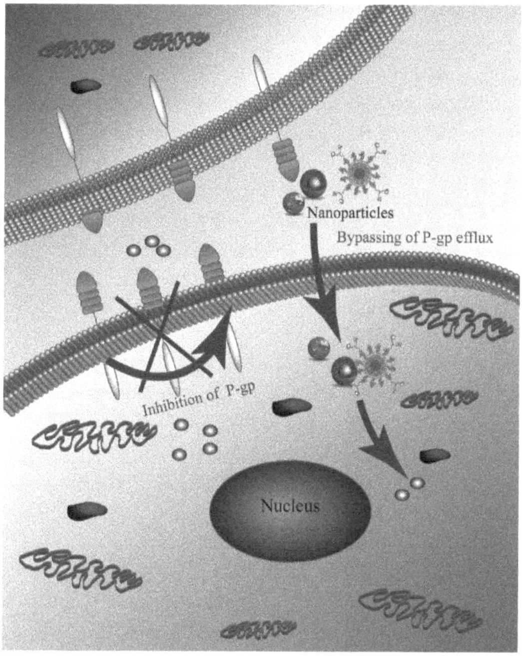

Fig. 2 Two major methods to overcome the P-gp.

various therapeutics to brain crossing the BBB (Kaur et al., 2014). Vast research has been done to treat tumor by inhibition of efflux pumps and the resistance caused due to the protein. The co-formulation of P-gp inhibitors with P-gp substrate in a single nanocarrier system can be helpful in treating various CNS disorders such as epilepsy as many of the antiepileptic drugs are P-gp substrates (Kaur et al., 2014).

References

Alam, M.I., Beg, S., Samad, A., Baboota, S., Kohli, K., Ali, J., et al., 2010. Strategy for effective brain drug delivery. Eur. J. Pharm. Sci. 40 (5), 385–403.

Aronica, E., Gorter, J.A., Redeker, S., van Vliet, E.A., Ramkema, M., Scheffer, G.L., et al., 2005. Localization of breast cancer resistance protein (BCRP) in microvessel endothelium of human control and epileptic brain. Epilepsia 46, 849–857.

Bangham, A.D., Horne, R.W., 1964. Negative staining of phospholipids and their structural modification by surface-active agents as observed in the electron microscope. J. Mol. Biol. 8, 660–668.

Batrakova, E.V., Kabanov, A.V., 2008. Pluronic block copolymers: evolution of drug delivery concept from inert nanocarriers to biological response modifiers. J. Control. Release 130, 98–106.

Cavaco, M.C., Pereira, C., Kreutzer, B., Gouveia, L.F., Silva-Lima, B., Brito, A.M., et al., 2017. Evading P-glycoprotein mediated-efflux chemoresistance using solid lipid nanoparticles. Eur. J. Pharm. Biopharm. 110, 76–84.

Chavanpatil, M.D., Khdair, A., Gerard, B., Bachmeier, C., Miller, D.W., Shekhar, M.P., et al., 2007. Surfactant-polymer nanoparticles overcome P-glycoprotein-mediated drug efflux. Mol. Pharm. 4 (5), 730–738.

Dallas, S., Miller, D.S., Bendayan, R., 2006. Multidrug resistance-associated proteins: expression and function in the central nervous system. Pharmacol. Rev. 58, 140–161.

Dassa, E., Bouige, P., 2001. The ABC of ABCs: a phylogenetic and functional classification of ABC systems in living organisms. Res. Microbiol. 152 (3–4), 211–229.

Deeken, J.F., Löscher, W., 2007. The blood-brain barrier and cancer: transporters, treatment, and Trojan horses. Clin. Cancer Res. 13 (6), 1663–1674.

Demeule, M., Régina, A., Jodoin, J., Laplante, A., Dagenais, C., Berthelet, F., et al., 2002. Drug transport to the brain: key roles for the efflux pump P-glycoprotein in the blood-brain barrier. Vasc. Pharmacol. 38, 339–348.

Du, J., Lu, W.L., Ying, X., Liu, Y., Du, P., Tian, W., et al., 2009. Dual-targeting topotecan liposomes modified with tamoxifen and wheat germ agglutinin significantly improve drug transport across the blood-brain barrier and survival of brain tumor-bearing animals. Mol. Pharm. 6 (3), 905–917.

Futscher, B.W., Foley, N.E., Gleason-Guzman, M.C., Meltzer, P.S., Sullivan, D.M., Dalton, W.S., 1996. Verapamil suppresses the emergence of P-glycoprotein-mediated multi-drug resistance. Int. J. Cancer 66 (4), 520–525.

Gazzin, S., Berengeno, A.L., Strazielle, N., Fazzari, F., Raseni, A., Ostrow, J.D., et al., 2011. Modulation of Mrp1 (ABCc1) and Pgp (ABCb1) by bilirubin at the blood-CSF and blood-brain barriers in the Gunn rat. PLoS One 6 (1), e16165.

Geldenhuys, W., Mbimba, T., Bui, T., Harrison, K., Sutariya, V., 2011. Brain-targeted delivery of paclitaxel using glutathione-coated nanoparticles for brain cancers. J. Drug Target. 19 (9), 837–845.

Gill, K.K., Kaddoumi, A., Nazzal, S., 2015. PEG-lipid micelles as drug carriers: physiochemical attributes, formulation principles and biological implication. J. Drug Target. 23, 222–231.

Gomes, M.J., Fernandes, C., Martins, S., Borges, F., Sarmento, B., 2017. Tailoring lipid and polymeric nanoparticles as siRNA carriers towards the blood-brain barrier—from targeting to safe administration. J. NeuroImmune Pharmacol. 12 (1), 107–119.

Hartz, A.M., Bauer, B., 2011. ABC transporters in the CNS—an inventory. Curr. Pharm. Biotechnol. 12, 656–673.

Huang, I.P., Sun, S.P., Cheng, S.H., Lee, C.H., Wu, C.Y., Yang, C.S., et al., 2011. Enhanced chemotherapy of cancer using pH-sensitive mesoporous silica nanoparticles to antagonize P-glycoprotein-mediated drug resistance. Mol. Cancer Ther. 10, 761–769.

Hugger, E.D., Novak, B.L., Burton, P.S., Audus, K.L., Borchardt, R.T., 2002. A comparison of commonly used polyethoxylated pharmaceutical excipients on their ability to inhibit P-glycoprotein activity in vitro. J. Pharm. Sci. 91, 1991–2002.

Huwyler, J., Cerletti, A., Fricker, G., Eberle, A.N., Drewe, J., 2002. By-passing of P-glycoprotein using immunoliposomes. J. Drug Target. 10, 73–79.

Kabanov, A.V., Batrakova, E.V., Alakhov, V.Y., 2002. Pluronic block copolymers as novel polymer therapeutics for drug and gene delivery. J. Control. Release 82 (2–3), 189–212.

Kakkar, V., Mishra, A.K., Chuttani Kaur, I.P., 2013. Proof of concept studies to confirm the delivery of curcumin loaded solid lipid nanoparticles (C-SLNs) to brain. Int. J. Pharm. 448 (2), 354–359.

Kaur, I.P., Bhandari, R., Bhandari, S., Kakkar, V., 2008. Potential of solid lipid nanoparticles in brain targeting. J. Control. Release 127 (2), 97–109.

Kaur, V., Garg, T., Rath, G., Goyal, A.K., 2014. Therapeutic potential of nanocarrier for overcoming to P-glycoprotein. J. Drug Target. 22 (10), 859–870.

Kumar, M., Kakkar, V., Mishra, A.K., Chuttani, K., Kaur, I.P., 2014. Intranasal delivery of streptomycin sulfate (STRS) loaded solid lipid nanoparticles to brain and blood. Int. J. Pharm. 461 (1–2), 223–233.

Liu, J., He, Y., Zhang, J., Li, J., Yu, X., Cao, Z., et al., 2016. Functionalized nanocarrier combined seizure-specific vector with P-glycoprotein modulation property for antiepileptic drug delivery. Biomaterials 74, 64–76.

Liu, J.S., Wang, J.H., Zhou, J., Tang, X.H., Xu, L., Shen, T., et al., 2014. Enhanced brain delivery of lamotrigine with Pluronic (®) P123-based nanocarrier. Int. J. Nanomedicine 9, 3923–3935.

Löscher, W., Potschka, H., 2005. Blood-brain barrier active efflux transporters: ATP-binding cassette gene family. NeuroRx 2 (1), 86–98.

Mahmoudzadeh, M., Fassihi, A., Emami, J., Davies, N.M., Dorkoosh, F., 2013. Physicochemical, pharmaceutical and biological approaches toward designing optimized and efficient hydrophobically modified chitosan-based polymeric micelles as a nanocarrier system for targeted delivery of anticancer drugs. J. Drug Target 21, 693–709.

Malmo, J., Sandvig, A., Vårum, K.M., 2013. Strand, nanoparticle mediated P-glycoprotein silencing for improved drug delivery across the blood-brain barrier: a siRNA-chitosan approach. PLoS One 8 (1), e54182.

Miller, D.S., Cannon, R.E., 2014. Signaling pathways that regulate basal abc transporter activity at the blood-brain barrier. Curr. Pharm. Des. 20 (10), 1463–1471.

Miller, D.S., Bauer, B., Hartz, A.M., 2008. Modulation of P-glycoprotein at the blood-brain barrier: opportunities to improve central nervous system pharmacotherapy. Pharmacol. Rev. 60, 196–209.

Miller, D.S., 2014. ABC transporter regulation by signaling at the blood-brain barrier: relevance to pharmacology. Adv. Pharmacol. 71, 1–24.

Miller, D.S., 2015. Regulation of ABC transporters at the blood-brain barrier. Clin. Pharmacol. Ther. 97, 395–403.

Moitra, K., Dean, M., 2011. Evolution of ABC transporters by gene duplication and their role in human disease. Biol. Chem. 392, 29–37.

Nagasaka, Y., Oda, K., Iwatsubo, T., Kawamura, A., Usui, T., 2012. Effects of aripiprazole and its active metabolite dehydroaripiprazole on the activities of drug efflux transporters expressed both in the intestine and at the blood-brain barrier. Biopharm. Drug Dispos. 33 (6), 304–315.

Niazi, M., Zakeri-Milani, P., Najafi Hajivar, S., Soleymani Goloujeh, M., Ghobakhlou, N., Shahbazi Mojarrad, J., et al., 2016. Nano-based strategies to overcome p-glycoprotein-mediated drug resistance. Expert Opin. Drug Metab. Toxicol. 12 (9), 1021–1033.

Pardridge, W., 2005. The blood-brain barrier: bottleneck in brain drug development. NeuroRx 2, 3–14.

Patel, N.R., Rathi, A., Mongayt, D., Torchilin, V.P., 2011. Multidrug resistance reversal by co-delivery of tariquidar (XR9576) and paclitaxel using long-circulating liposomes. Int. J. Pharm. 416 (1), 296–299.

Pinzón-Daza, M.L., Campia, I., Kopecka, J., Garzón, R., Ghigo, D., Riganti, C., 2013. Nanoparticle- and liposome-carried drugs: new strategies for active targeting and drug delivery across blood-brain barrier. Curr. Drug Metab. 14 (6), 625–640.

Qosa, H., Miller, D.S., Pasinelli, P., Trotti, D., 2015. Regulation of ABC efflux transporters at blood-brain barrier in health and neurological disorders. Brain Res. 1628 (Pt B), 298–316.

Reddy, J.S., Venkateswarlu, V., 2004. Novel delivery systems for drug targeting to the brain. Drugs Future 29, 63–83.

Riganti, C., Voena, C., Kopecka, J., 2011. Liposome-encapsulated doxorubicin reverses drug-resistance by inhibiting P-glycoprotein in human cancer cells. Mol. Pharm. 8 (3), 683–700.

Robey, R.W., Massey, P.R., Amiri-Kordestani, L., Bates, S.E., 2010. ABC transporters: unvalidated therapeutic targets in cancerand the CNS. Anti Cancer Agents Med. Chem. 10 (8), 625–633.

Sakata, A., Tamai, I., Kawazu, K., Deguchi, Y., Ohnishi, T., Saheki, A., Tsuji, A., 1994. In vivo evidence for ATP-dependent and P-glycoprotein mediated transport of cyclosporin A at the blood-brain barrier. Biochem. Pharmacol. 48 (10), 1989–1992.

Sharma, A.K., Garg, T., Goyal, A.K., Rath, G., 2016. Role of microemuslsions in advanced drug delivery. Artif. Cells Nanomed. Biotechnol. 44 (4), 1177–1185.

Sharom, F.J., 2008. ABC multidrug transporters: structure, function and role in chemoresistance. Pharmacogenomics 9, 105–127.

Shin, S.Y., Choi, B.H., Kim, J.R., Kim, J.H., Lee, Y.H., 2006. Suppression of P-glycoprotein expression by antipsychotics trifluoperazine in adriamycin-resistant L1210 mouse leukemia cells. Eur. J. Pharm. Sci. 28 (4), 300–306. (Epub 2006 Mar 17).

van Tellingen, O., Yetkin-Arik, B., de Gooijer, M.C., Wesseling, P., Wurdinger, T., de Vries, H.E., 2015. Overcoming the blood-brain tumor barrier for effective glioblastoma treatment. Drug Resist. Updat. 19, 1–12.

Varma, M.V., Ashokraj, Y., Dey, C.S., Panchagnula, R., 2003. P-glycoprotein inhibitors and their screening: a perspective from bioavailability enhancement. Pharmacol. Res. 48, 347–359.

Vasiliou, V., Vasiliou, K., Nebert, D.W., 2009. Human ATP-binding cassette (ABC) transporter family. Hum. Genomics. 3 (3), 281–290.

Wang, J.S., Zhu, H.J., Markowitz, J.S., Donovan, J.L., Yuan, H.J., Devane, C.L., 2008. Antipsychotic drugs inhibit the function of breast cancer resistance protein. Basic Clin. Pharmacol. Toxicol. 103 (4), 336–341.

Wang, W., Zheng, N., Zhang, J., Huang, X., Yu, S., 2017. Effect of efflux transporter inhibition on the distribution of fluconazole in the rat brain. Neurochem. Res. 42 (8), 2274–2281.

Weiss, J., Rose, J., Storch, C.H., Ketabi-Kiyanvash, N., Sauer, A., Haefeli, W.E., 2007a. Modulation of human BCRP (ABCG2) activity by anti-HIV drugs. J. Antimicrob. Chemother. 59 (2), 238–245.

Weiss, J., Theile, D., Ketabi-Kiyanvash, N., Lindenmaier, H., Haefeli, W.E., 2007b. Inhibition of MRP1/ABCC1, MRP2/ABCC2,and MRP3/ABCC3 by nucleoside, nucleotide, and non-nucleoside reverse transcriptaseinhibitors. Drug Metab. Dispos. 35 (3), 340–344.

Xiong, J., Mao, D.A., Liu, L.Q., 2015. Research progress on the role of ABC transporters in the drug resistance mechanism of intractable epilepsy. Biomed. Res. Int. 2015, 194541.

Zalipsky, S., Saad, M., Kiwan, R., 2007. Antitumor activity of new liposomal prodrug of mitomycin C in multidrug resistant solid tumor: insights of the mechanism of action. J. Drug Target. 15 (7–8), 518–530.

Zhou, Y., Zhang, G., Rao, Z., 2015. Increased brain uptake of venlafaxine loaded solid lipid nanoparticles by overcoming the efflux function and expression of P-gp. Arch. Pharm. Res. 38 (7), 1325–1335.

Physically open BBB

9

Rujing Chen, Xiao Zhao, Kaili Hu
Institute of Interdisciplinary Integrative Medicine Research, Shanghai University of Traditional Chinese Medicine, Shanghai, China

1 Introduction

The brain is a strategically placed, architecturally unique, and functionally complex regulatory organ. In order to regulate the body functions, information is transmitted to and from the brain by the neuronal cells which require a critically maintained microenvironment. In the brain, the appropriate stable environment required for optimal neuronal function is maintained by the "gateway" called the BBB (Jacob and Alexander, 2014). The BBB is an anatomical and biochemical barrier primarily characterized by tight junctions (TJs) between endothelial cells and the lack of endothelial fenestrations, providing the key mechanism for maintaining homeostasis of the environment milieu. Substances may cross the BBB by two primary pathways: one is the paracellular transport, which involves passing in between the endothelial cells, and the other is the transcellular transport, which involves passing across the luminal side of the endothelial cell, crossing the cytoplasm, and then passing across the abluminal side of the endothelial cell into the brain interstitium (Hersh et al., 2016).

The BBB maintains a delicate homeostatic environment by regulating ion and neurotransmitter concentrations, while simultaneously preventing the access of macromolecules, infectious agents, and potential neurotoxins from the peripheral circulatory system (Pardridge, 2005). While the functions, i.e., BBB regulating the transport of nutrients into the brain and assisting with removing waste products, are necessary for maintaining the health of the brain, the BBB prevents the access of therapeutic agents when brain diseases develop, making brain diseases treatment difficult. It has been estimated that the BBB prevents the access of over 98% of potential therapeutics from passing into the brain (Abbott et al., 2010).

The impermeability of the BBB is the result of a number of unique features. Firstly, the physical restriction imposed by TJs between endothelial cells greatly reduces paracellular permeability. Secondly, the transport system regulation of endothelial cells limits the number and types of molecules that undergo transcellular transport. Thirdly, the metabolic activity of endothelial cells, with powerful enzymes metabolizing many potentially harmful substances, adds to the difficulties faced by molecules trying to penetrate the BBB (Madsen and Hirschberg, 2010).

Due to the immense resistance of the BBB to the passage of compounds through it, numerous strategies have been developed to overcome the BBB to improve the delivery of therapeutic agents to the brain, which range from altering route of administration to modifying the transported agents and their carriers. An alternative strategy

Brain Targeted Drug Delivery Systems. https://doi.org/10.1016/B978-0-12-814001-7.00009-3

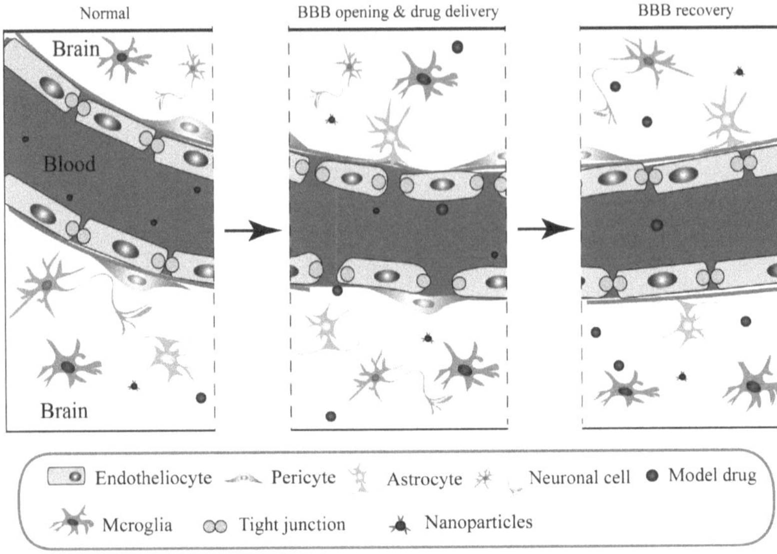

Fig. 1 Overview of brain drug delivery by working on the tight junctions to open the blood-brain barrier.

is to open the BBB (Moura et al., 2017) (Fig. 1). There are some methods that can temporarily work on TJs, either chemically or physically, and disrupt the barrier to increase delivery efficiency across the BBB. These include either pure physical methods or using certain chemicals. Physical methods use nonchemical substances to physically alter the structure of the BBB endothelial cells and their normal organization, to allow a higher permeability of compounds through the BBB (Moura et al., 2017). Focused ultrasound (FUS), osmotic disruption, photodynamic therapy (PDT), and photochemical internalization (PCI) are the representatives of physical methods to disrupt the BBB (Moura et al., 2017). Besides, chemicals like borneol, c-type natriuretic peptide, and lexiscan can also work on TJs to open the BBB.

There is also a growing list of CNS pathologies involving an element of BBB dysfunction, including multiple sclerosis, hypoxia and ischemia, edema, Parkinson's disease, Alzheimer's disease, epilepsy, tumors, glaucoma, and lysosomal storage diseases (Abbott et al., 2010). The barrier dysfunction can range from mild and transient TJ opening to chronic barrier breakdown, and changes in transport systems and enzymes can also occur (Abbott et al., 2010). For example, breaching of the BBB in vivo by triple-negative breast cancer cells results in increasing BBB permeability and changes in ZO-1 and claudin-5 TJ protein structures (Avraham et al., 2014).

In this chapter, both conventional and emerging strategies working on opening the BBB are discussed; some macromolecular molecules working on TJs are also included.

2 Small molecule compounds

Small molecule chemical agents are possible candidates to aid in BBB disruption. They are usually derived from plants or animals, after chemical separation and extraction. Many researchers studied small molecule compounds to open the BBB, which can offer values on different ways to increase the penetration of nanoparticles through the BBB.

2.1 *Hyperosmolar mannitol*

Mannitol ($C_6H_{14}O_6$) (Fig. 2) is a type of sugar alcohol, and it can be derived from a sugar (mannose) by reduction. It is a hyperosmolar, extracellular agent commonly used for the control of raised intracranial pressure (ICP) following brain injury (Gonzales-Portillo et al., 2014). Initially described in 1970 and first performed in a patient in 1980, intra-arterial infusion of mannitol for osmotic BBB opening has been performed in more than 4200 procedures in over 400 patients with brain tumors (Qin et al., 2017). Qin et al. have recently developed a method for precise and predictable opening of the BBB via the intra-arterial administration of mannitol, in a rabbit model, whose vascular anatomy facilitates the use of standard interventional neuroradiology techniques and devices (Qin et al., 2017). Youn et al. utilized autologous adipose tissue-derived pericytes with platelet-derived growth factor receptor β positivity to test the feasibility and safety of a cell delivery technique for clinical translation, specifically, intracarotid arterial delivery following mannitol-induced BBB opening in a moderate size animal model. Cells were administered 5 min after mannitol pretreatment. They found that intra-arterial cell infusion with mannitol pretreatment was a feasible and safe therapeutic approach in stable brain diseases such as chronic stroke (Youn et al., 2015).

Nanoparticles can serve as a promising drug delivery strategy by increasing drug bioavailability in the CNS due to their lower particle size and higher drug-loading capacity. Although different variables will influence the transport of nanoparticles, the penetration of nanoparticles through the BBB can be achieved through a direct disruption of the TJs in the BBB, diminishing the TJ effectiveness and opening TJs to the point that nanoparticles can be freely permeated (Moura et al., 2017). According to the researches mentioned above, mannitol can transiently disrupt the BBB, suggesting that it can be used to promote the efficiency of brain delivery of nanoparticle.

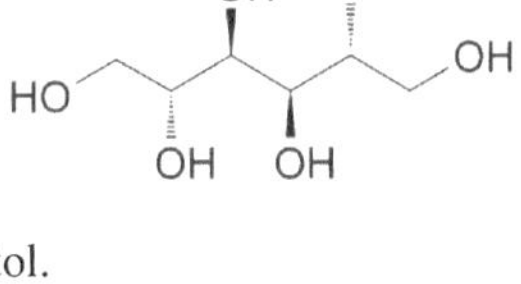

Fig. 2 The structure of D-mannitol.

The application of iron oxide nanoparticles (IONPs) as potential drug carriers has been explored actively over the last few years (Sun et al., 2014). However, under normal conditions, the permeability of IONPs across the BBB is restricted with little to no detectable penetration of IONPs reported with in vitro and in vivo models (Kenzaoui et al., 2012). The majority of studies reporting IONP delivery to the brain have been under conditions in which the BBB is compromised, such as in brain tumor models, where the enhanced permeability and retention effect of the tumor contribute to the accumulation of IONPs (Peer et al., 2007). As the extent of BBB disruption observed in brain tumor models is variable and is dependent on the stage of tumor development, other methods for delivery to the brain are required. In the study of Sun et al., they found that disruption of TJs by mannitol when paired with magnetic field-enhanced convective diffusion (MFECD) could significantly enhance IONP permeability in an in vitro model of the BBB (Sun et al., 2014).

To enhance the transport of the infused nanoparticles, Neeves et al. used co-infusion of nanoparticles and a hyperosmolar solution of mannitol to manipulate the brain extracellular matrix, resulting in an increase in the nanoparticle distribution volume of 50% (Neeves et al., 2007). Mannitol induces osmolarity-driven fluid movement from the cerebral tissue to the intravascular space (White et al., 2006). An increase in intravascular osmolarity causes the net movement of fluid out of the endothelial cells, thus shrinking them (Ikeda et al., 2002). This contraction stretches the TJs between the endothelial cells along the BBB, consequently increasing its permeability (Ikeda et al., 2002). This BBB permeabilization via intra-arterial infusion of mannitol is exploited as a drug and therapeutic agent delivery system, for it facilitates entrance of therapeutic biologics into the brain (Youn et al., 2015). However, this method also has some disadvantages. First, hypertonic solution is thought to osmotically pull water out of the endothelial cells, causing cell shrinkage, which may cause disengagement of the extracellular domains of the proteins forming and regulating the TJs. Second, it is nonselective under these circumstances, so albumin and excitatory neurotransmitters and other potentially damaging substances may gain entry from blood to brain (Begley, 2004).

2.2 Borneol

Borneol ($C_{10}H_{18}O$) (Fig. 3) is a monoterpenoid component derived from *Dryobalanops aromatica Gaertn f.* and *Blumea balsamifera DC*. It has been widely used in traditional Chinese medicine as a messenger drug, which facilitates the transport of multiple drugs to specific sites and harmonizes the effects of those drugs

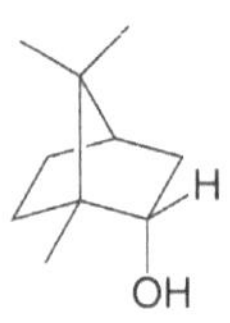

Fig. 3 Structure of borneol.

(Fan et al., 2015). Chen et al. showed borneol can significantly loosen the intercellular TJs and increase the number and volume of pinocytosis in in vitro BBB models (Chen et al., 2013). The results of Yu et al. suggested that borneol showed tissue-specific BBB-opening effect, which was associated with its regulation of the ultrastructure of brain tissues and the expressions of Mdr1a, Mdr1b, and Mrp1. They also indicated that borneol should be used in concert with drugs targeting hippocampus or hypothalamus to exert its synergistic effect to the maximum (Yu et al., 2013). Yin et al. found that L-borneol could induce transient disruption of the BBB after 20 min of oral administration, and the permeability of the BBB began to recover within 1 h (Yin et al., 2017). By decreasing the permeability of the BBB, L-borneol facilitated cisplatin penetration into the brain parenchyma and improved the survival of glioma-bearing mice, suggesting that it might be possible to target the delivery of cisplatin to the tumor at a suitable dose, thus enhancing the efficacy of the treatment (Yin et al., 2017). L-borneol could enhance epithelial junction permeability and then promoted paracellular drug transportation (Zhou et al., 2010). Within 5 min of L-borneol administration, borneol can open the BBB by increasing the levels of histamines and 5-hydroxytryptamine in the hypothalamus (Li et al., 2006).

Borneol has been proved to be capable of promoting drugs into the brain efficiently and, in recent years, it has been reported to increase the brain distribution of nanoparticles. The mechanisms of borneol's effect on improving the brain delivery of nanoparticles are still not clearly clarified. Zhang et al. evaluated the effect of borneol on the brain-targeting efficiency of aprotinin-conjugated nanoparticles (Apr-NP) and the effects of huperzine A (Hup A)-loaded nanoparticles on Alzheimer's disease (AD) rats, and they found the pharmacological effects of Hup A-loaded nanoparticles on improving the memory impairment of AD rats were greatly improved when combined with borneol. The results proved that borneol could improve the brain-targeting efficiency of the coadministered nanoparticles (Zhang et al., 2013a, b). Ren et al. studied whether borneol could enhance the transport of ganciclovir (GCV)-incorporated SLN to the brain in mice after intravenous administration, and they found GCV-SLN modified with borneol enhanced the transport of ganciclovir to the brain, which suggested that SLN modified with borneol was a potential delivery system for transporting drugs to the CNS (Ren et al., 2013).

Previous studies have shown that borneol could increase the permeability of BBB and enhance the therapeutic effect of drugs. At the same time, borneol can maintain the integrity of the BBB structure and cell composition, reduce the BBB permeability, and protect the BBB and brain tissue (Wang et al., 2017). The target spots and mechanisms of borneol's bidirectional regulation on the permeability of BBB are related to the structure and function of cerebral endothelial cells, the exocytosis effects of P-gp, and low pinocytosis internal transport effects. On one hand, borneol can down-regulate P-gp by inhibiting NF-κB to reduce the exocytosis effects of P-gp and promote the BBB pinocytosis to increase the permeability of BBB. On the other hand, borneol can reduce the degradation of basement membrane of blood vessels and TJs by inhibiting the expression of IL-1β, MMP-9 to decrease the permeability of BBB. Moreover, borneol influences the signaling pathways of Ca^{2+}-eNOS-NO and VEGF-eNOS-NO to have bidirectional regulation effects on BBB permeability.

However, the detailed mechanisms that borneol regulates and controls the permeability of BBB shall be further proved and clarified (Wang et al., 2017).

Borneol is a special promoter with a few pharmacological properties, such as acesodyne, sedation, anti-inflammation, antibiosis, etc. (Wei and Wu, 2010). The researches above showed that borneol was not only a good enhancer to deliver compounds into brain, but also a promising promoter for brain-targeting nanocarriers. Although the safety of borneol has been proved by numerous clinical applications (Zhao and Liu, 2002), the possible side effects of the use of borneol should not be ignored and need to be studied comprehensively. More safety of the application of borneol as a promoter for brain-targeting delivery is ongoing.

2.3 Lexiscan

Adenosine is a purine nucleoside that mediates its function through its 7-transmembrane G-protein-coupled receptors. Adenosine receptors (ARs) are of four different subtypes, A1, A2A, A2B, and A3 (Fredholm et al., 2011). Lexiscan (Fig. 4) is an A2A AR-specific agonist that was approved by the FDA as a coronary vasodilator for radionuclide myocardial perfusion imaging (Gao et al., 2014). And it was found to increase BBB permeability and support macromolecule delivery to the CNS in experimental setting (Carman et al., 2011). BBB permeability can be up-regulated by activating A2A adenosine receptor, which temporarily increases intercellular spaces between the brain capillary endothelial cells (Carman et al., 2011). Kim et al. reported that activation of the A2A AR on primary human brain endothelial cells triggered a rapid increase in Ras homolog gene family member A activity, reorganization of the actin cytoskeleton, and consequently disruption of the endothelial cell-to-cell junctions, leading to the increased paracellular permeability, and they used lexiscan as a BBB permeabilizing (or brain) drug-delivery tool (Kim and Bynoe, 2015). In the study of Carman et al., they found that AR signaling represented a novel endogenous mechanism for controlling BBB permeability and a potentially useful alternative to

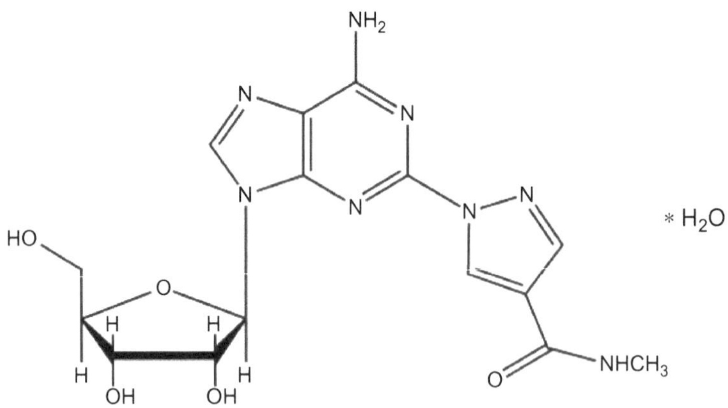

Fig. 4 The structure of lexiscan.

existing CNS drug-delivery technologies. Drugs like lexiscan, which increase BBB permeability and facilitate CNS entry of macromolecules like dextrans, represent a possible pathway toward future therapeutic applications in humans (Carman et al., 2011). It has been reported in the study of Jackson et al. that lexiscan might significantly increase the penetration of systemically administered chemotherapy into brain parenchyma. This agent is safe and its administration in an oncology outpatient setting is feasible given that it is routinely administered to outpatients who are unable to exercise for cardiac stress testing (Jackson et al., 2016).

AR agonist such as lexiscan-mediated TJ opening has attracted attention recently because of its ultrahigh efficiency (0.550 μg/kg) (Carman et al., 2011) and rapid TJ recovery, which attenuates potential side effects. However, the rapid excretion rate of the agonists leads to a narrow BBB-opening time-window and low brain drug delivery efficiency. Therefore, NAs with prolonged circulation lifetime and improved receptor signaling efficacy are the method of choice to address the above challenges (Gao et al., 2014). The strategy of brain drug delivery via the NA-mediated A2A AR signaling is achieved with three steps. First, the NAs specifically activate the A2A AR on brain capillary endothelial cells, which initiates intracellular signal transduction and leads to TJ opening. Second, drug is given when the BBB permeability is noninvasively imaged to reach its maximum. Third, the timely recovery of TJ integrity minimizes the side effects induced by uncontrollable BBB leakage (Gao et al., 2014). Han et al. proposed an innovative nanotechnology-based autocatalytic-targeting approach, in which lexiscan is encapsulated in nanoparticles to enhance BBB permeability and autocatalytically augment the brain stroke-targeting delivery efficiency of chlorotoxin-anchored nanoparticles. They found the nanoparticles efficiently and specifically accumulated in the brain ischemic microenvironment and the targeting efficiency autocatalytically increased with subsequent administrations, suggesting that the autocatalytic-targeting approach was a promising strategy for drug delivery to the ischemic microenvironment inside the brain. Nanoparticles developed in this study may serve as a new approach for the clinical management of stroke (Han et al., 2016).

2.4 Alkylglycerols

Alkylglycerols (AGs), (Fig. 5) the major component of shark liver oil, are glycerol ether lipids that have structural characteristics of an ether linkage between fatty acid and α-position of the glycerol backbone (Zhang et al., 2013a, b). Short-chain AGs are known to affect the physicochemical properties of biological membranes (Erdlenbruch et al., 2000), and the intra-arterial administration of short-chain AGs has been shown to increase delivery of a variety of drugs to the brain long time ago (Erdlenbruch et al., 2002; Unger et al., 1985). Studies show that the opening

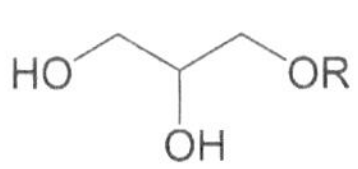

Fig. 5 The structure of alkylglycerols.

of the BBB in vivo is reversible and lasted for only a few minutes to about 1 h, depending on the AG concentration used, which suggest that the effect is concentration-dependent (Erdlenbruch et al., 2000). Variations in the chemical structure of the AGs allow the modification of the extent and the duration of BBB opening (Erdlenbruch et al., 2003). It has been reported that short-chain AGs have been successfully used to increase the access of both small drugs and macromolecules to the normal brain as well as to brain tumors (Erdlenbruch et al., 2005). In glioma-bearing rats, AGs open the BBB in the tumor tissue and the surrounding brain (Erdlenbruch et al., 2000). Due to their physicochemical properties and the lack of toxicity in long-term animal studies (Unger et al., 1985), these compounds are considered to be a promising tool to increase drug delivery to the CNS (Erdlenbruch et al., 2005). The research of Hülper et al. suggested that the properties of AGs might be suitable for opening the BBB to treat brain malignancies (Hülper et al., 2013). In their research, they examined the effects of two AGs, 1-O-pentylglycerol and 2-O-hexyldiglycerol, using an in vitro BBB model consisting of primary cultures of rat brain endothelial cells, cocultured with rat cerebral glial cells. Integrity of the paracellular, TJ-based, permeation route was analyzed by functional assays, such as immunostaining for junctional proteins, freeze-fracture electron microscopy, and analysis of claudin-claudin trans-interactions. The results showed that AG treatment (5 min) reversibly reduced transendothelial electrical resistance and increased BBB permeability for fluorescein accompanied by changes in cell morphology and immunostaining of claudin-5 and β-catenin. These short-term changes were not accompanied by alterations of inter-endothelial TJ strand complexity or the trans-interaction of claudin-5. They concluded that AG-mediated increase in brain endothelial paracellular permeability was short, reversible, and did not affect TJ strand complexity. Redistribution of junctional proteins and alterations in the cell shape indicated the involvement of the cytoskeleton in the action of AGs. These data confirmed the results from in vivo studies in rodents characterizing AGs as adjuvants that transiently open the BBB (Hülper et al., 2013).

Toman et al. reported on the formulation and physicochemical characterization of nanoparticulate nonviral vectors prepared from alkylglyceryl-dextrans and poly (lactic acid) and assessed their toxicity and permeability interaction with in vitro models of the BBB based on mouse and human brain capillary endothelial cells. The results of their studies using electric cell substrate impedance sensing suggested a transient decrease of the barrier function in an in vitro BBB model following incubation with these nanoformulations, and the in ovo study using 3-day chicken embryos indicated the absence of whole-organism acute toxicity effects. Their collective in vitro data suggested that these alkylglyceryl-modified dextran-poly nanoparticles were promising candidates for in vivo evaluations of their capability to transport therapeutic chemicals or fluorescent markers into the brain (Toman et al., 2015).

3 Macromolecular compound to open BBB

In addition to small molecular chemicals, macromolecular compounds that are studied by researchers all over the world can also open the BBB. They are usually produced by the human body or come from bacteria components. Most of them are generated by physiological or pathological factors to transiently increase the BBB permeability. However, there is a distinct lack of studies regarding their use concomitantly with nanoparticles, which may be because of a widespread disruption of the BBB and a rather long-lasting side effect caused by them.

3.1 Bradykinin and bradykinin analog

Bradykinin, a product of high-molecular-weight kininogen, is predominantly generated by the proteolytic action of kallikreins on kininogen precursors (Howl and Payne, 2003). Bradykinin is a short-lived peptide hormone that transmits its biological effects through increasing vascular permeability and enhancing vasodilatation (Chen et al., 2016a, b). It is found that among plasmin substrates including MK-801 (an inhibitor of NMDA-R), SCH-79797 (an inhibitor of protease-activated receptor-1), and CP-474471 (a large spectrum matrix metalloproteinase inhibitor), bradykinin and its related peptides are the most characterized and are able to permeabilize the BBB through β2 receptor activation on endothelial cells (Niego and Medcalf, 2014). Furthermore, growing lines of evidence suggest possible roles of bradykinin in altering the BBB's function (Chen et al., 2016a, b). Marcos et al. provided evidence that hyperfibrinolysis-induced BBB leakage was dependent on plasmin-mediated generation of bradykinin and subsequent activation of bradykinin β2 receptors (Marcos-Contreras et al., 2016).

RMP-7, a bradykinin analog with molecular weight of 1096 Da, has higher selectivity in binding to the BBB than bradykinin. RMP-7 can stimulate the expression of the β2 receptor expressed by endothelial cells and increase TJ permeability, but will also stimulate astrocytes to produce interleukin-6 (Bartus et al., 1996). The synergistic effect of these processes will further cause the opening of the BBB and increasing the probability of nanoparticles crossing it (Azad et al., 2015). The study of Kuo investigated the capability of methylmethacrylate–sulfopropylmethacrylate (MMA-SPM) nanoparticles (NPs) with grafted RMP-7 (RMP-7/MMA–SPM NPs) to deliver stavudine (D4T), delavirdine (DLV), and saquinavir (SQV) across the BBB. The BBB permeability coefficients of them evaluated by a coculture model containing human brain-microvascular endothelial cells (BMECs) and human astrocytes showed that the copolymeric MMA-SPM NPs grafted with RMP-7 could modulate endocytosis and TJ opening to improve the transport of antiretroviral drugs into the brain (Kuo and Lee, 2012). In their research, the mechanism by which RMP-7 to open TJ was discussed in the following portion. An exposure of RMP-7 to human BMECs yielded a rapid elevation of intracellular Ca^{2+}, which resulted from the hydrolysis of phospholipids to inositol phosphates. The fluxes of hydrolyzed Ca^{2+} led to a biochemical cascade and induced a contraction of HBMECs to deform TJ (Kuo and Lee, 2012).

RMP-7 is a good candidate to modify liposome. Both hydrophilic and hydrophobic drugs can be encapsulated into liposome and their properties may be cloaked, then they can be transported into the brain across BBB more easily than simply mixed together before injection. Zhang et al. found that both RMP-7 and DSPE (1,2-dioleoyl-sn-glycero-3-phosphoethanolamine)-PEG-RMP-7 could facilitate the transporting of liposome across the BBB, especially DSPE-PEG-RMP-7. The use of RMP-7 on transporting liposome could result in higher drug concentrations in the brain, thereby increasing the effectiveness of drug for brain disease (Zhang et al., 2003). Kuo et al. developed a drug delivery system of quercetin (QU)-encapsulated liposomes grafted with RMP-7 and lactoferrin (Lf) to permeate the BBB and rescue degenerated neurons. They found that surface RMP-7 and Lf enhanced the ability of QU to cross the BBB without inducing strong toxicity and disrupting the TJ (Kuo and Tsao, 2017).

3.2 C-type natriuretic peptide

C-type natriuretic peptide (CNP) belongs to the natriuretic peptide family, together with atrial natriuretic peptide (ANP) and brain natriuretic peptide (Sudoh et al., 1990). CNP is secreted from the heart (Lee et al., 2015) and can bind specifically to its receptor: natriuretic peptide receptor B (NPRB) (Potter et al., 2006). CNP promotes neurogenesis and connectivity within CNS structures, and intra-cerebroventricular administration of CNP has been shown to reduce food intake in rodents and lower arterial blood pressure in sheep (Wilson et al., 2015). Studies in rodents showed that CNP also increased the permeability of the BBB (Bohara et al., 2014). To clarify the effect of CNP on BBB permeability, Bohara et al., recently, performed research to examine this effect. They found that CNP could modulate and enhance BBB permeability by altering ZO-1 expression (Bohara et al., 2014). Herein, Wu et al. proposed that a novel type of nanocarrier, C-type natriuretic peptide-modified lipid vesicles, could be used to transport anticancer drugs across the BBB, and then eliminated brain glioma and destroyed neovasculatures. A coculture BBB model was established with BMECs seeded on the upper insert, whereas brain glioma (U87-MG) cells were seeded on the lower well to evaluate the transport effect across the BBB. The results showed the ranking of the transport ratio was CNP-modified vinorelbine lipid vesicles ($61.88 \pm 0.94\%$) > CNP-modified vinorelbine lipid vesicles incubated with a cyclic guanosine monophosphate (cGMP) inhibitor (Rp-8-CPT-cGMPS; $46.10 \pm 1.28\%$) > vinorelbine lipid vesicles ($49.84 \pm 1.41\%$) > free vinorelbine ($40.05 \pm 2.37\%$), suggesting that CNP-modified vinorelbine lipid vesicles could transfer across the BBB by disruption of TJs as well (Wu et al., 2017).

3.3 Lipopolysaccharide

The lipopolysaccharide (LPS), a component of the cell wall of gram-negative bacteria, mediates many of the alterations leading to endotoxic shock (Ruiz-Valdepeñas et al., 2011). LPS profoundly impairs endothelial functions, promoting intravascular coagulation, disruption of the endothelial wall, and intense vasodilation and hypotension. The therapeutic usefulness of potent antiinflammatory agents as steroids remains controversial (Russel, 2006). However, in some research, LPS was used to construct models of opening BBB on experimental animal. Mice receiving LPS showed a clear disruption of the BBB, as revealed by extravasation of the fluorescently labeled dextrane starting 45 min after administration (Ruiz-Valdepeñas et al., 2011). It has been found that local application of LPS on the tissue, rather than intravenously, does not systematically induce a disruption of the BBB (Ichikawa and Itoh, 2011). Chen et al. established an in vitro BBB model being composed of coculture with endothelial and astrocyte-like (ALT) cells to evaluate the toxicity and permeability of Ag nanoparticles (AgNPs) and TiO_2 nanoparticles (TiO_2NPs) in normal and inflammatory CNS, and they found that under the treatment of LPS, permeability coefficient of AgNPs was dramatically enhanced, which provided the new insight of toxic potency of AgNPs and TiO2NPs in BBB (Chen et al., 2016a, b).

4 Physical methods to open BBB

In the recent years, physical methods such as ultrasound-based techniques have also been shown to reversibly open the BBB. Physical methods use nonchemical substances to physically alter the structure of the BBB endothelial cells and their normal organization, to allow a high permeability of compounds through the BBB.

4.1 Focused ultrasound

Focused ultrasound (FUS) technique is a method of noninvasively inducing local biological effects deep inside the body without surgical intervention (Aryal et al., 2014). Several studies have shown that ultrasound-induced effects could result in localized blood-brain barrier disruption (BBBD), either accompanied by tissue necrosis or, in some cases, without any evident tissue damage at all (Vykhodtsev et al., 2008). A large number of clinical studies have found that FUS combined with microbubble contrast agents could achieve targeted, noninvasive, and transient opening of BBB (Hynynen et al., 2001; Kinoshita et al., 2006), meanwhile there was no obvious tissue damage or nerve damage to the surrounding brain tissue (Hynynen et al., 2005). FUS with the use of microbubbles can induce local and reversible BBBD by altering TJs in the cerebrovasculature. When the microbubbles interact with low-intensity ultrasound, mechanical forces on the endothelium can cause transient opening of the TJs (Fig. 6) (Rodriguez et al., 2015). These microbubbles are delivered intravenously and are composed of lipid-encased perfluorocarbon gas approximately 1–5 μm in

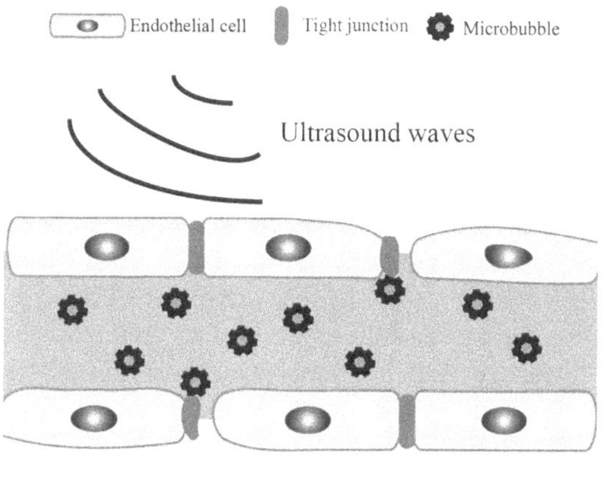

Fig. 6 Schematic of blood-brain barrier disruption by focused ultrasound. Disruption of the blood-brain barrier can be induced when microbubbles apply mechanical forces on endothelial cells that lead to openings of the tight junctions.

diameter (McDannold et al., 2006). Studies showed that the microbubble type and distribution could have significant effects on the FUS-induced BBB opening at lower, but less important at higher, pressure levels, possibly due to the stable cavitation that governed the former (Wang et al., 2014). To manipulate the area of BBBD, the size and resonance frequency of the microbubbles can be altered. With larger microbubbles, less acoustic pressure is needed to achieve BBB opening. With focused ultrasound, the BBB remains open for several hours and can be localized to the tumor region. The BBBD is transient and reversible (Rodriguez et al., 2015). This method has been reported to be widely used in routine targeting administration of CNS. The work of Etame et al. represented the first demonstration of focal enhanced delivery of AuNPs into the CNS using magnetic resonance imaging-guided focused ultrasound (MRgFUS) in a rat model both safely and effectively, and the results of it suggested a role for MRgFUS in the delivery of AuNPs with therapeutic potential into the CNS for targeting neurological diseases (Etame et al., 2012). Diaz et al. used magnetic resonance image-guided transcranial focused ultrasound (TcMRgFUS) to reversibly disrupt the BBB adjacent to brain tumor margins in rats, and they found BBB disruption permitted the delivery of surface-enhanced Raman scattering (SERS)-capable spherical 50 or 120nm gold nanoparticles to the tumor margins. They concluded that nanoparticles with SERS imaging capability could be delivered across the BBB noninvasively using TcMRgFUS and had the potential to be used as optical tracking agents at the invasive front of malignant brain tumors (Diaz et al., 2014).

Numerous studies have documented the use of FUS, coupled with circulating microbubbles, to reversibly open the BBB and safely facilitate the focal delivery of chemotherapy into the brain (Greene and Campbell, 2016). Recent advances in ultrasound-induced BBB-opening techniques have been used in clinical trials to treat brain tumors in human patients with good results. A recent study demonstrated the safety of this noninvasive, triggered, and targeted therapy, while another group demonstrated a simplified ultrasound (implantable rather than focused) with microbubbles to create a BBB opening, with no adverse effects found in a 17-patient clinical trial, which showed that inducing BBB opening by ultrasound with microbubbles was safe and reversible and had significant promise for applications in brain disease therapy (Fan et al., 2017).

4.2 Electromagnetic field exposure

Brain is a sensitive target of electromagnetic fields (EMFs). In a study on the penetration of horseradish peroxidase across BBB, Williams et al. observed horseradish peroxidase in the outer zone of BMEC after exposure to EMF for 2h and retrieved regular transport after termination of EMF for 1–2h. The results indicated temporary alteration in BBB behavior by EMF exposure (Williams et al., 1984). It has been widely known that an exposure to EMF could increase the permeability of CNS drug across the BBB (Kuo and Kuo, 2008). The rate of fluid-phase endocytosis has been concluded to increase about 1.5-fold when an EMF exposure was applied for 10min (Mahrour et al., 2005). In addition, evans blue (EB) complex and serum albumin would not extravasate into the brain via an EMF exposure, indicating that the BBB integrity was not disrupted by an EMF exposure (Cosquer et al., 2005). In the study of Kuo et al., permeability of saquinavir (SQV) across BBB under exposure to EMF was investigated in vitro. The in vitro BBB model was based on HBMEC, and SQV was incorporated in nanoparticulate carriers including PBCA, MMA-SPM, and SLN. The permeability of SQV was significantly enhanced by incorporation in the three carriers. These suggested that transport behavior of SQV across BBB was strongly influenced by the combination of nanoparticulate PBCA, MMA-SPM, and SLN with EMF exposure (Kuo and Kuo, 2008). In another research performed by the same group, the EMF-regulated transport of cationic solid lipid nanoparticles (CSLNs) across human BMECs was investigated. The experimental results showed that the permeability of SQV across the HBMEC monolayer increased about 17-fold when SQV was entrapped in CSLNs. Moreover, the permeability of SQV across the HBMEC monolayer increased about 22-fold by applying the CSLN encapsulation and EMF exposure. These results indicated that CSLNs and EMF could produce synergistic effect on improving the brain-targeting delivery (Kuo and Chen, 2010).

Electromagnetic pulse (EMP) is a particular EMF consisting of short pulse and high voltage with a rapid rise time, the spectral bandwidth of which is from 1 Hz to 1.5 GHz, which is a local, safe, and noninvasive therapeutic method. EMP is extensively used in many fields such as military campaigns (Merritt et al., 1995). It has been reported that exposure to EMP led to an increase in BBB permeability in rats, and the EMP-induced BBB opening was related to gelatinase-mediated ZO-1 degradation (Qiu et al., 2011). In the research of Zhang et al., they investigated BBB permeability after EMP exposure using EB. The results indicated that EMP exposure under 200 kV/m, 1 Hz, 200 pulses could transiently alter the permeability of BBB in rats. And they found that BBB permeability was selectively increased after exposure to EMP, which was related to the expression levels of occludin and ZO-1 which were selectively decreased, while MMP-2 and MMP-9 levels were increased (Zhang et al., 2012). Zhou et al. also studied the effect of EMP exposure on the permeability of in vitro BBB model. The in vitro BBB model, established by coculturing BMVEC and astroglial cells (AC) isolated from rat brain, was exposed to EMP at 100 kV/m and 400 kV/m, respectively. They measured the transendothelial electrical resistance (TEER) and the horseradish peroxidase (HRP) transmission at different time points to assay the permeability of the model. Levels of BBB TJ-related proteins were measured at 0, 1, 2, 4, 8, 12, 16, 20, 24 h after EMP exposure by western blotting. From the results, they concluded that EMP exposure at 100 kV/m and 400 kV/m can increase the permeability of in vitro BBB model and BBB TJ-related proteins such as ZO-1 and claudin-5 may defend against EMP-induced BBB permeability (Zhou et al., 2013).

Magnetic nanoparticles (MNPs) are being developed actively because of their unique ability to respond to magnetic fields, including magnetic hypothermia, controllable movements, and their use as magnetic resonance imaging (MRI) contrast agents (Qiao et al., 2012). Do et al. developed a novel nanotechnology-based strategy to deliver therapeutic electromagnetic-targeted agents to the brain via the BBB as a possible therapeutic approach for AD. In their study, mice were injected with fluorophore-labeled MNPs intravenously and the applied electromagnetic field was either kept constant or pulsed on and off to establish the ability of an external magnetic field to regulate the CNS distribution of MNPs. Their study results showed that a pulsed electromagnetic field facilitated the crossing of the BBB and accumulation of these magnetic nanoparticles in the brain parenchyma, indicating that a pulsed electromagnetic field could be used to optimize in vivo magnetically guided drugs or gene-targeting strategies for many potential clinical applications, such as the treatment of CNS diseases (Do et al., 2016).

4.3 Photodynamic therapy

Photodynamic therapy (PDT) is a technique that employs a photosensitizer agent, coupled with activation by light at a specific wavelength, to match the drug's, in question, peak absorbance (Dougherty et al., 1998). The resultant photochemical and photobiological events cause irreversible damage to tissues. Several studies have shown that PDT might prove useful in prolonging survival and improving the quality of life for glioma patients (Eljamel et al., 2008). Commonly, 5-aminolevulinic acid (ALA) is the prodrug employed, due to its usually rapid clearance and excellent tropism for tumors, especially glioblastomas (Madsen et al., 2003). PDT appears to have a two-fold effect: a direct antineoplastic effect on the remaining tumor cells as well as an effect that causes localized opening of the BBB (Madsen and Hirschberg, 2010). This technique is commonly used in tumors as it promotes irreversible damage to tissues. Hirschberg et al. reported the use of PDT-ALA on rats, showing that PDT-ALA was extremely efficient in opening the BBB at limited regions of the brain, with recuperation of normal function after 72 h (Hirschberg et al., 2008). Madsen et al. investigated the effects of PDT on the migration of systemically administered exogenous macrophages loaded with iron oxide nanoparticles in nontumor-bearing rats. Their results indicated that previously filtered nanoparticles at the BBB showed adequate iron oxide accumulation around brain capillaries, when preceded by PDT (Madsen et al., 2003).

Although the exact mechanisms by which PDT can accomplish transient BBB opening are still unknown, it is currently thought that PDT accomplishes the disruption of the BBB by promoting direct effects on the cytoskeleton of the endothelial cells of the BBB, causing configuration changes (Sporn and Foster, 1992).

4.4 Photochemical internalization

Photochemical internalization (PCI) is a novel BBB disrupting technology that employs the use of photosensitizers that tend to distribute themselves along the membranes of endocytic vesicles (Berg et al., 1999). After activation with light, the photosensitizer interacts with oxygen, damaging the vesicular membrane and promoting the release of the target molecules from said vesicles, instead of potentially being degraded by lysosomes (Madsen and Hirschberg, 2010). PCI has been shown to potentiate the biological activity of a large variety of macromolecules and other molecules that do not readily penetrate the plasma membrane, including proteins, peptides, DNA delivered as a complex with cationic polymers or incorporated in adenovirus or adeno-associated virus, peptide-nucleic acids, and chemotherapeutic agents (Hirschberg et al., 2009). Hirschberg et al. evaluated the ability of PCI to limit the effects of an agent known to broadly open the BBB to a target region of the brain. They treated nontumor-bearing inbred Fisher rats with photosensitizer and a nontoxic intraperitoneal dose of *Clostridium perfringens* epsilon prototoxin (ETXp) followed by light exposure. They used post-contrast T1 MRI scans to monitor the degree of BBB disruption. F98 tumor cells were implanted into the brains of other Fisher rats that were subsequently treated 24h later with ETXp-PCI BBB opening, followed by the i.p. administration of bleomycin (BLM).They found that the survival of Fisher rats implanted with F98 tumor cells was significantly extended following ETXp-PCI BBB opening and BLM therapy compared to controls, and PCI-delivered ETXp was effective in opening the BBB in a limited region of the brain, suggesting that ETXp-PCI-mediated BBB opening clearly increased the efficacy of BLM therapy (Hirschberg et al., 2009). Their research showed that the active toxin could promote reversible, although widespread, BBB disruption when coupled with photosensitizers to promote PCI. The mechanism seems to be similar to that presented for PDT, though there is still more to learn about the exact mechanism through which PCI accomplishes BBB disruption (Madsen and Hirschberg, 2010).

5 Conclusion and perspectives

BBB opening offers some advantages in brain disease therapy, such as rapid effect and reversibility which suited to short-term treatments (Begley, 2004). The disruption of the interactions between the endothelial cells and astrocytes/pericytes proves as a valuable tool in further increasing the permeability of nanoparticles across the BBB as it may result in a periodical opening of this barrier. However, barrier opening is a very nonspecific method of brain drug delivery, leading to the increased flux to the brain of not only drugs, but also other unwanted and potentially toxic molecules, e.g., albumin (Koziara et al., 2006), which will adversely affect CNS homeostasis and produce unwanted side effects (Begley, 2004), such as seizures, bradycardia, and hypotension (Meairs, 2015). Laboratory study even indicated that EMF exposure could increase the incidence of brain tumor (Hansson et al., 2003) and change the phenotype or electroencephalogram in animals (Hamblin et al., 2004). Besides, the approaches of BBB opening are usually relatively costly, require anaesthesia and hospitalization, and are non-patient friendly (Gabathuler, 2010). So we should pay close attention to the safety of opening BBB when using this strategy to facilitate nanoparticle brain delivery.

References

Abbott, N.J., Patabendige, A.A., Dolman, D.E., Yusof, S.R., Begley, D.J., 2010. Structure and function of the blood-brain barrier. Neurobiol. Dis. 37 (1), 13–25.

Aryal, M., Arvanitis, C.D., Alexander, P.M., McDannold, N., 2014. Ultrasound-mediated blood- brain barrier disruption for targeted drug delivery in the central nervous system. Adv. Drug Deliv. Rev. 72, 94–109.

Avraham, H.K., Jiang, S., Fu, Y., Nakshatri, H., Ovadia, H., Avraham, S., 2014. Angiopoietin-2 mediates blood–brain barrier impairment and colonization of triple-negative breast cancer cells in brain. J. Pathol. 232, 369–381.

Azad, T.D., Pan, J., Connolly, I.D., Remington, A., Wilson, C.M., Grant, G.A., 2015. Therapeutic strategies to improve drug delivery across the blood-brain barrier. Neurosurg. Focus. 38 (3), E9.

Bartus, R.T., Elliott, P.J., Hayward, N.J., Dean, R., McEwen, E.L., Fisher, S.K., 1996. Permeability of the blood brain barrier by the bradykinin agonist, RMP-7: evidence for a sensitive, auto-regulated, receptor-mediated system. Immunopharmacology 33 (1–3), 270–278.

Begley, D.J., 2004. Delivery of therapeutic agents to the central nervous system: the problems and the possibilities. Pharmacol. Ther. 104 (1), 29–45.

Berg, K., Selbo, P.K., Prasmickaite, L., 1999. Photochemical internalization: a novel technology for delivery of macromolecules into cytosol. Cancer Res. 59 (6), 1180–1183.

Bohara, M., Kambe, Y., Nagayama, T., Tokimura, H., Arita, K., Miyata, A., 2014. C-type natriuretic peptide modulates permeability of the blood-brain barrier. J. Cereb. Blood Flow Metab. 34, 589–596.

Carman, A.J., Mills, J.H., Krenz, A., Kim, D.G., Bynoe, M.S., 2011. Adenosine receptor signaling modulates permeability of the blood-brain barrier. J. Neurosci. 31 (37), 13272–13280.

Chen, I.C., Hsiao, I.L., Lin, H.C., Wu, C.H., Chuang, C.Y., Huang, Y.J., 2016a. Influence of silver and titanium dioxide nanoparticles on in vitro blood-brain barrier permeability. Environ. Toxicol. Pharmacol. 47, 108–118.

Chen, J.T., Lin, Y.L., Chen, T.L., Tai, Y.T., Chen, C.Y., Chen, R.M., 2016b. Ketamine alleviates bradykinin-induced disruption of the mouse cerebrovascular endothelial cell-constructed tight junction barrier via a calcium-mediated redistribution of occludin polymerization. Toxicology 368-369, 142–151.

Chen, Z.Z., Lu, Y., Du, S.Y., Shang, K.X., Cai, C.B., 2013. Influence of borneol and muscone on geniposide transport through MDCK and MDCK-MDR1 cells as blood–brain barrier in vitro model. Int. J. Pharm. 456, 73–79.

Cosquer, B., Vasconcelos, A.P., Fröhlich, J., Cassel, J.C., 2005. Blood–brain barrier and electromagnetic field: effects of scopolamine methylbromide on working memory after whole-body exposure to 2.45 GHz microwaves in rats. Behav. Brain Res. 161 (2), 229–237.

Diaz, R.J., McVeigh, P.Z., O'Reilly, M.A., Burrell, K., Bebenek, M., Smith, C., et al., 2014. Focused ultrasound delivery of Raman nanoparticles across the blood-brain barrier: potential for targeting experimental brain tumors. Nanomedicine 10 (5), 1075–1087.

Do, T.D., Ul Amin, F., Noh, Y., Kim, M.O., Yoon, J., 2016. Guidance of magnetic nanocontainers for treating Alzheimer's disease using an electromagnetic, targeted drug-delivery actuator. J. Biomed. Nanotechnol. 12 (3), 569–574.

Dougherty, T.J., Gomer, C.J., Henderson, B.W., Jori, G., Kessel, D., Korbelik, M., et al., 1998. Photodynamic therapy. J. Natl. Cancer Inst. 90 (12), 889–905.

Eljamel, M.S., Goodman, C., Moseley, H., 2008. ALA and Photofrin fluorescence-guided resection and repetitive PDT in glioblastoma multiforme: a single centre Phase III randomised controlled trial. Lasers Med. Sci. 23 (4), 361–367.

Erdlenbruch, B., Jendrossek, V., Eibl, H., Lakomek, M., 2000. Transient and controllable opening of the blood-brain barrier to cytostatic and antibiotic agents by alkylglycerols in rats. Exp. Brain Res. 135, 417–422.

Erdlenbruch, B., Jendrossek, V., Kugler, W., Eibl, H., Lakomek, M., 2002. Increased delivery of erucylphosphocholine to C6 gliomas by chemical opening of the blood–brain barrier using intracarotid pentylglycerol in rats. Cancer Chemother. Pharmacol. 50, 299–304.

Erdlenbruch, B., Kugler, W., Schinkhof, C., Neurath, H., Eibl, H., Lakomek, M., 2005. Blood-brain barrier opening with alkylglycerols: biodistribution of 1-O-pentylglycerol after intravenous and intracarotid administration in rats. J. Drug Target. 13, 143–150.

Erdlenbruch, B., Schinkhof, C., Kugler, W., Heinemann, D.E., Herms, J., Eibl, H., et al., 2003. Intracarotid administration of short-chain alkylglycerols for increased delivery of methotrexate to the rat brain. Br. J. Pharmacol. 139, 685–694.

Etame, A.B., Diaz, R.J., O'Reilly, M.A., Smith, C.A., Mainprize, T.G., Hynynen, K., et al., 2012. Enhanced delivery of gold nanoparticles with therapeutic potential into the brain using MRI-guided focused ultrasound. Nanomedicine 8 (7), 1133–1142.

Fan, C.H., Lin, C.Y., Liu, H.L., Yeh, C.K., 2017. Ultrasound targeted CNS gene delivery for Parkinson's disease treatment. J. Control. Release 261, 246–262.

Fan, X., Chai, L., Zhang, H., Wang, Y., Zhang, B., Gao, X., 2015. Borneol depresses P-glycoprotein function by a NF-kappaB signaling mediated mechanism in a blood–brain barrier in vitro model. Int. J. Mol. Sci. 16 (11), 27576–27588.

Fredholm, B.B., IJzerman, A.P., Jacobson, K.A., Linden, J., Müller, C.E., 2011. International union of basic and clinical pharmacology. LXXXI. Nomenclature and classification of adenosine receptors – an update. Pharmacol. Rev. 63 (1), 1–34.

Gabathuler, R., 2010. Approaches to transport therapeutic drugs across the blood–brain barrier to treat brain diseases. Neurobiol. Dis. 37 (1), 48–57.

Gao, X., Qian, J., Zheng, S., Changyi, Y., Zhang, J., Ju, S., et al., 2014. Overcoming the blood brain barrier for delivering drugs into the brain by using adenosine receptor nanoagonist. ACS Nano 8 (4), 3678–3689.

Gonzales-Portillo, G.S., Sanberg, P.R., Franzblau, M., Gonzales-Portillo, C., Diamandis, T., Staples, M., et al., 2014. Mannitol-enhanced delivery of stem cells and their growth factors across the blood-brain barrier. Cell Transplant. 23 (4–5), 531–539.

Greene, C., Campbell, M., 2016. Tight junction modulation of the blood brain barrier: CNS delivery of small molecules. Tissue Barriers 4 (1), e1138017.

Hamblin, D.L., Wood, A.W., Croft, R.J., Stough, C., 2004. Examining the effects of electromagnetic fields emitted by GSM mobile phones on human event-related potentials and performance during an auditory task. Clin. Neurophysiol. 115 (1), 171–178.

Han, L., Cai, Q., Tian, D., Kong, D.K., Gou, X., Chen, Z., et al., 2016. Targeted drug delivery to ischemic stroke via chlorotoxin-anchored, lexiscan-loaded nanoparticles. Nanomedicine 12 (7), 1833–1842.

Hansson, M.K., Hardell, L., Kundi, M., Mattsson, M.O., 2003. Mobile telephones and cancer: is there really no evidence of an association? Int. J. Mol. Med. 12 (1), 67–72.

Hersh, D.S., Wadajkar, A.S., Roberts, N., Perez, J.G., Connolly, N.P., Frenkel, V., et al., 2016. Evolving drug delivery strategies to overcome the blood brain barrier. Curr. Pharm. Des. 22 (9), 1177–1193.

Hirschberg, H., Uzal, F.A., Chighvinadze, D., Zhang, M.J., Peng, Q., Madsen, S.J., 2008. Disruption of the blood-brain barrier following ALA-mediated photodynamic therapy. Lasers Surg. Med. 40 (8), 535–542.

Hirschberg, H., Zhang, M.J., Gach, H.M., Uzal, F.A., Peng, Q., Sun, C.H., et al., 2009. Targeted delivery of bleomycin to the brain using photo-chemical internalization of *Clostridium perfringens* epsilon prototoxin. J. Neuro-Oncol. 95 (3), 317–329.

Howl, J., Payne, S.J., 2003. Bradykinin receptors as a therapeutic target. Expert Opin. Ther. Targets 7 (2), 277–285.

Hülper, P., Veszelka, S., Walter, F.R., Wolburg, H., Fallier-Becker, P., Piontek, J., et al., 2013. Acute effects of short-chain alkylglycerols on blood-brain barrier properties of cultured brain endothelial cells. Br. J. Pharmacol. 169 (7), 1561–1573.

Hynynen, K., McDannold, N., Sheikov, N.A., Jolesz, F.A., Vykhodtseva, N., 2005. Local and reversible blood-brain barrier disruption by noninvasive focused ultrasound at frequencies suitable for trans- skull sonications. NeuroImage 24 (1), 12–20.

Hynynen, K., McDannold, N., Vykhodtseva, N., Jolesz, F.A., 2001. Noninvasive MR imaging-guided focal opening of the blood–brain barrier in rabbits. Radiology 220 (3), 640–646.

Ichikawa, H., Itoh, K., 2011. Blood-arachnoid barrier disruption in experimental rat meningitis detected using gadolinium-enhancement ratio imaging. Brain Res. 1390, 142–149.

Ikeda, M., Bhattacharjee, A.K., Kondoh, T., Nagashima, T., Tamaki, N., 2002. Synergistic effect of cold mannitol and Na(+)/ Ca(2+) exchange blocker on blood–brain barrier opening. Biochem. Biophys. Res. Commun. 291, 669–674.

Jackson, S., Anders, N.M., Mangraviti, A., Wanjiku, T.M., Sankey, E.W., Liu, A., et al., 2016. The effect of regadenoson-induced transient disruption of the blood–brain barrier on temozolomide delivery to normal rat brain. J. Neuro-Oncol. 126 (3), 433–439.

Jacob, A., Alexander, J.J., 2014. Complement and blood–brain barrier integrity. Mol. Immunol. 61 (2), 149–152.

Kenzaoui, B.H., Bernasconi, C.C., Hofmann, H., Juillerat-Jeanneret, L., 2012. Evaluation of uptake and transport of ultrasmall superparamagnetic iron oxide nanoparticles by human brain-derived endothelial cells. Nanomedicine (London) 7 (1), 39–53.

Kim, D.G., Bynoe, M.S., 2015. A2A adenosine receptor regulates the human blood brain barrier permeability. Mol. Neurobiol. 52 (1), 664–678.

Kinoshita, M., McDannold, N., Jolesz, F.A., Hynynen, K., 2006. Noninvasive localized delivery of herceptin to the mouse brain by MRI-guided focused ultrasound- induced blood- brain barrier disruption. Proc. Natl. Acad. Sci. U. S. A. 103 (31), 11719–11723.

Koziara, J.M., Lockman, P.R., Allen, D.D., Mumper, R.J., 2006. The blood-brain barrier and brain drug delivery. J. Nanosci. Nanotechnol. 6 (9–10), 2712–2735.

Kuo, Y.C., Chen, H.H., 2010. Effect of electromagnetic field on endocytosis of cationic solid lipid nanoparticles by human brainmicrovascular endothelial cells. J. Drug Target. 18 (6), 447–456.

Kuo, Y.C., Kuo, C.Y., 2008. Electromagnetic interference in the permeability of saquinavir across the blood-brain barrier using nanoparticulate carriers. Int. J. Pharm. 351 (1–2), 271–281.

Kuo, Y.C., Lee, C.L., 2012. Methylmethacrylate–sulfopropylmethacrylate nanoparticles with surface RMP-7 for targeting delivery of antiretroviral drugs across the blood–brain barrier. Colloids Surf. B: Biointerfaces 90, 75–82.

Kuo, Y.C., Tsao, C.W., 2017. Neuroprotection against apoptosis of SK-N-MC cells using RMP-7- and lactoferrin-grafted liposomes carrying quercetin. Int. J. Nanomedicine 12, 2857–2869.

Lee, J., Than, M., Aldous, S., Troughton, R., Richards, M., Pemberton, C.J., 2015. CNP signal peptide in patients with cardiovascular disease. Front. Cardiovasc. Med. 2, 28.

Li, W.R., Yao, L.M., Mi, S.Q., 2006. Relation of openness of blood–brain barrier by borneol wih histamine and 5-hydroxytryptamine. Chin. J. Clin. Rehabil. 10, 167–169.

Madsen, S.J., Hirschberg, H., 2010. Site-specific opening of the blood-brain barrier. J. Biophotonics 3 (5–6), 356–367.

Madsen, S.J., Sun, C.H., Tromberg, B.J., Hirschberg, H., 2003. Repetitive 5-aminolevulinic acidmediated photodynamic therapy on human glioma spheroids. J. Neuro-Oncol. 62 (3), 243–250.

Mahrour, N., Pologea-Moraru, R., Moisescu, M.G., Orlowski, S., Levêque, P., Mir, L.M., 2005. In vitro increase of the fluid-phase endocytosis induced by pulsed radiofrequency electromagnetic fields: importance of the electric field component. Biochim. Biophys. Acta 1668 (1), 126–137.

Marcos-Contreras, O.A., Martinez, d., Lizarrondo, S., Bardou, I., Orset, C., Pruvost, M., Anfray, A., et al., 2016. Hyperfibrinolysis increases blood–brain barrier permeability by a plasmin- and bradykinin-dependent mechanism. Blood 128 (20), 2423–2434.

McDannold, N.J., Vykhodtseva, N.I., Hynynen, K., 2006. Microbubble contrast agent with focused ultrasound to create brain lesions at low power levels: MR imaging and histologic study in rabbits. Radiology 241 (1), 95–106.

Meairs, S., 2015. Facilitation of drug transport across the blood–brain barrier with ultrasound and microbubbles. Pharmaceutics 7 (3), 275–293.

Merritt, J.H., Kiel, J.L., Hurt, W.D., 1995. Considerations for human exposure standards for fast-rise-time highpeak-power electromagnetic pulses. Aviat. Space Environ. Med. 66 (6), 586–589.

Moura, R.P., Almeida, A., Sarmento, B., 2017. The role of non-endothelial cells on the penetration of nanoparticles through the blood brain barrier. Prog. Neurobiol. 159, 39–49.

Neeves, K.B., Sawyer, A.J., Foley, C.P., Saltzman, W.M., Olbricht, W.L., 2007. Dilation and degradation of the brain extracellular matrix enhances penetration of infused polymer nanoparticles. Brain Res. 1180 (1), 121–132.

Niego, B., Medcalf, R.L., 2014. Plasmin-dependent modulation of the blood-brain barrier: a major consideration during tPA-induced thrombolysis? J. Cereb. Blood Flow Metab. 34 (8), 1283–1296.

Pardridge, W.M., 2005. The blood-brain barrier: bottleneck in brain drug development. NeuroRx 2 (1), 3–14.

Peer, D., Karp, J.M., Hong, S., Farokhzad, O.C., Margalit, R., Langer, R., 2007. Nano-carriers as an emerging platform for cancer therapy. Nat. Nanotechnol. 2 (12), 751–760.

Potter, L.R., Abbey-Hosch, S., Dickey, D.M., 2006. Natriuretic peptides, their receptors, and cyclic guanosine monophosphate-dependent signaling functions. Endocr. Rev. 27, 47–72.

Qiao, R., Jia, Q., Hüwel, S., Xia, R., Liu, T., Gao, F., et al., 2012. Receptor-mediated delivery of magnetic nanoparticles across the blood–brain barrier. ACS Nano 6 (4), 3304–3310.

Qin, H., Janowski, M., Pearl, M.S., Malysz-Cymborska, I., Li, S., Eberhart, C.G., et al., 2017. Rabbit model of human gliomas: implications for intra-arterial drug delivery. PLoS One 12 (1), e0169656.

Qiu, L.B., Zhou, Y., Wang, Q., Yang, L.L., Liu, H.Q., Xu, S.L., et al., 2011. Sythenic gelatinases inhibitor attenuates electromagnetic pulse-induced blood-brain barrier disruption by inhibiting gelatinasesmediated ZO-1 degradation in rats. Toxicology 285 (1–2), 31–38.

Ren, J., Zou, M., Gao, P., Wang, Y., Cheng, G., 2013. Tissue distribution of borneol-modified ganciclovir-loaded solid lipid nanoparticles in mice after intravenous administration. Eur. J. Pharm. Biopharm. 83 (2), 141–148.

Rodriguez, A., Tatter, S.B., Debinski, W., 2015. Neurosurgical techniques for disruption of the blood–brain barrier for glioblastoma treatment. Pharmaceutics 7 (3), 175–187.

Ruiz-Valdepeñas, L., Martínez-Orgado, J.A., Benito, C., Millán, A., Tolón, R.M., Romero, J., 2011. Cannabidiol reduces lipopolysaccharide-induced vascular changes and inflammation in the mouse brain: an intravital microscopy study. J. Neuroinflammation 8 (1), 5.

Russel, J.A., 2006. Management of sepsis. N. Eng. J. Med. 355, 1699–1713.

Sporn, L.A., Foster, T.H., 1992. Photofrin and light induces microtubule depolymerization in cultured human endothelial cells. Cancer Res. 52 (12), 3443–3448.

Sudoh, T., Minamino, N., Kangawa, K., Matsuo, H., 1990. C-type natriuretic peptide (CNP): a new member of the natriuretic peptide family identified in porcine brain. Biochem. Biophys. Res. Commun. 168, 863–870.

Sun, Z., Worden, M., Wroczynskyj, Y., Yathindranath, V., van, L.J., Hegmann, T., et al., 2014. Magnetic field enhanced convective diffusion of iron oxide nanoparticles in an osmotically disrupted cell culture model of the blood–brain barrier. Int. J. Nanomedicine 20 (9), 3013–3026.

Toman, P., Lien, C.F., Ahmad, Z., Dietrich, S., Smith, J.R., An, Q., et al., 2015. Nanoparticles of alkylglyceryl-dextran-graft-poly(lactic acid) for drug delivery to the brain: Preparation and in vitro investigation. Acta Biomater. 23, 250–262.

Unger, C., Eibl, H., von Heyden, H.W., Krisch, B., Nagel, G.A., 1985. Blood-brain barrier and the penetration of cytostatic drugs. Klin. Wochenschr. 63 (12), 565–571.

Vykhodtsev, N., McDannold, N., Hynynen, K., 2008. Progress and problems in the application of focused ultrasound for blood-brain barrier disruption. Ultrasonics 48 (4), 279–296.

Wang, H.J., Wu, J.J., Xue, Q., Zhang, J.F., Xu, X.Y., 2017. Effect factors and mechanisms of borneol's bidirectional regulation on blood-brain barrier permeability. Zhongguo Zhong Yao Za Zhi. 42 (11), 2200–2207.

Wang, S., Samiotaki, G., Olumolade, O., Feshitan, J.A., Konofagou, E.E., 2014. Microbubble type and distribution dependence of focused ultrasound induced blood brain barrier opening. Ultrasound Med. Biol. 40 (1), 130–137.

Wei, C., Wu, G., 2010. Research advance in pharmacological effect of borneol and the underlying mechanism. Int. J. Pathol. Clin. Med. 5, 021.

White, H., Cook, D., Venkatesh, B., 2006. The use of hypertonic saline for treating intracranial hypertension after traumatic brain injury. Anesth. Analg. 102 (6), 1836–1846.

Williams, W.M., Del Cerro, M., Michaelson, S.M., 1984. Effect of 2450-MHz microwave energy on the blood–brain barrier to hydrophilic molecules: effect on the permeability toHRP. Brain Res. 319 (2), 171–181.

Wilson, M.O., Barrell, G.K., Prickett, T.C., Espiner, E.A., 2015. Sustained increases in plasma C-type natriuretic peptides fail toincrease concentrations in cerebrospinal fluid: evidence frompregnant sheep. Peptides 69, 103–108.

Wu, J.S., Mu, L.M., Bu, Y.Z., Liu, L., Yan, Y., Hu, Y.J., et al., 2017. C-type natriuretic peptide-modified lipid vesicles: fabrication and use for the treatment of brain glioma. Oncotarget 8 (25), 40906–40921.

Yin, Y., Cao, L., Ge, H., Duanmu, W., Tan, L., Yuan, J., et al., 2017. L-Borneol induces transient opening of the blood–brain barrier and enhances the therapeutic effect of cisplatin. NeuroReport 28, 506–513.

Youn, S.W., Jung, K.H., Chu, K., Lee, J.Y., Lee, S.T., Bahn, J.J., et al., 2015. Feasibility and safety of intra-arterial pericyte progenitor cell delivery following mannitol-induced transient blood–brain barrier opening in a canine model. Cell Transplant. 24 (8), 1469–1479.

Yu, B., Ruan, M., Dong, X., Yu, Y., Cheng, H., 2013. The mechanism of the opening of the blood–brain barrier by borneol: a pharmacodynamics and pharmacokinetics combination study. J. Ethnopharmacol. 150 (3), 1096–1108.

Zhang, L., Han, L., Qin, J., Lu, W., Wang, J., 2013a. The use of borneol as an enhancer for targeting aprotinin-conjugated PEG-PLGA nanoparticles to the brain. Pharm. Res. 30 (10), 2560–2572.

Zhang, M., Sun, S., Tang, N., Cai, W., Qian, L., 2013b. Oral administration of alkylglycerols differentially modulates high-fat diet-induced obesity and insulin resistance in mice. Evid. Based Complement. Alternat. Med. 2013, 834027.

Zhang, X.B., Jin, Y.G., Xie, Y., Xu, K., Hou, X.P., 2003. The effect of RMP-7 and its derivative on transporting evens blue liposomes into the brain drug delivery. Yao Xue Xue Bao. 38 (11), 867–870.

Zhang, Y.M., Zhou, Y., Qiu, L.B., Ding, G.R., Pang, X.F., 2012. Altered expression of matrix metalloproteinases and tight junction proteins in rats following PEMF induced BBB permeability change. Biomed. Environ. Sci. 25 (2), 197–202.

Zhao, B., Liu, Q., 2002. Comparison between borneol-induced opening of blood–brain barrier and its pathological opening. Tradit. Chin. Drug Res. Clin. Pharmacol. 5, 7.

Zhou, J.X., Ding, G.R., Zhang, J., Zhou, Y.C., Zhang, Y.J., Guo, G.Z., 2013. Detrimental effect of electromagnetic pulse exposure on permeability of in vitro blood-brain-barrier model. Biomed. Environ. Sci. 26 (2), 128–137.

Zhou, Y., Li, W., Chen, L., Ma, S., Ping, L., Yang, Z., 2010. Enhancement of intestinal absorption of akebia saponin D by borneol and probenecid in situ and in vitro. Environ. Toxicol. Pharmacol. 29, 229–234.

Nanoparticle systems for nose-to-brain delivery

10

Qingfeng Liu, Qizhi Zhang
Key Laboratory of Smart Drug Delivery, Ministry of Education (Fudan University), Shanghai, People's Republic of China, Department of Pharmaceutics, School of Pharmacy, Fudan University, Shanghai, People's Republic of China

1 Introduction

As an alternative to oral and parenteral routes, intranasal drug delivery has gained increasing attention in the last two decades. Due to the large surface area, porous endothelial membrane, high total blood flow, the avoidance of hepatic first-pass metabolism, and ready accessibility of the nasal mucosa, the intranasal route offers many advantages such as easy and needle-free drug application, good penetration of low molecular drugs, rapid absorption and fast onset of action, avoidance of chemical and enzymatic degradation, induction of local and distant mucosal immune responses after vaccination, and direct nose-to-brain delivery (Jadhav et al., 2007).

In most cases, the marketed intranasal products are small molecules and used for treatment of local diseases in the nose such as allergic rhinitis and nasal congestion due to high local drug concentration and rapid onset. These products include budesonide, mometasone furoate, ipratropium bromide, oxymetazoline hydrochloride, and so on. Another application of nasal administration is vaccination against respiratory infectious diseases. Compared with subcutaneous or intramuscular vaccination, nasal vaccination can induce much higher levels of mucosal immune response which is especially important in prevention against pathogen infection through mucosal surfaces (Davis, 2001). A representative product is Flumist® which is a nasal spray vaccine indicated for the active immunization of individuals against influenza disease caused by influenza virus subtypes A and B.

A novel application of intranasal route is rapidly delivering drugs directly from the nasal mucosa to the brain in a noninvasive way for the treatment of central nervous system (CNS) disorders while minimizing systemic exposure (Dhuria et al., 2010). Direct delivery of drugs to the brain via intranasal route was first proposed in 1989 by William H. Frey II of the Alzheimer's Research Center (Frey, 1991). It was reported that horseradish peroxidase (HRP) administered intranasally passed freely through intercellular junctions of the olfactory epithelia to reach the olfactory bulbs of the CNS within 45–90 min in rat and squirrel monkey, and wheat-germ agglutinin (WGA) conjugated to HRP (WGA-HRP) was transported to the brain within olfactory nerve axons, which were subsequently confirmed in a quantitative study by comparing intranasal and intravenous administration of WGA-HRP (Balin et al., 1986; Thorne

Brain Targeted Drug Delivery Systems. https://doi.org/10.1016/B978-0-12-814001-7.00010-X

et al., 1995). Since then, technologies and mechanism of nose-to-brain transport have been widely investigated and reported, which provides essential support to the development of intranasal formulations for therapy of CNS diseases.

The main obstacle of nose-to-brain transport is the limited bioavailability of drugs. Lipophilic drugs are usually able to easily cross the nasal mucosa with high bioavailabilities (>75%), for example, for drugs such as propranolol, fentanyl, and buprenorphine. However, hydrophilic drugs show poor absorption with a bioavailability of about 10% and the values for peptides and proteins are generally less than 1% (Casettari and Illum, 2014). The quantities of drugs transported directly from nose to brain via the olfactory or trigeminal nerves are further decreased, normally less than 0.1%, limiting the marketing of intranasally administrated drugs (Mistry et al., 2009). Several absorption enhancers such as chitosan, β-cyclodextrin derivatives, poly-L-arginine, and sodium caprate have been proved effective in intranasal delivery of hydrophilic drugs (Feng et al., 2011). Nevertheless, most of the absorption enhancers are toxic to the nasal mucosa, limiting their application in human. In particular, it is not suitable for the treatment of chronic diseases. Experiments in animal models have shown that nano-sized drug delivery systems can enhance nose-to-brain delivery of drugs compared to equivalent drug solution formulations, generating interest in previously abandoned drug compounds (Dhuria et al., 2010). This chapter will focus on nose-to-brain transport of nanoparticle drug carriers and provide feasible strategies for treatment of CNS diseases via intranasal route.

2 Anatomy of nasal cavity

The apparent external nose consists of a 5-cm high and 10-cm long dual chamber. The total surface area and total volume of nasal cavities is about 150 cm^2 and about 15 mL, respectively. The narrowest portion of the entire airway, the internal ostium (or nasal valve), is about 1.5 cm from the nares, with a cross-sectional area of about 30 mm^2 on each side. The nasal cavities are limited by the septal wall and the lateral wall, dominated by inferior, middle, and superior turbinates. The passages under and lateral to each of the turbinates are called the inferior, middle (and superior) meatuses, which receive the openings of the nasolacrimal duct and the paranasal sinuses. The nostrils are covered by skin, the anterior one third of the nasal cavity by a squamous and transitional epithelium, the upper part of the cavity by an olfactory epithelium, and the remaining portion by a typical respiratory epithelium, which is ciliated, pseudostratified, and columnar. The latter consists of four major cell types: basal cells, basement membrane, columnar cells, and goblet cells (Mygind and Dahl, 1998).

Basal cells are progenitors of the other cell types, lying on the basement membrane. Their main role is to help the adhesion of columnar cells to the airway basement membrane (Evans and Plopper, 1988). Columnar cells are related to neighboring cells by tight junctions apically and, in the uppermost part, by interdigitations of the cell membrane. The anterior one third of the nasal cavity is nonciliated. Cilia start occurring just behind the front edge of the inferior turbinate, and the posterior part of the nasal cavity, as well as the paranasal sinuses, is densely covered by cilia. The cilia have a typical ultrastructure, each ciliated cell containing about 100 cilia, 0.3 mm wide and 5 mm in length. Cilia beat about 1000 times per min. In the nose, the direction of ciliary beating is backwards and, in this way, cilia convey the mucus with its trapped inhaled particles to the throat where it is swallowed. Studies of normal subjects have shown that 80% exhibit clearance rates of 3–25 mm/min (average 6 mm/min), with slow rates in the remaining 20%. All columnar cells, ciliated and nonciliated, are covered by about 300 microvilli, uniformly distributed over the entire apical surface. These short and slender fingerlike cytoplasmic expansions increase the surface area of the epithelial cells, thus promoting exchange processes across the epithelium (Mygind and Dahl, 1998). Another cell type, characteristic of a respiratory epithelium, is the goblet cell. There are a larger number of goblet cells in the posterior than in the anterior part of the nasal cavity. The mean concentration of goblet cells is 4000–7000 cells/mm^2 (Tos, 1983). Ultrastructural studies have shown fragmentation and discontinuity of tight junctions around filled goblet cells, which may be of relevance for the absorption of aerosolized drugs, deposited on the airway epithelium.

A ciliated epithelium covers the upper part of the nasopharynx and a squamous epithelium the lower part. The change in type of epithelium generally occurs in the area where the uvula and the soft palate touch the posterior and lateral walls of the pharynx during the act of swallowing. The epithelium lining the adenoids has a loose structure which facilitates contact between inhaled antigens in the surface layer of mucus and the immune system of the adenoids. It is worth noting that most foreign particles, trapped in the nasal filter, by mucociliary transport are carried to the adenoidal region. The adenoids probably serve the same function in the nose as the bronchial-associated lymphoid tissue does in the lower airways (Mygind and Dahl, 1998).

The lamina propria in the nasal mucosa is rich in blood vessels, containing arterioles, capillaries, venous sinusoids, postcapillary venules, and arterio-venous anastomoses. The abundant blood vessels contribute most absorption of drugs administrated for systemic action.

There are two types of submucosal glands in the nose: anterior serous glands and seromucous glands. There are only 100–150 anterior serous glands on each side. Their long excretory ducts have large openings in the upper part of the internal ostium. There are about 100,000 seromucous glands in the human nose, which have a much larger secretory capacity (Tos, 1983). Secretions produced in the anterior part of the nose are waterier, having a considerably lower viscoelasticity, than secretions produced in the posterior part of the nose. These glands produce the main part of nasal secretions (mucus) and other sources such as goblet cells may contribute as well. Airway mucus is composed of water (95%), mucus glycoproteins (2%), other proteins including albumin, immunoglobulins, lysozyme and lactoferrin (1%), inorganic salts (1%), and lipids (<1%). And the mucus glycoproteins consist of a protein core (20%) with oligosaccharide side chains (80%), crosslinked by disulfide and hydrogen bonds (Kaliner et al., 1984). The mucus forms a double layer, consisting of an aqueous periciliary sol phase in which the cilia beat and a superficial blanket of gel which is moved forward by the tips of the cilia. Both layers are about 5 mm thick.

The nasal mucosa is innervated by olfactory and trigeminal nerves (Mistry et al., 2009). The olfactory neurons terminate at the apical surface of the olfactory epithelium as small bulbous knobs and are, hence, in direct contact with the environment in the nasal cavity. From here, the neurons pass through the lamina propria where they, in bundles with other neurons, pass through the cribriform place and reach synapse in the olfactory bulb. In contrast, the two branches of the trigeminal nerve that have nerve endings in the nasal cavity, the maxillary nerve and the mandibular nerve, are not directly exposed to the lumen of the nasal cavity, but lie in the epithelium near the apical surface terminating at the level of the tight junctions (Casettari and Illum, 2014).

3 Pathways of direct nose-to-brain transport

Due to the existence of blood-brain barrier (BBB), most of drugs cannot enter the brain through the vascular system. Fortunately, more and more evidences demonstrate that the nerves connecting the nasal passages to the brain tissue play an important role in the direct nose-to-brain transport, although the exact transport mechanisms are not entirely confirmed. Also, cerebrospinal fluid and the lymphatic system also participate in the transport process (Dhuria et al., 2010).

3.1 *Olfactory nerve pathways*

Olfactory nerve pathways are considered as a major component of nose-to-brain delivery. It was reported that the intranasally administrated 3 kDa fluorescein dextran was transferred in the connective tissue surrounding the olfactory nerve bundles to the olfactory bulb within 15 min (Jansson and Bjork, 2002). The drug concentrations in the olfactory bulbs are generally higher than other CNS parts (Graff et al., 2005; Thorne et al., 2008), and increase of the drug concentration in the olfactory bulbs results in simultaneous increase of drug concentrations in other CNS parts (Dhuria et al., 2009).

Olfactory pathways arise in the olfactory region, which contains four major cell types: ciliated olfactory receptor neurons, supporting cells, basal cells, and microvillar cells (Moran et al., 1982). Olfactory neurons mediate the sense of smell by conveying sensory information from the nasal cavity to the CNS. The dendrites of olfactory neurons extend into the mucous layer of the olfactory epithelium. The axons of these bipolar neurons extend along the lamina propria, pass through the cribriform plate of the ethmoid bone and the subarachnoid space containing cerebrospinal fluid (CSF), and terminate on mitral cells in the olfactory bulbs. Then the neural projections extend to multiple brain regions including the olfactory tract, anterior olfactory nucleus, piriform cortex, amygdala, and hypothalamus (Buck, 2000). Besides, chemosensory neurons in the Grueneberg ganglion project axons to glomeruli in the olfactory bulbs (Fuss et al., 2005).

Olfactory neurons in the olfactory epithelium regenerate every 3–4 weeks because of their direct and frequent contact with foreign toxins. Therefore, the proteolytic enzymes, tight junction proteins, and efflux transporters in the nasal passages may not be fully functional during the maturation of olfactory neurons, resulting in a "leaky" nasal barrier to the CNS (Balin et al., 1986). In addition, olfactory ensheathing cells envelope the axons of olfactory neurons, creating continuous, fluid-filled perineurial channels that remain open despite the degeneration and regeneration of olfactory neurons (Luzzati et al., 2004).

Given the unique characteristics of the olfactory mucosa and olfactory neurons, it is possible for intranasally administered drugs to reach the CNS via extracellular or intracellular mechanisms along olfactory nerves. Extracellular transport mechanisms involve the rapid movement of drugs between cells in the nasal epithelium, and only several minutes are needed for a drug to reach the olfactory bulbs and other CNS parts (Frey, 2002). Transport may involve bulk flow mechanisms within the channels created by the olfactory ensheathing cells (Thorne et al., 2004). Drugs may also be transported within these channels by the structural changes that occur during depolarization and axonal propagation of the action potential in adjacent axons (Luzzati et al., 2004). Intracellular transport mechanisms involve the uptake of drugs into olfactory neurons by passive diffusion, receptor-mediated endocytosis, or adsorptive endocytosis, followed by slower axonal transport, taking several hours to days for a drug to appear in the olfactory bulbs and other brain areas (Broadwell and Balin, 1985). It has been reported that small, lipophilic molecules such as gold particles (Gopinath et al., 1978) and aluminum salts (Perl and Good, 1987) can be transported through intracellular mechanisms. However, intracellular mechanisms may be not the dominating way of drug transport. Most of the published studies about nose-to-brain delivery showed rapid delivery of drugs to the CNS, almost immediately after or within an hour of intranasal administration, consistent with the rapid extracellular mechanisms (Charlton et al., 2008; Hanson et al., 2004). Further, receptor-mediated transport mechanisms cannot be the main way of transport because of the need of various kinds of specific receptors. Although some large molecules, such as galanin-like peptide, exhibit saturable transport pattern into the CNS (Nonaka et al., 2008), most of large molecules such as nerve growth factor and insulin-like growth factor-I (Thorne et al., 2004) are delivered into the brain in a nonsaturable and not receptor-mediated way.

3.2 Trigeminal nerve pathways

Another important pathway for nose-to-brain transport involves the trigeminal nerve. The trigeminal nerve innervates the respiratory and olfactory epithelium of the nasal passages and enters the CNS in the pons. Some trigeminal ganglion cells with sensory endings in the nasal epithelium also have branches reaching directly into the olfactory bulb (Schaefer et al., 2002). The trigeminal nerve conveys sensory information from the nasal cavity, the oral cavity, the eyelids, and the cornea to the CNS via the ophthalmic division, the maxillary division, or the mandibular division of the trigeminal nerve. The three branches come together at the trigeminal ganglion and extend centrally to enter the brain at the level of the pons, terminating in the spinal trigeminal nuclei in the brainstem. Branches from the ophthalmic division of the trigeminal nerve provide innervation to the dorsal nasal mucosa and the anterior portion of the nose, while branches of the maxillary division provide innervation to the lateral walls of the nasal mucosa (Dhuria et al., 2009). Therefore, the trigeminal nerve can enter the brain from the respiratory epithelium of the nasal cavity at two sites: through the anterior lacerated foramen near the pons to the caudal brain and through the cribriform plate near the olfactory bulbs to the rostral brain. In fact, it may be difficult to distinguish whether intranasally administered drugs reach the olfactory bulb and other rostral brain areas via the olfactory or trigeminal pathways or if both are involved (Thorne et al., 2004; Ahmad et al., 2017).

Thorne et al. first demonstrated that the trigeminal pathways involve the nose-to-brain transport of drugs, evidenced by the high levels of radioactivity in the trigeminal nerve branches, trigeminal ganglion, pons, and olfactory bulbs after intranasal administration of ^{125}I-insulin-like growth factor-I (Thorne et al., 2004). Intranasal studies with other proteins and nanoparticles, including hypocretin-1 (Dhuria et al., 2009) and wheat-germ agglutinin-conjugated poly(ethylene glycol)-poly(lactic acid) nanoparticles (WGA-NP) (Liu et al., 2012), found similar results of high levels of radioactivity in the trigeminal nerve, suggesting its pivotal role in nose-to-brain delivery.

3.3 Pathways involving the cerebrospinal fluid

CSF pathways connecting the subarachnoid space, perineurial spaces surrounding olfactory nerves, and the nasal lymphatics are important for CSF drainage (Boulton et al., 1996) and these same pathways also provide access for nose-to-brain delivery of drugs. Many intranasally administrated drugs gain direct access to the CSF from the nasal cavity, followed by subsequent distribution to the brain and spinal cord, and this transport is dependent on the lipophilicity, molecular weight, and degree of ionization of the drugs (Dhuria et al., 2009). However, the trigeminal nerve pathway also plays a role in distribution of intranasally administered drugs to the caudal brain areas, making it difficult to experimentally separate contributions of different pathways into the CNS.

The potential transport routes for substances from nasal cavity to the brain are summarized in Fig. 1.

4 Nanoparticle systems for nose-to-brain delivery

Nanoparticles may improve the nose-to-brain drug delivery since they are able to protect the encapsulated drugs from biological and/or chemical degradation and increase their penetration across biological barriers. Their small diameter potentially allows nanoparticles to be transported transcellularly through neurons to the brain via various endocytic pathways in the olfactory membrane (Mistry et al., 2009). These nano-sized systems mainly include chitosan-based nanoparticles, polyester-based nanoparticles, solid lipid nanoparticles, liposomes, nanoemulsions, micelles, nanocomplexes, and so on.

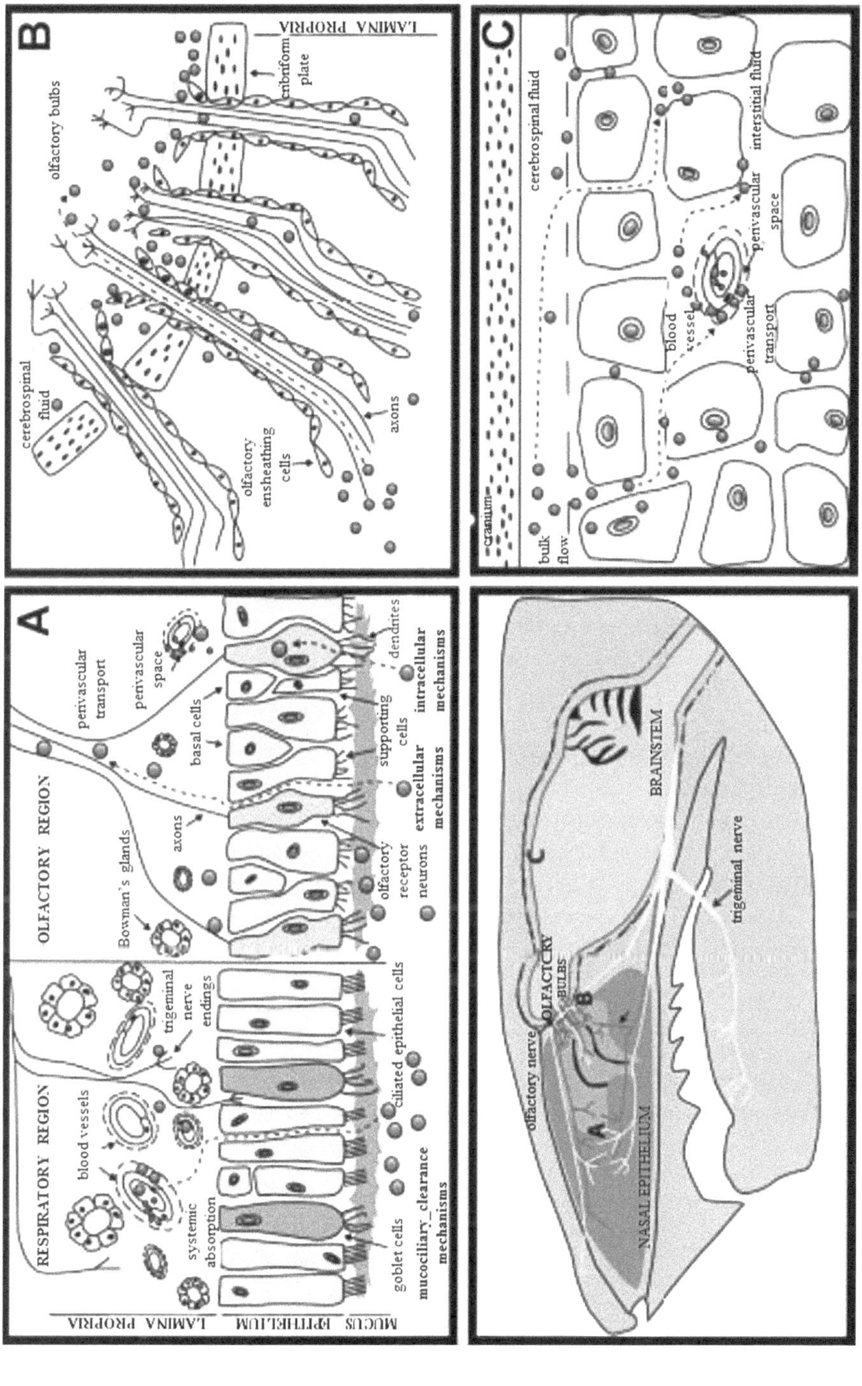

Fig. 1 See the legend on next page.

4.1 Chitosan-based nanoparticles

Chitosan is biocompatible polysaccharide derived from partial alkaline deacetylation of chitin mostly originating from crustacean shells. Chitosan and its derivatives are able to interact through their positively charged amino groups with the anionic counterpart present in the mucous layers, mainly sialic acid, and to affect the permeability of the epithelial membrane by the transient opening of the tight junctions in the epithelial cells, conferring both bioadhesion and absorption-enhancing capabilities to a formulation intended to deliver drugs from the nasal cavity to the CNS (Casettari and Illum, 2014). This is particularly important for brain targeting drugs, where there is a need to reach specific and confined nasal regions with increment in residence time and membrane permeation (Casettari and Illum, 2014).

Rivastigmine (RHT), an inhibitor of both acetylcholinesterase (AChE) and butrylcholinestrase (BuChE) enzyme, can be used for the treatment of Alzheimer's disease (AD). However, RHT shows restricted entry into brain due to its hydrophilicity, thereby necessitating frequent dosing resulting in severe cholinergic side effects. Therefore, Fazil et al. prepared RHT-loaded chitosan nanoparticles (CS-RHT NPs) by ionic gelation method to improve the bioavailability and enhance the uptake of RHT to the brain via intranasal delivery (Fazil et al., 2012). Using rhodamine-123 as a marker, brain targeting of the intranasally administrated chitosan nanoparticles was proved by the much stronger fluorescence signals in brain than the intravenously injected nanoparticles. The brain/blood ratio of RHT for intranasally administrated CS-RHT NPs at 10–480 min was 1.35–2.16, obviously higher than that of intranasally administrated RHT solution or intravenously injected CS-RHT NPs. The drug targeting efficiency (DTE) was 355% and direct transport percentage (DTP) was 71.8%, suggesting that the intranasally administrated CS-RHT NPs had a much better targeting efficiency.

Chitosan nanoparticles can also be used for delivery of peptides to the brain. Kumar et al. prepared leucine-enkephalin (Leu-Enk)-loaded N-trimethyl chitosan (TMC) nanoparticles by ionic gelation method as a brain delivery vehicle via nasal route (Kumar et al., 2013). The mean peptide encapsulation efficiency, mean particle size, and zeta potential of the optimized formulation were $78.28 \pm 3.8\%$, 443 ± 23 nm, and

Fig. 1, Cont'd Nose-to-brain transport pathways of drugs. Intranasally administrated drugs (*circles*) contact with the nasal mucosa, which is innervated by olfactory and trigeminal nerves. (A) Drugs can be transported to the brain by entering perivascular channels (*dashed lines* surrounding blood vessels) in the lamina propria or via extracellular or intracellular mechanisms involving olfactory and trigeminal nerves (*dashed arrows*). (B) Drugs in the lamina propria can enter channels created by olfactory ensheathing cells surrounding the olfactory nerves, and then access the CSF and olfactory bulbs (*dashed arrows*). (C) Drugs in CSF can be distributed via bulk flow mechanisms or enter perivascular spaces to be rapidly distributed throughout the brain.
Reproduced from Dhuria, S.V., Hanson, L.R., Frey, W.H. II, 2010. Intranasal delivery to the central nervous system: mechanisms and experimental considerations. J. Pharm. Sci. 99, 1654–1673, with permission from Elsevier.

+15 ± 2 mV, respectively. Permeability of Leu-Enk-loaded nanoparticles across the nasal mucosa was 35 folds improved as compared to Leu-Enk solution. Fluorescent microscopy of brain sections of mice showed higher accumulation of fluorescent marker NBD-F-labeled Leu-Enk, when administered nasally TMC nanoparticles compared to marker solution. The increased transport of Leu-Enk in nanoparticles resulted in significant improvement of antinociceptive effect of Leu-Enk in the hot plate and acetic acid induced writhing assay.

4.2 Polyester-based nanoparticles

Due to its biodegradability, excellent biocompatibility, and ease of encapsulation of different kinds of drugs, poly (lactic acid) (PLA)/poly (lactic-*co*-glycolic acid) (PLGA) becomes one of the most successfully used polymers in preparation of micro-/nano-carrier systems for controlled/targeted drug delivery.

Olanzapine is a second-generation atypical antipsychotic which selectively binds to central dopamine D_2 and serotonin receptors. However, it has poor bioavailability due to hepatic first-pass metabolism and low permeability into the brain due to efflux by P-glycoproteins (Seju et al., 2011). Seju et al. prepared olanzapine-loaded PLGA nanoparticles by the nanoprecipitation technique for direct nose-to-brain delivery to provide brain targeting and sustained release. in vitro drug release from nanoparticles showed an initial burst release (25.69% at 7 h) and then a sustained release (43.26% at 120 h), following the Fickian diffusion-based release mechanism. in vivo pharmacokinetic studies showed 6.35 and 10.86 times higher brain uptake of intranasally delivered nanoparticles than that of intravenous and intranasal olanzapine solution, respectively, proving that olanzapine could be transported directly to the brain after intranasal delivery of PLGA nanoparticles.

Nimodipine has important effects on neuroprotection and cognition, but its clinical application is limited by its high first-pass elimination in the liver, leading to poor oral bioavailability and low brain entry. Zhang et al. prepared nimodipine-loaded methoxy poly(ethylene glycol)-poly(lactic acid) nanoparticles (PEG-PLA-NPs) through an emulsion/solvent evaporation technique for nose-to-brain delivery (Zhang et al., 2006). The nanoparticles had a mean particle size of 76.5 nm, a negative surface charge, and a 5.2% nimodipine loading. Following intranasal administration, the olfactory bulb/plasma and CSF/plasma concentration ratios of nanoparticles were significantly higher ($P < .05$) than those of the nasal solution at 10–360 min. Furthermore, nasally administered nanoparticles yielded 1.6–3.3-fold greater DTP values in CSF, olfactory bulb, and other brain tissues compared to nasal solution, demonstrating its potential in the direct nose-brain transport for drugs.

Intranasally administrated PLA/PLGA nanoparticles may be rapidly cleared by nasal cilia, resulting in incomplete absorption. In order to prolong the retention time of nanoparticles on nasal mucosa and facilitate their absorption, various ligands such as lectins are used for modification of nanoparticles. Lectins are proteins or glycoproteins possessing at least one noncatalytic domain, which binds reversibly to specific mono- or oligosaccharides (Peumans and Van Damme, 1995). They specifically recognize and bind with carbohydrate residues on cell surface to initiate vesicular transport processes in cells (Goldstein and Hayes, 1978). Taking into account that the surface of nasal mucosa is rich in glycan, Gao et al. modified vasoactive intestinal peptide-loaded PEG-PLA nanoparticles with WGA and determined the biodistribution and efficacy of these nanoparticles after intranasal administration. The area under the concentration-time curve (AUC) of intact ^{125}I-vasoactive intestinal peptide in brain of mice for nanoparticles and WGA-conjugated nanoparticles was significantly enlarged by 3.5–4.7-folds and 5.6–7.7-folds, respectively, compared with that of intranasally applied drug solution. The increased concentrations of vasoactive intestinal peptide in brain also corresponded to improved memory function, as determined by the water maze behavioral test (Gao et al., 2006, 2007a). It was found that WGA-conjugated nanoparticles in the nasal cavity showed higher affinity to the olfactory mucosa than to the respiratory one, which may be attributed to slower removal of the olfactory mucosa, resulting in longer contact time of WGA-modified nanoparticles with the olfactory mucosa (Fig. 2, Gao et al., 2007a; Liu et al., 2012). Similar improvements were obtained after conjugation of nanoparticles with other lectins such as ulex europeus agglutinin I, odorranalectin, and solanum tuberosum lectin, proving the significant role of lectin modification in the nose-to-brain delivery (Gao et al., 2007b; Wen et al., 2011; Wu et al., 2012; Chen et al., 2012).

In addition, poly(ε-caprolactone) (PCL) is also widely used polyester material for preparation of nanoparticles. Sawant et al. prepared aripiprazole-loaded PCL nanoparticles using nanoprecipitation method (Sawant et al., 2016). The particle size, zeta potential, and encapsulation efficiency of optimized nanoparticles were 199.2 ± 5.65 nm, -21.4 ± 4.6 mV, and $69.2 \pm 2.34\%$, respectively. The nanoparticles could sustain drug release for about 8 h. The $AUC_{0\text{–}8h}$ of intranasally administered nanoparticles in rat brain was approximately two times higher than that of nanoparticles administered via intravenous route. A significant increase in maximum

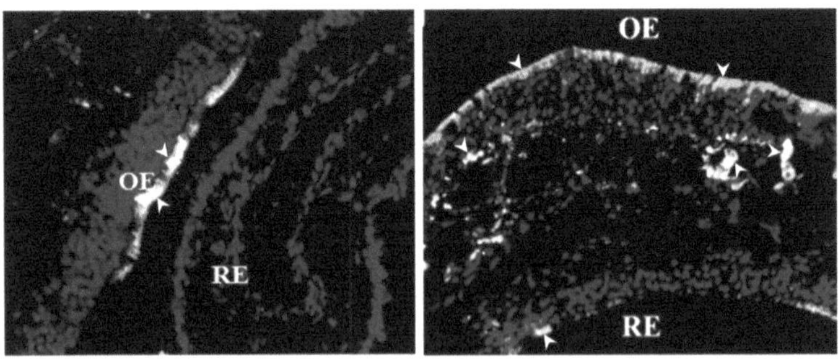

Fig. 2 Distribution of 6-counarin-loaded WGA-modified nanoparticles (*arrows*) in the nasal mucosa 30 min following intranasal administration. WGA-modified nanoparticles exhibited higher affinity to the olfactory mucosa than that to the respiratory one. *OE*: Olfactory epithelium, *RE*: respiratory epithelium (200 ×).
Reproduced from Liu, Q.F., Shen, Y.H., Chen, J., Gao, X.L., Feng, C.C., Wang, L., Zhang, Q.Z., Jiang, X.G., 2012. Nose-to-brain transport pathways of wheat germ agglutinin conjugated PEG-PLA nanoparticles. Pharm. Res. 29, 546–558, with permission from Springer Nature.

concentration (C_{max}) was observed in the intranasal group, which might help in dose reduction along with reduction in dose-related side effects. Modification of nanoparticles with ligands may further improve brain delivery of drugs. Liu et al. conjugated lactoferrin on PEG-PCL nanoparticle (Lf-NP) via a maleimide-thiol reaction for binding of nanoparticles on respiratory epithelial cells and neurons (Liu et al., 2013). Following intranasal administration, the AUC_{0-8h} of coumarin-6-loaded Lf-NP in rat cerebrum (with hippocampus removed), cerebellum, olfactory tract, olfactory bulb, and hippocampus was 1.36, 1.53, 1.70, 1.57, and 1.23 times higher than that of the unmodified nanoparticles, respectively. Using a neuroprotective peptide—NAPVSIPQ as the model drug, the neuroprotective and memory improvement effect of Lf-NP was observed even at lower dose than that of unmodified nanoparticles in a Morris water maze experiment. These studies prove PCL-based nanoparticles to be a feasible carrier for nose-to-brain delivery of drugs.

4.3 Solid lipid nanoparticles

Solid lipid nanoparticles (SLNs) are made up of a solid lipid core matrix that can solubilize lipophilic molecules and a surfactant outer shell. The lipid core typically consists of triglycerides (e.g., tristearin), diglycerides (e.g., glyceryl behenate), monoglycerides (e.g., glycerol monostearate), fatty acids (e.g., stearic acid), steroids (e.g., cholesterol), or waxes (e.g., cetyl palmitate) (Fonseca-Santos et al., 2015). SLNs have several advantages including targeted drug delivery, controlled drug release, increased bioavailability, good tolerability and biodegradability, lack of acute and chronic toxicity of the carrier, and easy to scale-up. SLNs may also improve nose-to-brain drug delivery due to increased nasal retention time caused by an occlusive effect and adhesion to mucous membranes (Yasir and Sara, 2014).

Haloperidol (HP) is a dopamine inverse agonist, used for certain psychiatric conditions including schizophrenia, manic states, medication-induced psychosis, and neurological disorders with hyperkinesias. After oral administration, the drug undergoes first-pass metabolism followed by systemic distribution, resulting in only a small portion being able to reach the brain through the blood. So, Yasir and Sara prepared haloperidol (HP)-loaded SLNs to increase the brain delivery of HP after intranasal administration (Yasir and Sara, 2014). This delivery system was prepared with glyceryl monostearate (GMS) and Tween 80 and lyophilized with 5% (*w/v*) mannitol as a cryoprotectant. The particle size was about 115 nm, with the encapsulation efficiency of 71.56%. After administration to albino Wistar rats, the brain/blood ratio at 0.5 h for HP-SLNs i.n., HP solution i.n., and HP solution i.v. was 1.61, 0.17, and 0.031, respectively, indicating direct nose-to-brain transport, bypassing the BBB. The C_{max} in brain achieved from i.n. administration of HP-SLNs (329.17 ± 20.89 ng/mL, T_{max} 2 h) was significantly higher than that achieved after i.v. (76.95 ± 7.62 ng/mL, T_{max} 1 h) and i.n. (90.13 ± 6.28 ng/mL, T_{max} 2 h) administration of HP solution. The highest DTE (2362.43%) and DTP (95.77%) was found with HP-SLNs, suggesting that HP-SLNs have better brain targeting efficiency as compared to other formulations.

Agomelatine is a novel antidepressant drug suffering from an extensive first-pass metabolism leading to a diminished absolute bioavailability. Fatouh et al. prepared agomelatine-loaded SLNs to enhance its absolute bioavailability and brain delivery (Fatouh et al., 2017). The SLNs were prepared using the emulsification solvent evaporation technique with Gelucire 43/01 and glyceryl tripalmitate. The optimum solid lipid nanoparticles had a particle size of 167.70 nm, zeta potential of -17.90 mV, polydispersity index of 0.12, entrapment efficiency of 91.25%, the percentage released after 1 h of 35.40%, and the percentage released after 8 h of 80.87%. The pharmacokinetic study of the optimized SLNs revealed a significant increase in each of the C_{max}, the $AUC_{0-360min}$ and, the absolute bioavailability compared to that of the oral suspension of Valdoxan® with the values of 759.00, 7805.69 ng min/mL, and 44.44%, respectively. The optimized SLNs had a DTE of 190.02% and a DTP of 47.37%, indicating a successful delivery of agomelatine using SLNs via the intranasal route.

4.4 Liposomes and cationic liposomes

As one of the earliest nano-formulations, liposomes present excellent characteristics such as good biocompatibility, suitability for hydrophobic and hydrophilic drugs, excellent penetrability across nasal mucosa, and easy industrialization. Several liposomal formulations such as Exparel (bupivacaine liposome injection), Doxil (doxorubicin hydrochloride liposome injection), Onivyde (irinotecan hydrochloride liposome injection), Marqibo (vincristine sulfate liposome injection), and Ambisome (amphotericin B liposome injection) have been approved by FDA for market sale.

Zheng et al. prepared a β-sheet breaker peptide, H102-loaded liposomes using a modified thin film hydration method for the treatment of AD. After intranasal administration, H102 peptide could be effectively delivered to the brain, and the $AUC_{0-90min}$ of the liposomes in the hippocampus was 2.92-folds larger than that of the solution containing the absorption enhancer chitosan (Fig. 3). H102 liposomes could excellently ameliorate spatial memory impairment of AD model rats, increase the activities of choline acetyltransferase and insulin degrading enzyme, and inhibit plaque deposition, even at a lower dosage compared with H102 solution (Zheng et al., 2015). In order to further increase the brain delivery of liposome after intranasal administration, functional ligands are often used to modify liposomes. Yang et al. modified liposomes with the cell-penetrating peptide (CPP) to improve rivastigmine distribution in brain (Yang et al., 2013). Rivastigmine concentrations of CPP-modified liposomes were significantly higher in hippocampus, cortex, and olfactory region at 15 min and 60 min than that of unmodified ones following intranasal administration, indicating that CPP can promote absorption of rivastigmine to brain through the nasal cavity.

Another strategy for improving brain delivery of intranasally administrated liposomes is cationization, increasing affinity of liposomes with negatively charged mucosal cells. Migliore et al. encapsulated glial cell line-derived neurotrophic factor (GDNF) by cationic liposomes (Migliore et al., 2014; Bender et al., 2015). They found that liposomes delivered 10-fold more GDNF to brain than GDNF solution. However, the liposomes and solution yielded similar neuroprotective efficacy in

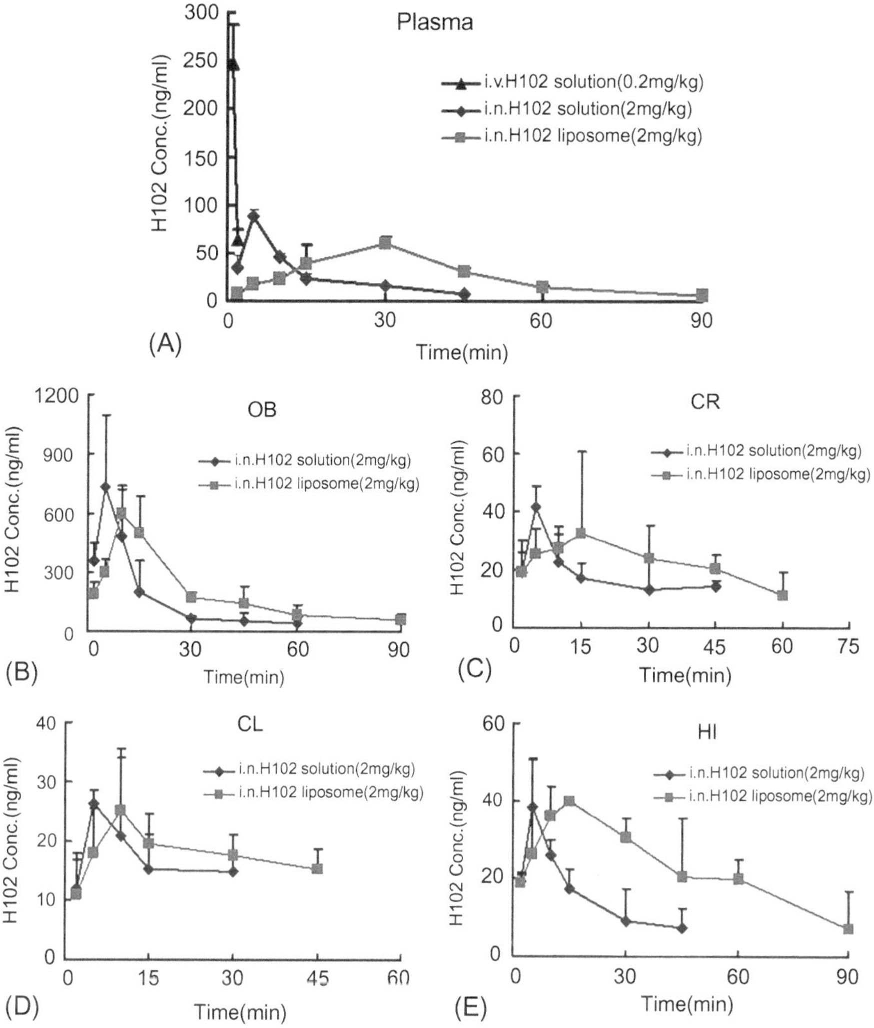

Fig. 3 Concentration-time profiles of H102 in plasma and brain tissue. (A), H102 in plasma following intranasal (i.n.) administration of H102 solution with 1% chitosan and 0.1% BSA (2 mg/kg); H102 liposomes (2 mg/kg) and intravenous (i.v.) administration of H102 solution with 0.1% BSA (0.2 mg/kg) to SD rats. (B–E); brain uptake of H102 following intranasal administration of H102 solution (containing 1% chitosan and 0.1% BSA, 2 mg/kg) and H102 liposomes (2 mg/kg) in the olfactory bulb (OB), cerebrum (CR), cerebellum (CL), and hippocampus (HI) (mean ± SD, $n=4$).
Reproduced from Zheng, X.Y., Shao, X.Y., Zhang, C., Tan, Y.Z., Liu, Q.F., Wan, X., Zhang, Q.Z., Xu, S.M., Jiang, X.G., 2015. Intranasal H102 peptide-loaded liposomes for brain delivery to treat Alzheimer's disease. Pharm. Res. 32, 3837–3849, with permission from Springer Nature.

the 6-hydroxydopamine model of Parkinson's disease, possibly due to the incomplete release of GDNF from liposomes in tissue. Although cationic liposomes can effectively increase penetration of drugs across nasal mucosa, their toxicity due to positive charges should be paid more attention in clinical use, especially in the treatment of chronic diseases.

4.5 Nanoemulsions and micelles

Surfactants-based nano-carriers such as nanoemulsions and micelles have been used to increase the solubility of poorly soluble drugs, improve drug stability, mucosal absorption, and brain delivery after intranasal administration. Abdel-Bar et al. prepared clonazepam nanoemulsions by mixing isopropyl myristate, Tween 80, Cremophor EL or lecithin, polyethylene glycol 200, propylene glycol, or ethanol in different ratios with water (Abdel-Bar et al., 2013). The particle size of nanoemulsions was 21.33–62.33 nm with narrow polydispersity indexes. Plasma T_{max} of clonazepam nanoemulsions varied from 10–30 min, while their brain T_{max} did not exceed 10 min, in comparison with 30 min for intravenous solution, indicating a rapid nose-to-brain transport of these nanoemulsions. The DTE and DTP were 459.6%–757.9% and 78.5–96.8%, respectively. The brain $AUC_{0-\infty}$ of different nasal formulations were 3.6–7.2-folds higher than that of the intravenous solution, confirming direct nose-to-brain transport of nanoemulsions via olfactory region.

Saquinavir mesylate (SQVM) is a protease inhibitor with activity against HIV-Type 1. The absolute bioavailability of SQVM is very low and it also shows poor brain permeability. Mahajan et al. encapsulated SQVM in nanoemulsions using the spontaneous emulsification method to increase its brain delivery after intranasal administration (Mahajan et al., 2014). In the in vivo biodistribution study, nanoemulsions showed much higher drug concentration in brain after intranasal administration than intravenous-delivered drug suspension. The higher DTE (2919.261% $\pm$ 5.68%) and DTP (96.57448% $\pm$ 0.76%) for optimized nanoemulsions indicated effective CNS targeting of SQVM via intranasal route.

Zolmitriptan, a structural analogue of 5-hydroxytryptamine, is prescribed for the treatment of acute migraine associated with menses, with or without aura and cluster headaches. However, oral zolmitriptan exhibits a short half-life of 1–2 h, with the drug undergoing first-pass metabolism and being rapidly cleared by the hepatic and the renal systems. In order to prolong the duration of action of zolmitriptan, Jain et al. prepared zolmitriptan-loaded micelles for nose-to-brain delivery with Transcutol P®, benzyl alcohol, Pluronic® F127, PEG-400, and TPGS (Jain et al., 2010). The micelles were around 23 nm with a spherical nature. in vivo biodistribution studies indicated that zolmitriptan micelles exhibited a significantly higher uptake ($P < .05$) in the brain when compared with the zolmitriptan nasal solution and zolmitriptan i.v. solution at all the time points tested. Autoradiography studies revealed a distinct and extensive brain distribution of zolmitriptan after intranasal administration of the micelles, confirming the potential of micelles for nose-to-brain delivery.

4.6 Nanocomplexes

Intranasal route can be used for direct delivery of nucleic acid drugs to the brain. Anionic nucleic acid drugs such as DNA and RNA often need cationic polymers to form nanocomplexes through electrostatic interaction so as to ensure their stability and transfection in vivo. Harmon et al. compacted single molecules of plasmid DNA encoding-enhanced green fluorescent protein (eGFP) with 10kDa PEG-substituted lysine 30-mers (CK30PEG10k) for nose-to-brain delivery (Harmon et al., 2014). Fluorescence microscopy, immunohistochemistry, and ELISA all demonstrated eGFP expression two days after intranasal delivery. eGFP-positive cells were found throughout the rostral-caudal axis of the brain, most often adjacent to capillary endothelial cells, indicating the distribution of the nanocomplexes via perivascular flow. Kanazawa et al. developed Tat-modified PEG-PCL nano-micelles for nose-to-brain delivery of small interfering RNA (siRNA) (Kanazawa et al., 2013). The particle size of the nanocomplexes was approximately 50–80nm, with a net positive charge. It was found that the model siRNA concentration in the rat brain following intranasal administration of nanocomplexes was significantly higher than that of intravenous nanocomplexes or intranasal solution, demonstrating the feasibility of transferring siRNA to brain via intranasal route (Fig. 4).

5 Problems to be resolved

5.1 Industrialization of nano-sized formulations

Although nano-sized formulations are easily prepared in lab, scale-up of nanoparticle production is a big challenge in most cases. There are several problems associated with scale-up of nanoparticle production. For examples, lack of industrial equipment and safe carrier materials, difficulty in optimization of process parameters, batch difference of materials, difficulty in the removal of organic solvents and balancing of multicomponent system at large scale. During scale-up, some desired features of nanoparticles may alter, even though the mechanism of large equipment is same to the lab ones. In addition, developing targeted and surface functionalized nanoparticles at large scale is more complexed and always encounters various problems (Paliwal et al., 2014).

5.2 Reproducibility of brain delivery after intranasal administration

A large variance between individuals often exists for nose-to-brain drug delivery. Various factors such as head position, delivery volume, device, and method of administration can influence the absorption of formulations within the nasal cavity and the transport pathways to the brain. Different head positions of the animal/patient can alter the transport of formulations into the CNS. The most promising position for brain targeting is with head down and forward position; however, this position is uncomfortable and inconvenient to patients. Different administration devices have been used

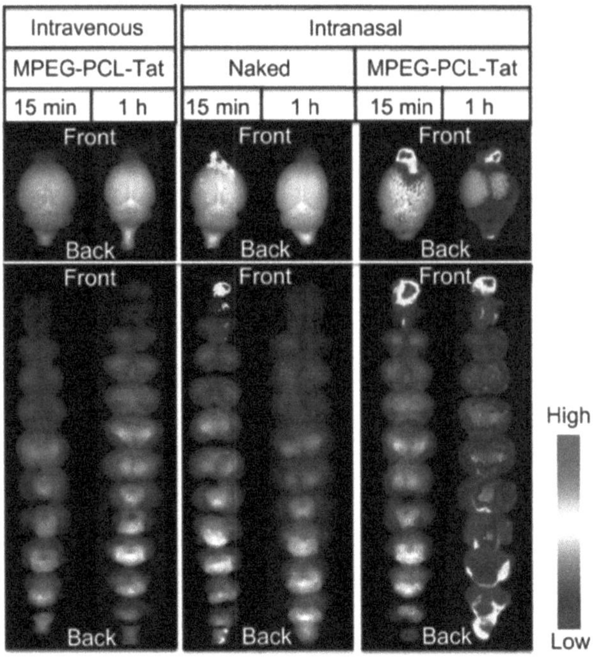

Fig. 4 Dynamics of PEG-PCL-Tat nanocomplex in brain tissue following i.n. or i.v. administration. Rats were sacrificed and each brain was enucleated at each point after i.n. or i.v. administration of naked Alexa-dextran or Alexa-dextran/PEG-PCL-Tat (dose = 40 μg as Alexa-dextran). Each sample was observed using Maestro™.
Reproduced from Kanazawa, T., Akiyama, F., Kakizaki, S., Takashima, Y., Seta, Y., 2013. Delivery of siRNA to the brain using a combination of nose-to-brain delivery and cell-penetrating peptide-modified nano-micelles. Biomaterials. 34, 9220–9226, with permission from Elsevier.

during intranasal administration, such as sprays, nose droppers, or needleless syringes, to target drug to different regions of the nasal cavity. Delivery volume is also an important factor to be considered for delivering therapeutics. Rats receive a total volume of 40–100 μL, mice receive a total volume of 5–10 μL, and in humans, the nasal cavity has a volume of 25 cm^3 and receives 400 μL resulting in CNS effects (Mittal et al., 2014). Efficient and reproducible delivery to the CNS may be achieved by selecting the right combination of head position, formulation, and delivery device to deliver the therapeutics to specific region of the nasal cavity (Dhuria et al., 2010).

5.3 Whether nanoparticles are transported intact to the brain and how are they cleared away?

Most of studies determined the concentrations of drugs or fluorescence probes in the brain tissue to reflect nose-to-brain transfer of nanoparticles. As we know, it may be difficult for nanoparticles larger than 100 nm to get access to the brain via the intraaxonal route because their diameter increasingly exceeds that of the axons in the filia olfactoria. The drugs in brain may come from a combination of nanoparticles and free drugs. However, it may need ingenious experimental design to determine whether: (i) intact particles are selectively taken into the olfactory epithelial cells and transported; or (ii) nanoparticles release the incorporated drug in vicinity of the apical surface of the olfactory cells (Mistry et al., 2009). This is because transport of nanoparticles from nose to brain is usually very limited and only a small amount of drug can be detected in the brain tissue. Also, visual observation is often limited by the low magnification of figures of tissue section (Mistry et al., 2009).

Furthermore, we still know little about how these nanoparticles are cleared from the brain. Although most nanoparticles are biodegradable, several weeks or months may be needed to degrade the polymers if they cannot be removed in some other ways. It was reported that soluble tracers could enter capillary basement membranes from the extracellular spaces and drain out of the brain along the basement membranes of cerebral capillaries and arteries as part of the rapid and direct lymphatic drainage of the brain parenchyma. But this pathway did not allow drainage of nanoparticles to regional lymph nodes. Nanoparticles are tracked along the pial-glial basement membrane and separated the glia limitans from the surface of arteries. It was speculated that this pathway also allowed nanoparticles to be cleared in an opposite direction (Morris et al., 2016). A possible way to tract nanoparticles is to label these polymers with isotopes and determine their concentrations in the brain, but no paper has reported this kind of results until now.

5.4 Are the nanoparticles toxic to the brain?

Some materials of nanoparticles and nanoemulsions, especially the cationic polymers and surfactants, are toxic to cells and tissues, but toxicity of therapeutic agents-loaded nanoparticles to the brain tissues is seldom studied. Liu et al. reported the in vivo toxicity and immunogenicity of WGA-NP to the brain in rats (Liu et al., 2011). It was found that WGA-NP showed slight toxicity to brain tissue, as evidenced by increased glutamate level in rat brain and enhanced LDH activity in rat olfactory bulb. No significant changes in acetylcholine level, acetylcholinesterase activity, GSH level, TNF-α level, IL-8 level, and WGA-specific antibodies were observed in rat olfactory bulb and brain, demonstrating the safety of this nano-carrier system to the brain. However, PLA is generally considered to be much safer than other polymers, so this research may not be representative enough to reflect the toxicity of most nanoparticles to the brain. Systematic studies are needed to evaluate the toxicity of nano-systems to the brain and nerves (e.g., olfactory nerve and trigeminal nerve), which may provide support for the clinical application of nanoparticles.

6 Future prospective

Effective noninvasive treatment of neurological diseases is often limited due to the presence of biochemical dynamic barriers: the BBB and blood-cerebrospinal fluid barrier (BCSFB) (Wong et al., 2012). BBB represents an insurmountable obstacle for a large number of drugs including antibiotics, antineoplastic agents, and various CNS-active drugs like neuropeptides. This creates a considerable threat for the therapy of cerebral diseases (Chakraborty et al., 2009). Therefore, treatment of neurological diseases has become one of the most significant challenges. The intranasal route bypasses the BBB and directly delivers drugs to the brain, providing a possible strategy for treatment of CNS diseases. Recent progresses in nanotechnology improve brain delivery of intranasally administrated drugs and may facilitate therapy for CNS disorders.

References

Abdel-Bar, H.M., Abdel-Reheem, A.Y., Awad, G.A., Mortada, N.D., 2013. Evaluation of brain targeting and mucosal integrity of nasally administrated nanostructured carriers of a CNS active drug, clonazepam. J. Pharm. Pharm. Sci. 16, 456–469.

Ahmad, E., Feng, Y., Qi, J., Fan, W., Ma, Y., He, H., Xia, F., Dong, X., Zhao, W., Lu, Y., Wu, W., 2017. Evidence of nose-to-brain delivery of nanoemulsions: cargoes but not vehicles. Nanoscale 9, 1174–1183.

Balin, B.J., Broadwell, R.D., Salcman, M., el-Kalliny, M., 1986. Avenues for entry of peripherally administered protein to the central nervous system in mouse, rat, and squirrel monkey. J. Comp. Neurol. 251, 260–280.

Bender, T.S., Migliore, M.M., Campbell, R.B., John Gatley, S., Waszczak, B.L., 2015. Intranasal administration of glial-derived neurotrophic factor (GDNF) rapidly and significantly increases whole-brain GDNF level in rats. Neuroscience 303, 569–576.

Boulton, M., Young, A., Hay, J., Armstrong, D., Fless-ner, M., Schwartz, M., Johnston, M., 1996. Drainage of CSF through lymphatic pathways and arachnoid villi in sheep: measurement of ^{125}I-albumin clearance. Neuropathol. Appl. Neurobiol. 22, 325–333.

Broadwell, R.D., Balin, B.J., 1985. Endocytic and exocytic pathways of the neuronal secretory process and trans-synaptic transfer of wheat germ agglutinin-horseradish peroxidase *in vivo*. J. Comp. Neurol. 242, 632–650.

Buck, L.B., 2000. The chemical senses. In: Kandel, E.R., Schwartz, J.H., Jessell, T.M. (Eds.), Principles of neural science. fourth ed. McGraw-Hill Companies, New York, pp. 625–652.

Casettari, L., Illum, L., 2014. Chitosan in nasal delivery systems for therapeutic drugs. J. Control. Release 190, 189–200.

Chakraborty, C., Sarkar, B., Hsu, C.H., Wen, Z.H., Lin, C.S., Shieh, P.C., 2009. Future prospects of nanoparticles on brain targeted drug delivery. J. Neurooncol. 93, 285–286.

Charlton, S.T., Whetstone, J., Fayinka, S.T., Read, K.D., Illum, L., Davis, S.S., 2008. Evaluation of direct transport pathways of glycine receptor antagonists and an Angiotensin antagonist from the nasal cavity to the central nervous system in the rat model. Pharm. Res. 25, 1531–1543.

Chen, J., Zhang, C., Liu, Q., Shao, X., Feng, C., Shen, Y., Zhang, Q., Jiang, X., 2012. Solanum tuberosum lectin-conjugated PLGA nanoparticles for nose-to-brain delivery: *in vivo* and *in vitro* evaluations. J. Drug Target. 20, 174–184.

Davis, S.S., 2001. Nasal vaccines. Adv. Drug Deliv. Rev. 51, 21–42.

Dhuria, S.V., Hanson, L.R., Frey II, W.H., 2009. Novel vasoconstrictor formulation to enhance intranasal targeting of neuropeptide therapeutics to the central nervous system. J. Pharmacol. Exp. Ther. 328, 312–320.

Dhuria, S.V., Hanson, L.R., Frey II, W.H., 2010. Intranasal delivery to the central nervous system: mechanisms and experimental considerations. J. Pharm. Sci. 99, 1654–1673.

Evans, M.J., Plopper, C.G., 1988. The role of basal cells in adhesion of columnar epithelium to airway basement membrane. Am. Rev. Respir. Dis. 138, 481–483.

Fatouh, A.M., Elshafeey, A.H., Abdelbary, A., 2017. Intranasal agomelatine solid lipid nanoparticles to enhance brain delivery: formulation, optimization and *in vivo* pharmacokinetics. Drug Des. Devel. Ther. 11, 1815–1825.

Fazil, M., Md, S., Haque, S., Kumar, M., Baboota, S., Sahni, J.K., Ali, J., 2012. Development and evaluation of rivastigmine loaded chitosan nanoparticles for brain targeting. Eur. J. Pharm. Sci. 47, 6–15.

Feng, C.C., Shao, X.Y., Zhang, C., Liu, Q.F., Chen, J., Shen, Y.H., Zhang, Q.Z., Jiang, X.G., 2011. Effect of absorption enhancers on nasal delivery of basic fibroblast growth factor. Afr. J. Pharm. Pharmaco. 5, 1070–1079.

Fonseca-Santos, B., Gremião, M.P., Chorilli, M., 2015. Nanotechnology-based drug delivery systems for the treatment of Alzheimer's disease. Int. J. Nanomedicine 10, 4981–5003.

Frey II, W.H., 2002. Bypassing the blood-brain barrier to delivery therapeutic agents to the brain and spinal cord. Drug Del. Tech. 2, 46–49.

Frey, W.H.I.I., 1991. WPTO. In: Neurologic agents for nasal administration to the brain. Chiron Corporation, US.

Fuss, S.H., Omura, M., Mombaerts, P., 2005. The Grueneberg ganglion of the mouse projects axons to glomeruli in the olfactory bulb. Eur. J. Neurosci. 22, 2649–2654.

Gao, X.L., Tao, W.X., Lu, W., Zhang, Q.Z., Zhang, Y., Jiang, X.G., Fu, S.K., 2006. Lectin-conjugated PEG-PLA nanoparticles: preparation and brain delivery after intranasal administration. Biomaterials 27, 3482–3490.

Gao, X., Wu, B., Zhang, Q., Chen, J., Zhu, J., Zhang, W., Rong, Z., Chen, H., Jiang, X., 2007a. Brain delivery of vasoactive intestinal peptide enhanced with the nanoparticles conjugated with wheat germ agglutinin following intranasal administration. J. Control. Release 121, 156–167.

Gao, X., Chen, J., Tao, W., Zhu, J., Zhang, Q., Chen, H., Jiang, X., 2007b. UEA I-bearing nanoparticles for brain delivery following intranasal administration. Int. J. Pharm. 340, 207–215.

Goldstein, I.J., Hayes, C.E., 1978. The lectins: Carbohydrate-binding proteins of plants and animals. Adv. Carbohydr. Chem. Biochem. 35, 127–340.

Gopinath, P.G., Gopinath, G., Kumar, A.T.C., 1978. Target site of intranasally sprayed substances and their transport across the nasal mucosa: A new insight into the intranasal route of drug delivery. Current Ther. Res. 23, 596–607.

Graff, C.L., Zhao, R., Pollack, G.M., 2005. Pharmacokinetics of substrate uptake and distribution in murine brain after nasal instillation. Pharm. Res. 22, 235–244.

Hanson, L.R., Martinez, P.M., Taheri, S., Kamsheh, L., Mignot, E., Frey II, W.H., 2004. Intranasal administration of hypocretin 1 (orexin A) bypasses the blood-brain barrier & targets the brain: A new strategy for the treatment of narcolepsy. Drug Del. Tech. 4, 66–70.

Harmon, B.T., Aly, A.E., Padegimas, L., Sesenoglu-Laird, O., Cooper, M.J., Waszczak, B.L., 2014. Intranasal administration of plasmid DNA nanoparticles yields successful transfection and expression of a reporter protein in rat brain. Gene Ther. 21, 514–521.

Jadhav, K.R., Gambhire, M.N., Shaikh, I.M., Kadam, V.J., Pisal, S.S., 2007. Nasal drug delivery system-Factors affecting and application. Curr. Drug Ther. 2, 27–38.

Jain, R., Nabar, S., Dandekar, P., Patravale, V., 2010. Micellar nanocarriers: potential nose-to-brain delivery of zolmitriptan as novel migraine therapy. Pharm. Res. 27, 655–664.

Jansson, B., Bjork, E., 2002. Visualization of *in vivo* olfactory uptake and transfer using fluorescein dextran. J. Drug Target. 10, 379–386.

Kaliner, M., Marom, Z., Patow, C., Shelhamer, J., 1984. Human respiratory mucus. J. Allergy Clin. Immunol. 73, 318–323.

Kanazawa, T., Akiyama, F., Kakizaki, S., Takashima, Y., Seta, Y., 2013. Delivery of siRNA to the brain using a combination of nose-to-brain delivery and cell-penetrating peptide-modified nano-micelles. Biomaterials 34, 9220–9226.

Kumar, M., Pandey, R.S., Patra, K.C., Jain, S.K., Soni, M.L., Dangi, J.S., Madan, J., 2013. Evaluation of neuropeptide loaded trimethyl chitosan nanoparticles for nose to brain delivery. Int. J. Biol. Macromol. 61, 189–195.

Liu, Q., Shao, X., Chen, J., Shen, Y., Feng, C., Gao, X., Zhao, Y., Li, J., Zhang, Q., Jiang, X., 2011. *In vivo* toxicity and immunogenicity of wheat germ agglutinin conjugated poly(ethylene glycol)-poly(lactic acid) nanoparticles for intranasal delivery to the brain. Toxicol. Appl. Pharmacol. 251, 79–84.

Liu, Q.F., Shen, Y.H., Chen, J., Gao, X.L., Feng, C.C., Wang, L., Zhang, Q.Z., Jiang, X.G., 2012. Nose-to-brain transport pathways of wheat germ agglutinin conjugated PEG-PLA nanoparticles. Pharm. Res. 29, 546–558.

Liu, Z., Jiang, M., Kang, T., Miao, D., Gu, G., Song, Q., Yao, L., Hu, Q., Tu, Y., Pang, Z., Chen, H., Jiang, X., Gao, X., Chen, J., 2013. Lactoferrin-modified PEG-*co*-PCL nanoparticles for enhanced brain delivery of NAP peptide following intranasal administration. Biomaterials 34, 3870–3881.

Luzzati, V., Benoit, E., Charpentier, G., Vachette, P., 2004. X-ray scattering study of pike olfactory nerve: Elastic, thermodynamic and physiological properties of the axonal membrane. J. Mol. Biol. 343, 199–212.

Mahajan, H.S., Mahajan, M.S., Nerkar, P.P., Agrawal, A., 2014. Nanoemulsion-based intranasal drug delivery system of saquinavir mesylate for brain targeting. Drug Deliv. 21, 148–154.

Migliore, M.M., Ortiz, R., Dye, S., Campbell, R.B., Amiji, M.M., Waszczak, B.L., 2014. Neurotrophic and neuroprotective efficacy of intranasal GDNF in a rat model of Parkinson's disease. Neuroscience 274, 11–23.

Mistry, A., Stolnik, S., Illum, L., 2009. Nanoparticles for direct nose-to-brain delivery of drugs. Int. J. Pharm. 379, 146–157.

Mittal, D., Ali, A., Md, S., Baboota, S., Sahni, J.K., Ali, J., 2014. Insights into direct nose to brain delivery: current status and future perspective. Drug Deliv. 21, 75–86.

Moran, D.T., Rowley 3rd, J.C., Jafek, B.W., Lovell, M.A., 1982. The fine structure of the olfactory mucosa in man. J. Neurocytol. 11, 721–746.

Morris, A.W., Sharp, M.M., Albargothy, N.J., Fernandes, R., Hawkes, C.A., Verma, A., Weller, R.O., Carare, R.O., 2016. Vascular basement membranes as pathways for the passage of fluid into and out of the brain. Acta. Neuropathol. 131, 725–736.

Mygind, N., Dahl, R., 1998. Anatomy, physiology and function of the nasal cavities in health and disease. Adv. Drug Deliv. Rev. 29, 3–12.

Nonaka, N., Farr, S.A., Kageyama, H., Shioda, S., Banks, W.A., 2008. Delivery of galanin-like peptide to the brain: Targeting with intranasal delivery and cyclodextrins. J. Pharmacol. Exp. Ther. 325, 513–519.

Paliwal, R., Babu, R.J., Palakurthi, S., 2014. Nanomedicine scale-up technologies: feasibilities and challenges. AAPS PharmSciTech. 15, 1527–1534.

Perl, D.P., Good, P.F., 1987. Uptake of aluminium into central nervous system along nasal-olfactory pathways. Lancet 1, 1028.

Peumans, W.J., Van Damme, E.J., 1995. Lectins as plant defense proteins. Plant Physiol 109, 347–352.

Sawant, K., Pandey, A., Patel, S., 2016. Aripiprazole loaded poly(caprolactone) nanoparticles: Optimization and *in vivo* pharmacokinetics. Mater. Sci. Eng. C Mater. Biol. Appl. 66, 230–243.

Schaefer, M.L., Böttger, B., Silver, W.L., Finger, T.E., 2002. Trigeminal collaterals in the nasal epithelium and olfactory bulb: a potential route for direct modulation of olfactory information by trigeminal stimuli. J. Comp. Neurol. 444, 221–226.

Seju, U., Kumar, A., Sawant, K.K., 2011. Development and evaluation of olanzapine-loaded PLGA nanoparticles for nose-to-brain delivery: *in vitro* and *in vivo* studies. Acta. Biomater. 7, 4169–4176.

Thorne, R.G., Emory, C.R., Ala, T.A., Frey 2nd., W.H., 1995. Quantitative analysis of the olfactory pathway for drug delivery to the brain. Brain Res. 692, 278–282.

Thorne, R.G., Hanson, L.R., Ross, T.M., Tung, D., Frey II, W.H., 2008. Delivery of interferon-b to the monkey nervous system following intranasal administration. Neuroscience 152, 785–797.

Thorne, R.G., Pronk, G.J., Padmanabhan, V., Frey II, W.H., 2004. Delivery of insulin-like growth factor-I to the rat brain and spinal cord along olfactory and trigeminal pathways following intranasal administration. Neuroscience 127, 481–496.

Tos, M., 1983. Distribution of mucus producing elements in the respiratory tract. Differences between upper and lower airway. Eur. J. Respir. Dis. Suppl. 128, 269–279.

Wen, Z., Yan, Z., Hu, K., Pang, Z., Cheng, X., Guo, L., Zhang, Q., Jiang, X., Fang, L., Lai, R., 2011. Odorranalectin-conjugated nanoparticles: preparation, brain delivery and pharmacodynamic study on Parkinson's disease following intranasal administration. J. Control. Release 151, 131–138.

Wong, H.L., Wu, X.Y., Bendayan, R., 2012. Nanotechnological advances for the delivery of CNS therapeutics. Adv. Drug Deliv. Rev. 64, 686–700.

Wu, H., Li, J., Zhang, Q., Yan, X., Guo, L., Gao, X., Qiu, M., Jiang, X., Lai, R., Chen, H., 2012. A novel small Odorranalectin-bearing cubosomes: preparation, brain delivery and pharmacodynamic study on amyloid-β(25-35)-treated rats following intranasal administration. Eur. J. Pharm. Biopharm. 80, 368–378.

Yang, Z.Z., Zhang, Y.Q., Wang, Z.Z., Wu, K., Lou, J.N., Qi, X.R., 2013. Enhanced brain distribution and pharmacodynamics of rivastigmine by liposomes following intranasal administration. Int. J. Pharm. 452, 344–354.

Yasir, M., Sara, U.V., 2014. Solid lipid nanoparticles for nose to brain delivery of haloperidol: *in vitro* drug release and pharmacokinetics evaluation. Acta. Pharm. Sin. B 4, 454–463.

Zhang, Q.Z., Zha, L.S., Zhang, Y., Jiang, W.M., Lu, W., Shi, Z.Q., Jiang, X.G., Fu, S.K., 2006. The brain targeting efficiency following nasally applied MPEG-PLA nanoparticles in rats. J. Drug Target. 14, 281–290.

Zheng, X.Y., Shao, X.Y., Zhang, C., Tan, Y.Z., Liu, Q.F., Wan, X., Zhang, Q.Z., Xu, S.M., Jiang, X.G., 2015. Intranasal H102 peptide-loaded liposomes for brain delivery to treat Alzheimer's disease. Pharm. Res. 32, 3837–3849.

Brain local delivery strategy

11

Raju Saka, Priyadarshini Sathe, Wahid Khan
Department of Pharmaceutics, National Institute of Pharmaceutical Education and Research (NIPER), Hyderabad, India

1 Introduction

Central nervous system (CNS) is the major control center of the human body. It is usually comprised of brain and spinal cord. The main function of CNS is to integrate information it receives from and coordinate and influence the activity of all parts of the bodies of bilaterally symmetric animals. Brain occupies the major portion of the CNS. The brain is responsible for controlling major activities of all the organs in the body. The brain is divided into various lobes, each of which has individual functions. Frontal lobe is associated with thinking, memory, behavior, and movement. Parietal lobe is responsible for touch and language. Hearing, learning, and feelings are controlled by temporal lobe. Occipital lobe is associated with sight and vision (Nieuwenhuys et al., 2013; Brodal, 2016). Brain stem is responsible for controlling breathing, heart rate, and temperature. Cerebellum is responsible for coordination and balance. Apart from basic sensory and cognitive functions, the brain also regulates the physiology of the body through hypothalamus and pituitary gland (Wilkins and King, 2002; Labrie, 2012). Efficient functioning of the brain is crucial to human health; care should be taken to maintain the functions of brain. Many diseases and disorders are localized in brain. These contribute to billions of healthcare costs in both developed and developing countries. These include infections like meningitis, encephalitis, brain abscess, etc., disorders like epilepsy, Alzheimer's disease (AD), Parkinson's disease, stroke, vasculitis, and multiple sclerosis, and proliferative diseases like glioma, meningioma, and glioblastoma multiforme (GBM) (Zigmond et al., 2014; Freedman, 2009). Of all the above diseases and disorders, neuro degenerative diseases along with proliferative diseases like tumors and cancers gathered extensive interest in scientific community from institutional level to industrial level. In terms of numbers affected, cerebrovascular diseases contribute highest number of cases. WHO report estimates that the brain disorders contribute for more than 12% of all the deaths by the end of year 2030. Diseases like AD itself contribute for around USD 605 billion in healthcare costs (World Health Organization, 2006). Advances in nanotechnology have led to improvement in maintaining the concentrations of drugs in brain at significant levels which cannot pass directly when injected into blood stream (Jain, 2012; Patel and Patel, 2017; Wong et al., 2012). Much of the research has been focused on design of nanocarriers to cross blood-brain barrier (BBB). Majority of the drugs have restricted access to BBB as the barrier is composed of various tight junctions and efflux proteins that prevent the transport of drugs through the

Brain Targeted Drug Delivery Systems. https://doi.org/10.1016/B978-0-12-814001-7.00011-1

membrane (Huber et al., 2001; Johansson, 1990). Nanotherapy has enabled drug transport through the BBB (Jo et al., 2015). This was made possible by use of various ligands that are substrate to the endothelial surface receptors (Hruby et al., 2015; Georgieva et al., 2014). Nanoparticles are also used in simultaneous diagnosis and therapy together called "theranostics" (Zhang et al., 2017; Singh and Sahoo, 2014). Other advantage of nanoparticles is that these particles protect the drug from external media and metabolizing enzymes; thus, increasing duration of action, thereby reducing dosing frequency (Reis et al., 2006; Woranuch and Yoksan, 2013). Nanotherapy is widely applied in the field of oncology. This was obvious as the nanoparticles can target the cancer tissue due to the leaky vasculature of the tumor (Greish, 2010; Maeda et al., 2009). Ligand-based approach has greatly improved the outcomes of majority of studies involving nanotherapeutic interventions (Das et al., 2009). This can be attributed to the unique features of nanoparticles. Majority of the nanoparticles targeting brain are administered either by intravenous (i.v.) route or intranasal (i.n.) route. Though these routes are advantageous, some amount of drug may reach other organs leading to toxicity. Also, some diseases are exclusively localized which need significant drug concentrations at specific site which is not possible with nanotherapeutics, except if these are targeted actively. Similarly, systemic delivery requires high doses of drugs which are also barriers during development. Hence, there is a need to develop local drug delivery strategies to brain which can treat various localize diseases.

1.1 Local drug delivery

Drug delivery includes formulation approaches that facilitate the entry and passage of therapeutic compounds in the body to elicit desired therapeutic effect. Local delivery to brain means direct administration of an official agent into the brain, or its surroundings, to produce a response, which allows direct access to site of action and avoids the adverse effects of standard systemic therapy (Jain, 2008).

Drugs when delivered by oral, parenteral, buccal, and inhalation routes get distributed into whole body and not to a specific target, where the effect is required. So as to reduce the detrimental effects of the systemic drug delivery, local delivery of drug is preferred. These routes have several limitations like poor biodistribution and high side effects. Moreover, biologics such as proteins, nucleic acids, enzymes, and genes get degraded and/or destabilized by enzymes and/or eliminated by the reticuloendothelial system before they reach their site of action (Morishita and Park, 2016). Furthermore, not all delivered drug can cross the biological barriers like BBB, capillary endothelial, or intestinal barrier or can circumvent first pass metabolism to show their activity at specific site at required concentration.

The development of local drug delivery systems is mainly beset by the shortcomings of the systemic drug delivery system. So as to address the limitations of the systemic drug delivery system, various approaches like targeted drug delivery and local drug delivery have been adopted. These provide high selectivity, efficiency, safety, and effectiveness with minimum risk of side effects to patients.

Advances in medicinal nano engineering, nano technology, and nano science have boosted the development of nanocarrier-based drug delivery systems. These delivery systems have been implemented for providing sustained, controlled, delayed, programmable, and localized delivery of drug at the site of action in host body (Losic et al., 2015). Local delivery of drug allows a greater concentration of drug to get accumulated at the site of action at low dose of drug. But the retention time of the drug at the site of action plays an important role here, which limits the use of rapidly metabolizing drugs. Numerous approaches are used to prolong the retention time of drug at target site; using nanotechnology-based endothelium targeting, or hydrophobic or lipophilic drug molecule having more residence time in cell (Domb and Khan, 2014).

1.1.1 Requirements

For a local delivery of drug, retention of drug at the target with proper dose and duration of time is of concern, to achieve therapeutic efficacy with fewer side effects. The formulations developed for local delivery should have following properties (Domb and Khan, 2014);

- Should be retained at the site of action for desired period of time
- Should offer programmed and continuous drug release at the site of action
- Should be easy to administer
- Should not cause any irritation or nuisance to the patient
- Should not alter normal physiological functions
- Should produce little or no systemic toxicity

1.1.2 Applications

Multifarious applications of pharmacotherapy to one specific site of action have been developed (Domb and Khan, 2014). These include the following points.

1.1.2.1 Stent therapy for arterial diseases

Drug eluting stents—These stents are basically bare metal stents, but modified through coating the surface of stent with polymer and/or drug. These stents overcome the problems associated with normal stents like in-stent neointimal hyperplasia, stent thrombosis, and inflammation (Kommineni et al., 2017).

1.1.2.2 Antimicrobial delivery for periodontitis

Local delivery of antimicrobial into the tooth pockets is essential to treat periodontitis; systemic delivery of antimicrobial limits its use because it is not accessible to the pathogens in periodontal pockets (Trombelli and Tatakis, 2003).

1.1.2.3 Ocular implants

Orbital implants (porous hydroxyapatite) are widely used in enucleation and in eviscerations. These implants have advantage of good prosthesis motility, less side effects, and is superior to others (Wong and Kochinke, 1995; Wong, 1992).

1.1.2.4 Dental implants

These implants are used for dental treatments in conditions like periodontitis, tooth caries, tooth infections, root canal, etc. Local delivery of drugs like analgesics and antibiotics from these implants makes them more effective (Pye et al., 2009).

1.1.2.5 Orthopedic implants

These are medical devices fabricated using stainless steel and titanium alloy (strength) with a plastic coat (artificial cartilage). These are used to replace bone or joints or to support damaged bone. These implants spread infection where they are placed, so now implants loaded with drugs like antibiotics are used which are coated with polymeric material (Anderson et al., 2005).

1.1.2.6 Skin diseases

For the treatment of skin diseases like psoriasis, pimples, vitiligo, and acne, local delivery of drug is of paramount importance. In these above specified conditions, the drug is to be applied over skin to show its activity; systemic delivery of drug is of very less importance in these types of conditions (Jain et al., 2016, 2017; Doppalapudi et al., 2017).

1.1.2.7 Brain delivery

For brain diseases like brain tumor and infections, and also to manage the severe pain, the drug is to be delivered directly to the brain. So in above specified conditions, drug is directly delivered to the site of action. The delivery to the site can be done by direct injection, implants, infusion pumps, chips, and by wafers (Guerin et al., 2004).

2 Local drug delivery to brain

Unlike topical drug delivery and local anesthesia, local drug delivery to brain is a challenging task. The administration is possible only by surgical interventions. Similarly, clearance of the drug from the brain is another challenge. Various conventional to novel strategies have been developed to locally deliver various drugs to brain (Fig. 1). These are discussed in the following sections.

2.1 Intracerebral injection

It is by far first used and is the simplest approach of local drug delivery to brain. Delivery of drugs directly to brain has numerous advantages. First, the intracerebral delivery eliminates the need for the drug to cross BBB, thereby reducing the dose of the drug that can be administered. Secondly, the drug will be available in the target at higher concentrations preventing systemic toxicities. In systemic drug delivery to brain, a large dose of the drug is needed to maintain optimum concentrations in brain. Only a fraction of dose reaches the target site and, hence, there is a scope for systemic toxicity. Hence, direct injection circumvents all these barriers. However, this technique is not widely used because the drug diffusion is directly dependent on molecular

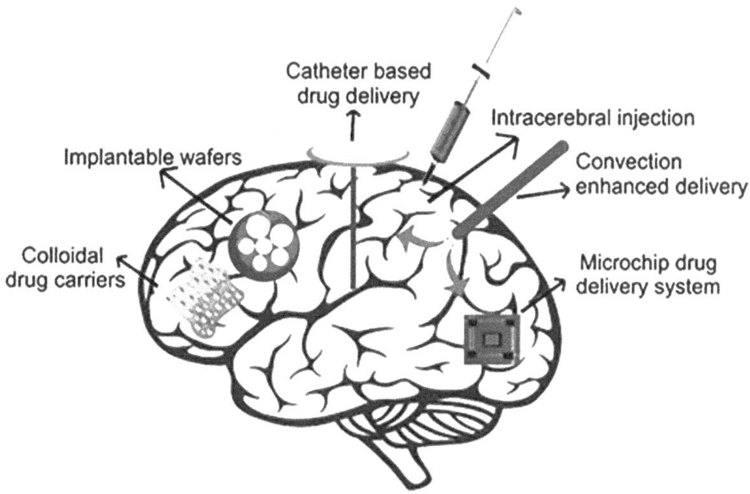

Fig. 1 Various strategies for local drug delivery to brain.

weight and concentration is dependent on rapid cerebrospinal fluid (CSF) exchange. This approach is applicable in cases where the target sites line ventricles or parenchymal surface (Scheld, 1989; Brasnjevic et al., 2009). Injection of simple solution containing active agent is not useful for chronic diseases. Fletcher et al. demonstrated that the intracerebral injection of DNA nanoparticles has provided long-term human glial cell line-derived neurotrophic factor (hGDNF) (Fletcher et al., 2011). Similarly, Yurek et al. have proved that intracerebral injection of nanoparticles encapsulating DNA encoding for hGDNF improved the gene expression and neuroprotection (Yurek et al., 2015).

2.2 Intrathecal and intraventricular administration

Drug delivery to brain via CSF is another approach where local drug delivery is possible. Blood-CSF barrier has fenestrated endothelium and multiple efflux transporters (Deeken and Löscher, 2007; Smith et al., 2004). Drug delivery through CSF bypasses both BBB and blood-CSF barriers. Delivery of drugs to CSF is done by three approaches: intrathecal, intraventricular, and intracavitary. The drug can be administered as bolus and infusion.

Intrathecal administration is usually done by injecting the drug into subarachnoid spaces in the lumbar region (Harbaugh et al., 1988). This method requires multiple procedures and the drug distribution from CSF is inefficient. Intraventricular injection can be done by direct puncturing of the skull followed by careful administration into the ventricles. Intraventricular administration results in improved volume of distribution throughout the CSF pathways (Tajes et al., 2014). Though well-tolerated, it has some limitations like meningitis, arachnoiditis, and focal neurologic injury. Restricted volume of distribution may arise due to CSF flow abnormalities. Hence, before initiating any CSF administration, CSF flow studies should be done to determine extent of variation (Blasberg et al., 1975).

2.2.1 Bolus administration

Bolus administration results in initial high CSF drug concentrations. However, the parenchymal penetration of drug was found to be less (Lee and Olszewski, 1960). Moreover, the bolus administration may be toxic to the patient. But still the drug penetrates into parenchyma and diffuses back into subarachnoid space when the CSF is cleared by bulk flow (Blasberg et al., 1977). To prevent toxicity, frequent smaller doses are recommended (Bleyer et al., 1978). Bolus injections are suitable in conditions where high concentrations in CSF and adjacent parenchyma are desired. These conditions include carcinomatous meningitis, spinal anesthesia, and chemical rhizotomy. Intrathecal bolus injection of tigecycline was used in the treatment of multidrug-resistant *Acinetobacter baumannii* meningitis (Wang et al., 2016). Intrathecal injection of antibiotics was found to be an effective alternative in treating various postoperative CNS infections. Long-term infusion has to be performed if the deeper diffusion of drug into parenchyma is desired (Rainov et al., 2001). Soderquist et al. studied the effect of DNA encoding for interleukin-10 loaded into poly-lacto glycolic acid (PLGA) microparticles for neuropathic pain. From the study, it was found that the administration of DNA as microparticles has reversed the neuropathic pain in rats (Soderquist et al., 2010). Nabhan et al. improved the half-life of mRNA coding for frataxin by formulating into lipid nanoparticles in treatment of Friedreich's ataxia. Other intrathecal nanoparticle-based gene delivery approaches have produced similar results such as long-term efficacy (Milligan et al., 2006).

2.2.2 Infusion using implantable pumps

The need for longer administration times to improve the drug penetration deeper into the brain has led to the development of infusion methods. As the exposure time increases, the depth of parenchymal penetration also increases. This was observed even in case of large protein molecules. Some compounds may need administration times from days to weeks to assess the effectiveness of the method. Parenchymal drug penetration occurs through both ependymal and pial surfaces (Rall, 1968; Rennels et al., 1985). Drugs administered into subarachnoid space as in case of intrathecal injection sometimes may not enter the ventricles in sufficient amounts (Bleyer, 1978). Intraventricular drug infusion results in more brain penetration when compared with intrathecal administration.

Intrathecal infusion is done by using various approaches. One approach is the use of percutaneous catheter connected to the external pump. Another approach includes use of totally implanted catheter provided with a subcutaneous injection port connected to an external pump. These are conventional approaches of infusing the drug intrathecally. Newer systems such as implantable fixed delivery rate pumps and implantable programmable delivery rate pumps are used to increase outcomes. External pumps are widely used as they are more economical option than using costlier implantable pumps (Govender et al., 2017). Implantable pumps for CNS infusion were first applied as potential treatment for chronic pain (Prager et al., 2014). Morphine was the first drug to be administered as CNS infusion. Morphine has been administered in cerebro ventricular system, lumbar subarachnoid space, and lumbar epidural space for treatment of chronic pain (Penn et al., 1984). It was then followed by various other drugs such as bupivacaine (Du Pen et al., 1992), clonidine (Ackerman et al., 2003), hydromorphone (Anderson et al., 2001), and analgesic peptides (Wermeling, 2005). CNS infusion has provided better pain relief when compared with other methods and was also found to be safe (Coombs et al., 1983). Similarly, the CNS infusion has been applied in treating spasticity. Morphine and baclofen were widely used for this purpose (Gatscher et al., 2002). Use of low-dose morphine was found to be effective in the management of spasticity. Baclofen, when administered orally, failed to reduce spasticity. This led to the development of intrathecal administration of baclofen to treat spasticity. When administered as intrathecal infusion, baclofen effectively reduced spasticity and associated pain in amyotrophic lateral sclerosis. Intrathecal infusion of baclofen reduced the dose from about 10–90 mg/day to 80–200 μg/day. Usually, baclofen is administered through subcutaneous implantable pumps. Most suitable pump used for baclofen delivery was Synchromed pump from Medtronic Inc. (Sindou and Mertens, 2000). Apart from the simple drug solutions, magnetic nanoparticles were intrathecally infused to target the drug for CNS disorders (Lueshen et al., 2015).

The main advantage of drug delivery through CSF is that the extent of protein binding and enzymatic activity is very less when compared with plasma. Other advantages like rapid diffusion of drug from CSF into brain extracellular fluid make it a suitable drug delivery platform (Schliep and Felgenhauer, 1978; Wood, 1980).

2.3 Convection-enhanced delivery

Brain interstitial fluid usually moves by both diffusion and convection. Convection in simple terms is defined as bulk flow which is a result of pressure gradient established in brain cavities and is independent of molecular weight (Lonser et al., 2015; Rosenberg et al., 1980; Fenstermacher and Kaye, 1988). Compounds generally travel by concentration gradient in any tissue. In brain, convection can be used to supplement the diffusion to improve the drug exposure to the deeper and inaccessible areas of brain where simple injection does not provide significant drug concentrations at the site. Interstitial infusion creates a pressure gradient which results in increased convection and improves drug delivery to brain without significant structural and functional damage (Bobo et al., 1994; Lieberman et al., 1995). This allows homogenous delivery of high molecular weight biomolecules with a potential to deliver these substances to surgically inaccessible brain tumors and far reaching regions in brain. Convection also plays a significant role in drug transport from the polymeric implants. Local cerebral edema caused by the implantation of polymer implant produces elevated pressure gradient that facilitates drug distribution to deeper tissues (Fung et al., 1996; Blakeley, 2008).

CED uses locally placed catheters to deliver the drugs into the target tissues. The general procedure involves insertion of stereotactically guided small-caliber catheter into brain parenchyma. The drug solution is pumped through the catheter into brain (Morrison et al., 1999). The drug then penetrates the interstitial spaces and the infusion is carried out for several days and catheter is removed at bedside. These interstitial pathways enable drug transport independent of its molecular weight. The infusion rates were varied from 0.1 to 10 μL/min. It was found that the penetration of drug into the brain parenchyma was about 2 cm with the CED approach which is very high when compared with the normal diffusion where the highest penetration was observed at 2 mm distances (Bobo et al., 1994; Gabathuler, 2010).

2.3.1 Factors influencing optimization of CED

Both design and procedural changes decide the fate of the CED therapy. Factors like cannula size, concentration of infusion, rate of infusion, position of catheter, and sealing time are critical in determining the success of the CED system (Chen et al., 1999). Of all these factors, infusion rate and cannula size affect the outcome the most. It was found that the increase in the infusion rate using radiolabelled albumin as a model drug increased the incidence of infusate leakage back along the delivery tract. This was attributed to the increase in the interstitial pressure due to high flow rates. Similarly, at low flow rate, the infusate was localized at the target site. Cannula size doesn't have effect on the drug distribution, but the increase in cannula diameter increases the susceptibility of leak back as it facilitates the low resistance pathway along the surface (Chen et al., 1999). For a CED system to be effective in conditions like brain tumors, high drug concentrations need to be maintained for extended period of time. Precise placement of catheter also affects the success of the CED system. Direction of flow is also critical in determining the success of CED therapy. This is in turn dependent on pressure gradient and resistance to flow. Resistance to flow depends on both direction and location. Also, white and gray matter properties determine the fate of the volume of distribution to volume of infusion ratio (Vd:Vi). White matter offers less resistance compared to gray matter, but in case of gray matter it is more homogenous when compared with white matter (Raghavan et al., 2006; Healy and Vogelbaum, 2015). Vd:Vi is also another key factor determining the efficiency of CED system. Usually, the Vd is approximately linear to infusion, but this tend to change in various conditions (Zhou et al., 2017). At higher flow rates, the Vd:Vi ratio gets altered; this may be due to the significant backflow which renders Vd independent of Vi (Chen et al., 2012).

2.3.2 Applications

CED therapy was widely used to treat various disorders like brain tumors, AD, Parkinson's, etc. Over a long period of time, many drugs have been used to treat brain tumors. These include paclitaxel (Lidar et al., 2004), carboplatin (Barua et al., 2016), doxorubicin (Xi et al., 2014), topotecan (Lopez et al., 2011), etc. Apart from simple solutions, novel formulations like nanodiamonds are also being administered via CED approach with considerable success rates in brain cancer therapy (Xi et al., 2014).

Similarly, glial-derived neurotropic factor was also delivered via CED for management of Parkinson's disease (Heiss, 2017). Advances in polymer science have led to the development of various polymeric nanoparticles. These were also used in conjunction with CED to improve therapeutic outcomes. Sawyer et al. prepared camptothecin-loaded polymeric nanoparticles and infused into rat brain by CED. The group treated with drug-loaded nanoparticles showed higher survival rates in rats with intracranial 9L tumors compared to the group treated with pain drug infusion (Sawyer et al., 2011). Similar study by Bernal et al. proved that the temozolomide coloaded with iron oxide in polymeric nanoparticles aided in image-guided therapy of malignant glioma (Bernal et al., 2014). Many studies have proved that combining nanoparticles with CED enhanced the penetration of dyes or radiolabelled agents into deeper tissues of brain (Weng et al., 2013; Saucier-Sawyer et al., 2016; Kenny et al., 2013). Further studies proved that the image-guided and tissue topology-dependent CED of nanocarriers is essential to improve the treatment outcomes (Foley et al., 2012; Saito et al., 2004). These advantages further expanded this field to efficient gene and protein delivery (Mastorakos et al., 2016). Salkmon et al. designed a formulation in which the drug, that is, methotrexate, was bound onto the maghemite nanoparticles coated with human serum albumin for CED treatments of gliomas. These nanoparticles as compared to plain drug showed good distribution and long clearance time and no drug-related toxicity was seen (Corem-Salkmon et al., 2011). Krauze et al. formulated and studied the effect of combination of topoisomerase I inhibitor CPT-11 and topoisomerase II inhibitor doxorubicin in nanoparticles and PEGylated liposomes, respectively. CED of these combination showed more efficacy than the drugs alone (Krauze et al., 2007).

2.3.3 Limitations

CED is associated with many physical limitations and also performance limitations. Backflow is one of the frequent problems associated with the CED therapy. It is commonly called as reflux of the infusate because of void formation caused by mechanical disruption of tissue. As a fluid-filled gap forms between the needle and the underlying tissue, the infusate escapes easily, thus preventing the drug penetration into the tissue. Other factors that cause backflow are presence of air bubbles, pressure spikes, deviation in catheter insertion procedure, and catheter design (Casanova et al., 2014; Sillay et al., 2014).

Air bubbles also pose problem during therapy as they contribute to backflow which has been described earlier. Air bubbles also act as obstacle for imaging during real time monitoring. These also disrupt the tissue altering the drug distribution (Sillay et al., 2014). Priming the cannula before insertion reduces air bubbles (Allard et al., 2009).

Pathological condition of the surrounding tissue also plays a spoil sport in the CED therapy. Conditions like active tumors and postoperative tissue alterations may present issues like increased interstitial pressure caused by edema and nonuniform blood vessel distribution. Excessive vasculature at tumor site may facilitate the loss of infusate to blood circulation (Mehta et al., 2017). In some cases, the infusate may follow the vasculature pattern, thus deviating from its intended distribution pattern (Allard et al., 2009). Hence, it is recommended that the catheters shall be placed 2 cm from any brain surface and 1 cm from any cavity.

2.3.4 Advances in CED

To address the major limitations, the improvements in the CED methodology and system designs have been introduced. Reflux-preventing catheters have been introduced to tackle backflow. These are designed in such a way that the cannula extends beyond the end by 5 mm to 10 mm (Debinski and Tatter, 2009). Multiple-hole catheters have been introduced which presented better pressure output and improved overall distribution. However, they failed in predicting the accurate flow pattern. To address this problem, hollow fiber catheters have been developed. These contain millions of pores along its wall which are very small, that is, in the magnitude of 0.45 μm (Bidros et al., 2010; Oh et al., 2007). These catheters have increased the amount of infusate transferred by threefold with improved distribution and reduced backflow. Other advances include balloon-tipped catheters and ultrafine catheters, which significantly reduced backflow and improved customized drug delivery which suits the relevant anatomy (Olson et al., 2008). Similarly, methodological changes like change from external pump infusion to subcutaneously implanted pump showed promising results as it prevented the increased risk of infection which is associated with the use of external catheters for prolonged periods of time (Yun et al., 2013; Bruce et al., 2011; Sonabend et al., 2011). Still, optimization needs to be done both in design and methodology to improve the treatment outcomes.

2.4 Implantable drug delivery systems

2.4.1 Implantable microchips

Microchips are novel devices that are effectively used for local drug delivery. These were generally applied for pulsatile delivery of drugs. The system is derived from solid state silicon microchip which provides programmed drug release from multiple reservoirs (Sutradhar and Sumi, 2016). Each micro-reservoir is an individual section of the microchip and can be loaded with different drugs. Usually, these reservoirs are covered by reservoir caps which, on stimuli, dissolve and release the drug. These systems were designed using micro-fabrication techniques. Santini et al. first developed solid state silicon drug delivery microchip at Massachusetts Institute of Technology (Santini et al., 1999). These microchips are capable of releasing either single or multiple drugs in a programmable manner.

2.4.1.1 Design of the system

The advances in the technological aspects in integrated circuit (IC) industry have enabled development of micro-machines. Conventionally in IC industry, microelectromechanical systems (MEMS) are employed in manufacturing micron scale devices like switches, sensors, gears, and filters from silicon which is the major component of the IC industry (Schulz, 1999; Sant et al., 2012). Basically, two methods were used in manufacture of ICs; these include surface and bulk micromachining. Surface micromachining involves design of micro-devices from the thin films of either polycrystalline silicon or other materials deposited on a surface. Bulk micromachining involves removal of considerable amounts of silicon from a substrate to form microstructures. Major techniques involved in microfabrication are photolithography, soft lithography, film deposition, etching, and bonding (Betancourt and Brannon-Peppas, 2006). These techniques provide accurate control on surface architecture, size, and topography of the device.

Conventional drug delivery systems do not provide many options to accurately tailor the shape for the purpose of controlled drug delivery (Santini et al., 2000). To overcome these drawbacks, microfabrication technology has been introduced in the field of drug delivery systems (Webb, 2004; Polla et al., 2000). This technology was used to create reservoirs to accommodate drugs. These reservoirs can be sealed with reservoir caps to protect and contain drugs. The device can be designed in such a way that the seal on individual reservoirs can be opened and drug can be released on specific command (Staples, 2010). With these features, a highly programmed and accurate drug release can be achieved which was cited as the important benefit of these microfabricated systems. One of the first developed microchip drug delivery system was an electrochemically activated solid state silicon drug delivery microchip. In this microchip, a thin gold membrane capping drug reservoir in silicon serves as anode in electrochemical reaction. The device was capable of storing and releasing multiple drugs. The device is composed of pyramidal reservoirs etched through silicon wafers (Dario et al., 2000). Each wafer can accommodate around 1000 reservoirs, each with a volume ~25 nL. The size of wafer and number of reservoirs in the wafer can be adjusted based on the treatment goals. This technology has been commercially pursued by Bedford MA where it was trademarked as MicroCHIPS Technology (Gardner, 2006). This company was the first to publish the preclinical data on the microchip drug delivery device. Microchips are usually divided into active systems and passive systems.

Active systems are basically solid state silicon microchips where the drug release can be controlled after implantation using electrical, magnetic, mechanical, or other stimuli. These silicon chip membranes consist of thin gold layers (Fig. 2A). Whenever a drug release is desired, voltage is applied to trigger dissolution of gold anode membrane by electrochemical reaction (Grayson et al., 2003). Passive devices are generally resorbable polymeric microchips where the controlled drug release is dependent on the polymer erosion (Fig. 2B). In passive systems, the drug release cannot be controlled after implantation. These contain biodegradable polymeric membranes. These systems exploit diffusion, osmotic potential, and concentration gradient as driving force for drug delivery. The drug delivery is directly dependent on composition, thickness, and molecular weight of the membrane forming material used to cap the reservoir (Daniel et al., 2009).

A typical microchip device is usually composed of a substrate, reservoir caps, therapeutic agent, and control circuitry and power source. The substrates are etched and machined reservoirs which serve as a support for the microchip. These are generally

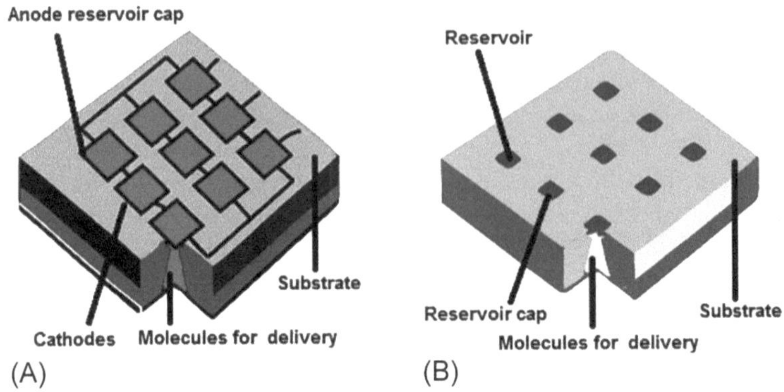

Fig. 2 Microchip drug delivery systems: (A) Silicon based and (B) Polymer based.

made up of polyethylene glycol (PEG), silicon, glass, and plastic materials (Santini et al., 2011). The material can be either nondegradable or degradable based on the design requirements. Therapeutic agents that can be used for localized delivery into brain through the microchips are commonly anticancer agents like carmustine (BCNU), lomustine (CCNU), and semustine (methyl-CCNU). Other drugs include antibiotics, analgesics, and anti-Alzheimer's drugs (Santini et al., 2011). Reservoir caps along with the reservoir matrix are the rate controlling substrates in the microchip device. In active devices, the reservoir caps act as anode and consist of thin films of conductive materials like copper, gold, silver, zinc, platinum or titanium, etc. Depending on the intended release pattern of drug, the cathode size and placement can be modified. In passive devices, the reservoir cap is usually composed of degradable polymeric material, which dissolves or degrades over time, but can be permeable for the molecules to be released (Santini et al., 1998; Tao and Desai, 2003). In active devices, the control circuitry is comprised of a timer, a demultiplexer, a microprocessor, and a memory source. Selection of power source is essential as the device should be able to perform intended role for predetermined period before the need for recharge. Most commonly used power sources for this purpose are lithium-based or rechargeable microbatteries. Though these are microdevices, these systems have considerable biocompatible issues due to the presence of silicon, gold, and other substrates. Only the external surface of microchip comes into contact with the tissue and, hence, necessary surface modifications should be done to improve biocompatibility (Shawgo et al., 2002; Chung et al., 2008). The major advantages of microchips include:

- These devices can be able to deliver drugs in all states
- These does not have any moving parts
- The loaded drug is protected from the harsh physiological environment and, hence, the dose required to elicit pharmacological effect can be less
- These devices can be used as both local and systemic drug delivery systems
- Multiple drugs can be loaded into a single microchip

However, these systems present significant challenges. There is considerable chance that only limited amount can be released from the reservoir; in such cases, expected effect may not be observed. Other challenge is that the drugs with high potency are more suitable for these devices. Similarly, a very stable formulation is ideal for this system as the device resides in the body for extended periods of time. High cost of the device is another limiting factor that reduced the effective use of this system.

2.4.1.2 Applications

Microchips are being evaluated for local brain delivery. US patent no. US8679093 B2 applied by MicroCHIPS Inc. has described in detail a multi-dose drug delivery device for potential application in local brain delivery. The device consists of at least two housing units connected in a linear orientation. In this, at least one housing unit is made of bioerodible polymer. In this device, the release is controlled by the in vivo disintegration of seal member (Farra, 2014). Similarly, US patent no. US 5797898 described the various design of microchip drug delivery design for potential application in local brain delivery. The patent has described both active and passive devices. The patent disclosed that the implantable microchip device can be used to locally deliver the chemotherapeutic agents which can be used in brain tumors (Santini Jr et al., 1998). US patent no. US6123861 has described fabrication of active and passive microchips formed by etching. In this patent, the authors described the design of reservoirs and subsequent filling by drug formulation followed by sealing. The authors suggested that the passive system is suitable for brain implantation as the material is biodegradable and, therefore, surgical removal of the implant is not needed. Hence, this system can also be explored for local brain delivery into tumors (Santini Jr et al., 2000). Kim et al. has designed a polymer-based microchip for local drug delivery to brain. They loaded BCNU in both microchip and polymer-based wafer. In this study, the authors compared the drug stability, pharmacokinetics, and antitumor efficacy. Drug stability was high in microchip when compared with wafer. Similarly, the half-life of the drug when administered in form of microchip has increased to greater extent. A gliosarcoma rat model was used to study the antitumor efficacy of BCNU microchips. From the study, it was observed that the dose-dependent decrease in tumor size was observed with BCNU microchips where 1.24 mg dose showed significant tumor reduction. This treatment showed similar efficacy to a BCNU-loaded polymeric wafer, but with high stability and better pharmacokinetic profile (Kim et al., 2007).

2.4.2 Implantable polymeric systems

Polymeric drug delivery systems were introduced to overcome the short duration of action of simple drug solutions. These systems provide controlled release of drugs for longer periods of time. Initially, during early days nonbiodegradable polymers were used for programmed drug release where it is due to slow diffusion of drug from the polymer matrix. However, use of nonbiodegradable polymers is not suitable for local drug delivery to sensitive organs like brain (Langer and Folkman, 1976). To prevent this, biodegradable polymers have been introduced in drug delivery systems. One of the first approved biodegradable polymers was poly-lacto glycolic acid (PLGA) for sutures (Craig et al., 1975; Conn et al., 1974; Austin et al., 1995). These polymers can be fabricated into various structures like microparticles, nanoparticles, gels, etc. to control the release of the drug (Benny et al., 2009; Tahara et al., 2011). One major advantage of the biodegradable polymer is that the drug release is controlled by both polymer degradation and drug diffusion through matrix. Other main advantage of polymeric systems is that these systems can achieve high local concentrations of therapeutic agents and eliminates/limits systemic toxicities.

2.4.2.1 Polymeric wafers

One of the first local drug delivery strategies to brain involving polymeric systems are implantable wafers. These were first developed for glioblastoma. The major rationale for use of degradable polymeric systems in local brain therapy is that there is no need for surgical removal of the implant after treatment. Poly (bis(p-carboxyphenoxy)-propane (PCPP):sebacic acid (SA) polymeric matrices were first evaluated for controlled release of therapeutic compounds in local drug delivery. The sustained release characteristics are due to formation of dicarboxylic acids during a spontaneous reaction with water. The polymer resists hydrolysis and enzymatic degradation due to its hydrophobic nature. The polymer degradation rate can be changed by modifying ratios of carboxyphenoxypropane (CPP) and SA. This polymer was found to be biocompatible in primates where they showed no symptoms regarding behavioral, neurological, and hematological complications. BCNU was one of the first chemotherapeutic agents to show efficacy in treatment of brain malignancies (Loo et al., 1966). Initially, BCNU was administered into systemic circulation for therapeutic benefit. However, clinical data showed no significant survival benefit to the patients undergoing systemic BCNU therapy (Walker et al., 1980). Since BCNU is an alkylating agent, their nonspecific targeting in systemic therapy may cause alkylation of DNA of healthy cells. These unwanted actions led to the development of diverse side effects like bone marrow suppression and pulmonary fibrosis. Even the drug has limited pharmacokinetic properties when injected as solution. The drug has very short half-life of less than 15 min, which is not ideal for chronic conditions like brain malignancies where long-term action is required for therapeutic benefit (Levin et al., 1978). For this purpose, the local delivery of BCNU with PCCP:SA polymer has been evaluated for potential treatment of brain tumors. This led to the development of first FDA-approved polymeric wafer for brain tumor, the Gliadel® wafer (2017c).

Gliadel® wafer is usually composed of BCNU impregnated into the PCCP:SA. The optimized ratio of PCCP:SA was adjusted to 20:80 in the marketed formulation. The drug, BCNU, was homogenously distributed into this copolymer matrix. The implantable system was designed in such a way that each wafer contains about 7.7 mg BCNU distributed in copolymer matrix of 192.3 mg (2017a). During initial development, the system was optimized into various PCPP:SA ratios (Leong et al., 1985). Initial preclinical studies were carried out at high PCCP to SA ratios (80:20) to evaluate the pharmacokinetic behavior of the drug in the system. In these studies, the delivery system increased the local drug exposure for more than a week. The system was able to maintain therapeutic levels of drug even at 4 cm distance from the site of implantation. This proved that drug retention in wafer was maintained for longer periods of time (Grossman et al., 1992). This study was followed by the pharmacodynamics comparison between polymeric BCNU group and systemic BCNU group in rat flank and intracranial 9 L gliosarcoma models. From the study, it was found that the polymer group increased the overall survival rates by 5.4 fold than control group. Systemic BCNU group only improved the survival by 2.4-fold (Tamargo et al., 1993). In other study, 20:80 PCPP:SA BCNU wafers were compared with intratumoral injection in equivalent doses. It was found that the median survival increased to up to 271% in comparison with control group (Buahin and Brem, 1995). Pharmacokinetic studies were performed to optimize the PCPP:SA ratio. Survival rates were higher with 20% PCPP. As the amount of PCPP reduces, the polymer blend becomes more hydrophobic, thus retaining drug release for extended period of time. Further studies found that the 20:80 PCPP:SA didn't lead to any systemic or local morbidities, even at 150th day after implantation. These encouraging results enabled the formulation to be carried out to the clinical stage (Sipos et al., 1997).

Multicenter phase I-II clinical trials were performed. Around 21 patients with a record of recurrent malignant glioma were enrolled for the study. Initial studies were conducted to assess the safety of the BCNU-loaded polymeric wafers. Each patient was administered with eight wafers of 200 mg weight each. The drug-polymer was administered at three different doses: 1.93, 3.85, and 6.35%. Results indicated that there was neither any systemic toxicity nor neurological degeneration after polymer implantation. Moreover, blood and urine analysis didn't reveal any bone marrow, renal, or hepatic injury. Treated patients showed median survival of 46 weeks. Of all patients, eight survived more than 1 year. These positive results paved way for phase III clinical trial (Brem et al., 1991). The study investigated the efficacy of 3.8% BCNU PCPP:SA polymers for treatment of recurrent malignant glioma. Survival rate for treatment group was 31 weeks when compared with the placebo group which showed 23 weeks survival rate. Fifty percent increase of survival in glioblastoma patients was observed in comparison with placebo group. These studies proved that the BCNU polymer treatment was safe and effective with absence of systemic toxicity (Brem et al., 1995). This study was pivotal for the FDA approval of 3.85% BCNU-loaded PCPP:SA wafer for the treatment of recurrent glioblastoma in 1996 (2017e).

The success of Gliadel® wafers led to the increased research in implantable wafers for brain malignancies. Drugs like mitoxantrone were also loaded into polymeric wafers and evaluated for their efficacy in treating malignant brain tumors. These wafers were implanted intracranially in 9L gliosarcoma in Fischer 344 rats. The combined median survival rate of rats at highest dose was found to be 50 days. This makes it a suitable candidate to treat brain malignancies (DiMeco et al., 2002). Similarly, the doxorubicin was loaded into PCPP:SA wafers and implanted in rats. The overall survival of doxorubicin wafers group was 45 days at the highest dose of 5% doxorubicin (Lesniak et al., 2005).

2.4.2.2 Implantable colloidal carriers

Apart from implantable polymeric wafers, colloidal drug carrier systems were also widely investigated for local delivery of therapeutics to brain. These formulations include microspheres/microparticles and nano formulations like nanofibres, nanorods, nanoparticles, etc. Various drugs like paclitaxel, BCNU, temozolomide, 5-fluorouracil, etc. were widely formulated into colloidal carrier systems for local delivery to brain malignancies. Apart from cancer applications, these systems were also utilized in delivery of drug which can treat neurodegenerative diseases (Tiwari et al., 2012; Zhou et al., 2013).

Microspheres/microparticles were the first choice for any controlled drug delivery applications. They are easy to formulate, requires less manpower, and can control drug release for longer periods of time. These systems are usually formulated using biodegradable polymers like PLGA, poly (lactic acid) (PLA), poly caprolactone (PCL), etc. (Nair and Laurencin, 2007). Common methods of formulating microspheres include single emulsion method and double emulsion methods (Rosca et al., 2004). Other methods like electrospray methods are also used for preparation of microspheres (Bock et al., 2011). In single emulsion method, the drug and polymer were dissolved in organic solvent. This organic phase is then added to aqueous solution containing a stabilizer and then homogenized. The organic solvent is then evaporated to recover drug-encapsulated microspheres. The drug loading, particle size, and morphology can be altered by changing parameters like polymer concentration, stabilizer concentration, homogenization speed, etc. (Rosca et al., 2004). This method is widely suitable for hydrophobic drugs, and hence, low encapsulation efficiency for hydrophilic compounds has been observed with this method. Double emulsion involves formation of water-in-oil-in-water (W/O/W) emulsion to encapsulate water-soluble drugs. The organic layer acts as barrier which prevents the hydrophilic drug to diffuse into the aqueous phase. The organic solvent is evaporated and the microspheres are recovered (Ghaderi et al., 1996). Other methods of preparation include spray drying and electro hydrodynamic atomization (EHDA) (Nie et al., 2010). Paclitaxel is a widely investigated compound for various types of cancers. It acts by promoting formation and stabilization of microtubules which inhibits mitotic cell division, thereby inducing apoptosis (Horwitz, 1994). Though the drug has been used to treat various types of cancers, it has found less benefit in systemic delivery for glioma therapy. The failure is because the drug was unable to cross BBB so as to reach at significant concentrations (Naraharisetti et al., 2007). Hence, the drug was formulated into microspheres for localized delivery to brain tumors. The paclitaxel microspheres were mostly studies in 9L gliosarcoma or C6 glioma tumors. In one study, the paclitaxel was loaded into PLGA microspheres by two methods: spray drying and EHDA. These microspheres were studies in BALB/c nude mice bearing C6 glioma tumor cells subcutaneously. The microspheres prepared by spray drying and EHDA inhibited tumor growth by 59% and 65%, respectively, when compared with placebo group. However, at longer time points, the spray-dried microspheres were found to be more effective than the EHDA microspheres (Naraharisetti et al., 2007). In a similar study, paclitaxel-encapsulated microspheres in alginate beads were evaluated in a similar animal model, but here the formulation is directly injected into tumors. Eighty-five percent tumor volume reduction was observed when compared with placebo group. Polilactofate microspheres, when compressed in wafer in presence of PEG, increased the median survival rates in rats when administered intracranially (Li et al., 2003). When the same system was studied at higher doses in higher animal models like canines, it was found that the formulation was safe which was evident by lack of systemic toxicity and myelosuppression. Adverse effects observed during study such as wound infections were easily treated with antibiotic therapy, thus concluding that the formulation is safe and effective (Pradilla et al., 2006). 5-Fluorouracil is a hydrophilic antimetabolite which has an effective record of being a powerful radio sensitizer. However, the drug does not cross BBB readily due to its hydrophobicity (Longley et al., 2003). Therefore, microsphere implantation was evaluated for their effective delivery to brain tumors. Studies involving 5-Fluorouracil-loaded PLGA microspheres showed sustained release profiles of 20 and 30 days (Chandy et al., 2000; Menei et al., 1999). These were also coloaded with antisense oligonucleotides for synergistic effects (Hussain et al., 2002). Intracranial study against C6 glioma cell line in Wistar and Sprague–Dawley rats was performed to compare the effect of the microspheres. The drug-loaded microsphere group significantly reduced the mortality in animals when compared with directly injected drug solution, which failed to show similar mortality as observed in reduction in mortality when compared with untreated group (Menei et al., 1996). Similar studies carried out for other drugs like carboplatin, BCNU, temozolomide, and protein-based endogenous inhibitors resulted in better treatment outcomes when compared with the control groups (Zhang and Gao, 2007; Ozeki et al., 2012; Rhines et al., 2003; Emerich et al., 2002).

Micro-colloidal systems were also used to locally deliver drugs into brain to treat neurodegenerative diseases. Bethanechol was formulated into microspheres for potential treatment of AD. Microspheres were formulated using 50:50 PCPP:SA copolymer. These were implanted in the denervated hippocampal region of rat brain and evaluated for improvement in behavioral studies. From the study, it was observed that the formulation was well-tolerated by rats. Similarly, the rats in the polymer group showed significant cognitive improvement, thus establishing this method as a novel localizing neurotransmitter delivery to reverse the memory deficits in rat brain (Howard III et al., 1989). These microspheres were also applied in treating Huntington's disease (HD). Nerve growth factor (NGF) has been widely reported for their effect in preventing neurodegeneration and behavioral characteristics in HD. However, their ability was limited to shorter period of time. This led to the development of controlled release formulations for NGF (Powell et al., 1990). In a study, the NGF-loaded PLGA microspheres were successfully synthesized by double emulsification method. These were administered stereotaxically into the striatum of rats. The formulation is administered one week prior to quinolinic acid (QA) infusion. Implanted microspheres released NGF over 75 days and were degraded in three months. These were proved to reduce the QA-induced lesions by 40% more than control group. This study proved that the implantable microspheres of NGF are neuroprotective against excitotoxic lesions, and thus, can serve as better alternative for HD therapy (Menei et al., 2000). Similar studies were performed in treatment of various CNS disorders like epilepsy, Parkinson's disease, and cerebral edema, where drug-loaded microspheres were found to improve the treatment outcomes when compared with simple drug solutions (Govender et al., 2017).

2.4.2.3 Hydrogels

Hydrogels are defined as hydrophilic three-dimensional polymeric networks which can absorb large volumes of water or physiological fluids without the dissolution of polymer. These have high thermodynamic compatibility with water, and hence, can swell in such environments (Bures et al., 2000). Hydrogels were termed as one of the excellent controlled release vehicles in field of targeted drug delivery. The major advantage of hydrogels is that it can be loaded with virtually any type of drug, that is, even loading of macromolecules can be done with ease (Milligan et al., 2006). The critical aspect of hydrogel formulation is "in-situ gelation." This gelation can be triggered by use of specific stimuli like pH, temperature, light, etc. (Van Tomme et al., 2008). The hydrogels are usually formed from the polymers which exhibit lower critical solubility temperature. These polymers include polyethylene oxides (PEO), hydroxypropyl acrylate, methyl cellulose, hydroxypropyl cellulose, hydroxypropyl methyl cellulose, polymethacrylic acid, and poly (N-isopropyl acrylamide) (pNIPAAm) (Hoffman, 1987). Hydrogels are investigated for their potential application in local drug delivery to brain to treat various diseases, especially brain malignancies. These can be implanted by intracerebral or intracerebroventricular injection. These can also be implanted intratumorally after surgical resection of the neoplasm. PLGA is one of the most successfully used biodegradable polymers in the field of drug delivery. The polymer is safe to use and has also been approved by major regulatory bodies like Food and Drug Administration (FDA) and European Medicine Agency (EMA) for systemic applications. PLGA-based hydrogels have limited water absorption capabilities (Danhier et al., 2012; Alexander et al., 2013). Nevertheless, these polymers were widely used in local delivery of anticancer agents in solid tumors. Akbar et al. developed a biodegradable gel matrix composed of temozolomide loaded in hydrogel of PLGA and plasticizers (40:60). The plasticizers used are acetyl triethyl citrate and triethyl citrate (1:1). Intracranial administration of the hydrogel in rats reduced the tumor growth significantly in the treatment group compared with blank group (Akbar et al., 2009). PLGA is also a major component of widely investigated hydrogel systems, ReGel™. ReGel™ is copolymer of PLGA and PEG and is a controlled release drug delivery system where the polymers are sensitive to external environment. It is supplied as a low viscous solution. At body temperatures, the solution becomes a viscous gel like structure which releases the drug in a controlled fashion. One of the formulations based on ReGel™ is Oncogel™. It is a paclitaxel-loaded hydrogel based on ReGel™ components (Vellimana et al., 2013; Tyler et al., 2010). Similarly, photopolymerizable hydrogels can also be used for application in local drug delivery to brain. These substances polymerize in presence of light to form a crosslinked structure. One of the studies involving photopolymerizable hydrogels was temozolomide hydrogel for potential treatment of glioblastoma. The drug was loaded into PEG-dimethacrylate and water (75:25). 0.5% of Lucirin-TPO® was used as photo initiator in the formulation. When irradiated for 15 s with light at 400 nm, the hydrogel spontaneously formed and appeared viscous. The in vitro release studies revealed that the formulation was able to control the drug release for more than a week. Tolerability studies in rat brain concluded that the formulation does not induce any apoptosis and damage to the brain cells. in vivo pharmacodynamics studies in tumor model resulted in reduced tumor growth in treatment group when compared with control group (Fourniols et al., 2015).

Apart from drug in solution form, the colloidal drug carriers can also be suspended into hydrogels to attain sustained release properties. One of such approach is suspending lipid nanocapsules into hydrogel. These nanocapsules are oily core of triglycerides surrounded by shell of surfactants. Nanocapsules-based hydrogel loaded with gemcitabine has been developed for local treatment of GBM. The formulation showed a significant reduction of tumor growth compared to free drug (Bastiancich et al., 2016; Moysan et al., 2014). Besides nanocapsules, polymeric nanoparticles/microparticles-loaded hydrogels were also widely evaluated for local brain delivery. These systems showed controlled local drug release (Baumann et al., 2010; Ranganath et al., 2009). Similarly, the hydrogels were also used for theranostic purpose for simultaneous imaging and delivery (Sun et al., 2016; Jiang et al., 2013). Though the system is very effective in localized drug delivery, it still has considerable challenges. Though the drug release was uniform in in vitro conditions, it is still unlikely that the delivery system will perform as expected. Tissue injury and pathological conditions contribute to most of the delivery system failure. Hence, it is essential to optimize and characterize the formulation considering all the in vivo exposure conditions.

3 Marketed products

With the increase in need for local drug delivery, many products were approved to improve treatment outcomes. Generally, these products were classified into infusion pumps (Table 1) and dosage forms (Table 2).

3.1 Safety concerns

For local drug delivery, one has to place the drug or a device at that site which will give a continuous supply of drug to maintain the effective concentration of drug to show its activity. These are the devices which are implanted to various sites of brain like intra thecal perfusion devices (baclofen perfusion), Giladel wafers, and catheters to deliver the drug at the site of action. These implants like intrathecal perfusion devices are used to deliver opioid analgesics (morphine) for management of chronic pain; when the management of pain fails by other routes, catheters are attached to the pumps which deliver the drug at the site from reservoir; Giladel wafers are used in conditions like brain tumor (Malheiro et al., 2015).

Complications related to these implants are relatively low, but still some are there (Teddy et al., 1992). These include problems related to devices, that is, mechanical problems associated to the pumps and catheters. These problems related to devices can be resolved by revision. Further serious complications include infection, overdose, skin necrosis, tissue damage, sensitivity reactions, CSF leak, and even epileptic seizures and acute withdrawal syndrome (Kofler et al., 1994; Siegfried et al., 1992). So, a clinician should be aware of all these complications before placing the implants

Table 1 List of approved implantable infusion pumps for brain delivery

S. No.	Product name	Manufacturer	Composition	Indication	References
1	Synchromed II	Medtronic	Tramadol Methadone	Certain types of severe pain	2017g
2	IsoMed pumps, continuous-flow pumps	Medtronic	Oxycodone	Severe pain	2017c
3	Codman 3000 constant-flow implantable pumps	Codman and Shurtleff	Hydromorphone	Severe pain	2017a
4	MedStream™ Programmable Pump	Codman and Shurtleff		Severe pain	2017e
5	Ommaya reservoirs	Medtronic	Methotrexate, Cytarabine	Carcinomatous meningitis, CNS lymphoma or leukemia intraventricular hemorrhage	2017f

and even after the placement of implant (Stetkarova et al., 2010; Stempien and Tsai, 2000).

A rare but most fatal complication of these implants or devices is infection at the site of placement because of the pumps and catheters which is in contact with the part of brain (Gilmartin et al., 2000). The cause behind these infections can be direct inoculation of microbes at the time of surgery and/or during refilling the reservoir or may be due to hematogenous contamination of device. The infectious organisms can be gram-positive or gram-negative (Wunderlich and Krach, 2006). Chances of other infections like urinary tract infection and pneumonia also increase. The infectious organism causing infection in a study was found to be methicillin-sensitive *Staphylococcus aureus*, *Pseudomonas aureus*, coagulase-negative Staphylococcus, enterobacteriacea like *Escherichia coli*, *K. pneumoniae* and *M. morgagnii*, *S. capitis*, *P. mirabilis*, and *S. epidermidis*. These organisms cause meningitis, cellulitis, and inflammation. Meningitis was seen due to the pumps and catheter; the mean time to develop meningitis was found to 2.2 months after placing the implants. These infection-causing organisms can be isolated from pump, blood, and catheter. *S. capitis*, *E. coli*, and *P. mirabilis* can be found in blood, *S. epidermidis* in CSF, and multi-drug-resistant organism such as methicillin-resistance *S. aureus*, *S. epidermidis*, *P. aeruginosa*, and enterobacteriacea (*E.coli*, *K. pneumoniae* and *M. morgagnii*) can be seen on catheter tips (Stempien and Tsai, 2000).

Table 2 **List of approved formulations for local brain delivery**

S. No.	Product name	Manufacturer	Composition	Indication	References
1	Lioresal	Medtronic	Baclofen	Muscle relaxant, antispastic	Lioresal ®INTRATHECAL [PACKAGE INSERT] (n.d.)
2	Baclofen injection	Sintetica SA, Mendrisic	Baclofen	Muscle relaxant, antispastic	2017f
3	Duramorph	WEST WARD	Morphine sulfate	Management of pain	
4	Isovue-M 200	Bracco diagnostics Inc.	Iopamidol	Neuroradiology thoraco-lumbar myelography	2017d
5	SPINRAZA (nusinersen) injection	Biogen Inc.	Nusinersen	Treatment of spinal muscular atrophy	Wood (1980)
6	Brineura	BioMarin	Cerliponase alfa	Neuronal ceroid lipofuscinosis type 2	Lonser et al. (2015)
7	Gliadel wafer	Eisai Inc	BCNU, Polifeprosan 20	Brain tumors	2017b
8	Exparel	PACIRA pharmaceuticals	Bupivacaine	Local infiltration, peripheral nerve block, sympathetic nerve block	Rosenberg et al. (1980)
9	DepoCyt(e)	PACIRA pharmaceuticals	Cytarabine	Lymphomatous meningitis	Fenstermacher and Kaye (1988)

Surgical site infections (SSI) are the second most common infectious complications. These infections are defined as small infections involving the suture, without pump exteriorization and small collections in pump pocket. Deep surgical site infections were defined as deep-incisional and organ space infection with large collection pump exteriorization or inflammatory signs in catheter tract. These infection symptoms are local inflammation and intraoperative traces of infection. To treat these conditions, oral antibiotic therapy is given with proper local wound care and sometimes the pump is also removed. The common antibiotic given is flucloxacillin which covers the potential to kill gram-positive organisms. Superficial-incisional surgical site infections are less severe; symptoms like fever and inflammation are only seen and no other systemic symptoms are seen. In case of severe surgical site infection such as deep-incisional and organ space infection, hospitalization is recommended in which intravenous antibiotics are given and pumps and catheters are removed. The drugs given in this case have varied spectrum of activity; generally vancomycin and meropenem are administered; the antibiotics selected for the activity are based on the intra-institutional resistance. The treatment starts with anti-staphylococcal agent. These infections have potential to cause meningitis. The other ways of treating the infection are intrapocket administration of antibiotic (Boviatsis et al., 2004), subfascial pump implantation (Kopell et al., 2001), or/and muscle flap wrap after effective local disinfection (Atiyeh et al., 2006).

Some organisms have unique features which aid colonization and ensuring pump infection. Colonization commences as early as the pump is implanted into the brain. At first, the pump gets rapidly covered with a film of connective tissue which are soluble containing fibronectin, collagen, fibrinogen, and other proteins (Stempien and Tsai, 2000). This coating attracts bacteria which have different binding sites for them, which allows irreversible bacterial adhesion. Slime production by cells facilitates colonization of surface by enabling bacteria to adhere together as a cell cluster and to facilitate exchange between cells (Fan-Havard and Nahata, 1987). Further, this layer acts as a barrier which protects the bacteria from the host defense mechanism and antibiotics which are given systemically. It even protects the organisms from the endogenous bactericidal compounds such as lysozymes.

The main reason for pump infection is breakdown of skin over device in spasticity patients. These patients are undernourished and are characterized by dearth of subcutaneous tissue. Spasticity patients have increased risk for preoperative infection, even without wound breakdown. The threshold of skin tolerance to breakdown is an inverse ratio of the intensity and duration of pressure. Some pumps are bulky in nature; insertion of such pumps leads to further continuous compression of the skin against pump and stretching, which impairs the blood supply and causes ulceration and necrosis. In case of undernourished patients, because of poor nutrition healing is impaired due to which wounds break down and the infection spreads (Stallings et al., 1993a, b).

Pump infections can be treated with and without removal of pumps. Infections without removal of pumps can be treated with therapeutic aspirations, pump disinfection, and local and systemic antibiotic treatment. It is difficult to treat infection without removal of pump. To remove a pump from brain, the patient has to go through two operations, that is, one for removal of the pump and second for pump replacement after eradicating the infection. This procedure increases the morbidity, hospitalization time, and cost (Boviatsis et al., 2004).

The time taken for infection to spread and cause varies from few days to several years. Early infections occur within 3 months after pump implantation, while the late infections are those which occur after 3 months or more after implantation. The infection can initiate from the time of pump or catheter implantation or, at the time of refilling, the reservoir. The surgical site infection and meningitis take first 3 months after the implantation of the device (Malheiro et al., 2015).

Several methods, approaches, and techniques are used to prevent the infections caused by the devices and implants. The techniques are use of sterile procedures, monitoring patient's condition after implanting the device or implant, and administering preoperative and intraoperative antibiotics to patient. The patients with risk of methicillin-resistant *Staphylococcus aureus* should be given nasal mupirocin and should obtain a pre-op nasal swab (Follett et al., 2004; Paice et al., 1996). Infection prevention during refilling of reservoirs can be reduced by maintaining proper skin hygiene, by sterilizing with chlorhexidine gluconate 4% topical liquid (hibiclens) before performing the operation, and by using the preprepared ampoules (Borrini et al., 2014).

In one of the cases, a lady was having cerebral palsy at the age of 26. She was suffering from pharmaceutically intractable spasticity located in the lower extremities from the age of 17. So as to conquer this situation, she has to implant a pump, but the pump was removed within 5 days because of Staphylococcal meningitis, which was treated with antibiotics. After this, she has to undergo second operation to implant a new pump with postoperative antibiotic treatment. After a week, she faced irritation, febrile (38.2°C), abdominal pain, and headache at the site of implantation. On clinical examination, it was found that the pocket in which the pump was placed was swollen. The fluid around the pump revealed *Pseudomonas aeruginosa*. So as to treat this infection, she was treated with amikacin i.v. and ciprofloxacin orally. Therapeutic aspiration and intrapocket antibiotic infusion were given for 2 weeks.

In another case, a man, 27 year old, had a 5-year history of quadriplegia and spinal cord injury at fourth cervical level. He was suffering from intractable spasticity causing extreme pain and abnormal posture. So, he has to undergo a surgery for implantation of baclofen pump. After 6 months till now, he has refilled the pump twice and the port of pump was explanted through the surgical scars; because of this, the patient has become febrile. For clinical examination, the pump puncture was avoided to prevent the possibility of iatrogenic contamination. The place around the pump showed the sign of local inflammation and serous discharge. The cultures revealed *Staphylococcus epidermidis*. Hence, immediate therapy of vancomycin i.v. and rifampicin orally was started. The pump was removed without replacement of catheter. Pump was cleaned and disinfected thoroughly with povidone-iodine solution and vancomycin solution and then placed again in deeper position.

4 Clinical trials

Various trials are being conducted to evaluate the effect of local drug delivery to brain in various conditions (Table 3). These include:

Table 3 **List of undergoing clinical trials for local drug delivery to brain**

S. No.	Title	Purpose	NCT No.	Phase	Status	References
1	Prometra Post-Approval Study	The Prometra Pump is approved by the FDA for use in the United States. The purpose of this study is to collect long-term safety data on the Prometra Pump	NCT01854229	Post-approval study	Recruiting	Matis (2018)
2	Intrathecal Rituximab in Progressive Multiple Sclerosis	The goal of investigators is to study the kinetics of action of a single dose of intrathecally infused rituximab upon cerebrospinal fluid (CSF) biological targets in progressive MS patients	NCT02545959	Phase 2	Recruiting	Bonnan (2017)
3	Patient registry of intrathecal pain management in Europe for prialt (Ziconotide Intrathecal Infusion) and alternative drugs for the management of severe, chronic pain. (PRIME)	The objective of this study is to monitor the long-term efficacy, safety, tolerability, and quality of life outcomes associated with Prialt and other analgesics utilized in the intrathecal management of severe chronic pain	NCT02268812	–	Completed	Zhou et al. (2017)
4	Clinical trial on the use of autologous bone marrow stem cells in amyotrophic lateral sclerosis (Extension CMN/ELA)	The purpose of this clinical trial is to assess the feasibility and the security of the intraspinal and intrathecal infusion of autologous bone marrow stem cells for the treatment of Amyotrophic Lateral Sclerosis patients	NCT01254539	Phase 1 Phase 2	Completed	Jiménez (2017)

5	Patient registry of intrathecal ziconotide management (PRIZM)	The objectives of this study are to evaluate the effectiveness, long-term safety, tolerability, satisfaction with treatment, and health-related quality of life (HRQoL) associated with Intrathecal PRIALT use for severe chronic pain of varying etiologies	NCT01888120		Completed	Huang (2017)
6	The effectiveness of pain management using the ARCHIMEDES® constant-flow infusion pump system for intrathecal delivery	The purpose of this observational registry is to collect a continuum of meaningful clinical data on the ARCHIMEDES implantable pump in pain management	NCT00196053	Phase 4	Completed	Ward (2017)
7	Wound infusion vs. spinal morphine for postcaesarean analgesia (Apcisaal)	The aim of this study is to compare effective analgesia with continuous wound infiltration of ropivacaine through multiholed catheter or with morphine 100 μg added intrathecally to spinal anesthesia, after elective caesarean delivery	NCT02264821	Phase 3	Completed	Linden (2017)
8	Safety study of 3 mg/mL baclofen injection (Intrathecal) using a programmable pump	Safety study to assess the 3 mg/mL baclofen injection (intrathecal) using a programmable pump	NCT01520545	Phase 3	Completed	Francisco (2017)

Continued

Table 3 **Continued**

S. No.	Title	Purpose	NCT No.	Phase	Status	References
9	Safety and exploratory efficacy study of NEUROSTEM® vs. placebo in patients with Alzheimer's disease	This combined phase 1/2a clinical trial is to investigate the safety, dose-limiting toxicity (DLT), and exploratory efficacy of three repeated intraventricular administrations of NEUROSTEM® (human umbilical cord blood-derived mesenchymal stem cells) vs. placebo via an Ommaya reservoir at 4-week intervals in patients with Alzheimer's disease	NCT02054208	Phase 1 Phase 2	Recruiting	Oh (2017)
10	Methotrexate and Etoposide infusions into the fourth ventricle in children with recurrent posterior fossa brain tumors	The goal of this clinical research study is to establish the safety of simultaneous infusions of methotrexate and etoposide into the fourth ventricle of the brain or resection cavity in patients with recurrent malignant posterior fossa brain tumors. These tumors include medulloblastoma, ependymoma, atypical teratoid/rhabdoid tumor, or	NCT02905110	Early Phase 1	Recruiting	Sandberg (2017a)

		other malignant brain tumor with recurrence or progression involving anywhere in the brain and/or spine. Patients' disease must have originated in the posterior fossa of the brain				
11	Phase II study of intraventricular methotrexate in children with recurrent or progressive malignant brain tumors	The purpose of this research study is to test an experimental treatment method for recurrent or progressive brain tumors in children aged from 0 to 22 years. The use of methotrexate and chemotherapy (topotecan and cyclophosphamide) is experimental in this study	NCT02684071	Phase 2	Recruiting	Khatib (2017)
12	A safety study of rituximab plus MTX injected into the cerebrospinal fluid in the treatment of brain lymphoma	Test the idea that the direct injection into the cerebrospinal fluid of Rituximab, a monoclonal antibody which attacks and kills lymphoma cells, is safe and when used in combination with methotrexate in patients with recurrent brain and intraocular lymphoma Also to test the idea that the	NCT00221325	Phase 1	Completed	Rubenstein (2017)

Continued

Table 3 **Continued**

S. No.	Title	Purpose	NCT No.	Phase	Status	References
		combination of rituximab plus methotrexate has activity and is effective in the treatment of recurrent brain and intraocular lymphoma				
13	Methotrexate infusion into fourth ventricle in children with recurrent malignant fourth ventricular brain tumors	The goal of this clinical research study is to establish the maximum tolerated dose (MTD) of direct administration of methotrexate into the fourth ventricle of the brain in patients with recurrent malignant brain tumors including medulloblastoma, primitive neuroectodermal tumors (PNET), atypical teratoid/rhabdoid tumors (AT/RT), and ependymoma	NCT02458339	Phase 1	Recruiting	Sandberg (2017d)
14	Mitigating cephalad fluid shifts: A NSBRI study (NSBRI)	This is a feasibility study to determine optimal thigh cuff design using a cephalad fluid shift protocol in patients who have an intraventricular catheter (such as Ommaya reservoir) placed for the delivery of central nervous	NCT03097523	–	Completed	Kesari (2017)

		system chemotherapy or for diagnosing potential elevation of ICP and monitoring its progression as part of standard medical care				
15	Intrathecal Mafosfamide	The purposes for this study are to (a) determine what dose of mafosfamide can be safely given into the cerebrospinal fluid through an Ommaya reservoir (surgically implanted catheters used to sample cerebrospinal fluid and to instill medication into the cerebrospinal fluid) and lumbar puncture (spinal tap) or lumbar reservoir; (b) look for side effects of drug treatment; (c) to study the pharmacology (how the human body handles the drug) when given directly into the spinal fluid; and (d) see if this drug is beneficial to the patient.	NCT00062881	Phase 1	Completed	Blaney et al. (2005)
16	Intrathecal therapy with monoclonal antibodies in progressive multiple sclerosis (ITT-PMS)	To study long-term stabilizing effects of neurological symptoms by regular intrathecal administered monoclonal antibodies in progressive multiple sclerosis	NCT01719159	Phase 2	Completed	Svenningsson et al. (2015)

Continued

Table 3 **Continued**

S. No.	Title	Purpose	NCT No.	Phase	Status	References
17	Intracerebral gene therapy for Sanfilippo Type A syndrome	The primary objective is to assess the tolerance and the safety associated to the proposed treatment through a one-year follow-up The secondary objective is to collect data to define exploratory tests that could become evaluation criteria for further clinical phase III efficacy studies	NCT01474343	Phase 1 Phase 2	Completed	Anon (2017e)
18	Intracerebral gene therapy for children with early onset forms of Metachromatic Leukodystrophy (TG-MLD)	The objective of this open-label, single arm, monocentric, phase I/II clinical study is to assess safety and efficacy of ARSA gene transfer in the brain of children affected with early onset forms of Metachromatic Leukodystrophy (MLD)	NCT01801709	Phase 1 Phase 2	active	Aubourg (2017)
19	A safety and tolerability Study of intracerebroventricular administration of sNN0031 to patients with Parkinson's disease	To evaluate the safety and tolerability of the drug product sNN0031, containing Platelet-Derived Growth Factor (PDGF), when administered directly into one of the fluid filled	NCT00866502	Phase 1 Phase 2	Completed	Pålhagen (2017)

		cavities in the brain using an implanted catheter and an implanted SynchroMed II pump. Patients with a diagnosis of Parkinson's disease will be enrolled				
20	A safety and tolerability study of Intracerebroventricular administration of sNN0029 to patients with amyotrophic lateral sclerosis	This study is conducted to evaluate the safety and tolerability of the drug product sNN0029, containing the growth factor VEGF165, when administered directly into one of the fluid filled cavities in the brain using an implanted catheter and an implanted SynchroMed II pump. Patients with Amyotrophic Lateral Sclerosis will be enrolled	NCT00800501	Phase 1 Phase 2	Completed	Robberecht (2017)
21	Methotrexate infusion into the fourth ventricle in children with malignant fourth ventricular brain tumors: a pilot study	To learn if it is safe to receive methotrexate through the fourth ventricle of the brain in patients with brain tumors	NCT01737671	Early Phase 1	Active	Sandberg (2017b)
22	Study of concurrent intravenous and intrathecal nivolumab for patients with leptomeningeal disease (LMD)	The goal of Phase 1 of this research study is to find the highest tolerable dose level of nivolumab that can be given both by intravenous (IV) infusion and intrathecal (IT) injection to patients	NCT03025256	Phase 1	Recruitment	Glitza (2017)

Continued

Table 3 **Continued**

S. No.	Title	Purpose	NCT No.	Phase	Status	References
		with leptomeningeal disease (LMD). IV infusions are given by vein, while IT injections are given directly into the cerebrospinal fluid (CSF)				
23	A dose ranging pilot study to assess intracerebroventricular (ICV) delivery of valproate in subjects with temporal seizures	Patients with medically refractory epilepsy will be treated by intracerebroventricular (ICV) delivery of valproate using an implantable drug pump system	NCT02899611	Phase 1 Phase 2	Recruiting	Zhou et al. (2017)

5 Conclusion and future perspective

Local drug delivery to brain is an efficient technique to treat localized brain disorders as it is easy to maintain therapeutic concentrations at low doses. Various case studies suggested that the field of local drug delivery is a promising strategy to treat various CNS diseases and disorders without significant toxicity. This was further catapulted by introduction of Gliadel® wafer. Introduction of Gliadel® wafer paved way for development of other implantable systems like microchips and hydrogels. Similarly, native techniques like intracerebral, intrathecal, and intraventricular infusion of drugs through implantable pumps were also proven to be effective when compared with intravenous administration. Hence, it can be inferred that the local brain delivery of drugs is a suitable strategy to overcome barriers that prevent drug permeation into brain when administered through parenteral route. One of the major safety concerns with this approach includes administration site infections, tissue damage, erratic release patterns, etc., which may limit the use of this approach. However, advances in the design of these implantable systems and administration technologies as in case of CED have reduced the safety burden. Still, there is a need to establish the design and safety of these devices and delivery technologies to improve the treatment outcomes. When all these issues get resolved, this local delivery strategy will be an ideal approach to deliver drugs for CNS disorders.

References

Ackerman, L.L., Follett, K.A., Rosenquist, R.W., 2003. Long-term outcomes during treatment of chronic pain with intrathecal clonidine or clonidine/opioid combinations. J. Pain Symptom Manag. 26, 668–677.

Akbar, U., Jones, T., Winestone, J., Michael, M., Shukla, A., Sun, Y., Duntsch, C., 2009. Delivery of temozolomide to the tumor bed via biodegradable gel matrices in a novel model of intracranial glioma with resection. J. Neuro-Oncol. 94, 203–212.

Alexander, A., Khan, J., Saraf, S., Saraf, S., 2013. Poly (ethylene glycol)–poly (lactic-*co*-glycolic acid) based thermosensitive injectable hydrogels for biomedical applications. J. Control. Release 172, 715–729.

Allard, E., Passirani, C., Benoit, J.-P., 2009. Convection-enhanced delivery of nanocarriers for the treatment of brain tumors. Biomaterials 30, 2302–2318.

Anderson, V.C., Cooke, B., Burchiel, K.J., 2001. Intrathecal hydromorphone for chronic nonmalignant pain: a retrospective study. Pain Med. 2, 287–297.

Anderson, K., Morrison, M., Dewey, J., Bruneau, A., Molz, F., Carls, T., Lange, E., 2005. Local Delivery of an Active Agent From an Orthopedic Implant. Google Patents.

Anon, 2017a. Codman 3000 constant-flow implantable pumps Codman & Shurtleff. Available: http://www.codmanpumps.com/PDFs/Chemo03.pdf. Accessed 5 September 2017.

Anon Giladel wafer[package insert] 2017b Available: http://arborpharma.com/docs/201241r1-gliadel-pi.pdf Accessed 05 September 2017.

Anon Isomed pump. 2017c Available: https://www.uhms.org/images/MEDFAQs/Intrathecal.pdf Accessed 05 September 2017.

Anon Isovue-M 200, Bracco diagnostics Inc. 2017d Available: http://medlibrary.org/lib/rx/meds/isovue-m-1/page/3/ Accessed 05 September 2017.

Anon MedStream™ Programmable Pump Codman & Shurtleff 2017e Available: Medstream%20Surgical%20Technique%20Guide%20(1).pdf Accessed 05 September 2017.
Anon Ommaya reservoir 2017f Available: http://pabrainspine.com/media/presentations/Customer%20Implant%20Therapy%20Presentation.pdf Accessed 05 September 2017.
Anon Synchromed I,II 2017g Available: http://www.medtronic.com/us-en/healthcare-professionals/products/neurological/drug-infusion-systems/synchromed-ii.html Accessed 05 September 2017.
Atiyeh, B.S., Hayek, S.N., Skaf, G.S., Araj, A.A., Chamoun, R.B., 2006. Baclofen pump pocket infection: a case report of successful salvage with muscle flap. Int. Wound J. 3, 23–28.
Aubourg, P. 2017. Intracerebral Gene Therapy for Children With Early Onset Forms of Metachromatic Leukodystrophy (TG-MLD) Available: https://clinicaltrials.gov/ct2/show/NCT01801709?term=intracerebral+injection&draw=1&rank=10 Accessed 31 August 2017.
Austin, P.E., Dunn, K.A., Eily-Cofield, K., Brown, C.K., Wooden, W.A., Bradfield, J.F., 1995. Subcuticular sutures and the rate of inflammation in noncontaminated wounds. Ann. Emerg. Med. 25, 328–330.
Barua, N.U., Hopkins, K., Woolley, M., O'sullivan, S., Harrison, R., Edwards, R.J., Bienemann, A.S., Wyatt, M.J., Arshad, A., Gill, S.S., 2016. A novel implantable catheter system with transcutaneous port for intermittent convection-enhanced delivery of carboplatin for recurrent glioblastoma. Drug Deliv. 23, 167–173.
Bastiancich, C., Vanvarenberg, K., Ucakar, B., Pitorre, M., Bastiat, G., Lagarce, F., PrÉat, V., Danhier, F., 2016. Lauroyl-gemcitabine-loaded lipid nanocapsule hydrogel for the treatment of glioblastoma. J. Control. Release 225, 283–293.
Baumann, M.D., Kang, C.E., Tator, C.H., Shoichet, M.S., 2010. Intrathecal delivery of a polymeric nanocomposite hydrogel after spinal cord injury. Biomaterials 31, 7631–7639.
Benny, O., Menon, L.G., Ariel, G., Goren, E., Kim, S.-K., Stewman, C., Black, P.M., Carroll, R.S., Machluf, M., 2009. Local delivery of poly lactic-co-glycolic acid microspheres containing imatinib mesylate inhibits intracranial xenograft glioma growth. Clin. Cancer Res. 15, 1222–1231.
Bernal, G.M., Lariviere, M.J., Mansour, N., Pytel, P., Cahill, K.E., Voce, D.J., Kang, S., Spretz, R., Welp, U., Noriega, S.E., 2014. Convection-enhanced delivery and in vivo imaging of polymeric nanoparticles for the treatment of malignant glioma. Nanomedicine 10, 149–157.
Betancourt, T., Brannon-Peppas, L., 2006. Micro-and nanofabrication methods in nanotechnological medical and pharmaceutical devices. Int. J. Nanomedicine 1, 483.
Bidros, D.S., Liu, J.K., Vogelbaum, M.A., 2010. Future of convection-enhanced delivery in the treatment of brain tumors. Future Oncol. 6, 117–125.
Blakeley, J., 2008. Drug delivery to brain tumors. Curr. Neurol. Neurosci. Rep. 8, 235–241.
Blaney, S.M., Balis, F.M., Berg, S., Arndt, C.A., Heideman, R., Geyer, J.R., Packer, R., Adamson, P.C., Jaeckle, K., Klenke, R., 2005. Intrathecal mafosfamide: a preclinical pharmacology and phase I trial. J. Clin. Oncol. 23, 1555–1563.
Blasberg, R., Patlak, C., Fenstermacher, J., 1975. Intrathecal chemotherapy: brain tissue profiles after ventriculocisternal perfusion. J. Pharmacol. Exp. Ther. 195, 73–83.
Blasberg, R., Patlak, C., Shapiro, W., 1977. Distribution of methotrexate in the cerebrospinal fluid and brain after intraventricular administration. Cancer Treat. Rep. 61, 633.
Bleyer, W.A., 1978. The clinical pharmacology of methotrexate. New applications of an old drug. Cancer 41, 36–51.

Bleyer, W.A., Poplack, D.G., Simon, R.M., 1978. "Concentration x time" methotrexate via a subcutaneous reservoir: a less toxic regimen for intraventricular chemotherapy of central nervous system neoplasms. Blood 51, 835–842.

Bobo, R.H., Laske, D.W., Akbasak, A., Morrison, P.F., Dedrick, R.L., Oldfield, E.H., 1994. Convection-enhanced delivery of macromolecules in the brain. Proc. Natl. Acad. Sci. 91, 2076–2080.

Bock, N., Woodruff, M.A., Hutmacher, D.W., Dargaville, T.R., 2011. Electrospraying, a reproducible method for production of polymeric microspheres for biomedical applications. Polymer 3, 131–149.

Bonnan, M. 2017. Intrathecal Rituximab in Progressive Multiple Sclerosis (EFFRITE) Available: https:/clinicaltrials.gov/ct2/show/NCT02545959?term=NCT02545959&recrs=a&rank=1 Accessed August 31 2017.

Borrini, L., Bensmail, D., Thiebaut, J.-B., Hugeron, C., Rech, C., Jourdan, C., 2014. Occurrence of adverse events in long-term intrathecal baclofen infusion: a 1-year follow-up study of 158 adults. Arch. Phys. Med. Rehabil. 95, 1032–1038.

Boviatsis, E., Kouyialis, A., Boutsikakis, I., Korfias, S., Sakas, D., 2004. Infected CNS infusion pumps. Is there a chance for treatment without removal? Acta Neurochir. 146, 463–467.

Brasnjevic, I., Steinbusch, H.W., Schmitz, C., Martinez-Martinez, P., Initiative, E.N.R., 2009. Delivery of peptide and protein drugs over the blood–brain barrier. Prog. Neurobiol. 87, 212–251.

Brem, H., Mahaley Jr., M.S., Vick, N.A., Black, K.L., Schold Jr., S.C., Burger, P.C., Friedman, A.H., Ciric, I.S., Eller, T.W., Cozzens, J.W., 1991. Interstitial chemotherapy with drug polymer implants for the treatment of recurrent gliomas. J. Neurosurg 74, 441–446.

Brem, H., Piantadosi, S., Burger, P.C., Walker, M., Selker, R., Vick, N.A., Black, K., Sisti, M., Brem, S., Mohr, G., 1995. Placebo-controlled trial of safety and efficacy of intraoperative controlled delivery by biodegradable polymers of chemotherapy for recurrent gliomas. Lancet 345, 1008–1012.

Brodal, P., 2016. The Central Nervous System. Oxford University Press.

Bruce, J.N., Fine, R.L., Canoll, P., Yun, J., Kennedy, B.C., Rosenfeld, S.S., Sands, S.A., Surapaneni, K., Lai, R., Yanes, C.L., 2011. Regression of recurrent malignant gliomas with convection-enhanced delivery of topotecan. Neurosurgery 69, 1272–1280.

Buahin, K.G., Brem, H., 1995. Interstitial chemotherapy of experimental brain tumors: comparison of intratumoral injection versus polymeric controlled release. J. Neuro-Oncol. 26, 103–110.

Bures, N.P.P., Leobandung, W., Ichikawa, H., 2000. Hydrogels in pharmaceutical formulations. Eur. J. Pharm. Biopharm. 50, 27.

Casanova, F., Carney, P.R., Sarntinoranont, M., 2014. Effect of needle insertion speed on tissue injury, stress, and backflow distribution for convection-enhanced delivery in the rat brain. PLoS One. 9e94919.

Chandy, T., Das, G., Rao, G., 2000. 5-Fluorouracil-loaded chitosan coated polylactic acid microspheres as biodegradable drug carriers for cerebral tumours. J. Microencapsul. 17, 625–638.

Chen, M.Y., Lonser, R.R., Morrison, P.F., Governale, L.S., Oldfield, E.H., 1999. Variables affecting convection-enhanced delivery to the striatum: a systematic examination of rate of infusion, cannula size, infusate concentration, and tissue—cannula sealing time. J. Neurosurg. 90, 315–320.

Chen, P.-Y., Ozawa, T., Drummond, D.C., Kalra, A., Fitzgerald, J.B., Kirpotin, D.B., Wei, K.-C., Butowski, N., Prados, M.D., Berger, M.S., 2012. Comparing routes of delivery

for nanoliposomal irinotecan shows superior anti-tumor activity of local administration in treating intracranial glioblastoma xenografts. Neuro-Oncology 15, 189–197.
Chung, A.J., Kim, D., Erickson, D., 2008. Electrokinetic microfluidic devices for rapid, low power drug delivery in autonomous microsystems. Lab Chip 8, 330–338.
Conn, J., Oyasu, R., Welsh, M., Beal, J.M., 1974. Vicryl (polyglactin 910) synthetic absorbable sutures. Am. J. Surg. 128, 19–23.
Coombs, D.W., Saunders, R.L., Gaylor, M.S., Block, A.R., Colton, T., Harbaugh, R., Pageau, M.G., Mroz, W., 1983. Relief of continuous chronic pain by intraspinal narcotics infusion via an implanted reservoir. JAMA 250, 2336–2339.
Corem-Salkmon, E., Ram, Z., Daniels, D., Perlstein, B., Last, D., Salomon, S., Tamar, G., Shneor, R., Guez, D., Margel, S., 2011. Convection-enhanced delivery of methotrexate-loaded maghemite nanoparticles. Int. J. Nanomedicine 6, 1595.
Craig, P., Williams, J., Davis, K., Magoun, A., Levy, A., Bogdansky, S., Jones Jr., J., 1975. A biologic comparison of polyglactin 910 and polyglycolic acid synthetic absorbable sutures. Surg. Gynecol. Obstet. 141, 1–10.
Danhier, F., Ansorena, E., Silva, J.M., Coco, R., Le Breton, A., PrÉat, V., 2012. Plga-based nanoparticles: an overview of biomedical applications. J. Control. Release 161, 505–522.
Daniel, K., Duc, H.L.H., Cima, M., Langer, R., 2009. Controlled release microchips. Chronopharmaceutics: Science and Technology for Biological Rhythm Guided Therapy and Prevention of Diseases, John Wiley & Sons. 187.
Dario, P., Carrozza, M.C., Benvenuto, A., Menciassi, A., 2000. Micro-systems in biomedical applications. J. Micromech. Microeng. 10, 235.
Das, M., Mohanty, C., Sahoo, S.K., 2009. Ligand-based targeted therapy for cancer tissue. Expert Opin. Drug Deliv. 6, 285–304.
Debinski, W., Tatter, S.B., 2009. Convection-enhanced delivery for the treatment of brain tumors. Expert. Rev. Neurother. 9, 1519–1527.
Deeken, J.F., Löscher, W., 2007. The blood-brain barrier and cancer: transporters, treatment, and Trojan horses. Clin. Cancer Res. 13, 1663–1674.
Dimeco, F., Li, K.W., Tyler, B.M., Wolf, A.S., Brem, H., Olivi, A., 2002. Local delivery of mitoxantrone for the treatment of malignant brain tumors in rats. J. Neurosurg. 97, 1173–1178.
Domb, A.J., Khan, W., 2014. Focal Controlled Drug Delivery. Springer, US.
Doppalapudi, S., Mahira, S., Khan, W., 2017. Development and in vitro assessment of psoralen and resveratrol co-loaded ultradeformable liposomes for the treatment of vitiligo. J. Photochem. Photobiol. B Biol. 174, 44–57.
Du Pen, S.L., Kharasch, E.D., Williams, A., Peterson, D.G., Sloan, D.C., Hasche-Klunder, H., Krembs, A.W., 1992. Chronic epidural bupivacaine-opioid infusion in intractable cancer pain. Pain 49, 293–300.
Emerich, D.F., Winn, S.R., Bartus, R.T., 2002. Injection of chemotherapeutic microspheres and glioma IV: Eradicating tumors in rats. Cell Transplant. 11, 47–54.
Fan-Havard, P., Nahata, M., 1987. Treatment and prevention of infections of cerebrospinal fluid shunts. Clin. Pharm. 6, 866–880.
Farra, R., 2014. Multi-Dose Drug Delivery Device and Method. Google Patents.
Fenstermacher, J., Kaye, T., 1988. Drug "diffusion" within the brain. Ann. N. Y. Acad. Sci. 531, 29–39.
Fletcher, A.M., et al., 2011. Transgene expression in the striatum following intracerebral injections of DNA nanoparticles encoding for human glial cell line-derived neurotrophic factor. Neuroscience 194, 220–226.

Foley, C.P., Nishimura, N., Neeves, K.B., Schaffer, C.B., Olbricht, W.L., 2012. Real-time imaging of perivascular transport of nanoparticles during convection-enhanced delivery in the rat cortex. Ann. Biomed. Eng. 40, 292–303.

Follett, K.A., Boortz-Marx, R.L., Drake, J.M., Dupen, S., Schneider, S.J., Turner, M.S., Coffey, R.J., 2004. Prevention and management of intrathecal drug delivery and spinal cord stimulation system infections. The Journal of the American Society of Anesthesiologists 100, 1582–1594.

Fourniols, T., Randolph, L.D., Staub, A., Vanvarenberg, K., Leprince, J.G., PrÉat, V., Des Rieux, A., Danhier, F., 2015. Temozolomide-loaded photopolymerizable PEG-DMA-based hydrogel for the treatment of glioblastoma. J. Control. Release 210, 95–104.

Francisco, G. 2017. Safety Study of 3 mg/mL Baclofen Injection (Intrathecal) Using A Programmable Pump Available: https://clinicaltrials.gov/ct2/show/NCT01520545?term=NCT01520545&rank=1 Accessed 01 September 2017.

Freedman, J., 2009. Brain Cancer: Current and Emerging Trends in Detection and Treatment. Rosen.

Fung, L.K., Shin, M., Tyler, B., Brem, H., Saltzman, W.M., 1996. Chemotherapeutic drugs released from polymers: distribution of 1, 3-bis (2-chloroethyl)-l-nitrosourea in the rat brain. Pharm. Res. 13, 671–682.

Gabathuler, R., 2010. Approaches to transport therapeutic drugs across the blood–brain barrier to treat brain diseases. Neurobiol. Dis. 37, 48–57.

Gardner, P., 2006. Microfabricated nanochannel implantable drug delivery devices: trends, limitations and possibilities. Expert Opin. Drug Deliv. 3, 479–487.

Gatscher, S., Becker, R., Uhle, E., Bertalanffy, H., 2002. Combined intrathecal baclofen and morphine infusion for the treatment of spasticity related pain and central deafferentiation pain. In: Functional Rehabilitation in Neurosurgery and Neurotraumatology. Springer.

Georgieva, J.V., Hoekstra, D., Zuhorn, I.S., 2014. Smuggling drugs into the brain: an overview of ligands targeting transcytosis for drug delivery across the blood–brain barrier. Pharmaceutics 6, 557–583.

Ghaderi, R., Sturesson, C., Carlfors, J., 1996. Effect of preparative parameters on the characteristics of poly d, l-lactide-*co*-glycolide microspheres made by the double emulsion method. Int. J. Pharm. 141, 205–216.

Gilmartin, R., Bruce, D., Storrs, B.B., Abbott, R., Krach, L., Ward, J., Bloom, K., Brooks, W.H., Johnson, D.L., Madsen, J.R., 2000. Intrathecal baclofen for management of spastic cerebral palsy: multicenter trial. J. Child Neurol. 15, 71–77.

Glitza, I. C. 2017. Study of Concurrent Intravenous and Intrathecal Nivolumab for Patients With Leptomeningeal Disease (LMD) Available: https://clinicaltrials.gov/ct2/show/NCT03025256?term=ommaya+reservoir+intrathecal&rank=6 Accessed 31 August 2017.

Govender, T., Choonara, Y.E., Kumar, P., Bijukumar, D., Du Toit, L.C., Modi, G., Naidoo, D., Pillay, V., 2017. Implantable and transdermal polymeric drug delivery technologies for the treatment of central nervous system disorders. Pharm. Dev. Technol. 22, 476–486.

Grayson, A.C.R., Choi, I.S., Tyler, B.M., Wang, P.P., Brem, H., Cima, M.J., Langer, R., 2003. Multi-pulse drug delivery from a resorbable polymeric microchip device. Nat. Mater. 2, 767.

Greish, K., 2010. Enhanced permeability and retention (EPR) effect for anticancer nanomedicine drug targeting. Cancer Nanotechnology: Methods and Protocols 25–37.

Grossman, S.A., Reinhard, C., Colvin, O.M., Chasin, M., Brundrett, R., Tamargo, R.J., Brem, H., 1992. The intracerebral distribution of BCNU delivered by surgically implanted biodegradable polymers. J. Neurosurg. 76, 640–647.

Guerin, C., Olivi, A., Weingart, J.D., Lawson, H.C., Brem, H., 2004. Recent advances in brain tumor therapy: local intracerebral drug delivery by polymers. Investig. New Drugs 22, 27–37.

Harbaugh, R.E., Saunders, R.L., Reeder, R.F., 1988. Use of implantable pumps for central nervous system drug infusions to treat neurological disease. Neurosurgery 23, 693–698.

Healy, A.T., Vogelbaum, M.A., 2015. Convection-enhanced drug delivery for gliomas. Surg. Neurol. Int. 6, S59.

Heiss, J. D. 2017. AAV2-GDNF for Advanced Parkinson s Disease Available: https://clinicaltrials.gov/ct2/show/Nct01621581?term=NCT01621581&rank=1 Accessed 05 September 2017.

Hoffman, A.S., 1987. Applications of thermally reversible polymers and hydrogels in therapeutics and diagnostics. J. Control. Release 6, 297–305.

Horwitz, S., 1994. Taxol (paclitaxel): mechanisms of action. Ann. Oncol. 5, S3–6.

Howard III, M.A., Gross, A., Grady, M.S., Langer, R.S., Mathiowitz, E., Winn, H.R., Mayberg, M.R., 1989. Intracerebral drug delivery in rats with lesion-induced memory deficits. J. Neurosurg. 71, 105–112.

Hruby, V.J., Yamamoto, T., Giri, A.K., Herman, D.S., Largent-Milnes, T., Vanderah, T., Porreca, F., 2015. Design of multivalent ligands that cross the blood brain barrier for the treatment of neuropathic pain without toxicities.Proceedings of the 24th American Peptide Symposium, 2015. American Peptide Society Orlando, FLpp. 43–44.

Huang, I.-Z. 2017. Patient Registry of Intrathecal Ziconotide Management(PRIZM) Available: https://clinicaltrials.gov/ct2/show/NCT01888120?term=NCT01888120&rank=1 Accessed 30 August 2017.

Huber, J.D., Egleton, R.D., Davis, T.P., 2001. Molecular physiology and pathophysiology of tight junctions in the blood–brain barrier. Trends Neurosci. 24, 719–725.

Hussain, M., Beale, G., Hughes, M., Akhtar, S., 2002. Co-delivery of an antisense oligonucleotide and 5-fluorouracil using sustained release poly (lactide-*co*-glycolide) microsphere formulations for potential combination therapy in cancer. Int. J. Pharm. 234, 129–138.

Jain, K.K., 2008. Drug Delivery Systems. Humana Press.

Jain, K.K., 2012. Nanobiotechnology-based strategies for crossing the blood–brain barrier. Nanomedicine 7, 1225–1233.

Jain, A., Doppalapudi, S., Domb, A.J., Khan, W., 2016. Tacrolimus and curcumin co-loaded liposphere gel: synergistic combination towards management of psoriasis. J. Control. Release 243, 132–145.

Jain, A., Pooladanda, V., Bulbake, U., Doppalapudi, S., Rafeeqi, T.A., Godugu, C., Khan, W., 2017. Liposphere mediated topical delivery of thymoquinone in the treatment of psoriasis. Nanomed.: Nanotechnol. Biol. Med. 13 (7), 2251–2262.

Jiang, L., Zhou, Q., Mu, K., Xie, H., Zhu, Y., Zhu, W., Zhao, Y., Xu, H., Yang, X., 2013. pH/temperature sensitive magnetic nanogels conjugated with Cy5. 5-labled lactoferrin for MR and fluorescence imaging of glioma in rats. Biomaterials 34, 7418–7428.

Jiménez, J. M. M. 2017. Clinical Trial on The Use of Autologous Bone Marrow Stem Cells in Amyotrophic Lateral Sclerosis (Extension Cmn/Ela) Available: https://clinicaltrials.gov/ct2/show/NCT01254539?term=NCT01254539&rank=1 Accessed 31 August 2017.

Jo, D.H., Kim, J.H., Lee, T.G., Kim, J.H., 2015. Size, surface charge, and shape determine therapeutic effects of nanoparticles on brain and retinal diseases. Nanomedicine 11, 1603–1611.

Johansson, B.B., 1990. The physiology of the blood-brain barrier. In: Circulating Regulatory Factors and Neuroendocrine Function. Springer.

Kenny, G.D., Bienemann, A.S., Tagalakis, A.D., Pugh, J.A., Welser, K., Campbell, F., Tabor, A.B., Hailes, H.C., Gill, S.S., Lythgoe, M.F., 2013. Multifunctional receptor-targeted nanocomplexes for the delivery of therapeutic nucleic acids to the brain. Biomaterials 34, 9190–9200.

Kesari, S. 2017. Mitigating Cephalad Fluid Shifts: A NSBRI Study (NSBRI) Available: https://clinicaltrials.gov/ct2/show/NCT03097523?term=NCT03097523&rank=1 Accessed 01 September 2017.

Khatib, Z. 2017. Phase II Study of Intraventricular Methotrexate in Children With Recurrent or Progressive Malignant Brain Tumors Available: https://clinicaltrials.gov/ct2/show/NCT02684071?term=ommaya+reservoir+intraventricular&rank=3 Accessed 31 August 2017.

Kim, G.Y., Tyler, B.M., Tupper, M.M., Karp, J.M., Langer, R.S., Brem, H., Cima, M.J., 2007. Resorbable polymer microchips releasing BCNU inhibit tumor growth in the rat 9L flank model. J. Control. Release 123, 172–178.

Kofler, M., Kronenberg, M., Rifici, C., Saltuari, L., Bauer, G., 1994. Epileptic seizures associated with intrathecal baclofen application. Neurology 44, 25–27.

Kommineni, N., Saka, R., Khan, W., Domb, A.J., 2017. Non-polymer drug-eluting coronary stents. Drug Deliv. Transl. Res. 1–15.

Kopell, B.H., Sala, D., Doyle, W.K., Feldman, D.S., Wisoff, J.H., Weiner, H.L., 2001. Subfascial implantation of intrathecal baclofen pumps in children. Neurosurgery 49, 753–757.

Krauze, M.T., Noble, C.O., Kawaguchi, T., Drummond, D., Kirpotin, D.B., Yamashita, Y., Kullberg, E., Forsayeth, J., Park, J.W., Bankiewicz, K.S., 2007. Convection-enhanced delivery of nanoliposomal CPT-11 (irinotecan) and PEGylated liposomal doxorubicin (Doxil) in rodent intracranial brain tumor xenografts. Neuro-Oncology 9, 393–403.

Labrie, F., 2012. Hypothalamus and Endocrine Functions. Springer, US.

Langer, R., Folkman, J., 1976. Polymers for the sustained release of proteins and other macromolecules. Nature 263, 797–800.

Lee, J., Olszewski, J., 1960. Penetration of radioactive bovine albumin from cerebrospinal fluid into brain tissue. Neurology 10, 814–822.

Leong, K., Brott, B., Langer, R., 1985. Bioerodible polyanhydrides as drug-carrier matrices. I: Characterization, degradation, and release characteristics. J. Biomed. Mater. Res. A 19, 941–955.

Lesniak, M.S., Upadhyay, U., Goodwin, R., Tyler, B., Brem, H., 2005. Local delivery of doxorubicin for the treatment of malignant brain tumors in rats. Anticancer Res. 25, 3825–3831.

Levin, V.A., Hoffman, W., Weinkam, R.J., 1978. Pharmacokinetics of BCNU in man: a preliminary study of 20 patients. Cancer Treat. Rep. 62, 1305–1312.

Li, K.W., Dang, W., Tyler, B.M., Troiano, G., Tihan, T., Brem, H., Walter, K.A., 2003. Polilactofate microspheres for Paclitaxel delivery to central nervous system malignancies. Clin. Cancer Res. 9, 3441–3447.

Lidar, Z., Mardor, Y., Jonas, T., Pfeffer, R., Faibel, M., Nass, D., Hadani, M., Ram, Z., 2004. Convection-enhanced delivery of paclitaxel for the treatment of recurrent malignant glioma: a phase I/II clinical study. J. Neurosurg. 100, 472–479.

Lieberman, D.M., Laske, D.W., Morrison, P.F., Bankiewicz, K.S., Oldfield, E.H., 1995. Convection-enhanced distribution of large molecules in gray matter during interstitial drug infusion. J. Neurosurg. 82, 1021–1029.

Linden, P. V. D. 2017. Wound Infusion vs Spinal Morphine for Post-caesarean Analgesia (Apcisaal) Available: https://clinicaltrials.gov/ct2/show/NCT02264821?term=NCT02264821&rank=1 Accessed 01 September 2017.

Lioresal ®INTRATHECAL[PACKAGE INSERT].n.d. *Cangene bioPharma, Inc., Baltimore MD* Available: https://www.accessdata.fda.gov/drugsatfda_docs/label/2010/022462s000lbl.pdf Accessed 01 September 2017.

Longley, D.B., Harkin, D.P., Johnston, P.G., 2003. 5-fluorouracil: mechanisms of action and clinical strategies. Nat. Rev. Cancer 3, 330.

Lonser, R.R., Sarntinoranont, M., Morrison, P.F., Oldfield, E.H., 2015. Convection-enhanced delivery to the central nervous system. J. Neurosurg. 122, 697–706.

Loo, T.L., Dion, R.L., Dixon, R.L., Rall, D.P., 1966. The antitumor agent, 1, 3-bis (2-chloroethyl)-1-nitrosourea. J. Pharm. Sci. 55, 492–497.

Lopez, K.A., Tannenbaum, A.M., Assanah, M.C., Linskey, K., Yun, J., Kangarlu, A., Gil, O.D., Canoll, P., Bruce, J.N., 2011. Convection-enhanced delivery of topotecan into a PDGF-driven model of glioblastoma prolongs survival and ablates both tumor-initiating cells and recruited glial progenitors. Cancer Res. 71, 3963–3971.

Losic, D., Aw, M.S., Santos, A., Gulati, K., Bariana, M., 2015. Titania nanotube arrays for local drug delivery: recent advances and perspectives. Expert Opin. Drug Deliv. 12, 103–127.

Lueshen, E., Venugopal, I., Soni, T., Alaraj, A., Linninger, A., 2015. Implant-assisted intrathecal magnetic drug targeting to aid in therapeutic nanoparticle localization for potential treatment of central nervous system disorders. J. Biomed. Nanotechnol. 11, 253–261.

Maeda, H., Bharate, G., Daruwalla, J., 2009. Polymeric drugs for efficient tumor-targeted drug delivery based on EPR-effect. Eur. J. Pharm. Biopharm. 71, 409–419.

Malheiro, L., Gomes, A., Barbosa, P., Santos, L., Sarmento, A., 2015. Infectious complications of intrathecal drug administration systems for spasticity and chronic pain: 145 patients from a tertiary care center. Neuromodulation: Technology at the Neural Interface 18, 421–427.

Mastorakos, P., Song, E., Zhang, C., Berry, S., Park, H.W., Kim, Y.E., Park, J.S., Lee, S., Suk, J.S., Hanes, J., 2016. Biodegradable DNA nanoparticles that provide widespread gene delivery in the brain. Small 12, 678–685.

Matis, K., 2018. Prometra Post-Approval Study. Available from: https://clinicaltrials.gov/ct2/show/NCT01854229 (Accessed 24 May 2018).

Mehta, A.M., Sonabend, A.M., Bruce, J.N., 2017. Convection-enhanced delivery. Neurotherapeutics 14 (2), 358–371.

Menei, P., Boisdron-Celle, M., Croué, A., Guy, G., Benoit, J.-P., 1996. Effect of stereotactic implantation of biodegradable 5-fluorouracil-loaded microspheres in healthy and C6 glioma-bearing rats. Neurosurgery 39, 117–124.

Menei, P., Venier, M.C., Gamelin, E., Saint-André, J.P., Hayek, G., Jadaud, E., Fournier, D., Mercier, P., Guy, G., Benoit, J.P., 1999. Local and sustained delivery of 5-fluorouracil from biodegradable microspheres for the radiosensitization of glioblastoma. Cancer 86, 325–330.

Menei, P., Pean, J., Nerriere-Daguin, V., Jollivet, C., Brachet, P., Benoit, J., 2000. Intracerebral implantation of Ngf-releasing biodegradable microspheres protects striatum against excitotoxic damage. Exp. Neurol. 161, 259–272.

Milligan, E.D., Soderquist, R.G., Malone, S.M., Mahoney, J.H., Hughes, T.S., Langer, S.J., Sloane, E.M., Maier, S.F., Leinwand, L.A., Watkins, L.R., 2006. Intrathecal polymer-based interleukin-10* gene delivery for neuropathic pain. Neuron Glia Biol. 2, 293–308.

Morishita, M., Park, K., 2016. Biodrug Delivery Systems: Fundamentals, Applications and Clinical Development. CRC Press.

Morrison, P.F., Chen, M.Y., Chadwick, R.S., Lonser, R.R., Oldfield, E.H., 1999. Focal delivery during direct infusion to brain: role of flow rate, catheter diameter, and tissue mechanics. Am. J. Phys. Regul. Integr. Comp. Phys. 277, R1218–R1229.

Moysan, E., GonzÁlez-FernÁndez, Y., Lautram, N., Béjaud, J., Bastiat, G., Benoit, J.-P., 2014. An innovative hydrogel of gemcitabine-loaded lipid nanocapsules: when the drug is a key player of the nanomedicine structure. Soft Matter 10, 1767–1777.

Nair, L.S., Laurencin, C.T., 2007. Biodegradable polymers as biomaterials. Prog. Polym. Sci. 32, 762–798.

Naraharisetti, P.K., Ong, B.Y.S., Xie, J.W., Lee, T.K.Y., Wang, C.-H., Sahinidis, N.V., 2007. In vivo performance of implantable biodegradable preparations delivering Paclitaxel and Etanidazole for the treatment of glioma. Biomaterials 28, 886–894.

Nie, H., Dong, Z., Arifin, D.Y., Hu, Y., Wang, C.H., 2010. Core/shell microspheres via coaxial electrohydrodynamic atomization for sequential and parallel release of drugs. J. Biomed. Mater. Res. A 95, 709–716.

Nieuwenhuys, R., Voogd, J., Van Huijzen, C., 2013. The Human Central Nervous System: A Synopsis and Atlas. Springer, Berlin Heidelberg.

Oh, W. 2017. Safety and Exploratory Efficacy Study of Neurostem® Versus Placebo in Patients With Alzheimer's Disease Available: https://clinicaltrials.gov/ct2/show/NCT02054208?term=ommaya+reservoir+intraventricular&rank=1 Accessed 31 August 2017.

Oh, S., Odland, R., Wilson, S.R., Kroeger, K.M., Liu, C., Lowenstein, P.R., et al., 2007. Improved distribution of small molecules and viral vectors in the murine brain using a hollow fiber catheter. J. Neurosurg. 107 (3), 568–577.

Olson, J.J., Zhang, Z., Dillehay, D., Stubbs, J., 2008. Assessment of a balloon-tipped catheter modified for intracerebral convection-enhanced delivery. J. Neuro-Oncol. 89, 159–168.

Ozeki, T., Kaneko, D., Hashizawa, K., Imai, Y., Tagami, T., Okada, H., 2012. Improvement of survival in C6 rat glioma model by a sustained drug release from localized PLGA microspheres in a thermoreversible hydrogel. Int. J. Pharm. 427, 299–304.

Paice, J.A., Penn, R.D., Shott, S., 1996. Intraspinal morphine for chronic pain: a retrospective, multicenter study. J. Pain Symptom Manag. 11, 71–80.

Pålhagen, S. 2017. A Safety and Tolerability Study of Intracerebroventricular Administration of sNN0031 to Patients With Parkinson's Disease Available: https://clinicaltrials.gov/ct2/show/NCT00866502?term=NCT00866502&rank=1 Accessed 01 September 2017.

Patel, M.M., Patel, B.M., 2017. Crossing the blood-brain barrier: recent advances in drug delivery to the brain. CNS Drugs 31 (2), 109–133.

Penn, R.D., Paice, J.A., Gottschalk, W., Ivankovich, A.D., 1984. Cancer pain relief using chronic morphine infusion: early experience with a programmable implanted drug pump. J. Neurosurg. 61, 302–306.

Polla, D.L., Erdman, A.G., Robbins, W.P., Markus, D.T., Diaz-Diaz, J., Rizq, R., Nam, Y., Brickner, H.T., Wang, A., Krulevitch, P., 2000. Microdevices in medicine. Annu. Rev. Biomed. Eng. 2, 551–576.

Powell, E.M., Sobarzo, M.R., Saltzman, W.M., 1990. Controlled release of nerve growth factor from a polymeric implant. Brain Res. 515, 309–311.

Pradilla, G., Wang, P.P., Gabikian, P., Li, K., Magee, C.A., Walter, K.A., Brem, H., 2006. Local intracerebral administration of paclitaxel with the Paclimer® delivery system: toxicity study in a canine model. J. Neuro-Oncol. 76, 131–138.

Prager, J., Deer, T., Levy, R., Bruel, B., Buchser, E., Caraway, D., Cousins, M., Jacobs, M., Mcglothlen, G., Rauck, R., 2014. Best practices for intrathecal drug delivery for pain. Neuromodulation: Technology at the Neural Interface 17, 354–372.

Pye, A., Lockhart, D., Dawson, M., Murray, C., Smith, A., 2009. A review of dental implants and infection. J. Hosp. Infect. 72, 104–110.

Raghavan, R., Brady, M.L., Rodríguez-Ponce, M.I., Hartlep, A., Pedain, C., Sampson, J.H., 2006. Convection-enhanced delivery of therapeutics for brain disease, and its optimization. Neurosurg. Focus. 20, E12.

Rainov, N.G., Heidecke, V., Burkert, W., 2001. Long-term intrathecal infusion of drug combinations for chronic back and leg pain. J. Pain Symptom Manag. 22, 862–871.

Rall, D.P., 1968. Transport through the ependymal linings. Prog. Brain Res. 29, 159–172.

Ranganath, S.H., Kee, I., Krantz, W.B., Chow, P.K.-H., Wang, C.-H., 2009. Hydrogel matrix entrapping Plga-paclitaxel microspheres: drug delivery with near zero-order release and implantability advantages for malignant brain tumour chemotherapy. Pharm. Res. 26, 2101–2114.

Reis, C.P., Neufeld, R.J., Ribeiro, A.J., Veiga, F., 2006. Nanoencapsulation II. Biomedical applications and current status of peptide and protein nanoparticulate delivery systems. Nanomedicine 2, 53–65.

Rennels, M.L., Gregory, T.F., Blaumanis, O.R., Fujimoto, K., Grady, P.A., 1985. Evidence for a 'paravascular'fluid circulation in the mammalian central nervous system, provided by the rapid distribution of tracer protein throughout the brain from the subarachnoid space. Brain Res. 326, 47–63.

Rhines, L.D., Sampath, P., Dimeco, F., Lawson, H.C., Tyler, B.M., Hanes, J., Olivi, A., Brem, H., 2003. Local immunotherapy with interleukin-2 delivered from biodegradable polymer microspheres combined with interstitial chemotherapy: a novel treatment for experimental malignant glioma. Neurosurgery 52, 872–880.

Robberecht, W. 2017. A Safety and Tolerability Study of Intracerebroventricular Administration of sNN0029 to Patients With Amyotrophic Lateral Sclerosis Available: https://clinicaltrials.gov/ct2/show/NCT00800501?term=NCT00800501&rank=1 Accessed 01 September 2017.

Rosca, I.D., Watari, F., Uo, M., 2004. Microparticle formation and its mechanism in single and double emulsion solvent evaporation. J. Control. Release 99, 271–280.

Rosenberg, G., Kyner, W., Estrada, E., 1980. Bulk flow of brain interstitial fluid under normal and hyperosmolar conditions. American Journal of Physiology-Renal Physiology 238, F42–F49.

Rubenstein, J. L. 2017. A Safety Study of Rituximab Plus MTX Injected Into the Cerebrospinal Fluid in the Treatment of Brain Lymphoma Available: https://clinicaltrials.gov/ct2/show/NCT00221325?term=ommaya+reservoir+intraventricular&rank=5 Accessed 31 August 2017.

Saito, R., Bringas, J.R., McKnight, T.R., Wendland, M.F., Mamot, C., Drummond, D.C., Kirpotin, D.B., Park, J.W., Berger, M.S., Bankiewicz, K.S., 2004. Distribution of liposomes into brain and rat brain tumor models by convection-enhanced delivery monitored with magnetic resonance imaging. Cancer Res. 64, 2572–2579.

Sandberg, D. 2017a. Methotrexate and Etoposide Infusions Into the Fourth Ventricle in Children With Recurrent Posterior Fossa Brain Tumors Available: https://clinicaltrials.gov/ct2/show/NCT02905110?term=ommaya+reservoir+intraventricular&rank=2 Accessed 31 August 2017.

Sandberg, D. 2017b. Methotrexate Infusion Into the Fourth Ventricle in Children With Malignant Fourth Ventricular Brain Tumors: A Pilot Study Available: https://clinicaltrials.gov/ct2/show/NCT01737671?term=ommaya+reservoir+intraventricular&rank=4 Accessed 31 August 2017.

Sandberg, D. I. 2017d. Methotrexate Infusion Into Fourth Ventricle in Children With Recurrent Malignant Fourth Ventricular Brain Tumors Available: https://clinicaltrials.gov/ct2/show/NCT02458339?term=ommaya+reservoir+intraventricular&rank=7 Accessed 31 August 2017.

Sant, S., Tao, S.L., Fisher, O., Xu, Q., Peppas, N.A., Khademhosseini, A., 2012. Microfabrication technologies for oral drug delivery. Adv. Drug Deliv. Rev. 64, 496–507.

Santini Jr., J.T., Cima, M.J., Langer, R.S., 1998. Microchip Drug Delivery Devices. Google Patents.

Santini Jr., J.T., Cima, M.J., Langer, R.S., 2000. Fabrication of Microchip Drug Delivery Devices. Google Patents.

Santini Jr., J.T., Cima, M.J., Langer, R.S., 2011. Method for Operating Microchip Reservoir Device. Google Patents.

Santini, J.T., Cima, M.J., Langer, R., 1999. A controlled-release microchip. Nature 397, 335–338.

Santini, J.T., Richards, A.C., Scheidt, R.A., Cima, M.J., Langer, R.S., 2000. Microchip Technology in Drug Delivery. Taylor & Francis.

Saucier-Sawyer, J.K., Seo, Y.-E., Gaudin, A., Quijano, E., Song, E., Sawyer, A.J., Deng, Y., Huttner, A., Saltzman, W.M., 2016. Distribution of polymer nanoparticles by convection-enhanced delivery to brain tumors. J. Control. Release 232, 103–112.

Sawyer, A.J., Saucier-Sawyer, J.K., Booth, C.J., Liu, J., Patel, T., Piepmeier, J.M., Saltzman, W.M., 2011. Convection-enhanced delivery of camptothecin-loaded polymer nanoparticles for treatment of intracranial tumors. Drug Deliv. Transl. Res. 1, 34–42.

Scheld, W.M., 1989. Drug delivery to the central nervous system: general principles and relevance to therapy for infections of the central nervous system. Rev. Infect. Dis. 11, S1669–S1690.

Schliep, G., Felgenhauer, K., 1978. Serum-Csf protein gradients, the blood-CSF barrier and the local immune response. J. Neurol. 218, 77–96.

Schulz, M., 1999. The end of the road for silicon? Nature 399, 729–730.

Shawgo, R.S., Grayson, A.C.R., Li, Y., Cima, M.J., 2002. BioMEMS for drug delivery. Curr. Opin. Solid State Mater. Sci. 6, 329–334.

Siegfried, R.N., Jacobson, L., Chabal, C., 1992. Development of an acute withdrawal syndrome following the cessation of intrathecal baclofen in a patient with spasticity. Anesthesiology 77, 1048.

Sillay, K.A., McClatchy, S.G., Shepherd, B.A., Venable, G.T., Fuehrer, T.S., 2014. Image-guided convection-enhanced delivery into agarose gel models of the brain. J. Vis. Exp. JoVE.

Sindou, M., Mertens, P., 2000. Neurosurgery for spasticity. Stereotact. Funct. Neurosurg. 74, 217–221.

Singh, A., Sahoo, S.K., 2014. Magnetic nanoparticles: a novel platform for cancer theranostics. Drug Discov. Today 19, 474–481.

Sipos, E.P., Tyler, B., Piantadosi, S., Burger, P.C., Brem, H., 1997. Optimizing interstitial delivery of BCNU from controlled release polymers for the treatment of brain tumors. Cancer Chemother. Pharmacol. 39, 383–389.

Smith, D.E., Johanson, C.E., Keep, R.F., 2004. Peptide and peptide analog transport systems at the blood–CSF barrier. Adv. Drug Deliv. Rev. 56, 1765–1791.

Soderquist, R.G., Sloane, E.M., Loram, L.C., Harrison, J.A., Dengler, E.C., Johnson, S.M., Amer, L.D., Young, C.S., Lewis, M.T., Poole, S., 2010. Release of plasmid DNA-encoding IL-10 from Plga microparticles facilitates long-term reversal of neuropathic pain following a single intrathecal administration. Pharm. Res. 27, 841–854.

Sonabend, A.M., Stuart, R.M., Yun, J., Yanagihara, T., Mohajed, H., Dashnaw, S., Bruce, S.S., Brown, T., Romanov, A., Sebastian, M., 2011. Prolonged intracerebral convection-enhanced delivery of topotecan with a subcutaneously implantable infusion pump. Neuro-Oncology 13, 886–893.

Stallings, V.A., Charney, E.B., Davies, J.C., Cronk, C.E., 1993a. Nutrition-related growth failure of children with quadriplegic cerebral palsy. Dev. Med. Child Neurol. 35, 126–138.

Stallings, V.A., Charney, E.B., Davies, J.C., Cronk, C.E., 1993b. Nutritional status and growth of children with diplegic or hemiplegic cerebral palsy. Dev. Med. Child Neurol. 35, 997–1006.

Staples, M., 2010. Microchips and controlled-release drug reservoirs. Wiley Interdiscip. Rev. Nanomed. Nanobiotechnol. 2, 400–417.

Stempien, L., Tsai, T., 2000. Intrathecal baclofen pump use for spasticity: a clinical survey. Am. J. Phys. Med. Rehabil. 79, 536–541.

Stetkarova, I., Yablon, S.A., Kofler, M., Stokic, D.S., 2010. Procedure-and device-related complications of intrathecal baclofen administration for management of adult muscle hypertonia: a review. Neurorehabil. Neural Repair 24, 609–619.

Sun, L., Joh, D.Y., Al-Zaki, A., Stangl, M., Murty, S., Davis, J.J., Baumann, B.C., Alonso-Basanta, M., Kao, G.D., Tsourkas, A., 2016. Theranostic application of mixed gold and superparamagnetic iron oxide nanoparticle micelles in glioblastoma multiforme. J. Biomed. Nanotechnol. 12, 347–356.

Sutradhar, K.B., Sumi, C.D., 2016. Implantable microchip: the futuristic controlled drug delivery system. Drug Deliv. 23, 1–11.

Svenningsson, A., Bergman, J., Dring, A., VÅgberg, M., Birgander, R., Lindqvist, T., Gilthorpe, J., Bergenheim, T., 2015. Rapid depletion of B lymphocytes by ultra-low-dose rituximab delivered intrathecally. Neurology-Neuroimmunology Neuroinflammation. 2e79.

Tahara, K., Kato, Y., Yamamoto, H., Kreuter, J., Kawashima, Y., 2011. Intracellular drug delivery using polysorbate 80-modified poly (D, L-lactide-co-glycolide) nanospheres to glioblastoma cells. J. Microencapsul. 28, 29–36.

Tajes, M., Ramos-FernÁndez, E., Weng-Jiang, X., Bosch-MoratÓ, M., Guivernau, B., Eraso-Pichot, A., Salvador, B., Fernandez-Busquets, X., Roquer, J., Munoz, F.J., 2014. The blood-brain barrier: structure, function and therapeutic approaches to cross it. Mol. Membr. Biol. 31, 152–167.

Tamargo, R.J., Myseros, J.S., Epstein, J.I., Yang, M.B., Chasin, M., Brem, H., 1993. Interstitial chemotherapy of the 9L gliosarcoma: controlled release polymers for drug delivery in the brain. Cancer Res. 53, 329–333.

Tao, S.L., Desai, T.A., 2003. Microfabricated drug delivery systems: from particles to pores. Adv. Drug Deliv. Rev. 55, 315–328.

Teddy, P., Jamous, A., Gardner, B., Wang, D., Silver, J., 1992. Complications of intrathecal baclofen delivery. Br. J. Neurosurg. 6, 115–118.

Tiwari, G., Tiwari, R., Sriwastawa, B., Bhati, L., Pandey, S., Pandey, P., Bannerjee, S.K., 2012. Drug delivery systems: An updated review. Int. J. Pharm. Investig. 2, 2.

Trombelli, L., Tatakis, D., 2003. Periodontal diseases: current and future indications for local antimicrobial therapy. Oral Dis. 9, 11–15.

Tyler, B., Fowers, K.D., Li, K.W., Recinos, V.R., Caplan, J.M., Hdeib, A., Grossman, R., Basaldella, L., Bekelis, K., Pradilla, G., 2010. A thermal gel depot for local delivery of paclitaxel to treat experimental brain tumors in rats. J. Neurosurg. 113, 210–217.

Van Tomme, S.R., Storm, G., Hennink, W.E., 2008. In situ gelling hydrogels for pharmaceutical and biomedical applications. Int. J. Pharm. 355, 1–18.

Vellimana, A.K., Recinos, V.R., Hwang, L., Fowers, K.D., Li, K.W., Zhang, Y., Okonma, S., Eberhart, C.G., Brem, H., Tyler, B.M., 2013. Combination of paclitaxel thermal gel depot with temozolomide and radiotherapy significantly prolongs survival in an experimental rodent glioma model. J. Neuro-Oncol. 111, 229–236.

Walker, M.D., Green, S.B., Byar, D.P., Alexander Jr., E., Batzdorf, U., Brooks, W.H., Hunt, W.E., Maccarty, C.S., Mahaley Jr., M.S., Mealey Jr., J., 1980. Randomized comparisons of radiotherapy and nitrosoureas for the treatment of malignant glioma after surgery. N. Engl. J. Med. 303, 1323–1329.

Wang, L., Zhang, J., Yu, X., Wang, J., Cheng, L., Hu, S., Han, G., 2016. Intrathecal injection of tigecycline in treatment of multidrug-resistant Acinetobacter baumannii meningitis: a case report. Eur. J. Hosp. Pharm. https://doi.org/10.1136/ejhpharm-2016-000972.

Ward, M. 2017. The Effectiveness of Pain Management Using the Archimedes® Constant-Flow Infusion Pump System for Intrathecal Delivery Available: https://clinicaltrials.gov/ct2/show/NCT00196053?term=NCT00196053&rank=1 Accessed 29 August 2017.

Webb, C., 2004. Implanted semiconductors will allow drugs to be delivered exactly when and where they are needed. IEEE Spectr. 37–41.

Weng, K.C., Hashizume, R., Noble, C.O., Serwer, L.P., Drummond, D.C., Kirpotin, D.B., Kuwabara, A.M., Chao, L.X., Chen, F.F., James, C.D., 2013. Convection-enhanced delivery of targeted quantum dot–immunoliposome hybrid nanoparticles to intracranial brain tumor models. Nanomedicine 8, 1913–1925.

Wermeling, D.P., 2005. Ziconotide, an Intrathecally Administered N-Type Calcium Channel Antagonist for the Treatment of Chronic Pain. Pharmacotherapy: The Journal of Human Pharmacology and Drug Therapy 25, 1084–1094.

Wilkins, L.W., King, J., 2002. Anatomy and Physiology. Lippincott Williams & Wilkins.

Wong, V.G., 1992. Biodegradable Ocular Implants. Google Patents.

Wong, V.G., Kochinke, F., 1995. Biocompatible Ocular Implants. Google Patents.

Wong, H.L., Wu, X.Y., Bendayan, R., 2012. Nanotechnological advances for the delivery of Cns therapeutics. Adv. Drug Deliv. Rev. 64, 686–700.

Wood, J.H., 1980. Physiology, pharmacology, and dynamics of cerebrospinal fluid. In: Wood, J.H. (Ed.), Neurobiology of Cerebrospinal Fluid 1. Boston, Ma, Springer.

Woranuch, S., Yoksan, R., 2013. Eugenol-loaded chitosan nanoparticles: I. Thermal stability improvement of eugenol through encapsulation. Carbohydr. Polym. 96, 578–585.

World Health Organization, 2006. Neurological Disorders: Public Health Challenges. World Health Organization.

Wunderlich, C.A., Krach, L.E., 2006. Gram-negative meningitis and infections in individuals treated with intrathecal baclofen for spasticity: a retrospective study. Dev. Med. Child Neurol. 48, 450–455.

Xi, G., Robinson, E., Mania-Farnell, B., Vanin, E.F., Shim, K.-W., Takao, T., Allender, E.V., Mayanil, C.S., Soares, M.B., Ho, D., 2014. Convection-enhanced delivery of nanodiamond drug delivery platforms for intracranial tumor treatment. Nanomedicine 10, 381–391.

Yun, J., Rothrock, R.J., Canoll, P., Bruce, J.N., 2013. Convection-enhanced delivery for targeted delivery of antiglioma agents: the translational experience. J. Drug Deliv. 2013.

Yurek, D., Hasselrot, U., Cass, W., Sesenoglu-Laird, O., Padegimas, L., Cooper, M., 2015. Age and lesion-induced increases of Gdnf transgene expression in brain following intracerebral injections of DNA nanoparticles. Neuroscience 284, 500–512.

Zhang, H., Gao, S., 2007. Temozolomide/PLGA microparticles and antitumor activity against glioma C6 cancer cells in vitro. Int. J. Pharm. 329, 122–128.

Zhang, K., Yang, P.-P., Zhang, J.-P., Wang, L., Wang, H., 2017. Recent advances of transformable nanoparticles for theranostics. Chin. Chem. Lett. 28 (9), 1808–1816.

Zhou, J., Patel, T.R., Sirianni, R.W., Strohbehn, G., Zheng, M.-Q., Duong, N., Schafbauer, T., Huttner, A.J., Huang, Y., Carson, R.E., 2013. Highly penetrative, drug-loaded nanocarriers improve treatment of glioblastoma. Proc. Natl. Acad. Sci. 110, 11751–11756.

Zhou, Z., Singh, R., Souweidane, M.M., 2017. Convection-enhanced delivery for diffuse intrinsic pontine glioma treatment. Curr. Neuropharmacol. 15, 116–128.

Zigmond, M.J., Coyle, J.T., Rowland, L.P., 2014. Neurobiology of Brain Disorders: Biological Basis of Neurological and Psychiatric Disorders. Elsevier Science.

Further reading

Blaney, S. 2017. Intrathecal Gemcitabine to treat Neoplastic Meningitis, IT Gemcitabine Available: https://clinicaltrials.gov/ct2/show/NCT00074607?term=ommaya+reservoir+intrathecal&rank=5 Accessed 31 August 2017.

Bogdahn, U. 2017. Phase IIb Clinical Trial With TGF-β2 Antisense Compound AP 12009 for Recurrent or Refractory High-Grade Glioma Available: https://clinicaltrials.gov/ct2/show/NCT00431561?term=NCT00431561&rank=1 Accessed 01 September 2017.

Elder, J. 2017. *Carboplatin in Treating Patients With Recurrent High-Grade Gliomas* Available: https://clinicaltrials.gov/ct2/show/NCT01644955?term=NCT01644955&rank=1 Accessed 01 September 2017.

Khatua, S. 2017. Fourth Ventricle Infusions of Autologous ex vivo Expanded NK Cells in Children With Recurrent Posterior Fossa Tumors Available: https://clinicaltrials.gov/ct2/show/NCT02271711?term=NCT02271711&rank=1 Accessed 01 September 2017.

Maestro, R. D. 2017. Efficacy and Safety of AP 12009 in Patients With Recurrent or Refractory Anaplastic Astrocytoma or Secondary Glioblastoma (SAPPHIRE) Available: https://clinicaltrials.gov/ct2/show/NCT00761280?term=NCT00761280&rank=1 Accessed 01 September 2017.

Michael Saulino, M. S. T. 2017. Measuring Signatures in the Fluid Surrounding the Spinal Cord in Patients Who Have Problems With Intrathecal Drug Delivery Available: https://clinicaltrials.gov/ct2/show/NCT01117090?term=implantable+drug+delivery+systems+for+brain&draw=1&rank=1 Accessed 31 August 2017.

Patchell, R. A. 2017. Radiation Therapy Followed by Bleomycin in Treating Adult Patients With Newly Diagnosed Supratentorial Glioblastoma Multiforme Available: https://clinicaltrials.gov/ct2/show/NCT00006916?term=NCT00006916&rank=1 Accessed 01 September 2017.

Sandberg, D. I. 2017c. Infusion of 5-Azacytidine (5-AZA) Into the Fourth Ventricle in Children With Recurrent Posterior Fossa Ependymoma (5-AZA) Available: https://clinicaltrials.gov/ct2/show/NCT02940483?term=NCT02940483&rank=1 Accessed 01 September 2017.

Vles, J. S. 2017. Dutch National ITB Study in Children With Cerebral Palsy Available: https://clinicaltrials.gov/ct2/show/NCT00367068?term=NCT00367068&rank=1 Accessed 01 September 2017.

Yurek, D., Hasselrot, U., Sesenoglu-Laird, O., Padegimas, L., Cooper, M., 2017. Intracerebral injections of DNA nanoparticles encoding for a therapeutic gene provide partial neuroprotection in an animal model of neurodegeneration. Nanomedicine 13, 2209–2217.

Part III

Nanoparticles-based brain targeting delivery for CNS disorder management

Glioma targeted delivery systems 12

*Shanshan Wang**,†, Chengyi Li*, Min Qian*, Rongqin Huang**
*Department of Pharmaceutics, School of Pharmacy, Key Laboratory of Smart Drug Delivery, Ministry of Education, Fudan University, Shanghai, China,
†Department of Pharmacy, Zhongshan Hospital, Fudan University, Shanghai, China

Glioma, which arises from glial cells, is by far the most frequent and lethal brain tumor, accounting for ~80% of malignant tumors in central nervous systems (CNS) (Agnihotri et al., 2013; Alifieris and Trafalis, 2015). According to the growing speed and the infiltration extent to nearby brain tissues, glioma can be categorized to low-grade [World Health Organization (WHO) grade I and II) as well as high-grade (WHO grade III and IV] (Paw et al., 2015). Even in combination with current most effective therapies including surgery, radiotherapy, and chemotherapy, median survival for high-grade glioma still remains gloomy (14.6 months) (Li et al., 2014; Stupp et al., 2005). This might be attributed to specific properties of glioma, such as the highly infiltrative nature and lack of clear margins. The physical and chemical constraints of several barriers, such as blood-brain barrier (BBB) and blood-brain tumor barrier (BBTB), are also tough obstacles to the multimodality therapies for glioma (Cornago et al., 2014; de Boer and Gaillard, 2007; Parrish et al., 2015; Van Tellingen et al., 2015). In addition, glioma stem cells (GSC), with a capacity for self-renewal, multipotency, and induction of tumorigenesis, have been considered as the main factor for glioma relapse and an important target for glioma therapy (Binello and Germano, 2011).

As a particular barrier with the body, BBB is made up of brain capillary endothelial cells (BCECs) which are joined together by tight junctions. It plays an important role as a selective barrier and a critical regulator of brain homeostasis, separating the brain from circulating toxins and potentially harmful chemicals and allowing access of a small subset of molecules with the appropriate size (400–600 Da), charge, and lipid solubility (Abbott et al., 2006; Aryal et al., 2015; Manich et al., 2013; Van Tellingen et al., 2015). Besides, drug delivery to the brain is also restricted by a range of active efflux transporters present on the BBB and other contributing structures (Van Tellingen et al., 2015). Hence, more than 98% small molecular drugs and almost all large molecules are hindered from the brain tissues (Pardridge, 2015). It has been reported that the BBB dysfunction is related to the increasing histological grade of glioma, which implies that the BBB is grossly intact at the early stage and gradually disrupted with the progress of glioma (Azad et al., 2015). Based on this occasion, the glioma targeted drug delivery systems are mainly divided into two categories. When the BBB is intact, the systems which must deliver drugs across the BBB for tumortargeting are defined as cascade targeting systems. Other drug delivery systems utilized in high-grade glioma are designated as glioma targeted systems, which mainly

Brain Targeted Drug Delivery Systems. https://doi.org/10.1016/B978-0-12-814001-7.00012-3

accumulate in the glioma by enhanced permeation retention (EPR) effect and then enter glioma cells via overcoming different barriers.

In recent years, plenty of strategies have been developed for glioma targeted, which are mainly divided as passive and active targeting. Many nanocarriers (such as liposomes, nanoparticles (NPs), polymeric micelles, dendrimers, and polymersomes) are used for glioma targeted delivery. In this chapter, both passive and active targeting delivery systems to glioma will be introduced.

1 Passive targeting delivery systems

Passive targeting is achieved based on the theory of EPR effect. Cancerous tissues undergo rapid angiogenesis, thus yield poorly organized and nonuniform vasculature and produce irregular blood flow. The leaky vasculature, coupled with poor lymphatic drainage, allows large macromolecules or nanoparticles to extravasate from the tumor vasculature and remain within the tumor mass (Perry et al., 2017). This phenomenon, well-known as EPR effect, has been witnessed more than 30 years (Matsumura and Maeda, 1986). And this has been applied as a passive targeting pattern while designing drug delivery systems. There exist several important influential factors affecting the accumulation efficiency from the nanotechnology aspect, including nanoparticle size, charge, and shape (Bertrand et al., 2014). Some other aspects, such as tumor model, location, and biology, would also have impact on the EPR effect.

Till now, many researches have been carried out for glioma therapy via a passive targeting strategy based on the EPR effect. Huynh and colleagues incorporated long chains of PEG (DSPE-mPEG2000) on the surface of lipid nanocapsules (LNCs) by postinsertion technique (Huynh et al., 2011). The results showed that in a subcutaneous gliosarcoma model, a single intravenous injection of FcdiOH-LNCs (400 μL, 2.4 mg/rat) considerably inhibited tumor growth when compared to the control. DSPE-mPEG2000-FcdiOH-LNCs exhibited a strong antitumor effect by nearly eradicating the tumor by the end of the study. This study indicated that coating DSPE-mPEG2000 to the surface of LNCs confers long-circulating properties, leading to the passive accumulation of PEGylated LNCs at the tumor site (Huynh et al., 2011). Lainé et al. (2014) further used the stealth ansa-FcdiOH LNCs to treat ectopic glioma-bearing rats via repeated intravenous injections. The results also showed that this kind of stealth LNCs induced a significant tumor growth inhibition, supported by a reduced number of proliferative cells in tumors compared to control group. Additionally, no liver damage was observed in treated animals, indicating the adequate passive targeting accumulation based on the EPR effect (Lainé et al., 2014). Besides researches in animal models, drug delivery systems have also been demonstrated in preclinical and clinical studies. Matsumura (2011) reported NK012, an SN-38-loaded polymeric micelle constructed in an aqueous milieu by the self-assembly of an amphiphilic block copolymer, PEG-PGlu (SN-38, biologically active metabolite of CPT-11). The antitumor activity was evaluated in several orthotopic tumor models including glioma, renal cancer, stomach cancer, and pancreatic cancer. Two independent phase I clinical trials were conducted in Japan and the United States.

According to data of preclinical studies, NK012 showing enhanced distribution with prolonged SN-38 release may be ideal for cancer treatment because the antitumor activity of SN-38 is time-dependent. Clinical studies showed that NK012 was well-tolerated and had antitumor activity including partial responses and several occurrences of prolonged stable disease across a variety of advanced refractory cancers. The data from several preclinical studies shows that the formulation appears to accumulate selectively and remains for a long time in solid tumor tissues by utilizing the EPR effect (Matsumura, 2011). However, some other researchers argue that, although the EPR effect has been observed and studied in many rodent models using subcutaneous and orthotopic xenografts, as well as genetically engineered mouse models, its prevalence in human primary and metastatic tumors requires further investigations (Lammers et al., 2012; Taurin et al., 2012). Animal models, especially xenograft models, used to study NPs at the preclinical stage seem to offer limited predictive value of the clinical outcome in humans (Zamboni et al., 2012). Furthermore, in most real cases, patients might receive surgery as the first step, thus most tumor tissues are extracted. That means patients can't wait for the cancer therapy based on the EPR effect. Thus, in real biomedical application, more efficient targeting strategy should be developed.

2 Active targeting delivery systems

In contrast to passive targeting delivery systems, active targeting delivery systems are considered to be rather effective for glioma targeted delivery. Active targeting increases the affinity of the delivery systems for tumor cells and their tumor residence time and allows the delivery systems to efficiently enter the cells through specific process (Bertrand et al., 2014). That means, for effective drug delivery, the vehicles should not only be able to accumulate within the tumor regions via the EPR effect, but also to target specific cell populations and get internalized. For glioma targeted delivery, the vehicles might overcome the BBB and/or target to glioma via receptor-, transporter-, or adsorptive-mediated drug delivery according to different transport mechanisms (Beduneau et al., 2007; Gabathuler, 2010).

2.1 *Receptor-mediated glioma targeted drug delivery*

As one of the major approaches, receptor-mediated drug delivery has been extensively studied over the past decade. This kind of drug delivery systems are comprised of nanocarriers (such as liposomes, NPs, polymeric micelles, dendrimers, and polymersomes) and various ligands targeting to different receptors including transferrin receptor (TfR), lactoferrin receptor (LfR), low-density lipoprotein receptor (LDLR), and folate receptor (FR) (Chen et al., 2014a, b; Cui et al., 2013; Hayavi and Halbert, 2005; Su et al., 2014). In this part, recent progresses on receptor-mediated drug delivery systems targeting to glioma are summarized according to the amount and type of the targeting moieties.

2.1.1 With BBB overcoming

Some receptor-mediated glioma targeted delivery systems are designed to overcome the BBB as the first step and then target to glioma, realizing the cascade targeting function. These systems could be characterized as single or dual ligand-modified ones. The single ligand-modified drug delivery systems are conjugated with just one ligand that could target to both BBB and glioma. For dual ligands-modified targeting systems, the two ligands are binding to specific receptors on the BBB and glioma, respectively.

2.1.1.1 Single ligand-modified targeting systems

Some receptors have been reported to be highly expressed on both BBB and glioma, which provide the cascade targeting sites for receptor-mediated drug delivery systems. The single targeting ligand that could mediate both transportation of drugs across the BBB and their internalization into glioma cells is referred figuratively as "multistage rocket," which represents the simplest approach for secondary targeting delivery. Some representative examples of the single ligand-modified targeting systems are summarized in Table 1.

TfR-mediated targeting systems As an essential element of human body, cellular iron plays a crucial role in cell proliferation (Ganz and Nemeth, 2015; Liu et al., 2015). The best characterized mechanism for iron uptake is mediated by the cell surface TfR, which is classified as TfR1 and TfR2 (Daniels et al., 2012; Dixit et al., 2015; Neves et al., 2011; Sakurai et al., 2014). Both TfR1 and TfR2 are overexpressed in some proliferating cells such as BCECs and many malignant tumor cells (Liu et al., 2013; Zhang et al., 2012). In addition, TfR is also highly expressed in some normal tissues such as liver, which limits other specific targeting efficiency in vivo to some extent (Daniels et al., 2012). Lots of studies have reported that TfR could be used for mediating drug delivery systems to the glioma. These systems are designed to utilize various targeting moieties such as transferrin (Tf), antibodies, or specific peptides to lead carriers directly to the diseased sites.

Since TfR was found as a highlighted target for mediating drugs across the BBB, many targeting moieties aiming at TfR have been discovered. As an innate ligand, Tf is a naturally existing protein possessing high affinity for TfR (Zhang et al., 2012). Liu et al. (2013) constructed Tf-conjugated doxorubicin (DOX)-encapsulated PEGylated nanoscaled graphene oxide (GO) (Tf-PEG-GO-DOX) as a BBB targeting antiglioma drug delivery system. Quantitative determination revealed that a faster transport rate and a 4.63 intensification of cell inhibition to C6 glioma cell were achieved with the conjugation of Tf. Consistent with these results, Tf-PEG-GO-DOX also exhibited stronger inhibitory effect on tumor growth. In addition, Cui et al. (2013) studied the Tf-conjugated magnetic silica poly(D,L-lactic-*co*-glycolic acid) (PLGA) NPs loading DOX and paclitaxel (PTX) (DOX-PTX-NPs-Tf) to bypass the BBB and subsequently target to the glioma. It is showed that U87 glioma cells treated by the Tf-conjugated NPs have higher intracellular accumulation of drugs than unconjugated counterparts. Besides, the in vivo antiglioma studies demonstrated that DOX-PTX-NPs-Tf

Table 1 Representative single ligand-modified cascade targeting systems (Wang et al., 2015a, b)

Target targeting site	BCECs	Glioma	Targeting moiety	Nanocarrier	References
TfR	√	√	Tf	PEGylated nanoscaled GO	Liu et al. (2013)
				Magnetic silica PLGA NPs	Cui et al. (2013)
			OX26	Immunomicelles	Yue et al. (2012)
			T7	Dendrigraft poly-L-lysine	Liu et al. (2012)
				Dendrigraft poly-L-lysine	Kuang et al. (2013)
			TfR-lytic hybrid peptide	TfR-lytic hybrid peptide	Kawamoto et al. (2011) and Kawamoto et al. (2013)
LR	√	√	Lf	Superparamagnetic iron oxide NPs	Xie et al. (2011)
LDLR	√	√	nLDL	nLDL	Nikanjam et al. (2007)
			Peptide-22	PEG-PLA NPs	Zhang et al. (2013)
LRP	√	√	Angiopep-2	Gold NPs	Ruan et al. (2015)
				PEG-PCL NPs	Xin et al. (2012)
			MTf	–	Gabathulera et al. (2005)
FR	√	√	Folate	MnO NPs	Leamon and Low (2001)
				PEGylated PEI	Chen et al. (2014a, b)
Insulin receptor	√	√	83–14 murine monoclonal antibody	PEGylated immunoliposomes	Fan et al. (2016)

treatments resulted in a substantial reduction in tumor size compared to Tf-unconjugated NPs. More recently, the use of Tf in preparation of cascade targeting antiglioma drug delivery systems has risen sharply, which is related to the high affinity for TfR and the effective treatments in the past studies (Dixit et al., 2015; Jeong et al., 2015; Liu et al., 2013). Such conjugates with Tf have demonstrated enhanced cellular uptake via Tf-mediated mechanisms and increased selective cytotoxicity in glioma cells and tumor xenograft animal models.

However, it has been reported that high concentration of endogenous Tf (2250 nM) may produce competitive inhibition to the Tf-modified drug delivery systems (Chen et al., 2014a, b). Therefore, some alternatives with similar affinity for TfR were developed. Many studies have demonstrated the capacity of anti-TfR antibodies to inhibit cell growth, especially for some malignant cells (Inoue et al., 2012). For example, OX26, a mouse monoclonal antibody against rat TfR1, has been developed as a targeting moiety for delivering drugs into the brain. The first use of OX26 for the delivery of therapeutic agents across the BBB was reported in the early 1990s (Yoshikawa and Pardridge, 1992). Recently, Yue et al. (2012) have prepared OX26 covalently linked immunomicelles and demonstrated a twofold increase in intracellular drug concentration with the conjugation of OX26, indicating that the OX26 modification can increase the brain uptake of micelles through TfR-mediated endocytosis. Some other anti-TfR antibodies including Ri7, 8D3, and 7579 also have great potential for cascade targeting delivery. Although these antibodies have not been verified in this field, many related achievements opened the door for Ri7, 8D3, or 7579-mediated drug delivery systems. For example, the brain distribution of Ri7 and 8D3 was characterized by Paris-Robidas et al. (2011). They proved that fluorolabeled anti-TfR antibodies could readily be accumulated into BCECs and the antibodies were able to attach to the TfR via measuring fluorescence in brain homogenates (Paris-Robidas et al., 2011). Despite the potentials of TfR targeting antibodies for drug delivery, the fact that preparation of these antibodies is difficult within rigorous laboratory conditions makes it hard to control their quality and limit their developments in real applications.

Recently, some peptides have been greatly impressed by considerable researchers due to their facile synthesis methods and high affinity for TfR. A 7 peptide (HAIYPRH, T7) has been reported to specifically bind to TfR (Du et al., 2013, 2015; Han et al., 2011). Its high affinity for TfR is comparable to that of Tf, with the Kd of $\sim$10 nM (Han et al., 2011). Furthermore, T7 binding site on TfR was reported to be different from that of Tf, which might avoid interference of endogenous Tf. Interestingly, the cellular uptake of T7-conjugated drug delivery systems was found to be accelerated when endogenous Tf bound with TfR (Han et al., 2011). Based on these researches, Jiang's group prepared a T7-modified co-delivery system loading DOX and antiglioma gene medicine pORF-hTRAIL (DGDPT/pORF-hTRAIL) (Liu et al., 2012). Results showed that T7-modified co-delivery system enhanced the cellular uptake of DOX and pORF-hTRAIL, increased their brain accumulation, and prolonged the survival time of tumor-bearing mice, compared to the system without T7 modification. Further studies demonstrated better RNA interference effect of T7-functionalized siRNA-encapsulated NPs compared to the unmodified counterparts

(Kuang et al., 2013). Consensus were reached by others, suggesting that the T7-modified nano-enabled drug delivery systems could cross the BBB, reach the glioma, and be internalized by glioma cells (Wang et al., 2015a, b; Zong et al., 2014a, b). Besides T7, another targeting peptide used to bind with TfR is TfR-lytic hybrid peptide, a combination of the TfR-binding peptide and a lytic peptide. An intriguing study designed by Kawamoto et al. (2011, 2013) has drawn researchers' attention recently. The results showed that the peptide itself was a drug delivery system which could cross the BBB and target to the glioma via the TfR-binding peptide and further lead to cancer cell death via lysis by the lytic peptide. Cytotoxic and binding activity of the TfR-lytic hybrid peptide were verified in murine glioma GL261 cells and human glioma U251 cells, and significant inhibited effect of tumor growth was observed in in vivo antitumor studies. As mentioned above, both the T7 and the hybrid peptide can be exploited as appropriate candidates for clinical application owing to their advantage of small steric hindrance, stability, and good mediators for crossing the BBB.

LfR-mediated targeting systems As a member of the Tf family, lactoferrin (Lf) is a single-chain cationic iron-binding glycoprotein (Yu et al., 2014a, b). The high concentration of endogenous Lf in human milk and its capacity to bind to the iron in breast milk suggested that Lf has a physiological function in the newborn infant (Almond et al., 2013; Raei et al., 2015). Multiple biological activities of Lf are mediated by LfR (Pandey et al., 2015). According to some investigations on binding kinetics of Lf to target cells, different tissues or cell types seem to express their own LfR, and their characteristics vary among different cell types. Several proofs including the results of immunohistochemistry and reverse transcriptase-polymerase chain reaction (RT-PCR) have demonstrated the presence of specific LfR in the brain (Suzuki and Lonnerdal, 2004; Talukder et al., 2003). Moreover, LfR has been proved not only existing on the BBB in different species, but also on the cell surface of glioma, which makes it a potential cascade targeting ligand (Fang et al., 2014; Huang et al., 2007). Compared to Tf, Lf possesses two main advantages as a braintargeting ligand. First, the plasma concentration of Lf is much lower ($\sim$5 nM), avoiding the interference of endogenous Lf (Huang et al., 2008). Second, the transport of Lf across the BBB is unilateral, decreasing the reverse transport of Lf-modified drug delivery systems from the brain to the blood circulation (Fillebeen et al., 1999). A number of studies have demonstrated LfR-mediated enhancement in therapeutic effects against glioma. Su et al. (2014) have successfully developed Lf-modified NPs as a targeting carrier for facilitating the uptake of DOX in brain tissue and treating glioma. In addition, Fang et al. have developed an Lf-modified targeting magnetic polydiacetylene nanocarriers (PDNCs) delivery system. It has been proved that this system can effectively decrease the progression of brain tumors in vivo (Fang et al., 2016).

Apart from their therapeutic benefits, these receptor-mediated systems can also play a crucial role in diagnosis of glioma. The group of Yang explored Lf-conjugated superparamagnetic iron oxide NPs (Lf-SPIONs) as a MRI contrast agent for glioma detection in vivo (Xie et al., 2011). The MR images of rats' brains after injection with Lf-SPIONs displayed more significant contrast enhancement in the tumor area compared to SPIONs, indicating that Lf-SPIONs selectively accumulated in the tumor tissues with the help of Lf and could be used for the preoperative MRI diagnosis of the glioma.

To sum up, Lf can be exploited as a targeting ligand conjugated to some nano-enabled carriers to yield an efficient gliomatargeting vector.

LDLR-mediated targeting systems Low-density lipoprotein receptor (LDLR), which is able to prompt the internalization of lipoprotein, has been reported to be highly expressed on the BBB and glioma cells (Bertato et al., 2012; Zhang et al., 2013). Moreover, some studies on the distribution of LDLR suggested that normal brain tissues, particularly neurons, have relatively low LDLR numbers (Huang et al., 2015). All results indicated that the LDLR is a potential molecular target for the selective delivery of antitumor agents to glioma (Jain, 2013). Interestingly, as a natural ligand of the LDLR, LDL once was an ideal carrier for loading and delivering cancer therapeutic and diagnostic agents to targeting sites due to its structure characteristics and chemical properties. First, the size of LDL particles is precisely controlled by its apolipoprotein B-100 (ApoB-100) component through a complex network of amphipathic a-helix protein-lipid interactions (Kader and Pater, 2002). Second, the native LDL is made up of 4563 amino acid residues, which serves as the binding domain for the LDLR and also keeps them soluble in aqueous environment (Chakraborty et al., 2014). Most of all, LDL has a highly hydrophobic core that is surrounded by a hydrophilic shell which can make LDL possess multimodal loading capability for embedding drugs with different affinities into the shell or the core (Chu et al., 2001). However, many studies argued that native LDL is not suitable to act as an appropriate targeting agent because it is difficult to be isolated in large scale and is variable in composition and size. Moreover, large batches of reconstituted LDL cannot be accomplished due to the hard purification of ApoB. Thus, increasing synthetic LDL analogues are developed as replacements of native LDL. Hayavi et al. created a synthetic LDL particle using a lipid emulsion and a peptide composed of LDLR binding domain of ApoB (Hayavi and Halbert, 2005). This synthetic particle can support cell growth by delivering cholesterol to cells via the LDLR. In addition, Nikanjam and coworkers developed a synthetic nano-LDL (nLDL) particle containing a lipid emulsion and a unique bifunctional peptide, which could be internalized by glioma cell lines (including SF-767 cells) (Nikanjam et al., 2007). After loaded with a lipophilic prodrug, paclitaxel oleate (PO), the glioma-internalizing ability, was maintained and glioma cell killing effects were apparently enhanced compared to free drug. What's more, the cell killing effect could be significantly inhibited by suramin, a LDLR inhibitor. These results suggested the LDLR-mediated mechanism of nLDL.

Some targeting moieties such as ApoB, apolipoprotein E (ApoE), or some peptides corresponding to the LDLR-binding domain of ApoE or ApoB have been proven to be effective in LDLR-targeted therapy of neoplastic diseases (Sarkar et al., 2011; Spencer and Verma, 2007). However, they are not promising candidates as targeting moieties due to some inherent drawbacks such as protein instability, competition with endogenous LDL, and so on. The group of Jiang proposed that peptide-22, a peptide which showed high affinity for LDLR without competition with endogenous LDL, could be used to transport PTX-loaded NPs across the BBB and subsequently target to brain tumors (Zhang et al., 2013). The peptide-22-decorated NPs proved its targeting capacity on monolayer BBB model, glioma cells, and a BCECs/C6 glioma coculture model in vitro. In the meantime, the NPs exhibited stronger brain permeation, glioma targeted, and enhanced chemotherapeutic effect compared to other groups in vivo. These results revealed the feasibility of peptide-22 as a cascade targeting moiety for LDLR.

LRP-mediated targeting systems Low-density lipoprotein receptor-related protein (LRP) is a type of transmembrane proteins belonging to the LDL receptor family (Bell et al., 2007; Bertrand et al., 2011). The ubiquitous LRP has been detected up-regulated in numerous human diseases including glioma (Donahue et al., 2006; Hendrickx et al., 2013; Pires et al., 2012). It has been reported that LRP is not only overexpressed on glioma cancerous cells, but also on the BBB (Xin et al., 2012). Moreover, LRP can serve as a common receptor of multiple ligands across the BBB such as melanotransferrin (MTf), Lf, and receptor-associated protein (Gabathulera et al., 2005; Pan et al., 2004). These findings confirmed the role of LRP as an ideal target that can be used for direct delivery of antitumor agents to tumor cells. Angiopep-2 peptide, the most famous ligand of LRP, was derived from the common peptidic sequence of the LRP protein ligands and has shown transcytosis capacity in an in vitro BBB model and the ability to cross the BBB in vivo by LRP-mediated pathway (Demeule et al., 2008a, b). In recent years, more and more nano vehicles have been fabricated with angiopep-2 to target therapeutic agents to cross the BBB and accumulate in glioma. Ruan and colleagues developed angiopep-2-conjugated DOX-loaded gold NPs to target both BBB and glioma cells (Ruan et al., 2015). The enhanced cellular uptake and antiglioma activity of the gold NPs are achieved because angiopep-2 could mediate glioma targeted by specific interaction with LRP. At even earlier time, Fang's group used angiopep-2 to modify PTX-loading poly(ethylene gly*co*l)-*co*-poly(ε-caprolactone) (PEG-PCL) NPs (Xin et al., 2012). The conjugation of angiopep-2 mediated higher inhibitory effect to U87 MG glioma spheroid and larger amount of NPs in the solid glioma, demonstrating the transportation ability of angiopep-2 across the BBB and enrichment of NPs in glioma selectively. What's exciting is that a paclitaxel-angiopep-2 conjugate, GRN1005, has shown safety, fairly well tolerance in Phase I clinical trial (Drappatz et al., 2013). Although the preliminary efficacy of GRN1005 in patients with recurrent glioma is modest, the success of brain penetration increased the probability for further clinical trials. MTf, also known as a human melanoma-associated antigen p97, is a homologue of Tf (Suryo et al., 2012). It is identified as another potential targeting moiety to LRP due to its high affinity. In addition, the specific structure and functions of MTf suggest that it might be an ideal vehicle to transport drug conjugates into the brain (Karkan et al., 2008). Gabathuler and colleagues reported that the MTf-adriamycin conjugate significantly increased the survival of mice implanted with C6 glioma cells compared to injections of free Adriamycin (Gabathulera et al., 2005). In addition, the brain's uptake of conjugate was over eightfold higher than that of bovine serum albumin (BSA) or Lf. Taken together, p97 may have potential to deliver therapeutic drugs to the glioma as a viable effective carrier.

FR-mediated targeting systems Folate is a low-molecular-weight pterin-based vitamin. FR is essential to capture exogenous folate and various derivatives into the cell cytosol due to the lack of key enzymes of the folate biosynthetic pathway in animal cells (Leamon and Low, 2001). Studies demonstrated that FR is significantly overexpressed on both the BBB and glioma cells, but is subexpressed in normal brain tissues (Chen et al., 2014a, b). These intriguing studies inspired researchers to develop folate-configured nano-enabled carriers as solid tumor targeting vehicles. Cheng and colleagues studied the combined DOX and BCL-2 siRNA therapy using the FR-targeted multifunctional nanopaticle for penetrating BBB and targeting glioma (Cheng et al., 2012). The results indicated that FA-conjugated multifunctional nanocarrier could effectively deliver DOX and siRNA into C6 cells in vitro. in vivo experiments showed significant antiglioma effect and improvement in the survival time of tumor-bearing mice when compared with other formulations like nontargeting nanocarrier. Moreover, Chen and coworkers fabricated FA-conjugated *N*-(trimethoxysilylpropyl) ethylene diamine triacetic acid (TETT)-modified MnO NPs (MnO-TETT-FA) as tumor-specific MRI contrast agents for glioma detection (Chen et al., 2014a, b). MR images showed that the accumulation of MnO-TETT-FA NPs was more than that of MnO-TETT NPs in the brain of giloma-bearing mice. This additionally illustrated the role of FA in effective drug delivery to the glioma. Besides, increasing studies give high priority to FR targeting systems as possible therapeutics for glioma (Chen et al., 2015; Lee et al., 2014; Smith and Gumbleton, 2006).

IL-6R-mediated targeting systems Interleukin-6 receptor (IL-6R) is also expressed on both brain capillary endothelial cells and glioma cells, which consists of the ligand-binding IL-6Rα chain and the signal-transducing GP130 chain (Sturzu and Heckl, 2010; Vallières and Rivest, 1997). Its natural ligand, interleukin-6 (IL-6), is one of the most important cytokines. Growing evidences have shown that the IL-6/IL-6R signal pathway promotes the tumor growth in various cancers, especially for glioma (Yu et al., 2014a, b). Hence, IL-6R not only can be used as a target site for transporting drugs, but also as a therapeutic site. Recently, a heptapeptide (N- to C-terminus: LSLITRL), designated as I_6P_7, which can specifically bind to IL-6R, has been proved to inhibit the binding between IL-6 and IL-6R, thereby retarding the tumor growth (Sturzu and Heckl, 2010; Su et al., 2005). In this regard, the interaction of I_6P_7 and IL-6R could not only be utilized to increase the BBB transporting efficiency and concentrate therapeutic agents in glioma, but also inhibit the glioma growth and progression. In a study of Huang's group, I_6P_7 was covalently conjugated to polymer-coated nitrogen-doped carbon nanodot (pCD) to construct a simple nanocarrier (pCDPI) for encapsulating DOX via π-π stacking, yielding a multifunctional nano drug delivery system (pCDPID) (Wang et al., 2017a, b). The in vivo and in vitro evaluation results both showed that I_6P_7 can mediate the BBB transportation, the targeted glioma recognition, and the biological therapy (Fig. 1). Meanwhile, the assessment of the in vivo antiglioma efficacy illuminated a synergistic-targeted chemo-biotherapeutic effect of pCDPID, suggesting a high potential for practical cancer treatment. Another study of Huang's group developed I_6P_7 peptide-modified

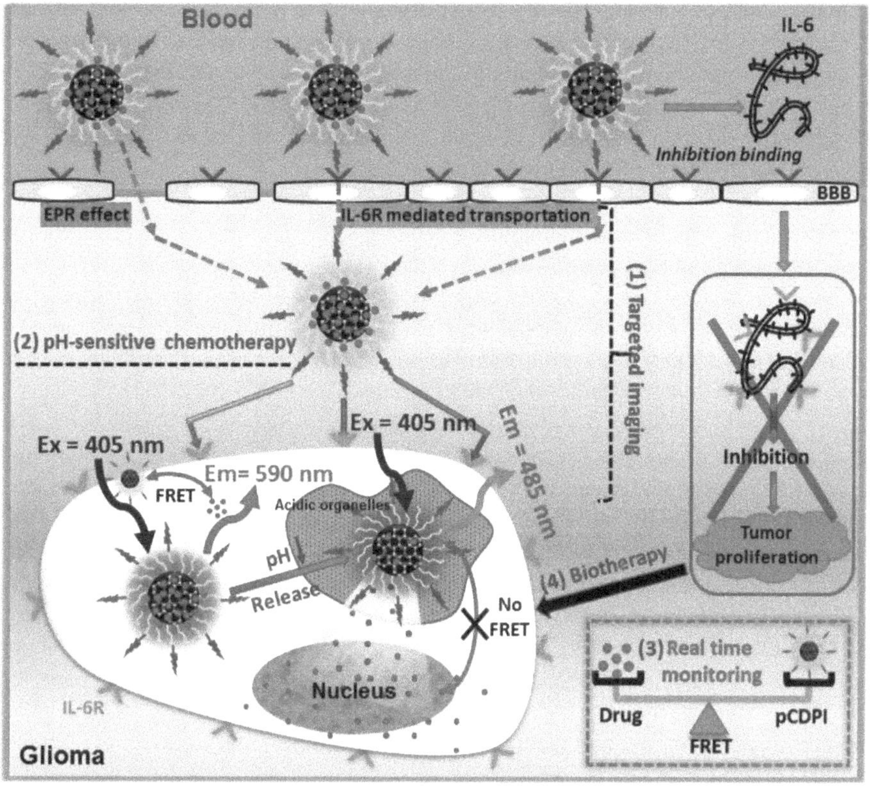

Fig. 1 Schematic diagrams of in vivo delivery process of multifunctional pCDPID and its application for targeted imaging, pH-sensitive chemotherapy, real time monitoring, and biotherapy.

gene-loaded nanoparticles (NPs) (Wang et al., 2017a, b). This study also confirmed the possibility and superiority of I_6P_7 peptide as a ligand of glioma.

Other receptor-mediated targeting systems Beyond the receptors listed above, there are still several receptors being referred as targeting sites for therapeutic agents highly expressed on the BCECs and glioma. One example is the insulin receptor, a membrane glycoprotein present in BCECs as well as glioma cells (Fan et al., 2016). Zhang and colleagues reported that PEGylated immunoliposomes (PILs) modified with 83–14 murine monoclonal antibody, an antibody to the human insulin receptor, could target the gene formulation to brain tumors in vivo (Zhang et al., 2002). Many studies suggested that humanized 83–14 murine monoclonal antibody had the potential to be used in clinical treatments. Another potential targeting site is the membrane-bound precursor of heparin-binding epidermal growth factor (HB-EGF), which is expressed on both BBB and neuroglial cells and also known as the diphtheria toxin receptor (DTR) (Kuo and Liu, 2014). Gaillard and colleagues utilized a nontoxic mutant of diphtheria toxin (known as CRM197) as the receptor-specific carrier protein, which conjugated directly to horseradish peroxidase. Results demonstrated that the DTR seemed to be a human applicable, safe, and effective uptake receptor which could mediate drugs targeting to the brain (Gururangan and Friedman, 2002).

2.1.1.2 Dual ligands-modified targeting systems

Two ligands in this kind of systems may play independent functions to different targeting sites, which then mediate drug delivery systems to overcome different barriers for final glioma targeted.

The first strategy of the cascade targeting systems is to fabricate the nanocarriers modified with two kinds of ligands, with one targeting across the BBB and the other targeting tumor cells. Gao's group came up with a cascade targeting strategy in order to achieve high and precise brain glioma targeted (Gao et al., 2012). They employed PEG-PCL NPs modified with two kinds of targeting ligands. The cellular uptake results suggested that the first stage targeting ligand only targeted to endothelial cells which are the major cellular structure of the BBB, and the second stage ligand only delivered NPs to neuroglial cells that are involved in the majority of CNS diseases including glioma. Another study of them further indicated that this strategy could increase tumor accumulation and decrease the normal brain distribution (Gao et al., 2011).

Also, the second strategy of the cascade targeting systems is to build nanocarriers modified with two kinds of ligands, with one targeting to the BBB and tumor cells, and the other promoting the targeting effect. The former ligands are usually some targeting moieties binding to their corresponding receptors, and the latter ligands may be some cell-penetrating peptides or some targeting moieties binding to the corresponding receptors, transporters, and so on. Drug delivery system, G4-DOX-PEG-Tf-TAM, was synthesized with Tf conjugated on the exterior and Tamoxifen (TAM) in the interior of polyamidoamine (PAMAM) dendrimer by Li et al. (2012). In this system, Tf was conjugated to mediate the dual targeting carrier to transport across the BBB and enhance its internalization in glioma. Another targeting moiety, TAM, is an estrogen receptor modulator which was used to improve the BBB permeability. The uptake ability of C6 glioma cells followed the order of G4-DOX-PEG-Tf-TAM > G4-DOX-PEG-Tf > G4-DOX-PEG, indicating that the dual ligands-modified carrier mediated the highest cellular uptake than single ligand-modified or nontargeting carriers. Further study verified the strongest transport efficiency of G4-DOX-PEG-Tf-TAM (6.06%) across the in vitro BBB model compared to that of G4-DOX-PEG-Tf (4.93%) and G4-DOX-PEG (4.62%). He and coworkers developed another dual ligands-mediated cascade targeting DOX-loaded NPs conjugated with Tf and wheat germ agglutinin (WGA), which has the potential to transfer drugs across the BBB and further target glioma cells (He et al., 2011). The PAMAM-PEG-WGA-Tf-DOX showed great inhibitory effect to C6 cells after crossing the BBB, compared to PAMAM-PEG-Tf-DOX, PAMAM-PEG-WGA-DOX, and free DOX, indicating better effect by treatments with dual ligands-modified system. Based on their work, Chen and coworkers prepared polymersomes conjugated with des-octanoyl ghrelin and folate as novel BBB-penetrating and cancer targeting delivery system

Table 2 **Representative dual ligands-modified cascade targeting systems (Wang et al., 2015a, b)**

Nanocarrier	Targeting moiety	Targeting site	Payload	References
PAMAM dendrimer	Tf WGA	TfR WGA receptor	DOX	He et al. (2011)
PAMAM dendrimer	Tf TAM	TfR ABC transporter transporters ABC transporters	DOX	Li et al. (2012)
PEG-PLA NPs	Lf tLyP-1	LfR Neuropilin-1	PTX	Miao et al. (2014)
Liposomes	Angiopep-2 tLyP-1	LRP Neuropilin-1	VEGF siRNA, docetaxel	Yang et al. (2014)
Liposomes	Tf TAT	TfR –	DOX	Zheng et al. (2015)
PEG-PCL NPs	Angiopep-2 EGFP-EGF1	LRP Specific tissue factor	DOX	Gao et al. (2011)
Polymer-lipid hybrid NPs	Folate RGD	FR Integrin	PTX	Agrawal et al. (2015)
PEGylated Liposomes	OX26 CTX	TfR Matrix metalloproteinase-2	PC27	Yue et al. (2014)

(Chen et al., 2014a, b). As a 28 residue peptide hormone, des-octanoyl ghrelin was identified as an endogenous ligand of the growth hormone secretagogue receptor, which was observed to transport only in the blood-to-brain direction. Uptake of drugs by the C6 glioma cells through the in vitro BBB model and glioma in in vivo experiments showed that this bifunctional polymersome could enhance BBB transport and tumor accumulation. In addition, a mass of dual cascade targeting drug delivery systems including daunorubicin-loaded liposome conjugated with *p*-aminophenyl-α-D-manno-pyranoside (MAN) and Tf, liposome co-modified with T7 and TAT, has been proved to possess stronger BBB-crossing and glioma-accumulating capability compared with single ligand-modified systems (Zitzmann et al., 2002; Zong et al., 2014a, b). Some representative dual targeting systems are summarized in Table 2.

2.1.2 *Without BBB overcoming*

Usually, with the aggravation of glioma, the proliferation and invasion of cancer cells will cause a local disruption of the BBB and produce various mediators which can increase the permeability of the capillary endothelium (Azad et al., 2015; Zhan and Lu, 2012). On this occasion, BBB is no longer the main barrier for the drug delivery and some new barriers form. Also, some specific receptors on glioma and/or neovasculatures will play crucial roles.

2.1.2.1 Single ligand-modified targeting systems

ILR-mediated targeting systems It has been reported that some interleukin receptors (ILRs) are highly expressed in many tumorous cells because they can contribute to malignant progression and apoptosis resistance of various cancer types including glioma (Kioi et al., 2008). Among these ILRs, interleukin-13 receptor (IL-13R) has already been used as a targeting site for mediating nano-enabled delivery systems to glioma.

As one of the inflammatory cytokines, interleukin 13 (IL-13) can bind to two receptor chains, IL-13Rα1 and IL-13Rα2 (Gao et al., 2013; Geskin et al., 2015). IL-13Rα2 is reported to be overexpressed on human tumors including glioma cell lines and with a high affinity for IL-13, which makes IL-13Rα2 an attractive target (Gao et al., 2013; Suzuki et al., 2014). In recent years, a few attempts have been reported to utilize IL-13 to enhance therapeutic effect of glioma (Thaci et al., 2014). However, as a targeting ligand, several disadvantages like large molecular weight and easy denaturation still remain the major challenges of IL-13 (Wang et al., 2012). As replacements, some peptides have been developed as targeting ligands for IL-13Rα2. IL-13 peptide (IP), which is consistent with the residues within IL-13 protein, has been demonstrated to possess high affinity for IL-13Rα2. Huang's group developed IP-modified mesoporous silica NPs (MSN-PEG-IP) as a novel vehicle for delivering DOX to glioma cell lines for the first time (Wang et al., 2012). The cellular uptake of MSN-PEG-IP/DOX in U251 glioma cells was significantly higher than that of unmodified NPs, indicating that IP is a potential ligand for fabricating glioma targeted drug delivery systems. In order to further verify the targeting ability of IP, Huang and colleagues synthesized IP-modified mesoporous silica-coated graphene nanosheets (GSPI) to load DOX for combined therapy of glioma (Fig. 2and Wang et al., 2013, 2015a, b). The novel multifunctional drug delivery system showed higher cellular uptake and cytotoxicity against glioma cells than those of unmodified counterparts. All these results cemented the fact that IP is promising to target nano-enabled theranostic systems to glioma. Besides IP, other peptides such as IL-13p and Pep-1 have also shown great targeting ability to glioma (Kioi et al., 2008; Wang et al., 2014).

Integrin-mediated targeting systems As known, integrin is a member of cell adhesion receptors' family, playing an important role in tumor growth, invasion and metastasis (Park et al., 2015). It is composed of α and β subunits. In mammals, 18 α subunits and 8 β subunits assemble into 24 integrin receptors (Hood and Cheresh, 2002). Several integrins have been reported to be highly expressed on the surface of glioma cells and the tumor neovasculatures, but minimally expressed on epithelial and mature endothelial cells (Zhan and Lu, 2012). These integrins support some docking sites for drug delivery systems to target to the glioma. Among these receptors, αvβ3, αvβ5, and α5β1 can specifically recognize an RGD motif, which is an exogenous peptide ligand composed by an Arg-Gly-Asp amino acid sequence (Zitzmann et al., 2002). In the past several years, RGD and its analogs have been

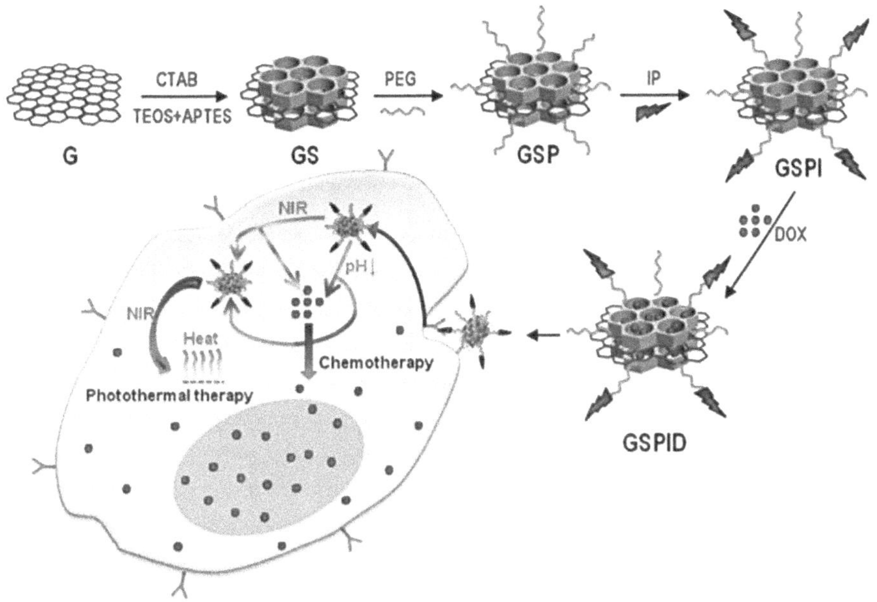

Fig. 2 Design of GSPID as a multifunctional drug delivery system for combined chemo-photothermal-targeted glioma therapy.

widely investigated for glioma targeted as integrin ligands. Slegerova and colleagues prepared cyclic RGD-modified fluorescent nanodiamonds for targeting drug delivery to glioblastoma cells (Slegerova et al., 2015). Results showed that the fluorescent nanodiamonds possessed high internalization efficacy into U87 cells with conjugation of a cyclic RGD peptide. Furthermore, Peiris et al. (2015) used a cyclic RGD peptide to conjugate the chain-like NPs (nanochain). After loaded with DOX, the nanochain exhibited a 2.6-fold higher deposition in brain tumors than nontargeting counterpart, illustrating the targeting ability of the cyclic RGD peptide to glioma and the therapeutic efficacy of the nanochain treatment. Therefore, RGD has been identified as a potential targeting ligand for glioma.

2.1.2.2 Dual ligands-modified targeting systems

Similar to single ligand-modified gliomatargeting systems, the dual ligands-conjugated systems can specifically target to receptors on the glioma and/or neovasculatures. Gao's group utilized RGD and IP as ligands to modify polymeric NPs (IRNPs) (Gao et al., 2014). The modification of IP and RGD could increase the uptake amount within C6 cells through corresponding receptors and the in vivo study revealed that the fluorescent intensity of DiR-loaded IRNPs in glioma was 3.82-fold of that of unmodified NPs. These results demonstrated that the co-modification of RGD and IP could increase the glioma targeted effect, which proved the superiority of dual ligands-modified targeting delivery systems. Although lots of dual ligands-modified targeting systems showed more satisfactory targeting effect, the systems with a single ligand are also another choice which could simplify the preparation of therapeutics. Thus, different researches may choose the best way in accordance with requirements in the further applications.

2.2 Adsorptive-mediated glioma targeted drug delivery

2.2.1 The concept and mechanism of adsorptive-mediated transcytosis

The transcytosis of cerebral endothelial cells can be divided into specific process (e.g., receptor-mediated transcytosis, RMT) and nonspecific process (e.g., adsorptive-mediated transcytosis, AMT) (Chen and Liu, 2012; Neuwelt et al., 2008). RMT is mainly based on specific receptors that express abundantly on the cell membranes of cerebral endothelial cells. The most studied receptors are insulin receptors, TfR and LDLR (Rip et al., 2009). Drug delivery systems integrated with the three ligands could greatly enhance their permeability through the BBB and glioma uptake efficiency. Nevertheless, there only exist several limited types of receptors enriched in the cerebral endothelial cells, which would greatly restrict the improvement and clinical application of drug delivery strategy for glioma therapy. In comparison, glioma drug delivery via AMT has various routes aiming at different specific situations.

AMT was originated with the observation that cationic proteins can cross the BBB with a much higher efficiency compared with neutral or negative-charged proteins (Herve et al., 2008). Many researches have indicated that not only cationic proteins, but also proteins mixed with cationic macrmolecules could increase the BBB permeability and further improve the glioma drug delivery efficiency (Lu, 2012). These phenomena can be elucidated by the electrostatic interaction between negatively charged cerebral endothelial cell membrane with those cationic proteins. Structural researches further proved that there existed a negative-charged barrier both in the luminal and abluminal surface of cerebral endothelial cell membrane, and their constitutions have some differences (Abbott et al., 2010). The sialic acid-containing glycoproteins with a less degree of heparan sulfate proteoglycans are the main anionic components in luminal membrane. As for the abluminal membrane, the negative-charged barrier was constituted mainly by heparan sulfates. Furthermore, in vitro and in vivo studies also showed that glioma drug delivery across the BBB via AMT is a time-, concentration- and energy-dependent process (Deli et al., 2005). It spends minutes to transport proteins across the cerebral endothelial cells, which is much longer than the carrier-mediated transport. And the AMT is also a saturable transport process with micromolar half-saturation constants. To make use of this AMT process to increase the glioma uptake efficiency, two kinds of strategy were developed, including protein cationization and cell-penetrating peptides.

2.2.2 Protein cationization

Cationization of proteins is a useful modified method that endows proteins with the ability to cross the BBB. By amidating their carboxylic groups with polyamine, some proteins could be positively charged. The most widely used polyamine molecules in the case of BBB transfer include hexamethylenediamine, putrescine, spermidine, and spermine, which could facilitate those modified proteins with BBB transport ability. For some drug proteins, like albumin, immunoglobulin G, or monoclonal antibody, polyamine modification could change their charge characteristics and hence greatly enhance their BBB-crossing ability. Lu et al. (2005a, b) have pioneeringly modified PEG-PLA nanoparticles with cationic bovine serum albumin, which indicated a much more enhanced BBB-crossing and glioma drug delivery efficiency with low toxicity. Nevertheless, since majority of drugs cannot be cationized, drug delivery systems that connected with cationized proteins turn out to be an alternative way for their BBB transportation. The most studied cationized proteins that are used to combine with other drug delivery systems or to form chimeric proteins include cationized human serum albumin, cationized histone, avidin, and so forth.

Although cationization may bring the attractive characteristics of the BBB-crossing ability, some drawbacks are unavoidable. No matter if cationization happens in a heavy or mild degree, potential activity of proteins might be influenced after the amidation. Because the anionic sites exist in nearly all living cells, cationized proteins also have a tendency that adsorb to all other normal cells, other than guidance toward glioma. This will undoubtfully increase a random tissue distribution of cationized proteins or their combined drug delivery systems. Moreover, even injected with a low dose of modified drugs, the undirected organ distribution and enhanced normal cell adsorption of cationized proteins might cause some gravely toxic or adverse effects. Besides, if the cationized proteins are heterologous, some undesired strong immunoreaction might happen and yield damage to human body.

2.2.3 *Cell-penetrating peptides*

Another pathway that opens up an even more extensive application prospect for glioma transportation is cell-penetrating peptides, which were discovered in some small peptides stem from protein-transduction domains. Numerous researches indicated that these proteins have the ability to translocate even the tight conjunction existing in the BBB and into the interior of glioma (Wong et al., 2010). Although those cell-penetrating peptides derive from various families and are different in size and sequence, they have some vital features in common that feature them with the penetrating ability, like amphipathic, ability to interact with lipid membranes, and most of all, positive charges. It was surmised that positively charged cell-penetrating peptides firstly get in touch with the lipid bilayer through electrostatic interaction, then form an inverted micelle, and passively transfer through the lipid bilayers of cell membrane. Hence, this kind of character could be used to enhance the BBB-crossing efficiency and glioma drug delivery. In recent studies, Tat, Syn-B, penetratin, and some other peptides are the mostly investigated cell-penetrating peptides.

Tat-derived peptide Originated from a transcription factor serving for the replication of HIV-1, the Tat peptide could rapidly be absorbed by cells and accumulated around nucleus (Rao et al., 2008). It has been showed that the cell-penetrating domain located in the residues from 49 to 58. Further studies indicated that fragment Tat

(38–60 or 48–60), which contain a cell-penetrating and nuclear localization domain, could easily cross the cell membrane and concentrate in the nucleus (Vives et al., 1997). Hence, making use of its penetrating property, no matter the full-length Tat peptide or derived Tat peptide (48–60) could all be used to feature other drugs or drug delivery systems with the property of adsorptive-mediated transcytosis (Tahrir et al., 2017). After conjugating of Tat peptide with drugs or drug delivery systems, the drug uptake in glioma has been measured with a much higher concentration than that without modification. Researches further proved that the heparan sulfate proteoglycans in cell surface play an important role for the Tat-mediated transcytosis cross BBB.

Syn-B Syn-B peptide family could be traced to a natural antimicrobial peptide (protegrin 1, PG-1), which was firstly found to form pores in the lipid membrane of bacteria (Drin et al., 2003). Based on this natural peptide, membrane disrupting activity was eliminated by the removal of cysteine residues, while excellent membrane-penetrating property was preserved at the same time, and the final optimization peptide was called Syn-B peptide (Hussain et al., 2016). According to researches, the Syn-B-associated transport is an energy-dependent and saturable process, which takes advantage of electrostatic interaction between Syn-B peptide and cell membrane (Martin et al., 1978). Several researches have exhibited a well glioma uptake of drugs after conjugated with Syn-B peptides.

There also have been many other peptides including poly-arginine peptide, Penetratin (43–58), Transportan, Amphipathic model peptide, and so forth, which all have been demonstrated to yield great potentials for the future endeavor in the field of brain drug delivery.

2.2.4 Drawbacks

Although these cell-penetrating peptides have indicated excellent BBB-crossing and glioma targeted potential, some pitfalls still leave them much space to be improved (Patel et al., 2007). The first problem needed to be considered is their instability. Since these peptides aim at in vivo drug delivery, they must have long enough half-life to enable them reach target site with sufficient dose. Hence, methods are needed to improve their stability to make full use of their cell-penetrating property. Another tough issue is their toxicity and immunogenicity. Studies have indicated a neuron toxicity of Tat peptide in mouse, for which the degree of toxicity depends on the length of Tat peptide. Besides, majority of these cell-penetrating peptides are all sourced from nonhuman; they own a high probability to cause immunogenicity when used in human body.

2.3 Transporter-mediated glioma targeted drug delivery

Brain tissue and tumors both require a large number of nutrients to maintain physiological functions. Substances can easily go through the BBB and actively target to cancers via those transporters highly expressed on brain capillary endothelial cells and cancer cells. Among those transporters, glucose transporter (GLUT), large amino acid transporter 1 (LAT1), and albumin transporters (e.g., SPARC and gp60) are the focus of researchers in recent years.

2.3.1 Glucose transporter-mediated delivery systems

As one of important nutrient transporters, D-Glucose transporter protein (GLUT) has a considerable high concentration in brain microvessels. In contrast to TfR, a brain-special target which has been widely utilized for active drug delivery, the concentration of GLUT is ~100-fold more (Wiley et al., 2013). In addition, GLUT is also found to be overexpressed on brain tumor cells (Gorin et al., 2004). Binding with glucose, the drug delivery systems endowed encephalic glioma targeted property through facilitative glucose metabolism by the glucose transporters highly expressed on glioma cancerous cells (Ying et al., 2010). Thus, glucose targeting ligands have received extensive attention on the capability for both enhanced delivery across the BBB and active glioma targeted. Based on these, Jiang and coworkers developed 2-deoxy-D-glucose-modified poly(ethylene gly*co*l)-*co*-poly(trimethylene carbonate) nanoparticles (DGlu-NP) for potent glioblastoma targeting therapy. In comparison with nonglucosylated nanoparticles, a significantly higher amount of DGlu-NP was internalized by RG-2 glioma cells through caveolae-mediated and clathrin-mediated endocytosis. Results showed that both the transport ratios of DGlu-NP/PTX across the in vitro BBB model and the cytotoxicity of RG-2 cells via GLUT were significantly greater than that of unmodified counterpart. The antiglioblastoma efficacy of DGlu-NP/PTX was significantly improved compared with that of Taxol and unmodified control (Jiang et al., 2014). Meanwhile, Niu et al. synthesized glucose transporter and folic acid (FA) receptor-mediated Pluronic P105 polymeric micelles loaded with DOX (GF-DOX) for optimizing the BBB transportation and improving the drug accumulation in the glioma cells. They verified that GF-DOX exhibited higher BBB transportation ability with the transporting ratio of 21.47% in 4h (Niu et al., 2014).

2.3.2 LAT1-mediated delivery systems

Amino acid metabolism is reprogrammed due to its important role in energy metabolism abnormity in tumor cells. Being the most prominent part in tumor-specific amino acid metabolic pathways, glutamine, the second important energy resource of tumor cells, produces abundant ATP for tumor growth (Bhutia et al., 2015). At the same time, other amino acids related to tumor growth are all exceedingly indispensable to sustain tumor cells along with the rapid and unlimited proliferation (Wise and Thompson, 2010). For the sake of the fast-growing transport requirement for amino acids of tumor, relative genetic changes are naturally tailored and correspondent amino acid transporters, such as LAT1, ASCT2 (system ASC amino acid transporter-2), amd xCT (cysteine/glutamate antiporter), are up-regulated (Bröer, 2002). Thus, amino acid transporters which overexpressed in tumor cells have become drug targets for cancer therapy. An et al. (2016) incorporated 3CDIT, a better substrate of LAT1 which is highly expressed both in BBB and glioma tumor cells, into pOEI/DOX/ATP aptamer NP for elevated accumulation and rapid GSH & ATP dual-responsive DOX release in glioma. Results showed that more efficient therapeutic effects came with 3CDITtargeting pOEI/DOX/ATP aptamer NP than free DOX and no systemic toxicity was observed. What's more, Li et al. (2016) applied docetaxel-loaded glutamate-D-tocopherol polyethylene glycol 1000 succinate copolymer (Glu-TPGS)-functionalized LAT1targeting liposomes (DTX-TGL) to achieve the reformative BBB penetration and glioma targeted accumulation. Compared with unmodified liposomes, a significant higher cellular uptake and cell cytotoxicity was found in TGL-treated group.

2.3.3 Albumin transporter-mediated delivery systems

Albumin, a momentous nutrient source for the body, is normally excluded from entering the brain. Due to rapid growth of metabolically active tumors, albumin intake into tumor tissues is greatly increased as a source of amino acids and energy for cancer cells (Stehle et al., 1997; Wunder et al., 1997). Like SPARC (secreted protein acidic and rich in cysteine) and glycoprotein 60 (gp60), albumin-binding proteins are the dominating pathways for tumor albumin uptake, a process including transcytosis across endothelium and endocytosis in tumor cells (Merlot et al., 2014). Since SPARC has been reported to be overexpressed in brain tumors, serving as a facilitator to glioma progression and invasion, its potential therapeutic value is worthy of the wait (Rempel et al., 2001; Shi et al., 2007). Thus, Lin et al. explored the possibility of using SPARC and gp60 as medium for brain targeting biomimetic delivery. The results showed that the albumin nanoparticles could penetrate the BBB and target glioma cells via the mechanisms of SPARC- and gp60-mediated transport. Interestingly, by modification with the cell-penetrating peptide LMWP, the albumin nanoparticles exhibited improved treatment outcomes in both subcutaneous and intracranial glioma models, with reduced toxic side effects (Lin et al., 2016).

2.4 Glioma targeted drug delivery via nasal pathway

2.4.1 Glioma targeted drug delivery via nasal pathway

The BBB is an important sentry ward that prevents toxic substances flow into brain, hence providing a stable micro-environment for the operation of nervous systems. However, this tight junction barrier also prevents drugs from transporting into brain to achieve glioma therapeutic effects. Therefore, researchers have developed numerous methods to overcome the BBB and gain enough concentrations of drugs in brain for the cure of glioma, mainly including RMT and AMT, which take advantage of biological or physical characters of the cerebral endothelial cells. And, some invasive techniques that are even making use of some artificially means to disrupt the BBB and form a hole in the BBB for drug transport into brain. Those are methods that aim at increasing drug delivery efficiency cross the BBB. In this section, intranasal pathway would be introduced, which could bypass the BBB and directly deliver drugs into brain for therapy of glioma.

The nasal passage can be categorized into three parts, nasal vestibule, olfactory region, and respiratory region (Dhuria et al., 2010). Nasal vestibule has barely no adsorptive function. Drugs go through respiratory region, mainly get adsorbed into blood vessel, and then undergo systemic circulation, with the BBB still remaining the major difficulty for brain uptake. Only small part of trigeminal distributed in this region that drugs deliver toward brain could take advantage of. However, the last olfactory region would be the key zone for drug delivery to bypass the BBB and target toward brain focus (Thorne et al., 2004). Since olfactory nerve and trigeminal are concentrated within olfactory region, the olfactory region offers a direct passage for drugs delivered to CNS. Moreover, the adsorptive pathway through olfactory region can be further divided into two accesses, nerve pathway and mucosa pathway, where drugs firstly are taken up by nerve cells or mucosa cells in olfactory region and further be transported into CNS through intra or intercellular pathway (Illum, 2000).

2.4.2 Nerve pathway

Olfactory nerve In the olfactory region, the center processes of olfactory cells form unmyelinated olfactory nerve fibers, named fila olfactory, which pass through olfactory foramina and terminate in olfactory bulb within the brain (Mistry et al., 2009) Drugs administrated by nasal passage could make use of this nerve pathway to greatly enhance their glioma uptake efficiency. Drugs adsorbed in olfactory region enter nerve cells through phagocytosis or pinocytosis. After that, drugs were transported through the axone of olfactory nerve or linking tissues surrounding the olfactory nerves toward cerebral spinal fluid or brain. Researches also indicated that majority of viruses by nasal passage were infected through olfactory nerves, which is the same as drugs absorbed through olfactory nerves. Shingaki and colleagues indicated an obviously improved methotrexate intake of glioma through this pathway (Shingaki et al., 2010). Moreover, Kanazawa and co-workers even connected a cell-penetrating peptide upon the drug delivery system to further enhance the delivery efficiency toward glioma by this nasal nerve pathway (Kanazawa et al., 2014).

Trigeminal The embranchment of trigeminal is elongated with one end connected to respiratory region and olfactory region, while the other end passes through pons and links with CNS, including nuclei tractus spinalis nervi trigemini in brain stem and olfactory bulb. Many researches use fluorescence-labeled protein drugs to investigate this pathway, and strong fluorescence feedback was observed within the CNS.

2.4.3 Mucosa pathway

Other than being transported by olfactory nerve cells, drugs could also be absorbed through olfactory mucosa cells and be delivered into brain. This pathway can be further divided into two subtypes, trans-cellular and para-cellular pathways. By transcellular transport method, drugs are delivered into glioma through carrier transport, pinocytosis, or passive diffusion. Besides, drugs could also infiltrate through interval between sustentacular cells and olfactory cells into intercellular fluid and further be delivered into the CNS. Mucosa pathway is a fast transport pathway compared with olfactory nerve pathway, which could take effect within even several minutes. By injecting neural cells through nasal pathway, Reitz et al. (2012) discovered a rapid and enriched distribution of neural cells in the nasal mucosa and glioma.

2.4.4 Factors influence glioma drug delivery through nasal pathway

Although nasal-brain pathway is a shortcut that body offers for the brain drug delivery, there also exists several factors that limit the absorption of drugs, including nasal ciliary elimination, cellular excretion mechanism, enzyme metabolism, and blood vessel absorption (Alpar et al., 2005; Gao et al., 2006; Misra and Kher, 2012). In order to gain a high brain delivery efficiency, drugs must obtain appropriate properties to overcome these troubles. Numerous nasal cilium is grown upon the surface of nasal mucosa; this physiological character has provided a clean and safe environment for nasal passage. Hence, drugs with higher and proper viscosity would have a longer adhesive time and higher adsorptive efficiency. In order to decrease the influence of transport proteins expressed in nasal mucosa (like P-gp), which could increase the excretion of drugs, some transporter inhibitors are used at the same time. This modification could greatly enhance the adsorption of drugs and its content in brain. Besides, some enzyme inhibitors are also combined with those drugs to improve the stability of drugs and extended their halftime in nasal cavity. Moreover, because of the abundant distribution of blood capillary in nasal passage, drugs might be adsorbed quickly through blood vessels and further undergo the body circulation and the BBB before the brain uptake. Hence, vasoconstrictor is also an alternative choice for increasing the drug uptake by nasal mucosa or nerve cells.

3 Conclusions

For glioma diagnosis and therapy, a growing number of strategies based on passive and/or active targeting have been and are being proposed. Compared with other strategies, receptor-mediated drug delivery is most extensively studied lying on several advantages. These systems possess a vital component: nanocarriers modified with targeting moieties. Till now, lots of targeting moieties which are ligands of the receptors on the BBB or glioma have been exploited for BBB-crossing and/or glioma targeted drug delivery, such as potential peptide ligands. In addition, more and more researches have proved that BBB/glioma-specific targeting nanocarrier can help drugs selectively target to the glioma, thus providing higher therapeutic efficiency while simultaneously decreasing systemic toxicity. It seems that the strategy has developed quite well, but so far all the systems except GRN1005 were just used for preclinical studies and none of them has completed its Phase III Clinical Trials. This reminds us that the strategy is still a long way off. It is particularly gratifying that increasing receptors are being found on the BBB and glioma cells, which provide possible targeting sites for developing new receptor-mediated targeting systems. Therefore, extensive researches are still required to identify new receptors and corresponding ligands. Most importantly, great efforts should be made to explore and facilitate potential delivery systems for glioma theragnosis in future clinical applications.

References

Abbott, N.J., Ronnback, L., Hansson, E., 2006. Astrocyte-endothelial interactions at the blood-brain barrier. Nat. Rev. Neurosci. 7, 41–53.

Abbott, N.J., Patabendige, A.A.K., Dolman, D.E.M., Yusof, S.R., Begley, D.J., 2010. Structure and function of the blood-brain barrier. Neurobiol. Dis. 37, 13–25.

Agnihotri, S., Burrell, K.E., Wolf, A., Jalali, S., Hawkins, C., Rutka, J.T., et al., 2013. Glioblastoma, a brief review of history, molecular genetics, animal models and novel therapeutic strategies. Arch. Immunol. Ther. Exp. (Warsz). 61, 25–41.

Agrawal, U., Chashoo, G., Sharma, P.R., Kumar, A., Saxena, A.K., Vyas, S.P., 2015. Tailored polymer-lipid hybrid nanoparticles for the delivery of drug conjugate: dual strategy for brain targeting. Colloids Surf. B 126, 414–425.

Alifieris, C., Trafalis, D.T., 2015. Glioblastoma multiforme: pathogenesis and treatment. Pharmacol. Ther. 152, 63–82.

Almond, R.J., Flanagan, B.F., Antonopoulos, A., Haslam, S.M., Dell, A., Kimber, I., et al., 2013. Differential immunogenicity and allergenicity of native and recombinant human lactoferrins: role of glycosylation. Eur. J. Immunol. 43, 170–181.

Alpar, H.O., Somavarapu, S., Atuah, K.N., Bramwell, V., 2005. Biodegradable mucoadhesive particulates for nasal and pulmonary antigen and DNA delivery. Adv. Drug Deliv. Rev. 57, 411–430.

An, S., Lu, X., Zhao, W., Sun, T., Zhang, Y., Lu, Y., Jiang, C., 2016. Amino acid metabolism abnormity and microenvironment variation mediated targeting and controlled glioma chemotherapy. Small 12, 5633–5645.

Aryal, M., Vykhodtseva, N., Zhang, Y.Z., McDannold, N., 2015. Multiple sessions of liposomal doxorubicin delivery via focused ultrasound mediated blood-brain barrier disruption: a safety study. J. Control. Release 204, 60–69.

Azad, T.D., Pan, J., Connolly, I.D., Remington, A., Wilson, C.M., Grant, G.A., 2015. Therapeutic strategies to improve drug delivery across the blood-brain barrier. Neurosurg. Focus. 38, E9.

Beduneau, A., Saulnier, P., Benoit, J.P., 2007. Active targeting of brain tumors using nanocarriers. Biomaterials 28, 4947–4967.

Bell, R.D., Sagare, A.P., Friedman, A.E., Bedi, G.S., Holtzman, D.M., Deane, R., et al., 2007. Transport pathways for clearance of human Alzheimer's amyloid beta-peptide and apolipoproteins E and J in the mouse central nervous system. J. Cerebr. Blood F. Met. 27, 909–918.

Bertato, M.P., Oliveira, C.P., Wajchenberg, B.L., Lerario, A.C., Maranhao, R.C., et al., 2012. Plasma kinetics of an LDL-like nanoemulsion and lipid transfer to HDL in subjects with glucose intolerance. Clinics (Sao Paulo) 67, 347–353.

Bertrand, Y., Currie, J.C., Poirier, J., Demeule, M., Abulrob, A., Fatehi, D., et al., 2011. Influence of glioma tumour microenvironment on the transport of ANG1005 via low-density lipoprotein receptor-related protein 1. Br. J. Cancer 105, 1697–1707.

Bertrand, N., Wu, J., Xu, X., Kamaly, N., Farokhzad, O.C., 2014. Cancer nanotechnology: the impact of passive and active targeting in the era of modern cancer biology. Adv. Drug Deliv. Rev. 66, 2–25.

Bhutia, Y.D., Babu, E., Ramachandran, S., Ganapathy, V., 2015. Amino acid transporters in cancer and their relevance to "glutamine addiction": novel targets for the design of a new class of anticancer drugs. Cancer Res. 75, 1782–1788.

Binello, E., Germano, I.M., 2011. Targeting glioma stem cells: a novel framework for brain tumors. Cancer Sci. 102, 1958–1966.

Bröer, S., 2002. Adaptation of plasma membrane amino acid transport mechanisms to physiological demands. Pflugers Arch. 444, 457–466.
Chakraborty, S., Cai, Y., Tarr, M.A., 2014. In vitro oxidative footprinting provides insight into apolipoprotein B-100 structure in low-density lipoprotein. Proteomics 14, 2614–2622.
Chen, Y., Liu, L., 2012. Modern methods for delivery of drugs across the blood–brain barrier. Adv. Drug Deliv. Rev. 64, 640–665.
Chen, Y.C., Chiang, C.F., Chen, L.F., Liang, P.C., Hsieh, W.Y., Lin, W.L., 2014a. Polymersomes conjugated with des-octanoyl ghrelin and folate as a BBB-penetrating cancer cell-targeting delivery system. Biomaterials 35, 4066–4081.
Chen, N., Shao, C., Qu, Y., Li, S., Gu, W., Zheng, T., et al., 2014b. Folic acid-conjugated MnO nanoparticles as a T1 contrast agent for magnetic resonance imaging of tiny brain gliomas. ACS Appl. Mater. Interfaces 6, 19850–19857.
Chen, Y.C., Chiang, C.F., Wu, S.K., Chen, L.F., Hsieh, W.Y., Lin, W.L., 2015. Targeting microbubbles-carrying TGFbeta1 inhibitor combined with ultrasound sonication induce BBB/BTB disruption to enhance nanomedicine treatment for brain tumors. J. Control. Release 211, 53–62.
Cheng, D., Cao, N., Chen, J., Yu, X., Shuai, X., 2012. Multifunctional nanocarrier mediated co-delivery of doxorubicin and siRNA for synergistic enhancement of glioma apoptosis in rat. Biomaterials 33, 1170–1179.
Chu, A.C., Tsang, S.Y., Lo, E.H., Fung, K.P., 2001. Low density lipoprotein as a targeted carrier for doxorubicin in nude mice bearing human hepatoma HepG2 cells. Life Sci. 70, 591–601.
Cornago, M., Garcia-Alberich, C., Blasco-Angulo, N., Vall-Llaura, N., Nager, M., Herreros, J., Comella, J.X., et al., 2014. Histone deacetylase inhibitors promote glioma cell death by G2 checkpoint abrogation leading to mitotic catastrophe. Cell Death Dis. 5, e1435.
Cui, Y., Xu, Q., Chow, P.K., Wang, D., Wang, C.H., 2013. Transferrin-conjugated magnetic silica PLGA nanoparticles loaded with doxorubicin and paclitaxel for brain glioma treatment. Biomaterials 34, 8511–8520.
Daniels, T.R., Bernabeu, E., Rodriguez, J.A., Patel, S., Kozman, M., Chiappetta, D.A., et al., 2012. The transferrin receptor and the targeted delivery of therapeutic agents against cancer. Biochim. Biophys. Acta 1820, 291–317.
de Boer, A.G., Gaillard, P.J., 2007. Drug targeting to the brain. Annu. Rev. Pharmacol. 47, 323–355.
Deli, M.A., Abraham, C.S., Kataoka, Y., Niwa, M., 2005. Permeability studies on in vitro blood–brain barrier models: physiology, pathology, and pharmacology. Cell. Mol. Neurobiol. 25, 59–127.
Demeule, M., Regina, A., Che, C., Poirier, J., Nguyen, T., Gabathuler, R., et al., 2008a. Identification and design of peptides as a new drug delivery system for the brain. J. Pharmacol. Exp. Ther. 324, 1064–1072.
Demeule, M., Currie, J.C., Bertrand, Y., Che, C., Nguyen, T., Regina, A., et al., 2008b. Involvement of the low-density lipoprotein receptor-related protein in the transcytosis of the brain delivery vector angiopep-2. J. Neurochem. 106, 1534–1544.
Dhuria, S.V., Hanson, L.R., Frey, W.H., 2010. Intranasal delivery to the central nervous system: mechanisms and experimental considerations. J. Pharm. Sci. 99, 1654–1673.
Dixit, S., Novak, T., Miller, K., Zhu, Y., Kenney, M.E., Broome, A.M., 2015. Transferrin receptor-targeted theranostic gold nanoparticles for photosensitizer delivery in brain tumors. Nanoscale 7, 1782–1790.
Donahue, J.E., Flaherty, S.L., Johanson, C.E., Duncan, J.R., Silverberg, G.D., Miller, M.C., et al., 2006. RAGE, LRP-1, and amyloid-beta protein in Alzheimer's disease. Acta Neuropathol. 112, 405–415.

Drappatz, J., Brenner, A., Wong, E.T., Eichler, A., Schiff, D., Groves, M.D., et al., 2013. Phase I study of GRN1005 in recurrent malignant glioma. Clin. Cancer Res. 19, 1567–1576.
Drin, G., Cottin, S., Blanc, E., Rees, A.R., Temsamani, J., 2003. Studies on the internalization mechanism of cationic cell-penetrating peptides. J. Biol. Chem. 278, 31192–31201.
Du, W., Fan, Y., Zheng, N., He, B., Yuan, L., Zhang, H., et al., 2013. Transferrin receptor specific nanocarriers conjugated with functional 7peptide for oral drug delivery. Biomaterials 34, 794–806.
Du, W., Fan, Y., He, B., Zheng, N., Yuan, L., Dai, W., et al., 2015. Bionano interactions of mcf-7 breast tumor cells with a transferrin receptor targeted nanoparticle. Mol. Pharm. 12, 1467–1476.
Fan, C.H., Chang, E.L., Ting, C.Y., Lin, Y.C., Liao, E.C., Hung, C.Y., et al., 2016. Folate-conjugated gene-carrying microbubbles with focused ultrasound for concurrent blood-brain barrier opening and local gene delivery. Biomaterials 106, 46–57.
Fang, J.H., Lai, Y.H., Chiu, T.L., Chen, Y.Y., Hu, S.H., Chen, S.Y., 2014. Magnetic core-shell nanocapsules with dual-targeting capabilities and co-delivery of multiple drugs to treat brain gliomas. Adv. Healthc. Mater. 3, 1250–1260.
Fang, J.H., Chiu, T.L., Huang, W.C., Lai, Y.H., Hu, S.H., Chen, Y.Y., et al., 2016. Dual-targeting lactoferrin-conjugated polymerized magnetic polydiacetylene-assembled nanocarriers with self-responsive fluorescence/magnetic resonance imaging for in vivo brain tumor therapy. Adv. Healthc. Mater. 5, 688–695.
Fillebeen, C., Descamps, L., Dehouck, M.P., Fenart, L., Benaissa, M., Spik, G., et al., 1999. Receptor-mediated transcytosis of lactoferrin through the blood-brain barrier. J. Biol. Chem. 274, 7011–7017.
Gabathuler, R., 2010. Approaches to transport therapeutic drugs across the blood-brain barrier to treat brain diseases. Neurobiol. Dis. 37, 48–57.
Gabathulera, R., Arthura, G., Kennarda, M., Chena, Q., Tsaia, S., Yanga, J., et al., 2005. Development of a potential protein vector (NeuroTrans) to deliver drugs across the blood-brain barrier. Int. Congr. Ser. 1277, 171–184.
Ganz, T., Nemeth, E., 2015. Iron homeostasis in host defence and inflammation. Nat. Rev. Immunol. 15, 500–510.
Gao, X.L., Tao, W.X., Lu, W., Zhang, Q.Z., Zhang, Y., Jiang, X.G., et al., 2006. Lectin-conjugated PEG-PLA nanoparticles: preparation and brain delivery after intranasal administration. Biomaterials 27, 3482–3490.
Gao, H., Pan, S., Yang, Z., Cao, S., Chen, C., Jiang, X., et al., 2011. A cascade targeting strategy for brain neuroglial cells employing nanoparticles modified with angiopep-2 peptide and EGFP-EGF1 protein. Biomaterials 32, 8669–8675.
Gao, H., Qian, J., Cao, S., Yang, Z., Pang, Z., Pan, S., et al., 2012. Precise glioma targeting of and penetration by aptamer and peptide dual-functioned nanoparticles. Biomaterials 33, 5115–5123.
Gao, H., Yang, Z., Zhang, S., Cao, S., Pang, Z., Yang, X., et al., 2013. Glioma-homing peptide with a cell-penetrating effect for targeting delivery with enhanced glioma localization, penetration and suppression of glioma growth. J. Control. Release 172, 921–928.
Gao, H., Xiong, Y., Zhang, S., Yang, Z., Cao, S., Jiang, X., 2014. RGD and interleukin-13 peptide functionalized nanoparticles for enhanced glioblastoma cells and neovasculature dual targeting delivery and elevated tumor penetration. Mol. Pharm. 11, 1042–1052.
Geskin, L.J., Viragova, S., Stolz, D.B., Fuschiotti, P., 2015. Interleukin-13 is overexpressed in cutaneous T-cell lymphoma cells and regulates their proliferation. Blood 125, 2798–2805.
Gorin, F., Harley, W., Schnier, J., Lyeth, B., Jue, T., 2004. Perinecrotic glioma proliferation and metabolic profile within an intracerebral tumor xenograft. Acta Neuropathol. 107, 235–244.

Gururangan, S., Friedman, H.S., 2002. Innovations in design and delivery of chemotherapy for brain tumors. Neuroimaging Clin. N. Am. 12, 583–597.

Han, L., Li, J., Huang, S., Huang, R., Liu, S., Hu, X., et al., 2011. Peptide-conjugated polyamidoamine dendrimer as a nanoscale tumor-targeted T1 magnetic resonance imaging contrast agent. Biomaterials 32, 2989–2998.

Hayavi, S., Halbert, G.W., 2005. Synthetic low-density lipoprotein, a novel biomimetic lipid supplement for serum-free tissue culture. Biotechnol. Prog. 21, 1262–1268.

He, H., Li, Y., Jia, X.R., Du, J., Ying, X., Lu, W.L., et al., 2011. PEGylated poly(amidoamine) dendrimer-based dual-targeting carrier for treating brain tumors. Biomaterials 32, 478–487.

Hendrickx, D.A., Koning, N., Schuurman, K.G., van Strien, M.E., van Eden, C.G., Hamann, J., et al., 2013. Selective upregulation of scavenger receptors in and around demyelinating areas in multiple sclerosis. J. Neuropathol. Exp. Neurol. 72, 106–118.

Herve, F., Ghinea, N., Scherrmann, J.M., 2008. CNS delivery via adsorptive transcytosis. AAPS J. 10, 455–472.

Hood, J.D., Cheresh, D.A., 2002. Role of integrins in cell invasion and migration. Nat. Rev. Cancer 2, 91–100.

Huang, R.Q., Ke, W.L., Qu, Y.H., Zhu, J.H., Pei, Y.Y., Jiang, C., 2007. Characterization of lactoferrin receptor in brain endothelial capillary cells and mouse brain. J. Biomed. Sci. 14, 121–128.

Huang, R., Ke, W., Liu, Y., Jiang, C., Pei, Y., 2008. The use of lactoferrin as a ligand for targeting the polyamidoamine-based gene delivery system to the brain. Biomaterials 29, 238–246.

Huang, C.L., Hsiao, I.L., Lin, H.C., Wang, C.F., Huang, Y.J., Chuang, C.Y., 2015. Silver nanoparticles affect on gene expression of inflammatory and neurodegenerative responses in mouse brain neural cells. Environ. Res. 136, 253–263.

Hussain, M.A., Haile, A., Ahmad, T., 2016. Infestation of two tephritid fruit flies, *Bactrocera dorsalis* (syn. B. invadens) and *Ceratitis capitata*, in guava fruits from selected regions of Eritrea. Afr. Entomol. 1, 265.

Huynh, N.T., Morille, M., Bejaud, J., Legras, P., Vessieres, A., Jaouen, G., et al., 2011. Treatment of 9L gliosarcoma in rats by ferrociphenol-loaded lipid nanocapsules based on a passive targeting strategy via the EPR effect. Pharm. Res. 28, 3189–3198.

Illum, L., 2000. Transport of drugs from the nasal cavity to the central nervous system. Eur. J. Pharm. Sci. 11, 1–18.

Inoue, S., Patil, R., Portilla-Arias, J., Ding, H., Konda, B., Espinoza, A., et al., 2012. Nanobiopolymer for direct targeting and inhibition of EGFR expression in triple negative breast cancer. PLoS One 7, e31070.

Jain, A.J.K.J., 2013. Low density lipoproteins mediated nanoplatforms for cancer targeting. J. Nanopart. Res. 15, e1888.

Jeong, G.W., Park, S.C., Choi, C., Nam, J.P., Kim, T.H., Choi, S.K., et al., 2015. Anticancer effect of gene/peptide co-delivery system using transferrin-grafted LMWSC. Int. J. Pharm. 488, 165–173.

Jiang, X., Xin, H., Ren, Q., Gu, J., Zhu, L., Du, F., et al., 2014. Nanoparticles of 2-deoxy-D-glucose functionalized poly(ethylene glycol)-co-poly(trimethylene carbonate) for dual-targeting drug delivery in glioma treatment. Biomaterials 35, 518–529.

Kader, A., Pater, A., 2002. Loading anticancer drugs into HDL as well as LDL has little affect on properties of complexes and enhances cytotoxicity to human carcinoma cells. J. Control. Release 80, 29–44.

Kanazawa, T., Morisaki, K., Suzuki, S., Takashima, Y., 2014. Prolongation of life in rats with malignant glioma by intranasal siRNA/drug codelivery to the brain with cell-penetrating peptide-modified micelles. Mol. Pharm. 11, 1471–1478.

Karkan, D., Pfeifer, C., Vitalis, T.Z., Arthur, G., Ujiie, M., Chen, Q., et al., 2008. A unique carrier for delivery of therapeutic compounds beyond the blood-brain barrier. PLoS One 3, e2469.

Kawamoto, M., Horibe, T., Kohno, M., Kawakami, K., 2011. A novel transferrin receptor-targeted hybrid peptide disintegrates cancer cell membrane to induce rapid killing of cancer cells. BMC Cancer 11, 359.

Kawamoto, M., Kohno, M., Horibe, T., Kawakami, K., 2013. Immunogenicity and toxicity of transferrin receptor-targeted hybrid peptide as a potent anticancer agent. Cancer Chemother. Pharmacol. 71, 799–807.

Kioi, M., Seetharam, S., Puri, R.K., 2008. Targeting IL-13RA2-positive cancer with a novel recombinant immunotoxin composed of a single-chain antibody and mutated Pseudomonas exotoxin. Mol. Cancer Ther. 7, 1579–1587.

Kuang, Y., An, S., Guo, Y., Huang, S., Shao, K., Liu, Y., et al., 2013. T7 peptide-functionalized nanoparticles utilizing RNA interference for glioma dual targeting. Int. J. Pharm. 454, 11–20.

Kuo, Y.C., Liu, Y.C., 2014. Cardiolipin-incorporated liposomes with surface CRM197 for enhancing neuronal survival against neurotoxicity. Int. J. Pharm. 473, 334–344.

Lainé, A.L., Clavreul, A., Rousseau, A., Tétaud, C., Vessieres, A., Garcion, E., et al., 2014. Inhibition of ectopic glioma tumor growth by a potent ferrocenyl drug loaded into stealth lipid nanocapsules. Nanomedicine 10, 1667–1677.

Lammers, T., Kiessling, F., Hennink, W.E., Storm, G., 2012. Drug targeting to tumors: principles, pitfalls and (pre-) clinical progress. J. Control. Release 161, 175–187.

Leamon, C.P., Low, P.S., 2001. Folate-mediated targeting: from diagnostics to drug and gene delivery. Drug Discov. Today 6, 44–51.

Lee, K.D., Choi, S.H., Kim, D.H., Lee, H.Y., Choi, K.C., 2014. Self-organized nanoparticles based on chitosan-folic acid and dextran succinate-doxorubicin conjugates for drug targeting. Arch. Pharm. Res. 37, 1546–1553.

Li, Y., He, H., Jia, X., Lu, W.L., Lou, J., Wei, Y., 2012. A dual-targeting nanocarrier based on poly(amidoamine) dendrimers conjugated with transferrin and tamoxifen for treating brain gliomas. Biomaterials 33, 3899–3908.

Li, X.T., Ju, R.J., Li, X.Y., Zeng, F., Shi, J.F., Liu, L., et al., 2014. Multifunctional targeting daunorubicin plus quinacrine liposomes, modified by wheat germ agglutinin and tamoxifen, for treating brain glioma and glioma stem cells. Oncotarget 5, 6497–6511.

Li, L., Di, X., Zhang, S., Kan, Q., Liu, H., Lu, T., et al., 2016. Large amino acid transporter 1 mediated glutamate modified docetaxel-loaded liposomes for glioma targeting. Colloids Surf. B 141, 260–267.

Lin, T., Zhao, P., Jiang, Y., Tang, Y., Jin, H., Pan, Z., et al., 2016. Blood-brain-barrier-penetrating albumin nanoparticles for biomimetic drug delivery via albumin-binding protein pathways for anti-glioma therapy. ACS Nano 10, 9999–10012.

Liu, S., Guo, Y., Huang, R., Li, J., Huang, S., Kuang, Y., et al., 2012. Gene and doxorubicin co-delivery system for targeting therapy of glioma. Biomaterials 33, 4907–4916.

Liu, G., Shen, H., Mao, J., Zhang, L., Jiang, Z., Sun, T., et al., 2013. Transferrin modified graphene oxide for glioma-targeted drug delivery: in vitro and in vivo evaluations. ACS Appl. Mater. Interfaces 5, 6909–6914.

Liu, L., Wei, Y., Zhai, S., Chen, Q., Xing, D., 2015. Dihydroartemisinin and transferrin dual-dressed nano-graphene oxide for a pH-triggered chemotherapy. Biomaterials 62, 35–46.

Lu, W., 2012. Adsorptive-mediated brain delivery systems. Curr. Pharm. Biotechnol. 13, 2340–2348.

Lu, W., Tan, Y.Z., Hu, K.L., Jiang, X.G., 2005a. Cationic albumin conjugated pegylated nanoparticle with its transcytosis ability and little toxicity against blood-brain barrier. Int. J. Pharm. 295, 247–260.

Lu, W., Zhang, Y., Tan, Y.Z., Hu, K.L., Jiang, X.G., Fu, S.K., 2005b. Cationic albumin-conjugated pegylated nanoparticles as novel drug carrier for brain delivery. J. Control. Release 107, 428–448.

Manich, G., Cabezon, I., Del, V.J., Duran-Vilaregut, J., Camins, A., Pallas, M., et al., 2013. Study of the transcytosis of an anti-transferrin receptor antibody with a Fab' cargo across the blood-brain barrier in mice. Eur. J. Pharm. Sci. 49, 556–564.

Martin, K., Freitag, J., Conrades, M., Hruska, K., Klahr, S., Slatopolsky, E., 1978. Selective uptake of synthetic amino terminal PTH fragment (Syn B-PTH 1-34) by isolated perfused bone. Clin. Res. 3, A562.

Matsumura, Y., 2011. Preclinical and clinical studies of NK012, an SN-38-incorporating polymeric micelles, which is designed based on EPR effect. Adv. Drug Deliv. Rev. 63, 184–192.

Matsumura, Y., Maeda, H., 1986. A new concept for macromolecular therapeutics in cancer chemotherapy: mechanism of tumoritropic accumulation of proteins and the antitumor agent smancs. Cancer Res. 46, 6387–6392.

Merlot, A.M., Kalinowski, D.S., Richardson, D.R., 2014. Unraveling the mysteries of serum albumin-more than just a serum protein. Front. Physiol. 5, 299.

Miao, D., Jiang, M., Liu, Z., Gu, G., Hu, Q., Kang, T., et al., 2014. Co-administration of dualtargeting nanoparticles with penetration enhancement peptide for anti-glioblastoma therapy. Mol. Pharm. 11, 90–101.

Misra, A., Kher, G., 2012. Drug delivery systems from nose to brain. Curr. Pharm. Biotechnol. 13, 2355–2379.

Mistry, A., Stolnik, S., Illum, L., 2009. Nanoparticles for direct nose-to-brain delivery of drugs. Int. J. Pharm. 379, 146–157.

Neuwelt, E., Abbott, N.J., Abrey, L., Banks, W.A., Blakley, B., Davis, T., et al., 2008. Strategies to advance translational research into brain barriers. Lancet Neurol. 7, 84–96.

Neves, J.V., Caldas, C., Wilson, J.M., Rodrigues, P.N., 2011. Molecular mechanisms of hepcidin regulation in sea bass (Dicentrarchus labrax). Fish Shellfish Immunol. 31, 1154–1161.

Nikanjam, M., Gibbs, A.R., Hunt, C.A., Budinger, T.F., Forte, T.M., 2007. Synthetic nano-LDL with paclitaxel oleate as a targeted drug delivery vehicle for glioblastoma multiforme. J. Control. Release 124, 163–171.

Niu, J., Wang, A., Ke, Z., Zheng, Z., 2014. Glucose transporter and folic acid receptor-mediated Pluronic P105 polymeric micelles loaded with doxorubicin for brain tumor treating. J. Drug Target. 22, 712–723.

Pan, W., Kastin, A.J., Zankel, T.C., van Kerkhof, P., Terasaki, T., Bu, G., 2004. Efficient transfer of receptor-associated protein (RAP) across the blood-brain barrier. J. Cell Sci. 117, 5071–5078.

Pandey, V., Gajbhiye, K.R., Soni, V., 2015. Lactoferrin-appended solid lipid nanoparticles of paclitaxel for effective management of bronchogenic carcinoma. Drug Deliv. 22, 199–205.

Pardridge, W.M., 2015. Blood-brain barrier endogenous transporters as therapeutic targets: a new model for small molecule CNS drug discovery. Expert Opin. Ther. Tar. 19, 1059–1072.

Paris-Robidas, S., Emond, V., Tremblay, C., Soulet, D., Calon, F., 2011. In vivo labeling of brain capillary endothelial cells after intravenous injection of monoclonal antibodies targeting the transferrin receptor. Mol. Pharmacol. 80, 32–39.

Park, E.J., Yuki, Y., Kiyono, H., Shimaoka, M., 2015. Structural basis of blocking integrin activation and deactivation for anti-inflammation. J. Biomed. Sci. 22, 51.

Parrish, K.E., Sarkaria, J.N., Elmquist, W.F., 2015. Improving drug delivery to primary and metastatic brain tumors: strategies to overcome the blood-brain barrier. Clin. Pharmacol. Ther. 97, 336–346.
Patel, L.N., Zaro, J.L., Shen, W.C., 2007. Cell penetrating peptides: intracellular pathways and pharmaceutical perspectives. Pharm. Res. 24, 1977–1992.
Paw, I., Carpenter, R.C., Watabe, K., Debinski, W., Lo, H.W., 2015. Mechanisms regulating glioma invasion. Cancer Lett. 362, 1–7.
Peiris, P.M., Abramowski, A., Mcginnity, J., Doolittle, E., Toy, R., Gopalakrishnan, R., et al., 2015. Treatment of invasive brain tumors using a chain-like nanoparticle. Cancer Res. 75, 1356–1365.
Perry, J.L., Reuter, K.G., Luft, J.C., Pecot, C.V., Zamboni, W., DeSimone, J.M., 2017. Mediating passive tumor accumulation through particle size, tumor type, and location. Nano Lett. 17, 2879–2886.
Pires, L.A., Hegg, R., Freitas, F.R., Tavares, E.R., Almeida, C.P., Baracat, E.C., et al., 2012. Effect of neoadjuvant chemotherapy on low-density lipoprotein (LDL) receptor and LDL receptor-related protein 1 (LRP-1) receptor in locally advanced breast cancer. Braz. J. Med. Biol. Res. 45, 557–564.
Raei, M., Rajabzadeh, G., Zibaei, S., Jafari, S.M., Sani, A.M., 2015. Nano-encapsulation of isolated lactoferrin from camel milk by calcium alginate and evaluation of its release. Int. J. Biol. Macromol. 79, 669–673.
Rao, K.S., Reddy, M.K., Horning, J.L., Labhasetwar, V., 2008. TAT-conjugated nanoparticles for the CNS delivery of anti-HIV drugs. Biomaterials 29, 4429–4438.
Reitz, M., Demestre, M., Sedlacik, J., Meissner, H., Fiehler, J., Kim, S.U., et al., 2012. Intranasal delivery of neural stem/progenitor cells: a noninvasive passage to target intracerebral glioma. Stem Cells Transl. Med. 1, 866–873.
Rempel, S.A., Golembieski, W.A., Fisher, J.L., Maile, M., Nakeff, A., 2001. SPARC modulates cell growth, attachment and migration of U87 glioma cells on brain extracellular matrix proteins. J. Neuro-Oncol. 53, 149–160.
Rip, J., Schenk, G.J., de Boer, A.G., 2009. Differential receptor-mediated drug targeting to the diseased brain. Expert Opin. Drug Deliv. 6, 227–237.
Ruan, S., Yuan, M., Zhang, L., Hu, G., Chen, J., Cun, X., et al., 2015. Tumor microenvironment sensitive doxorubicin delivery and release to glioma using angiopep-2 decorated gold nanoparticles. Biomaterials 37, 425–435.
Sakurai, K., Sohda, T., Ueda, S., Tanaka, T., Hirano, G., Yokoyama, K., et al., 2014. Immunohistochemical demonstration of transferrin receptor 1 and 2 in human hepatocellular carcinoma tissue. Hepatogastroenterol 61, 426–430.
Sarkar, G., Curran, G.L., Mahlum, E., Decklever, T., Wengenack, T.M., Blahnik, A., et al., 2011. A carrier for non-covalent delivery of functional beta-galactosidase and antibodies against amyloid plaques and IgM to the brain. PLoS One 6, e28881.
Shi, Q., Bao, S., Song, L., Wu, Q., Bigner, D.D., Hjelmeland, A.B., et al., 2007. Targeting SPARC expression decreases glioma cellular survival and invasion associated with reduced activities of FAK and ILK kinases. Oncogene 26, 4084–4094.
Shingaki, T., Inoue, D., Furubayashi, T., Sakane, T., Katsumi, H., Yamamoto, A., et al., 2010. Transnasal delivery of methotrexate to brain tumors in rats: a new strategy for brain tumor chemotherapy. Mol. Pharm. 7, 1561–1568.
Slegerova, J., Hajek, M., Rehor, I., Sedlak, F., Stursa, J., Hruby, M., et al., 2015. Designing the nanobiointerface of fluorescent nanodiamonds: highly selective targeting of glioma cancer cells. Nanoscale 7, 415–420.
Smith, M.W., Gumbleton, M., 2006. Endocytosis at the blood-brain barrier: from basic understanding to drug delivery strategies. J. Drug Target. 14, 191–214.

Spencer, B.J., Verma, I.M., 2007. Targeted delivery of proteins across the blood-brain barrier. Proc. Natl. Acad. Sci. USA 104, 7594–7599.

Stehle, G., Sinn, H., Wunder, A., Schrenk, H.H., Stewart, J.C., Hartung, G., et al., 1997. Plasma protein (albumin) catabolism by the tumor itself–implications for tumor metabolism and the genesis of cachexia. Crit. Rev. Oncol. Hematol. 26, 77–100.

Stupp, R., Mason, W.P., van den Bent, M.J., Weller, M., Fisher, B., Taphoorn, M.J., et al., 2005. Radiotherapy plus concomitant and adjuvant temozolomide for glioblastoma. New Engl. J. Med. 352, 987–996.

Sturzu, A., Heckl, S., 2010. Magnetic resonance imaging of human glioma cells by means of an interleukin-6 receptor-targeted contrast agent. Chem. Biol. Drug Des. 75, 369–374.

Su, J., Lai, K., Chen, C., Yang, C., Chen, P., Chang, C., et al., 2005. A novel peptide specifically binding to interleukin-6 receptor (gp80) inhibits angiogenesis and tumor growth. Cancer Res. 65, 4827–4829.

Su, Z., Xing, L., Chen, Y., Xu, Y., Yang, F., Zhang, C., et al., 2014. Lactoferrin-modified poly(ethylene glycol)-grafted BSA nanoparticles as a dual-targeting carrier for treating brain gliomas. Mol. Pharm. 11, 1823–1834.

Suryo, R.Y., Bal, S., Loh, K.H., Yu, Y., Richardson, D.R., 2012. Melanotransferrin: search for a function. Biochim. Biophys. Acta 1820, 237–243.

Suzuki, Y.A., Lonnerdal, B., 2004. Baculovirus expression of mouse lactoferrin receptor and tissue distribution in the mouse. Biomaterials 17, 301–309.

Suzuki, A., Leland, P., Kobayashi, H., Choyke, P.L., Jagoda, E.M., Inoue, T., et al., 2014. Analysis of biodistribution of intracranially infused radiolabeled interleukin-13 receptor-targeted immunotoxin IL-13PE by SPECT/CT in an orthotopic mouse model of human glioma. J. Nucl. Med. 55, 1323–1329.

Tahrir, F.G., Shanmughapriya, S., Ahooyi, T.M., Knezevic, T., Gupta, M.K., Kontos, C.D., et al., 2017. Dysregulation of mitochondrial bioenergetics and quality control by HIV-1 Tat in cardiomyocytes. J. Cell. Physiol. (2), 748.

Talukder, M.J., Takeuchi, T., Harada, E., 2003. Receptor-mediated transport of lactoferrin into the cerebrospinal fluid via plasma in young calves. J. Vet. Med. Sci. 65, 957–964.

Taurin, S., Nehoff, H., Greish, K., 2012. Anticancer nanomedicine and tumor vascular permeability, where is the missing link? J. Control. Release 164, 265–275.

Thaci, B., Brown, C.E., Binello, E., Werbaneth, K., Sampath, P., Sengupta, S., 2014. Significance of interleukin-13 receptor alpha 2-targeted glioblastoma therapy. Neuro-Oncology 16, 1304–1312.

Thorne, R.G., Pronk, G.J., Padmanabhan, V., Frey, W.H., 2004. Delivery of insulin-like growth factor-I to the rat brain and spinal cord along olfactory and trigeminal pathways following intranasal administration. Neuroscience 127, 481–496.

Vallières, L., Rivest, S., 1997. Regulation of the genes encoding interleukin-6, its receptor, and gp130 in the rat brain in response to the immune activator lipopolysaccharide and the proinflammatory cytokine interleukin-1 β. J. Neurochem. 69, 1668–1683.

Van Tellingen, O., Yetkin-Arik, B., de Gooijer, M.C., Wesseling, P., Wurdinger, T., de Vries, H.E., 2015. Overcoming the blood-brain tumor barrier for effective glioblastoma treatment. Drug Resist. Updat. 19, 1–12.

Vives, E., Brodin, P., Lebleu, B., 1997. A truncated HIV-1 Tat protein basic domain rapidly translocates through the plasma membrane and accumulates in the cell nucleus. J. Biol. Chem. 272, 16010.

Wang, Y., Shi, W., Song, W., Wang, L., Liu, X., Jiang, C., et al., 2012. Tumor cell targeted delivery by specific peptide-modified mesoporous silica nanoparticles. J. Mater. Chem. 22, 14608–14616.

Wang, Y., Wang, K., Zhao, J., Liu, X., Bu, J., Yan, X., et al., 2013. Multifunctional mesoporous silica-coated graphene nanosheet used for chemo-photothermal synergistic targeted therapy of glioma. J. Am. Chem. Soc. 135, 4799–4804.
Wang, B., Lv, L., Wang, Z., Zhao, Y., Wu, L., Fang, X., et al., 2014. Nanoparticles functionalized with Pep-1 as potential glioma targeting delivery system via interleukin 13 receptor alpha2-mediated endocytosis. Biomaterials 35, 5897–5907.
Wang, Y., Lin, T., Zhang, W., Jiang, Y., Jin, H., He, H., et al., 2015a. A prodrug-type, MMP-2targeting nanoprobe for tumor detection and imaging. Theranostics 5, 787–795.
Wang, S., Meng, Y., Li, C., Qian, M., Huang, R., 2015b. Receptor-mediated drug delivery systems targeting to glioma. Nanomaterials 6, 3–19.
Wang, S., Li, C., Qian, M., Jiang, H., Shi, W., Chen, J., et al., 2017a. Augmented glioma-targeted theranostics using multifunctional polymer-coated carbon nanodots. Biomaterials 141, 29–39.
Wang, S., Reinhard, S., Li, C., Qian, M., Lächelt, U., Wagner, E., et al., 2017b. Antitumoral cascade-targeting ligand for IL-6 receptor-mediated gene delivery to glioma. Mol. Ther. 25, 1556–1566.
Wiley, D.T., Webster, P., Gale, A., Davis, M.E., 2013. Transcytosis and brain uptake of transferrin-containing nanoparticles by tuning avidity to transferrin receptor. Proc. Natl. Acad. Sci. USA 110, 8662–8667.
Wise, D.R., Thompson, C.B., 2010. Glutamine addiction: a new therapeutic target in cancer. Trends Biochem. Sci. 35, 427–433.
Wong, H.L., Chattopadhyay, N., Wu, X.Y., Bendayan, R., 2010. Nanotechnology applications for improved delivery of antiretroviral drugs to the brain. Adv. Drug Deliv. Rev. 62, 503–517.
Wunder, A., Stehle, G., Sinn, H., Schrenk, H., Hoffbiederbeck, D., Bader, F., et al., 1997. Enhanced albumin uptake by rat tumors. Int. J. Onocl. 11, 497–507.
Xie, H., Zhu, Y., Jiang, W., Zhou, Q., Yang, H., Gu, N., et al., 2011. Lactoferrin-conjugated superparamagnetic iron oxide nanoparticles as a specific MRI contrast agent for detection of brain glioma in vivo. Biomaterials 32, 495–502.
Xin, H., Sha, X., Jiang, X., Zhang, W., Chen, L., Fang, X., 2012. Anti-glioblastoma efficacy and safety of paclitaxel-loading Angiopep-conjugated dual targeting PEG-PCL nanoparticles. Biomaterials 33, 8167–8176.
Yang, Z.Z., Li, J.Q., Wang, Z.Z., Dong, D.W., Qi, X.R., 2014. Tumor-targeting dual peptides-modified cationic liposomes for delivery of siRNA and docetaxel to gliomas. Biomaterials 35, 5226–5239.
Ying, X., Wen, H., Lu, W.L., Du, J., Guo, J., Tian, W., et al., 2010. Dual-targeting daunorubicin liposomes improve the therapeutic efficacy of brain glioma in animals. J. Control. Release 141, 183–192.
Yoshikawa, T., Pardridge, W.M., 1992. Biotin delivery to brain with a covalent conjugate of avidin and a monoclonal antibody to the transferrin receptor. J. Pharmacol. Exp. Ther. 263, 897–903.
Yu, Y., Jiang, X., Gong, S., Feng, L., Zhong, Y., Pang, Z., 2014a. The proton permeability of self-assembled polymersomes and their neuroprotection by enhancing a neuroprotective peptide across the blood-brain barrier after modification with lactoferrin. Nanoscale 6, 3250–3258.
Yu, H., Lee, H., Herrmann, A., Buettner, R., Jove, R., 2014b. Revisiting STAT3 signaling in cancer: new and unexpected biological functions. Nat. Rev. Cancer 14, 736–746.
Yue, J., Liu, S., Wang, R., Hu, X., Xie, Z., Huang, Y., et al., 2012. Fluorescence-labeled immunomicelles: preparation, in vivo biodistribution, and ability to cross the blood-brain barrier. Macromol. Biosci. 12, 1209–1219.

Yue, P.J., He, L., Qiu, S.W., Li, Y., Liao, Y.J., Li, X.P., et al., 2014. OX26/CTX-conjugated PEGylated liposome as a dual-targeting gene delivery system for brain glioma. Mol. Cancer 13, 191.

Zamboni, W.C., Torchilin, V., Patri, A.K., Hrkach, J., Stern, S., Lee, R., et al., 2012. Best practices in cancer nanotechnology: perspective from NCI nanotechnology alliance. Clin. Cancer Res. 18, 3229–3241.

Zhan, C., Lu, W., 2012. The blood-brain/tumor barriers: challenges and chances for malignant gliomas targeted drug delivery. Curr. Pharm. Biotechnol. 13, 2380–2387.

Zhang, Y., Jeong, L.H., Boado, R.J., Pardridge, W.M., 2002. Receptor-mediated delivery of an antisense gene to human brain cancer cells. J. Gene Med. 4, 183–194.

Zhang, P., Hu, L., Yin, Q., Zhang, Z., Feng, L., Li, Y., 2012. Transferrin-conjugated polyphosphoester hybrid micelle loading paclitaxel for brain-targeting delivery: synthesis, preparation and in vivo evaluation. J. Control. Release 159, 429–434.

Zhang, B., Sun, X., Mei, H., Wang, Y., Liao, Z., Chen, J., et al., 2013. LDLR-mediated peptide-22-conjugated nanoparticles for dual-targeting therapy of brain glioma. Biomaterials 34, 9171–9182.

Zheng, C., Ma, C., Bai, E., Yang, K., Xu, R., 2015. Transferrin and cell-penetrating peptide dual-functioned liposome for targeted drug delivery to glioma. Int. J. Clin. Exp. Med. 8, 1658–1668.

Zitzmann, S., Ehemann, V., Schwab, M., 2002. Arginine-glycine-aspartic acid (RGD)-peptide binds to both tumor and tumor-endothelial cells in vivo. Cancer Res. 62, 5139–5143.

Zong, T., Mei, L., Gao, H., Shi, K., Chen, J., Wang, Y., et al., 2014a. Enhanced glioma targeting and penetration by dual-targeting liposome co-modified with T7 and TAT. J. Pharm. Sci. 103, 3891–3901.

Zong, T., Mei, L., Gao, H., Cai, W., Zhu, P., Shi, K., et al., 2014b. Synergistic dual-ligand doxorubicin liposomes improve targeting and therapeutic efficacy of brain glioma in animals. Mol. Pharm. 11, 2346–2357.

Nanotherapeutic strategies for the treatment of neurodegenerative diseases

13

Meng Huang, Xiao Gu, Xiaoling Gao
Department of Pharmacology and Chemical Biology, Faculty of Basic Medicine, Shanghai Jiao Tong University School of Medicine, Shanghai, China

1 Introduction

Neurodegenerative disease is an umbrella term for a range of diseases including Alzheimer's disease (AD), Parkinson's disease (PD), Huntington's disease (HD), etc. Neurodegenerative diseases occur when neurons in the central or peripheral nervous system progressively lose functions and eventually die. Available treatments at present only help relieve some of the physical or mental symptoms associated with neurodegenerative diseases, while there is currently no cure to slow disease progression. With relatively long disease course and high cost for medical care, neurodegenerative disease has become a tremendous burden for both families and society.

AD is the most common form of dementia as well as neurodegenerative disease. According to the World Alzheimer Report 2014, the number of people living with dementia is around 44 million worldwide and estimated to double in 2030 and triple by 2050. PD is the second common type of neurodegenerative disease. The number of individuals with PD over age 50 in world's 10 most populous nations countries was 4.1–4.6 million in 2005 and will double to 8.7–9.3 million by 2030 (Dorsey et al., 2007). The risk of being affected by AD and PD increases dramatically with age. As worldwide health improvements have increased life expectancy, more and more people may be affected by age-related neurodegenerative diseases in coming decades. This creates an urgent need to improve our understanding of pathogenesis of neurodegenerative diseases and develop new approaches for treatment and prevention.

Another major obstacle for the treatment of brain disease is the existence of blood-brain barrier (BBB), a physical barrier that protects brain from potential detrimental substances in circulation, significantly impeding most of the potential drugs from entering into the central nervous system (CNS). Hence, there is an urgent need to develop new therapeutic modalities that can overcome BBB and improve efficacy.

Many delivery strategies have been developed to solve this problem, among which nanoparticles (NPs) are of particular interest (Gregori et al., 2015). Nanoparticles have good stability, small size (3–200 nm), and can be mono or multi-functionalized by surface modification, which offer special advantages over free drug by increasing drug concentration at the target sites, reducing side effects to normal tissues, and improving

Brain Targeted Drug Delivery Systems. https://doi.org/10.1016/B978-0-12-814001-7.00013-5

the pharmacokinetic and pharmacodynamics profile of the marketed or clinically potential therapeutics; thereby enabling their promising application in brain drug delivery for the treatment of neurodegenerative diseases.

In this contribution, we briefly overview the nanotherapeutic strategies that have been developed to overcome BBB and review the recent advances in the application of nanotherapeutics for the treatment of AD and PD based on the understanding of pathogenesis of these two diseases.

2 Nanotherapeutic strategies to overcome blood-brain barrier

The BBB is composed of brain capillary endothelial cells (BCECs), basal lamina, pericytes, and astrocytes end feet (Zlokovic, 2008) (Fig. 1A). The translocation of molecules from circulation into brain parenchyma is very difficult due to the presence of tight junction formed by BCECs and active efflux pump like P-glycoprotein in BCECs. Several approaches have been studied to tackle this difficulty and are generalized as two major types, namely invasive and noninvasive approaches. The invasive approaches include intracerebroventricular injection/infusion (ICV), intracerebral implants, convection-enhanced diffusion (CED), and BBB disruption; the noninvasive approaches include lipid-mediated drug transport, carrier-mediated transcytosis (CMT), receptor-mediated transcytosis (RMT), adsorptive-mediated transcytosis (AMT), and intranasal administration (Bhaskar et al., 2010).

It is worth noting that alteration of BBB under disease condition has been reported by many studies. Such BBB disruption may include increased BBB permeability (Fig. 1B), transporter dysfunction, and decreased cerebral blood flow (Lacalle-Aurioles et al., 2014; Zlokovic, 2008). The altered BBB in neurodegenerative disease might be both beneficial and harmful for drug delivery. On the one hand, due to the increased BBB permeability and the reduced expression of efflux transporter, BBB under disease conditions might allow more brain entrance of substances, which is normally excluded, and increase their retention. On the other hand, the decreased cerebral blood flow as a function of the disease progress could greatly reduce brain drug distribution (McDade et al., 2014), especially for those drugs with high BBB permeability (Banks, 2012). Therefore, the pathological features of BBB in the different stages of neurodegenerative disease should be taken into concern when designing nanotherapeutic strategies to cross BBB.

2.1 *Invasive strategies*

ICV, intracerebral injection, and intracerebral implantation provide straightforward ways to overcome the BBB. But diffusion of drug into the brain parenchyma is minimal, leaving the injection site with a high drug concentration which might induce neurotoxicity. In contrast to diffusion, convection, which is driven by fluid pressure gradients that exist within tissue, is an effective delivery technique. Convection-enhanced delivery (CED), a bulk flow-driven process, possesses the advantages that

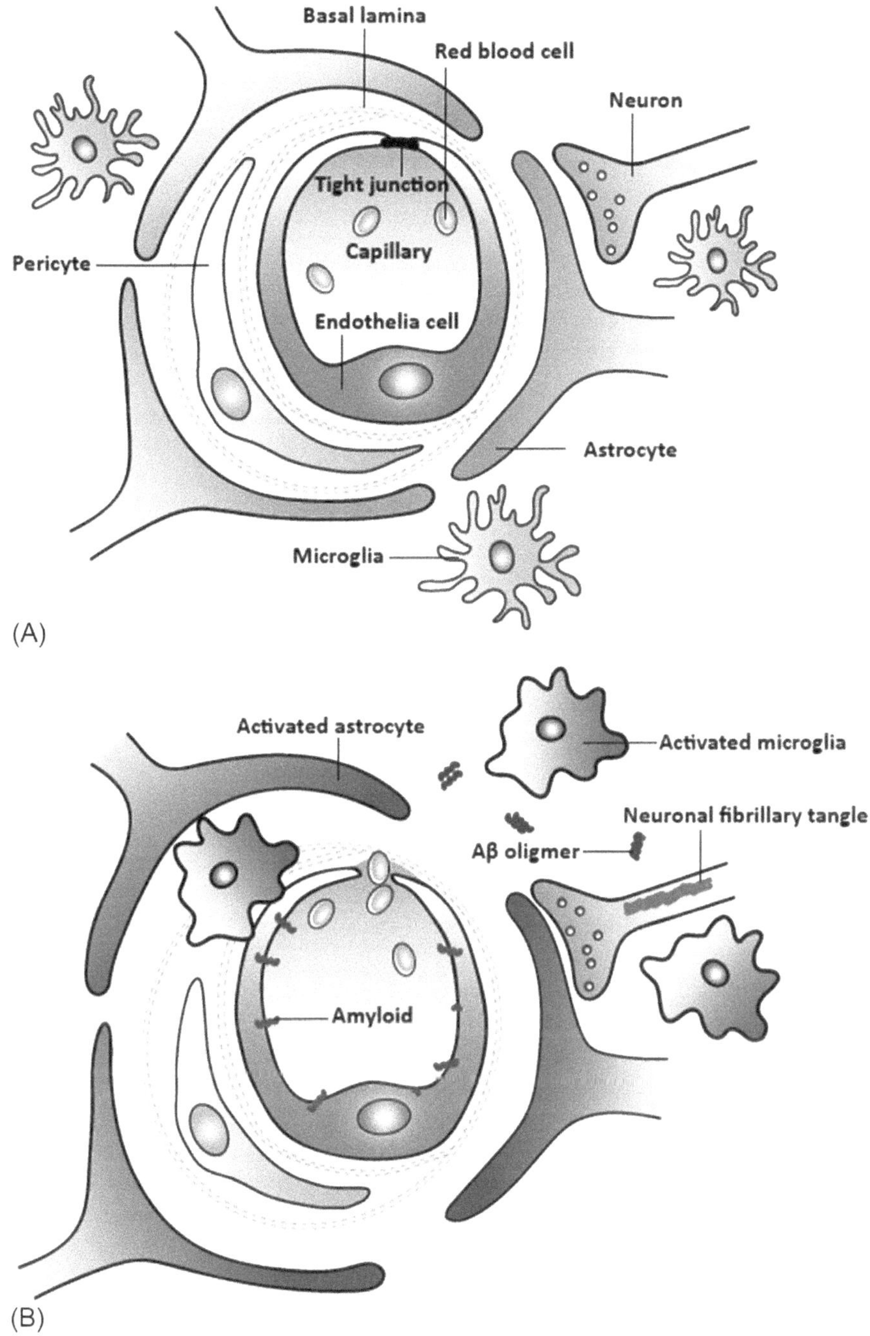

Fig. 1 Cellular constituents of blood-brain barrier under physical state (A) and AD pathological state (B). The barrier is formed by capillary endothelial cells, surrounded by basal lamina and astrocytic perivascular end feet. In AD, neurotoxic amyloid-β oligomers accumulated in the interstitial fluid (ISF), and BBB dysfunction leads to microhaemorrhages, increased deposition of perivascular amyloid, and activation of microglia and astrocytes.

include bypassing the BBB, targeted delivery, and reproducible diffusion (Lonser et al., 2015). This approach has been used for the brain delivery of peptide, siRNA, and NPs such as liposome, polymeric NP, and magnetite NP (Barua et al., 2012; Peng and Masliah, 2010; Perlstein et al., 2008; MacKay et al., 2005). CED enables targeted drug delivery to the disease-associated brain area with minimal systemic side effects. However, for the treatment of neurodegenerative diseases, drug delivery to the widespread lesions remains a severe challenge (Barua et al., 2014).

Besides, MRI-guided ultrasound-mediated BBB opening provides an alternative strategy for brain drug delivery by the reversible disruption of BBB integrity. In this case, microbubbles (ultrasound contrast agent) are injected into the blood stream, following the exposure to ultrasound, the BBB temperately opens, and therapeutic agents are administered during the period of BBB opening (Hynynen et al., 2006; Kinoshita et al., 2006). This approach has been applied to increase the brain delivery efficiency of small molecular compounds, large biomolecules, and even nanoparticles (Yao et al., 2014).

Although various therapeutic agents have been delivered into the brain by the aforementioned invasive approaches, these approaches suffer from high risk of side effects such as infection, edema, and neuron damage (Gabathuler, 2010; Pardridge, 2003). The safety concern, inconvenience, and relatively high expense have hindered their applications as standard therapeutic strategies for those CNS diseases which have relatively long disease process and need repeated administration.

2.2 Noninvasive strategies

To enable noninvasive brain drug delivery, liposomes, polymeric NPs, and solid-lipid NPs (SLN) are the most studied NPs, due to their biocompatibility, stability, limited antigenicity, and biodegradability. Moreover, they can be functionalized through surface modification and are suitable for delivery of both hydrophilic and hydrophobic drugs. The most common approach to facilitate the transportation of NPs from circulation to CNS is by taking advantage of the physiological mechanisms such as RMT and AMT. NPs aiming at crossing BBB through these two mechanisms require surface functionalization with targeting ligands or cationic molecules.

RMT is a well-studied mechanism for BBB crossing of NPs. There are three commonly targeted receptors on the BBB to mediate NPs transportation: transferrin receptor (TfR), lactoferrin receptor (LfR), and low-density lipoprotein receptor (LDLR). Ligands for these three receptors range from peptides screened via phage display, whole length, or specific binding fragment of their endogenous ligands to antibodies. For TfR targeting, Liu et al. utilized a peptide named B6 peptide (CGHKAKGPPK) selected from phage display as a substitute for transferrin and conjugated it to the poly(ethylene glycol)-poly(lactic acid) block copolymer (PEG-PLA) nanoparticles via a maleimide-thiol coupling. B6-modified PEG-PLA nanoparticles exhibited much higher brain accumulation comparing to unmodified nanoparticles after being intravenously injected to BALB/c nude mice (Liu et al., 2013b). The authors used this functionalized NP to deliver a neuroprotective peptide called NAP (NAPVSIPQ) for the treatment of AD. Administration of B6-NP-encapsulated NAP via tail vein injection into AD mouse models showed excellent amelioration in learning impairments, cholinergic disruption, and loss of hippocampal neurons (Liu et al., 2013b). Mourtas et al. synthesized a multifunctional liposome with lipid-PEG-curcumin derivative and decorated the liposome with a transferrin monoclonal antibody named OX26 for the treatment of AD. The OX26 functionalization significantly improved their intake by human brain capillary endothelial cells (Mourtas et al., 2014).

Lactoferrin is an endogenous ligand for LfR. Meng et al. reported a lactoferrin-modified low-density lipoprotein (LDL)-mimic nanostructured lipid carrier (NLC) for the brain-targeted delivery of curcumin. Lactoferrin was adsorbed onto the surface of NLC via electrostatic interaction with the negatively charged carboxylated PEG (100) monostearate (S100-COOH), which was previously anchored onto the surface of NLC. Such lactoferrin modification increased the cellular uptake by 1.39 folds in an in vitro BBB model (BCECs cell line) through an LfR-mediated process. Also, ex vivo imaging studies showed that lactoferrin-modified NLC effectively permeated the BBB and preferentially accumulated in the brain of Sprague-Dawley rats after intravenous injection (Meng et al., 2015).

For targeting LDLR, the endogenous ligand apoE and its derivatives are usually used. ApoE plays an important role in AD etiology and pathology, although the specific mechanism remains to be elucidated. For the treatment of AD, apoE can be used to target LDLR on BBB to facilitate BBB transport of NPs. For instance, Zensi et al. manufactured a human serum albumin nanoparticle, with recombinant apoE3 bound on the surface via a bifunctional Mal-PEG-NHS crosslinker. At 15 min or 30 min after intravenous injection in SV 129 mice, it was found that only the apoE-functionalized nanoparticles were detected in brain capillary endothelial cells and neurons, whereas nanoparticles without apoE was undetectable in the brain (Zensi et al., 2009). The LDLR targeting ability of apoE-derived peptide was reported by Ru et al. They showed that decorating liposomes with the monomer or the tandem dimer of mApoE, which was derived from the receptor-binding domain (a.a. residues 141-150) of human ApoE, enhanced their permeability across BBB both in vitro and in vivo (Bana et al., 2014; Re et al., 2011).

Coating NPs with polysorbate 80 (P-80) also facilitated BBB permeability (Kreuter, 2001). Wilson et al. showed that, in healthy rats, the brain concentration of intravenously injected rivastigmine can be enhanced by 3.82-fold when loaded in the poly(n-butylcyanoacrylate) nanoparticles coated with 1% P-80 (Wilson et al., 2008a). Mittal et al. further extended the usage of P-80 by showing that, compared with the incoated ones, orally administered P-80-coated estradiol-loaded PLGA nanoparticles resulted in significantly higher brain estradiol levels at 24 h after administration in the ovariectomized rat model that mimics the postmenopausal conditions (Mittal et al., 2011). The mechanisms of P-80 to facilitate BBB permeability are estimated to be related to its absorption of apolipoproteins (Kreuter et al., 2002) in the circulation and inhibition of the brain efflux system, especially P-glycoprotein (Kreuter, 2012). The apolipoproteins absorbed on P-80-coated NPs can mimic natural lipoprotein particles and interact with and then be taken up by the brain capillary endothelial cells via receptor-mediated endocytosis (Kreuter et al., 2002).

Manipulating the NPs surface charge toward positive has also been used to promote BBB transcytosis. The rationality is that the positively charged NPs trigger adsorptive-mediated transcytosis by interacting with the negatively charged endothelial cell surface. Chitosan is a biocompatible and biodegradable polymer that can enhance positive charge density on the NP surface at physiological pH. Jaruszewski et al. showed that chitosan enhanced the targeting capacity of immuno-nanovehicles to cerebrovascular amyloid deposits (Jaruszewski et al., 2012). As adsorptive-mediated transcytosis might also result in disruption of the BBB (Lockman et al., 2004), despite chitosan being relatively nontoxic and biocompatible (Kean and Thanou, 2010), the safety issue should be concerned when using this material.

Beside the above mechanisms, nasal administration offers an alternative approach for direct drug delivery to the brain bypassing the BBB via the nose-to-brain pathway. However, this strategy still needs improvement in absorption/retention of NPs on nasal mucosa as well as enhancement of the permeability. The aforementioned positively charged chitosan has also been used to facilitate NPs absorption following intranasal administration. Hanafy et al. synthesized galantamine hydrobromide/chitosan complex nanoparticles (CX-NP2) and showed that nasal-administrated CX-NP2 induced a significant decrease in AChE protein level and activity in rat brains than the oral- and nasal-dosed galantamine hydrobromide solutions (Hanafy et al., 2016). Wheat germ agglutinin (WGA) specifically binds to N-acetyl-d-glucosamine and sialic acid, which are abundant in the nasal cavity, and triggers absorptive-mediated transcytosis. Thus, WGA makes a good functional ligand to enhance the retention and permeability of NPs in nasal cavity (Berger et al., 2005). Gao et al. linked WGA to PLA-PEG NPs and found that, following intranasal administration, the brain accumulation of WGA-modified NPs in Sprague-Dawley rats was 100% higher than that of the unmodified ones (Gao et al., 2006, 2007a, b).

3 Pathology and therapeutic targets of neurodegenerative diseases

3.1 Pathology and therapeutic targets of AD

AD is clinically characterized by progressive loss of memory and impaired cognitive functions and histologically characterized by intracellular neurofibrillary tangles (NFTs) and extracellular amyloid plaques (Scheltens et al., 2016). NFTs are aggregates of hyperphosphorylated tau protein, which is a microtubule-associated protein (MAP), and amyloid plaques are aggregated proteins whose main component is a peptide with 40–42 amino acids named amyloid β (Aβ). Whether these histological changes are the causes or consequences of AD remains unclear, and the pathogenesis of AD is still unrevealed. Several hypotheses have been proposed to explain the pathogenesis of AD, including the Aβ cascade hypothesis, tau hypothesis, cholinergic hypothesis, oxidative stress hypothesis, metal hypothesis, neurovascular hypothesis, and so on, among which amyloid cascade hypothesis is the most popular one (Hardy and Selkoe, 2002; Mondragon-Rodriguez et al., 2013; ManafiRad et al., 2014).

3.1.1 Damage of cholinergic neuron

The current first-line therapy mainly comes from the cholinergic hypothesis, which is based on the presynaptic deficits found in the brains of patients with AD and studies of the role of acetylcholine in animal and human behavior (Bartus, 2000). Actually, a perturbation of cholinergic innervation is likely to be present even in the very early stages of AD. Although the pathological lesion of cholinergic neuron is unlikely to be a major determinant of the clinical symptoms, it certainly contributes to the severity of the cognitive and behavioral deficits, especially in the areas of memory and attention. The therapeutic strategy based on cholinergic hypothesis focuses much on the necessity to restore acetylcholine (Ach) to treat cognitive decline (Ferreira-Vieira et al., 2016). Following this, some therapeutic approaches for AD have been developed, among which the most developed one is cholinesterase inhibitors (ChEI), including donepezil, rivastigmine, and galantamine on market. They were the first type of pharmacotherapeutic agents to be approved for AD treatment, and still the first-line drugs currently (Camps and Munoz-Torrero, 2002). However, the therapeutic strategy to target cholinergic system is only a symptomatic treatment and cannot stop or slow the disease progression.

3.1.2 Amyloid cascade

Amyloid cascade hypothesis regards Aβ as a primary cause of AD, in which the accumulation of soluble Aβ into toxic oligomers and amyloid plaques initiates the pathogenic cascade, leading to tau protein hyperphosphorylation, intracellular neurofibrillary tangles, synaptic dysfunction, neuronal death, and, ultimately, loss of cognitive function (Hardy and Selkoe, 2002). Genetic, pathological, and biochemical evidence suggested that Aβ accumulation in the brain is induced by an imbalance between its production and clearance. Aβ are the hydrolysis products of amyloid precursor protein (APP) after the cleavage by β- and γ-secretase (Haass et al., 2012). $A\beta_{40}$ and $A\beta_{42}$ are the two major forms (Storey and Cappai, 1999): $A\beta_{40}$ accounts for almost 90% of the most abundant cleaved form of APP, which is nearly tenfold of $A\beta_{42}$, while $A\beta_{42}$ has a greater propensity to aggregate compared to $A\beta_{40}$. Based on the amyloid cascade hypothesis, therapeutics that can reduce Aβ production, prevent Aβ aggregation into plaques, promote Aβ clearance, lower its soluble levels in the brain, and dissemble the established plaques have been actively pursued as main strategies in the treatment of AD. Some therapeutics have been developed and tested preclinically or clinically, including β- or γ-secretase inhibitors that can prevent amyloidogenic cleavage of APP, peptide inhibitors that can inhibit Aβ fibrillogenesis, and anti-Aβ antibodies that can facilitate Aβ clearance (Graham et al., 2017).

Although Aβ is the most focused target for AD treatment, there are still some doubts about its role in AD pathology, especially after the clinical trials involving Aβ interference failed (ManafiRad et al., 2014).

3.1.3 Tau hyperphosphorylation

The tau hypothesis of AD pathogenesis is another widely accepted hypothesis. Tau hypothesis suggests that tau hyperphosphoralation, which results in the formation of neurofibrillary tangles, plays a central role in the progression of AD. The aggregation of Tau can be initiated or accelerated by the addition of seeds, and the seed can be transported from one neuron to another along the neural network of axons, resulting in the formation of new tangles at new locations, even throughout the brain in theory (Goedert et al., 2017). Due to the important role of tau in neurodegeneration, tau-targeted strategies including inhibition of tau phosphorylation, inhibition of tau aggregation, reduction of tau levels, tau immunization, and microtubule stabilization are of high interests to develop disease-modifying treatments for AD (Spillantini and Goedert, 2013).

3.1.4 Oxidative stress

Oxidative hypothesis of AD pathogenesis suggested that an increased reactive oxygen species (ROS) production and/or the decreased endogenous pool of antioxidants during aging has a strong relationship with the onset of AD. The excess oxygen species can damage various cellular structures including cellular membranes and cellular contents such as DNA, proteins, and carbohydrates, resulting in damage of cell function and viability (Padurariu et al., 2013). According to this, antioxidants like polyphenols and metal redox agents such as ceria have been studied for AD treatment (Massaad, 2011).

3.1.5 Metal ions

The transition metals such as copper, iron, and zinc play both supportive and toxic roles in the CNS (Dong et al., 2003). In AD patients, normal metal ion distribution in the CNS has been enormously altered (Ehmann et al., 1986). Compared with that in normal age-matched samples, concentrations of copper, zinc, and iron elevated by several-folds in AD brains (Bush, 2003). Copper, zinc, and iron are found enriched in senile plaques, which implicates that these metal ions are involved in Aβ aggregation and Aβ-associated toxicity (Bolognin et al., 2011). And after binding with oligomers and fibrils, these metal ions produced H_2O_2 and contributed to Aβ-induced oxidative stress in the CNS (Opazo et al., 2002). Based on this evidence, clioquinol, a hydrophobic Cu/Zn chelator, has been tested as a therapeutic strategy for AD by modulating metals level (Barcia et al., 2011).

3.1.6 Neurovascular pathways

Not only in the brain parenchyma, Aβ also deposit on the cerebral vascular wall to form cerebral amyloid angiopathy (CAA) (Fig. 1B) (Blennow et al., 2006). Epidemiological observations and experimental studies discovered that CAA was found in both AD and cerebral atherosclerosis and was associated with the development of cognitive deficits (Iadecola, 2010; Stanimirovic and Friedman, 2012). These studies challenged the common view that pathology of AD starts from neuron and brought out the two-hit vascular hypothesis of AD pathogenesis. This hypothesis proposes that cerebrovascular damage (hit 1) can lead to accumulation of neurotoxins and hypoperfusion, resulting in neuronal injury, and influence the amyloidogenic pathway, leading to elevated Aβ levels in the brain (hit 2) (Nelson et al., 2016). These two pathways can work independently and/or synergistically on the AD pathogenesis. According to this hypothesis, vasculoprotective approaches that can restore neurovascular functions or protect the neurovascular system from pathological changes may have potential for the disease-modifying intervention of AD. The supposed strategies include the pharmacological regulation of key receptors or proteins such as LRP1 to restore Aβ transport on BBB and activated protein C (APC) to stabilize the microvessel, etc.

3.1.7 Microglia

One of the histological features of AD is the presence of a group of reactive astrocytes and microglia around Aβ plaques, which is characterized as microgliosis and astrogliosis. Microglia are resident phagocytes in the brain and have been recognized to participate in brain maintenance through scavenging cellular debris and plagues, releasing neurotrophic factors, and also play an important role in shaping synaptic connection. Considering AD is an age-related disease, aging-associated weakening of these function have been paid attention to in AD pathogenesis. The direct evidence to link microglia with AD pathogenesis comes from the genome-wide association study (GWAS) that identified loss-of-function variants of *TREM2* (which encodes triggering receptor expressed on myeloid cells 2, TREM2) as a major genetic risk for AD (Guerreiro et al., 2013; Jonsson et al., 2013). In the brain, TREM2 is expressed highly and exclusively by microglial cells (Zhang et al., 2014c). Studies on AD model mice showed that *TREM2*-deficient microglia appeared to be unresponsive to the Aβ plaques around them (Wang et al., 2015), which may exacerbate the Aβ pathology. Although some progress has been made, how *TREM2* variants lead to the onset of AD still remains to be elucidated. The current understanding of the role which microglia plays in AD pathogenesis suggests that enhancing microglial function may have therapeutic benefit at the early stage.

Overall, AD is likely to be caused by copathogenic interactions with multiple factors involved. It has been widely accepted that the secondary pathological processes such as dysfunction of synapse and neuron loss could independently aggravate the severity of AD. Hence, the development of novel multifunctional therapeutics that can address the varied pathological aspects of the disease represents a promising strategy for AD therapy.

3.2 Pathology and therapeutic targets of PD

The symptomatology of PD is recognized to be heterogeneous, with motor features including bradykinesia, rigidity, and rest tremor, and nonmotor features including olfactory dysfunction, sleep disorders, and cognitive impairment (Kalia and Lang, 2015).

The loss of dopamine (DA) neurons within substantia nigra pars compacta (SNpc), a basal ganglia structure located in the midbrain, and the Lewy pathology are thought to be the hallmarks of PD. Lewy pathology is characterized by proteinaceous inclusions mainly composed of abnormally folded and aggregated α-synuclein within the neuronal cell body (Lewy bodies) and neurites (Lewy neurites).

The loss of dopaminergeric neurons in SNpc can lead to reduced supplement of the neurotransmitter dopamine to the brain striatum, resulting in the major motor symptoms in PD patients. The current available and the first-line therapy for PD, dopamine replacement therapy, is to decrease the degradation of dopamine and increase the stimulation of dopamine receptors in the brain in order to relief the motor symptoms. As dopamine does not cross the BBB, the therapeutic strategies are to use the dopamine precursor. Medications include levodopa, dopamine agonist, and MAO B inhibitors. However, long-term use of these drugs is associated with side effects such as dyskinesia and wearing-off effects, and these drugs are just symptomatic treatments that are unable to slow or stop the neurodegeneration process. The ultimate goal is to develop disease-modifying therapy for the treatment of PD and the understanding of pathogenesis can provide the potential therapeutic targets for this purpose.

Two centuries after the first description by James Parkinson, PD is now considered to be a complex neurodegenerative disease while the etiology and pathogenesis are still not fully understood. With the aid from recent advancement in sequencing technology, the disease is now considered to be resulted from a combination of genetic and environmental factors (Kalia and Lang, 2015). The elucidation of predisposing genes of PD has given some insights on the pathogenesis of PD. At present, α-synuclein transmission, loss of trophic support, neuroinflammation, and several cellular processes like mitochondrial dysfunction, disrupted autophagy or lysosomal process, and dysregulation of calcium homeostasis have been considered to be related to the pathogenesis of PD (Lotharius and Brundin, 2002). Some of them that are considered to be therapeutic targets will be discussed below.

3.2.1 α-synuclein

The α-synuclein is the main protein accumulated and aggregated in Lewy bodies (LBs) and Lewy neurites (LNs). As mutations or multiplications of the gene encoding α-synuclein (*SNCA*) have been associated with familial forms and even some sporadic forms of PD (Tofaris and Spillantini, 2007), the pathogenic role of this protein in its aggregated forms has been proposed (Lashuel et al., 2013). The oligomerization (Conway et al., 1998) and fibril growth (Taschenberger et al., 2012) of α-synuclein are considered to be toxic. However, the molecular mechanisms by which α-synuclein aggregation contributes to neuronal cell loss and cellular processes affected by α-synuclein remain unknown. Still, therapeutic approaches targeting α-synuclein have been pursued as the disease-modifying therapy of PD. The possible therapeutic strategies include inhibiting the transmission, production, and aggregation and enhancing α-synuclein clearance.

Lewy pathology in PD is hypothesized to progress in a pattern called Braak staging, starting in the peripheral nervous system and progressively affecting the central nervous system in a caudal-to-rostral direction within the brain (Kalia and Lang, 2015). This may partially be explained by the in vitro and in vivo findings that α-synuclein can transmit between neurons, which bring the presumption that PD is a prion-like disease (Visanji et al., 2013). Inhibiting α-synuclein transmission seems to be promising to stop neurodegeneration; however, there is no effective strategy to prevent its propagation currently. Instead, inhibition of α-synuclein production via gene therapy has been tested in the treatment of PD, and nanotechnology may aid to it by constructing delivery system with higher safety/efficiency than traditional viral vectors.

Enhancement of α-synuclein clearance via immune system by immunization against α-synuclein or via its physiological pathways is another promising strategy. Studies on transgenic mice overexpressing human α-synuclein showed that both active and passive immunization with monoclonal antibodies against α-synuclein facilitated reduction and clearance of α-synuclein and rescued behavioral deficits in these mice (Masliah et al., 2005, 2011).

The physiological pathways to clear intracellular α-synuclein are through the ubiquitin-proteasome or autophagy-lysosomal systems. As revealed by genetic and pathological discoveries, defects in these systems have been identified in patients with PD (Kalia and Lang, 2015). Therefore, therapeutic modulation of some of the components in these two systems is promising in PD treatment: (1) Parkin is an E3 ubiquitin ligase that is involved in the degradation of misfolded or damaged proteins by the ubiquitin-proteasome pathway (Doherty et al., 2013; Giasson and Lee, 2001). The mutation in *parkin* (or *PARK2*), which encode parkin, is the most common cause of autosomal recessive PD with a mean age of onset of about 28 years (Doherty et al., 2013). Therapeutic strategies to correct this pathology have been proposed (Tardiff et al., 2013); (2) Chaperone-mediated autophagy (CMA) is possibly responsible for degradation of α-synuclein via autophagy-lysosomal pathway. Reduced expression of lysosomal-associated membrane protein type 2A (LAMP2A) and hsc70, both of which are the main components in CMA process, in dopaminergic cell lines leads to reduced level of chaperone-mediated autophagy and decreased clearance of wild-type α-synuclein (Alvarez-Erviti et al., 2010). Furthermore, pathogenic mutants of α-synuclein block CMA and impair its own degradation (Martinez-Vicente et al., 2008). These studies support the idea that stimulation of CMA pathway may enhance α-synuclein clearance; (3) Mutations in the glucocerebrosidase gene (*GBA*), which encode β-glucocerebrosidase (GCase) that is involved in regulation of lysosomal function and α-synuclein folding, are observed in up to 25% of patients with early-onset PD (Duran et al., 2013). The GCase targeting therapeutic strategies were encouraged by the finding that restoration of activity in *GBA*-knockout mice through adeno-associated viral vector reduced α-synuclein levels (Sardi et al., 2013).

3.2.2 Oxidative stress

Similar with that in AD, oxidative stress also plays an important role in the pathogenesis of PD. The dopaminergic neurons seem to be especially venerable to oxidative stress, as being supported by the finding that 6-hydroxydopamine (6-OHDA) destroys dopaminergic neurons following stereotaxic injection into the substantia nigra (Ungerstedt et al., 1974). The oxidative stress in PD results from the failure of or defect in endogenous antioxidative protection, dopamine metabolism, mitophagy, and accumulation of mutation mitochondrial DNA (Athauda and Foltynie, 2015). Reduction of the oxidative stress may represent promising disease-modifying strategies for PD. The antioxidants such as rasagiline, vitamin E, resveratrol, urate, etc. are of interests. Besides, dopamine can be transformed by monoamine oxidase (MAO) into the nontoxic metabolite and hydrogen peroxide (Lotharius and Brundin, 2002). Prevention of this process by MAO inhibitors may reduce the oxidative stress results from dopamine metabolism. Actually, the MAO B inhibitors are among the current first-line drugs for the treatment of PD, with the main purpose to suppress the degradation and increase the concentration of dopamine. Iron accumulation may also contribute to the oxidative stress in PD, as suggested by the finding of excessive iron accumulation in the SNpc of some PD patients (Sian-Hulsmann et al., 2011). And iron chelator showed neuroprotective activity in 6-OHDA-induced animal model of PD (Dexter et al., 2011). Metal analysis showed that the use of calcium channel blockers is associated with reduced risk of PD (Noyce et al., 2012), which could balance the disturbed calcium homeostasis in SNpc and reduce the oxidative stress in mitochondria (Surmeier and Schumacker, 2013). Thus, calcium channel blockers may also benefit PD patients.

3.2.3 Mitochondrial function

The mitochondrial dysfunction is linked to PD as evidenced by discoveries from postmortem, animal, and genetic studies: complex I deficiency in the substantia nigra was found in patients died with PD (Schapira et al., 1990); mitotoxic drugs such as 1-methyl-4-phenyl-1,2,3,6-tetrahydropyridine (MPTP) can cause parkinsonism; and mutations in *parkin*, *DJ-1* (also as *PARK7*), and *PINK1*, which encode proteins that are all related to mitochondrial heath, can cause autosomal recessive forms of PD. Parkin, as mentioned before, and PINK1 are the major components in mitophagy, and DJ-1 is presumed to be protective against oxidative stress (Guzman et al., 2010). Thus, elevating the mitochondrial levels or enhancing the mitochondrial function may meet the energy demand of neurons and slow the neurodegenerative process in PD. The activation of PGC-1α-PPARγ-SIRT1 network to control mitochondrial function and upregulate its biogenesis is of particular interests for the treatment of PD (Carta and Pisanu, 2013).

3.2.4 LRRK2 kinase

Leucine-rich repeat kinase 2 (LRRK2), which is encoded by *LRRK2* (or *PARK8*), is a multifunctional protein kinase that includes a GTPase domain. Mutation in *LRRK2* is the most common cause of autosomal dominant PD (Kalia and Lang, 2015) and is also associated with sporadic PD. Although some progress on the understanding of LRRK2 function has been made, the specific role of LRRK2 in PD pathogenesis has yet to be identified. LRRK2 is now recognized to participate in the autophagy-lysosomal pathway, endosome formation by interacting with Rab GTPases, mitochondria fission and fusion process, microtubule dynamics, and upregulation of microglial inflammation via the nuclear factor kappa-B (NF-κB) pathway (Chan and Tan, 2017). The most prevalent pathogenic mutations of *LRRK2* can cause increased phosphorylation of LRRK2. Thus, inhibition of LRRK2 kinase has now been pursued as a promising strategy to modify the defected function with LRRK2 mutations. Studies on pluripotent cells derived from patients with mutations in LRRK2 and PINK1 showed that LRRK2 kinase inhibitors can protect these neurons from toxins-induced mitochondrial deficits (Cooper et al., 2012).

3.2.5 Trophic factors

Trophic factors are proteins that can promote cell growth and viability. The glial cell line-derived neurotrophic factor (GDNF) is of particular interest in PD treatment since the landmark observation demonstrated that GDNF could support the viability of midbrain dopaminergic neurons in tissue culture (Lin et al., 1993a) and several in vivo studies confirmed the ability of GDNF to prevent degeneration of dopaminergic neurons in 6-OHDA- and MPTP-lesioned animals (Kordower and Bjorklund, 2013). However, double-blind clinical trials in which growth factors or their genes were administered or delivered directly into the cerebral ventricle or putamen did not show any benefit (Nutt et al., 2003; Marks et al., 2010). The possible explanation is the limit distribution of therapeutics to the target region or their impaired transportation from the injection site to the substantia nigra pars compacta because of axonal degeneration or dysfunction, etc. (Schapira et al., 2014). Strategies to overcome such drawbacks are of high potential for the disease-modifying therapy of PD.

4 Nanotherapeutic strategies for the treatment of AD

4.1 Nanotherapeutic strategies targeting cholinergic system

The progress of AD is followed by degeneration of cholinergic neurons and the associated loss of cholinergic neurotransmission (Francis et al., 1999). Cholinesterase inhibitors (ChEIs) including donepezil, rivastigmine, and galantamine, which can reduce the hydrolysis of ACh and increase the availability of ACh consequently, have been approved by FDA for AD treatment (Standridge, 2004). They were the first type of therapeutic agents to be approved for AD treatment and still the first-line drugs now (Camps and Muñoz-Torrero, 2002). However, the poor pharmacokinetics of ChEIs as well as their limited BBB permeability limits their efficacy. For example, rivastigmine has extensive first-pass metabolism and the plasma elimination half-life is of 1.5 h, which lead to its low oral bioavailability (Tse and Laplanche, 1998). To overcome such drawbacks, different types of nanoparticles have been studied for brain delivery of ChEIs.

In order to increase the brain concentration of intravenously injected tacrine and rivastigmine, Wilson et al. constructed polysorbate 80-coated poly(n-butylcyanoacrylate) nanoparticles for drug delivery. It was found that in the brain a significant increase in rivastigmine/tacrine distribution was achieved compared to the free drug (Wilson et al., 2008a,b). In another study, in order to increase the bioavailability of galantamine at the target site, solid-lipid nanoparticles were developed to deliver galantamine hydrobromide (GH) (Misra et al., 2016). The obtained nanoparticles offered approximately twice bioavailability to that of free drug and demonstrated significant improved memory restoration capability in cognitive deficit rats.

4.2 Nanotherapeutic strategies targeting Aβ metabolism

Based on the Aβ cascade hypothesis, several Aβ-targeted nanotherapeutic strategies have been pursued, including modulation of Aβ production, inhibition of Aβ aggregation, and enhancement of Aβ clearance.

4.2.1 Strategies for Aβ-binding nanoparticles

A successful therapeutic strategy should specifically direct to the pathological sites to improve drug efficacy and reduce potential side effects. Giving that Aβ aggregation is a major hallmark as well as the key pathogenic cascade in AD, nanotherapeutic strategies with high affinity for Aβ are actively sought after. Through the direct interaction between Aβ and its ligand co-delivered with drugs, drugs can accumulate at the surrounding of Aβ aggregates and resist to the diffusion throughout the brain, and Aβ aggregation/disaggregation features may be interfered in a therapeutic way. The ligands for Aβ include antibodies, peptides, lipids, and even small molecules such as curcumin.

Immunotherapy against Aβ can inhibit Aβ deposition and clear already existing Aβ plaques in different transgenic AD mouse models (DeMattos et al., 2001). Antibody-decorated liposomes can thus act as promising vehicles for AD treatment with their relatively high stability and specific targeting profile. Canovi et al. developed a nanoparticle by conjugating nanoliposomes with an anti-Aβ monoclonal antibody (Aβ-MAb) (Canovi et al., 2011), in which the liposomes were prepared from DSPC, phosphatidylcholine, and DSPE-PEG_{2000} via thin film hydration, and then attached with Aβ monoclonal antibody (Aβ-MAb) to the surface through the biotin-streptavidin interaction. The binding affinity (indicated by K_D) of these immunoliposomes with $Aβ_{42}$ monomers and fibrils was 2.1 and 1.6 nM, respectively. Moreover, in postmortem AD brain samples, these Aβ-MAb-liposomes were found to be able to bind amyloid deposits, indicating that these immunoliposomes have the potential to target $Aβ_{42}$ for diagnostic or therapeutic applications.

Zhang et al. utilized QSHYRHISPAQV (QSH), a D-enantiomeric peptide with high affinity to $Aβ_{42}$, screened using a mirror-image phage display, for the development of a dual-functional nanoparticle drug delivery system (Zhang et al., 2014a,b; Zheng et al., 2017). This nanoparticle (denoted as TQNP) was prepared from maleimide-PEG-PLA and methoxy-PEG-PLA via the emulsion/solvent evaporation method, followed by the conjugation with two targeting peptides, TGN and QSH. TGN acted as a ligand for targeting the BBB, while QSH recognized $Aβ_{42}$. TQNP was found to exhibit improved and precise targeted delivery to amyloid depositions in the brain of AD model mice (Zhang et al., 2014a).

It has been shown that curcumin, a polyphenol compound and a major component of the yellow curry spice turmeric, presents potent antioxidant and anti-inflammatory activities (Shen and Yu, 2008) and is also able to bind Aβ and disaggregate Aβ plaques, as well as prevent fibril and oligomer formation (Lim et al., 2001; Durairajan et al., 2008; Reinke and Gestwicki, 2007). Taylor et al. reported that liposomes decorated (on their surface) with curcumin derivatives with planar structure showed very high binding affinity to fibrillary $A\beta_{42}$ (1-5 nM) in vitro (Mourtas et al., 2011). Moreover, these decorated liposomes were able to inhibit the formation of fibrillary and/or oligomeric Aβ in vitro (Taylor et al., 2011).

Monosialoteterahexosyl ganglioside (GM1) was found to bind Aβ with high affinity (Yanagisawa et al., 1995). Such observation led to investigation of whether other anionic lipids can interact with Aβ. Gobbi et al. identified phosphatidic acid (PA) and cardiolipin (CL), both are anionic phospholipids as suitable $A\beta_{42}$ ligands (Gobbi et al., 2010). Liposomes and solid-lipid nanoparticles functionalized with PA or CL and showed affinity for $A\beta_{42}$ fibrils (22–60 nM) (Gobbi et al., 2010). Interestingly, it is noted that lower percentage of (2.5–5 mol%) PA or CL incorporation allows better interaction with Aβ than higher percentage (20 mol% of the same lipid) (Ahyayauch et al., 2012).

4.2.2 Targeting Aβ production

The amyloidogenic Aβ monomer is derived from proteolytic processing of APP. The β-secretase BACE1 (β-site APP-cleaving enzyme 1) is a protease for the cleavage of APP. BACE1 and γ-secretase work together to produce β amyloid peptide, which can aggregate terminally. Targeting Aβ production by the secretase inhibitors is one way widely pursued for AD treatment. Although γ-secretase inhibitors can remarkably reduce Aβ production, they are not suitable for clinical application as APP is not the only substrate of γ-secretase and they have been found to result in serious gastrointestinal and immunological side effects (Aguzzi and O'Connor, 2010). In contrast, the deletion of BACE1 does not induce an overt effect on phenotype in mice (Luo et al., 2001), suggesting that BACE1 inhibitors might serve as potent therapeutic candidates for AD treatment without noticeable toxicity.

BACE1 siRNA has been investigated to silence BACE1 mRNA and reduced the expression of BACE1 protein. To realize its therapeutic potential, efficient, tissue-specific, and nonimmunogenic delivery technologies must be developed. Shyam et al. utilized a linear polyethyleneimine (LPEI)-*g*-PEG copolymer-based micellar nanoparticle system for intraventricular delivery of siRNA targeting BACE1 and APP. The encapsulation of siRNA by LPEI-*g*-PEG carriers, with different grafting degrees of PEG, leads to the formation of micellar nanoparticles with distinct morphologies. They found that the rod-shaped nanoparticles achieved the most efficient knockdown of BACE1 in the brain following ICV (Shyam et al., 2015).

Modified exosomes have also been used as nanocarriers for brain-targeting delivery of BACE1 siRNA (Alvarez-Erviti et al., 2011). Exosomes are membrane-bound nano-vesicles secreted by most cell types, with a dimension ranging from 40 to 100 nm. The content of exosomes varies and can include mRNAs, proteins, and lipids, which can be transported from host to recipient cells to affect cellular function. The capability of exosomes to serve as vesicles for bioactive molecules and their role in intercellular communication make them a potential platform for drug delivery. Exosomes are able to be used in their native forms isolated from cultured cells as well as being used with modification (Ferguson and Nguyen, 2016). Alvarez-Erviti et al. harvested bone marrow from inbred C57BL/6 mice and selected immature dendritic cells to produce nonimmunogenic exosomes. Targeting was achieved by engineering the dendritic cells to express Lamp2b, an exosomal membrane protein, fused to the neuron-specific rabies viral glycoprotein peptide. Purified exosomes were loaded with exogenous siRNA by electroporation. The therapeutic potential of exosome-mediated siRNA delivery was demonstrated by the strong mRNA (60%) and protein (62%) knockdown of BACE1 in C57BL/6 mice (Alvarez-Erviti et al., 2011). Such exosome-mediated in vivo siRNA delivery showed exciting potential in modulation of Aβ production.

Liu et al. showed another example to modulate Aβ production by targeting Rho-associated kinas-II (ROCK-II). ROCK is a serine/threonine kinase involved in many aspects of neuronal function such as axon regeneration (Yang et al., 2010). ROCK includes two types of isomers: ROCK-I and ROCK-II, while ROCK-II is abundantly expressed in the brain. Targeted knockdown of ROCK-II with siRNA decreases LR11 ectodomain shedding and simultaneously increases intracellular LR11 protein levels, which results in a decrease of Aβ production (Herskowitz et al., 2011). Liu et al. utilized PEG-PEI co-polymer to overcome the poor intracellular uptake and limited blood stability of siRNA and to mediate the delivery of ROCK-II-siRNA into C17.2 neural stem cells in vitro, finding that PEG-PEI/ROCK-II-siRNA complexes effectively suppressed ROCK-II mRNA expression (Liu et al., 2013a). However, the potential of PEG-PEI/ROCK-II-siRNA complexes for AD treatment still need further in vivo verification.

4.2.3 Targeting Aβ clearance

The imbalance between the production and clearance is suggested to cause Aβ deposition. Especially, recent studies found that the common late-onset form of AD is characterized by an overall impairment in Aβ clearance, but not in Aβ production (Mawuenyega et al., 2010). Such evidences suggested that the enhancement of Aβ clearance may represent a promising strategy for AD therapy (Cramer et al., 2012). One therapeutic approach proposed for the reduction of CNS Aβ is immunotherapy, which is to utilize Aβ-specific antibodies passively administrated (Bard et al., 2000) or actively raised by Aβ vaccination (Morgan et al., 2000). Another approach is through "sink effect", which means that by peripheral sequestration of Aβ, the equilibrium between brain and plasma Aβ pools may be pulled toward the peripheral blood circulation, eventually drawing out the excess Aβ from the brain and/or from the brain vessels. DeMattos et al. reported that peripheral administration of a monoclonal anti-Aβ antibody to transgenic AD mice models resulted in an increase of Aβ in the plasma, despite minimal entry of the antibody into the brain (DeMattos et al., 2001). Matsuoka et al. further showed that certain compounds that are unrelated to antibodies, but have the ability to bind Aβ in the periphery, also effectively reduced brain Aβ via altering the periphery/brain dynamics (Matsuoka et al., 2003). Because there are several safety issues associated with immunotherapy (Liu et al., 2012), non-antibody compounds with high affinity to Aβ might become a promising therapeutic candidate for AD treatment. Re et al. constructed liposomes from sphingomyelin and cholesterol, bi-functionalized them with phosphatidic acid and a peptide (CWG-LRKLRKRLLR) that was derived from the receptor-binding domain (a.a. residues 141–150) of human apoE, and named them mApoE-PA-LIP (Mancini et al., 2016). In a transwell BBB cell culture model, they observed a strongly enhanced (5-fold) efflux of Aβ oligomers, but not of Aβ fibrils, from the "brain" side to the "blood" side in presence of mApoE-PA-LIP. In contrast, the Aβ oligomer efflux was limited when mApoE-PA-LIP was loaded in the brain side, which suggested that the enhanced efflux of Aβ oligomer could be due to peripheral mApoE-PA-LIP by sink effect. They further showed that intraperitoneal administration of mApoE-PA-LIP significantly increased the plasma Aβ level in APP/PS1 mice (Mancini et al., 2016). Moreover, mApoE-PA-LIP has been showed by the same group to cross the BBB and affect Aβ aggregation/disaggregation features (Bana et al., 2014).

4.2.4 *Targeting Aβ aggregation*

Aggregation of Aβ monomer into toxic oligomeric and insoluble aggregates has been shown to be highly related with the progression of AD. Blocking the formation of these Aβ aggregates could potentially slow and even prevent AD progression (Heffern et al., 2014; Churches et al., 2014).

Peptide and peptide mimetics are two main types of Aβ inhibitors (Tjernberg et al., 1996; Frydman-Marom et al., 2009). Short peptides containing the core sequence KLVFF, the $A\beta_{16\text{-}20}$ amino acid sequence, can act as anti-amyloid agents. However, the rapid degradation of the peptides in plasma and poor BBB permeability are the major challenges for their application (Liu et al., 2009b). Polyoxometalates (POMs) are a class of early-transition-metaloxygen-anion nanoclusters that can also inhibit Aβ aggregation. However, this inhibition is a non-specific electrostatic interaction, which might also inhibit the aggregation of larger Aβ assemblies and aggravate soluble oligomer-derived toxicity. To solve this problem, Li et al. developed a novel strategy by preparing polyoxometalate-peptide (POM@P) hybrid particles from POMs and $A\beta_{15\text{-}20}$ peptide via a straightforward self-assembly process (Li et al., 2013). The obtained two-in-one bifunctional POM@P nanoparticles showed enhanced targeted inhibition of Aβ-peptide aggregation in vitro.

As previously mentioned, curcumin presents potent antioxidant and anti-inflammatory activities (Shen and Yu, 2008) and is also able to bind Aβ and prevent fibril and oligomer formation (Lim et al., 2001; Durairajan et al., 2008; Reinke and Gestwicki, 2007). However, due to its poor aqueous solubility and propensity of being degraded in acidic, basic, and oxidative conditions, the poor bioavailability of curcumin following oral administration remained an obstacle for its application

(Sharma et al., 2005). To overcome such drawbacks, Mathew et al. synthesized water-soluble curcumin-loaded nanoparticles by using PLGA as the polymer matrix (Mathew et al., 2012). Nanoparticle was conjugated with Tet-1 peptide which possesses the affinity to neurons and the ability of retrograde transportation. The obtained curcumin-encapsulated nanoparticles were found to destroy amyloid aggregates and show antioxidative activity without inducing cytotoxicity in vitro.

AuNPs have also shown the ability to inhibit Aβ aggregation, but lacking specificity. In a study performed by Kogan et al., AuNPs were linked to the peptide H-Cys-Leu-Pro-Phe-Phe-AspNH2 (Cys-PEP) which can selectively attach to the Aβ aggregates (Kogan et al., 2006). This AuNP-Cys-PEP nanoparticle was applied to dissolve $A\beta_{42}$ aggregates and interfere with their growth, by using the local heat dissipated by AuNP attached to the Aβ aggregates and irradiated with low gigahertz electromagnetic fields. This method can be manipulated locally and remotely without any bulk heating. However, further investigations in real biosystems are needed.

4.3 Nanotherapeutic strategies targeting transition metal ions

Metal chelators can bind to metal ions and convert the metal ions into an inert form, thus reducing the total pool of bioavailable metals and lessen their interaction with Aβ. Results from postmortem AD brain tissues showed that following proper incubation, metal chelators can resolubilize Aβ depositions to the aqueous form (Cherny et al., 2000). However, the hepatotoxicity, poor BBB penetration, and potential neurotoxicity limit the utility of chelators for AD therapy (Liu et al., 2005).

Liu et al. synthesized a nanoparticle-chelator conjugate (Nano-N2PY) by conjugating an iron chelator 2-methyl-N-(2′-aminoethyl)-3-hydroxyl-4-pyridinone (MAEHP) with carboxylic-functionalized polystyrene nanoparticles (Liu et al., 2009a). The Nano-N2PY was showed to inhibit Aβ-associated cytotoxicity in human cortical neuronal cells and exhibit no significant adverse effects on cell growth/proliferation. In another study, Cui et al. covalently conjugated D-Penicillamine, a FDA-approved copper chelator for the treatment of Wilson's disease and rheumatoid arthritis, to 1,2-Dioleoyl-sn-glycero-3-phosphoethanolamine-N-[4-(p -maleimidophenyl)butyramide] (MPB-PE) and 1,2-dioleoyl-sn-glycero-3-phosphoethanolamine-N-[3-(2-pyridyldithio)propionate] (PDP-PE) NPs via a disfide bond or a thioether bond (Cui et al., 2005). These NP formulations showed long circulation in the blood (Lockman et al., 2003b) and efficient brain uptake in situ and in vivo with no significant changes to the BBB integrity (Lockman et al., 2003a). The D-penicillamine-conjugated NPs effectively resolubilized copper-$A\beta_{42}$ aggregates under reducing conditions in vitro. However, the above studies are preliminary and further investigations in real biosystems are needed to determine the exact outcomes.

4.4 Nanotherapeutic strategies targeting oxidative stress

Oxidative stress reflects an imbalance between the overproduction/incorporation of reactive oxygen species (ROS) and the ability of a body to detoxify them. ROS affects both the structure and function of neurons and contributes to a wide range of neurodegenerative diseases, including PD and AD (Padurariu et al., 2013). Based on this oxidative stress hypothesis, antioxidants like ceria nanoparticles and polyphenols have been studied for AD treatment.

4.4.1 Ceria nanoparticles targeting oxidative stress

Ceria (CeO_2) nanoparticles are known to exhibit ROS-scavenging activity in a recyclable way by reversible binding of oxygen atoms and shuttling between the Ce^{3+} (reduced) and Ce^{4+} (oxidized) states on their surface (Karakoti et al., 2009). In order to reduce abnormal generation of ROS resulted from mitochondrial dysfunction, Kwon et al. synthesized triphenylphosphonium-conjugated ceria nanoparticles (TPP-ceria NPs) (Kwon et al., 2016). TPP is a lipophilic cation that is capable of targeting mitochondria by taking advantage of negative mitochondrion membrane potential. Both in vitro and in vivo experiments showed that TPP-ceria NPs were biocompatible and can reduce oxidative stress by scavenging mitochondrial ROS. The authors further studied the effects of TPP-Ceria NPs for AD treatment in a 5XFAD transgenic AD mouse model, finding that the TPP-ceria NPs efficiently mitigated the reactive gliosis and suppressed neuronal death. In another study, Guan et al. combined the antioxidative ability of ceria and Aβ aggregates degradation features of polyoxometalates (POMs) and synthesized CeONP@POMs nanoparticles (Guan et al., 2016). in vitro studies showed that CeONP@POMs efficiently degraded Aβ aggregates, reduced intracellular ROS, promoted PC12 cell proliferation, inhibited Aβ-induced BV2 microglial cell activation, and also crossed the BBB. in vivo studies in normal mice further indicated that CeONP@POMD possessed good biocompatibility.

4.4.2 Nanoparticles to deliver polyphenolic compounds

Polyphenols are the most abundant antioxidants in diet. In the past two decades, the neuroprotective effects of polyphenols have attracted considerable attention. These compounds are able to protect neurons in various in vivo and in vitro models. Polyphenols, especially epigallocatechin gallate (EGCG), curcumin, resveratrol, and α-mangostin (α-M), become the new therapeutic options for AD treatment. It has become clear that the neuroprotective effects of polyphenols in AD are not only due to their antioxidant activity, but also rely on their different targets on various pathways in AD pathology. The main obstacles for the use of polyphenols as AD therapeutics are their rapid elimination in body and difficulty to cross BBB. Nanotechnology presents imaginative approaches to solve these problems.

Alpha-mangostin, a polyphenolic xanthone derivative from mangosteen (Wang et al., 2012), has been shown to have antioxidative (Fang et al., 2016) and anti-inflammation (Franceschelli et al., 2016) activity. Our group also found that α-M could up-regulate low-density lipoprotein receptor (LDLR) expression in microglia and liver cells and efficiently facilitated Aβ clearance, thus α-M could serve as a potential therapeutic for AD (Fig. 2) (Yao et al., 2016). For improving the bioavailability of α-M, we encapsulated α-M into the core of PEG-PLA nanoparticles

[NP(α-M)] (Yao et al., 2016). Both in vitro and in vivo experiments showed that NP(α-M) improved the biodistribution of α-M in both the brain and liver, enhancing the brain clearance of $A\beta_{42}$ in an LDLR-dependent manner. Further studies on two AD model mice (SAMP8 and APP/PS1 transgenic mice) demonstrated that NP(α-M) reduced Aβ deposition, attenuated neuroinflammatory responses, ameliorated neurologic changes, and reversed behavioral deficits. These findings not only validated the concept that polyphenol-mediated modulation of LDLR expression might serve as a safe and efficient disease-modifying therapy for AD by accelerating Aβ clearance, but also presented the potential of nanotechnology in modulating the biodistribution of drug to improve its therapeutic efficacy in AD.

Resveratrol is a polyphenol found in grapes, cranberries, and peanuts (Mancuso et al., 2007). Several studies have demonstrated the antioxidative, anticancer, anti-inflammatory, and estrogenic activities of resveratrol (Baur and Sinclair, 2006). Like α-M, the therapeutic application of resveratrol suffers from its poor pharmacokinetics. Aiming at overcoming this limitation, Lu et al. developed resveratrol-loaded polymeric micelles based on amphiphilic block copolymer which consisted polycaprolactone (PCL) as the hydrophobic core and PEG as the hydrophilic shell (Lu et al., 2009). This formulation didn't show any toxicity to PC12 cells and protected PC12 cells from Aβ-induced damage in a dose-dependent manner by attenuating intracellular oxidative stress and caspase-3 activity.

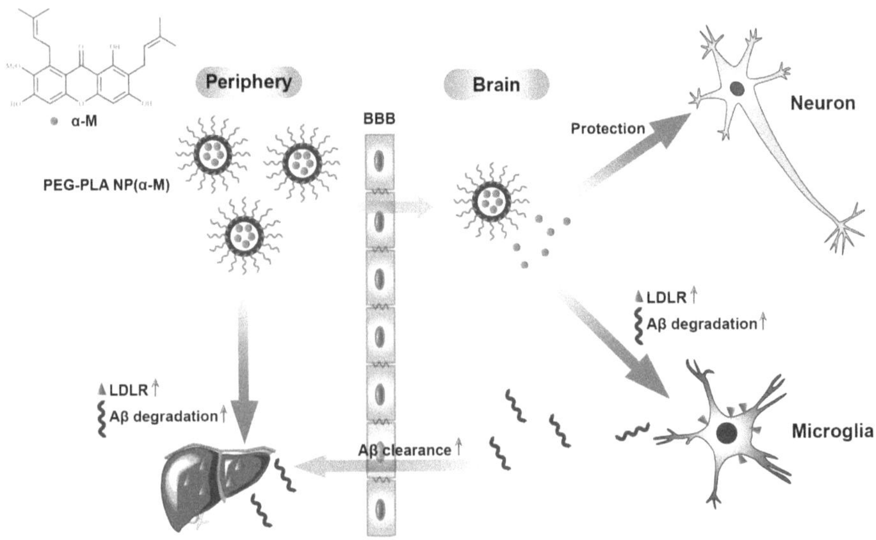

Fig. 2 Nanoformulated α-mangostin up-regulated LDLR expression in microglia and liver cells and efficiently facilitated Aβ clearance.
Reproduced with permission from Yao, L., Gu, X., Song, Q., Wang, X., Huang, M., Hu, M., et al., 2016. Nanoformulated alpha-mangostin ameliorates Alzheimer's disease neuropathology by elevating LDLR expression and accelerating amyloid-beta clearance. J. Control. Release, 226, 1–14.

EGCG is a green tea polyphenol known for its antioxidant properties and being able to modulate APP processing by upregulating α-secretase (Rezai-Zadeh et al., 2005), thereby processing great therapeutic potential for AD. To enhance the oral bioavailability and achieve maximum neuroprotective bioactivity of EGCG, Smith et al. developed nanolipidic EGCG particles (Smith et al., 2010). This formulation improved the neuronal α-secretase activity by up to 91% in SweAPP N2a cells and doubled the oral bioavailability of EGCG in rats.

4.5 Multifunctional nanoparticles for the treatment of AD

For the intriguing diseases such as AD that manifest different features in different stages, the use of a single therapeutic strategy is not sufficient to obtain the expected treatment success. Thus, the development of multifunctional nanocarriers that simultaneously possess more than one property to increase delivery specificity or therapeutic effects has been proposed as further evolution of drug delivery systems (Singh et al., 2014). It has been proposed that the secondary pathological processes such as dysfunction of synapse and neuron loss could independently aggravate the severity of AD, once initiated by Aβ (Hyman, 2011). Thus, the development of novel multifunctional therapeutics that can not only accelerate Aβ clearance, but also inhibit the subsequent pathological cascades represents a promising strategy for AD therapy (Mansoori and Nazem, 2014; Prada et al., 2007).

Lipoproteins, which are natural nanoparticles, play an important biological role and are highly suitable as a nanoplatform for medical diagnostics and therapeutics. High-density lipoprotein (HDL), the smallest lipoprotein, is of particular interest due to their ultrasmall size and favorable surface properties. Specifically, HDL subtype with apoE as the apolipoprotein component exhibits high binding affinity to Aβ and has been demonstrated to facilitate the degradation of Aβ in an apoE isoforms-dependent manner (E2 > E3 > E4) (Castellano et al., 2011). It is worth noting that, as mentioned previously, apoE can be used to target LDLR on BBB to facilitate BBB transport of NPs. For the combination treatment of AD, the nanoparticulate drug delivery system that possesses both BBB permeability and high Aβ-binding affinity is of special interest. Furthermore, considering that reconstituted high-density lipoprotein (rHDL) is a versatile class of biologically inspired nanostructures that can also carry both hydrophobic and hydrophilic agents (Bricarello et al., 2011), it holds great potential to be developed into a multifunctional nanoplatform for the combination therapy of AD. Our group designed a biologically inspired nanostructure for facilitating Aβ clearance (Song et al., 2014). This lipoprotein-based nanoparticle, apoE3-reconstituted high-density lipoprotein (ApoE3-rHDL), was prepared by self-assembly of apoE3 and phospholipid vesicles. It showed BBB permeability and high affinity to both Aβ monomer and oligomer and accelerated Aβ clearance by enhancing microglial, astroglial, and liver cellular uptake and degradation of Aβ. ApoE3-rHDL decreased Aβ deposition, attenuated microgliosis, ameliorated neurologic changes, and rescued memory deficits in an AD animal model (SAMP8 mice). The findings of this work provided the direct evidence of a biomimetic nanostructure crossing the BBB, capturing Aβ, and facilitating its degradation by glial cells, indicating the capability of ApoE3-rHDL for disease modification in AD by accelerating Aβ clearance, which also justified the concept that nanostructures with Aβ-binding affinity might provide a novel nanoplatform for AD therapy (Song et al., 2014).

In order to realize the combination therapy of AD, we further designed an rHDL-based multifunctional nanocarrier (GM1-rHDL), in which ganglioside GM1 was inserted into the lipid membrane of rHDL to increase Aβ-binding affinity and accelerate Aβ clearance. The NAP peptide, which is showed by others to improve memory (Liu et al., 2013c), was incorporated following fusion with α-helix peptide (αNAP) to inhibit Tau phosphoration and provide neuroprotection (Fig. 3) (Huang et al., 2015). GM1-rHDL was found to possess antibody-like high binding affinity to Aβ and facilitated Aβ clearance both in vitro and in vivo. Moreover, the αNAP-loaded GM1-rHDL was found to be able to reduce Aβ deposition, ameliorate neurologic changes, and rescue memory loss more efficiently than both αNAP solution and GM1-rHDL in AD model mice following intranasal administration (Huang et al., 2015). We further explored the drug loading capability and therapeutic efficacy of ApoE3-rHDL with siRNA (Huang et al., 2017) and polyphenols (Song et al., 2016). The above work provides a versatile nanoplatform, especially for the combinational therapy of AD.

Other multifunctional approaches have also been developed for the treatment of AD. For example, Liu et al. synthesized PEGylated dendrigraft poly-L-lysines (DGLs) as nanocarrier for brain co-delivery of BACE1 shRNA and a therapeutic peptide which can disrupt phosphorylated tau (p-tau)-associated fibril formation

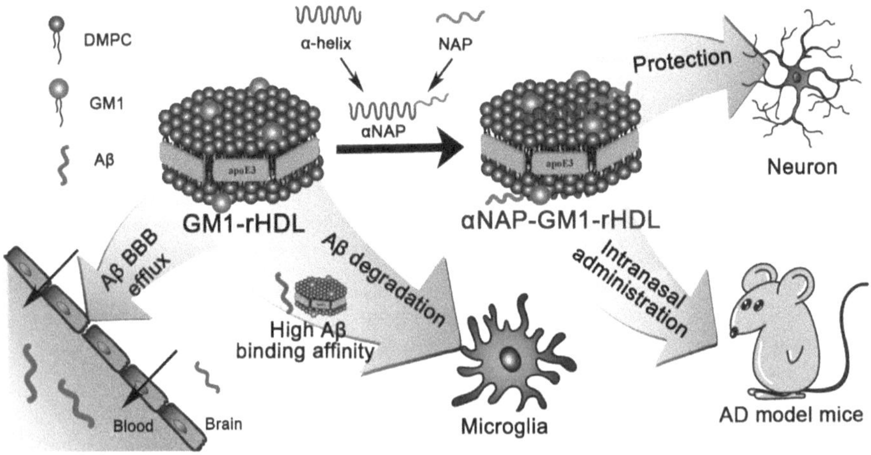

Fig. 3 Monosialotetrahexosyl ganglioside-incorporated reconstituted high-density lipoprotein (GM1-rHDL) possesses antibody-like high binding affinity to Aβ, facilitates Aβ degradation by microglia, and Aβ efflux across the blood-brain barrier (BBB), and simultaneously allows the efficient loading of neuroprotective agents, serving as a nanoparticulate drug delivery system for the combination therapy of AD.
Reproduced with permission from Huang, M., Hu, M., Song, Q., Song, H., Huang, J., Gu, X., et al., 2015. GM1-modified lipoprotein-like nanoparticle: multifunctional nanoplatform for the combination therapy of Alzheimer's disease. ACS Nano, 9, 10801–10816.

(Liu et al., 2016). Both in vitro and in vivo studies demonstrated the simultaneous efficacy of gene therapy targeting the BACE1 noncoding RNA in concert with peptide therapy targeting the p-tau-related fibril formation.

5 Nanotherapeutic strategies for the treatment of PD

5.1 Nanoparticles for dopamine replacement therapy

Dopamine replacement therapy is now the first-line choice for PD. Because of the incapability of dopamine to cross the BBB, this therapy includes or is in association with dopamine precursor levodopa, dopamine receptor agonists, and MAO inhibitors, among which levodopa is currently considered as the most effective medication for PD. However, as the disease progresses, many levodopa-take patients suffered from dyskinesia and fluctuations, which are thought to be partially induced by the inconstant level of central dopamine stimulation provided by levodopa (Chase et al., 1989; Pilleri and Antonini, 2014). As some studies demonstrated that it is beneficial to maintain stable concentrations of dopamine (Khor and Hsu, 2007), several studies have focused on using nanoparticulate drug delivery system to achieve this goal.

Pahuja et al. designed dopamine-loaded PLGA nanoparticles (DA NPs) to deliver dopamine to the brain (Pahuja et al., 2015). These NPs slowly and constantly released dopamine, leading to reduced quinone adduct formation and decreased dopamine autoxidation. After systemic intravenously administrated, DA NPs significantly increase dopamine levels in the striatum of a 6-hydroxydopamine (6-OHDA)-induced rat model of PD and recover neurobehavioral abnormalities in these animals. In another study, by taking advantage of the mucoadhesive properties of glycol chitosan (GCS), Di Gioia et al. synthesized glycol chitosan/sulfobutylether-β-cyclodextrin-based nanoparticles (DA GCS/DA-CD NPs) to deliver dopamine to striatum through the nasal route (Di Gioia et al., 2015). Sulfobutylether-β-cyclodextrin was used as crosslinking agent to stabilize DA. It was showed that repeated intranasal administration of DA GCS/DA-CD NPs into the right nostril of rats significantly increased DA in the ipsilateral striatum.

Nanoparticles to delivery MAO inhibitors and dopamine receptor agonists have also been developed. Mittal et al. synthesized chitosan glutamate nanoparticles (RAS-CG-NPs) for intranasal delivery of rasagiline (RAS) (Mittal et al., 2016), a second-generation MAO-B inhibitor with dopamine receptor agonist activity. RAS-CG-NPs were prepared via ionic gelation of chitosan glutamate with tripolyphosphate anions. It was found that the brain drug concentrations following intranasal administration of RAS-CG-NPs were significantly higher at all the time points than both intranasal delivery of free drugs and intravenous administration of RAS-CG-NPs. Jafarieh et al. also developed chitosan nanoparticles for nasal delivery of ropinirole hydrochloride, a non-ergot D2/D3 dopamine agonist (Jafarieh et al., 2015). These nanoparticles were prepared with an ionic gelation method, showed sustained drug release for up to 18 h, and achieved significantly higher drug concentration in the brain than free drugs at all the time points following intranasal administration. However, pharmacodynamic studies on PD animal models are still needed to verify the efficacy of the aforementioned nanoparticulate drug delivery systems.

5.2 Nanoparticles to deliver neurotrophic factors

GDNF is regarded as a drug candidate for the treatment of PD due to its strong trophic effect on the dopaminergic neurons (Lin et al., 1993b). Garbayo et al. reported controlled GDNF delivery using biodegradable PLGA microspheres in an animal model with partial dopaminergic lesion induced by 6-OHDA (Garbayo et al., 2009). The GDNF-loaded microspheres were unilaterally injected into the model rats, released biologically active GDNF for up to 5 weeks in vivo, and improved rotational behavior in model rats without developing antibodies against GDNF developed.

The approaches for brain delivery of GDNF-encoding gene delivery have also been investigated. Huang et al. synthesized an angiopep-conjugated dendrigraft poly-L-lysine (DGL)-based gene delivery system to deliver human GDNF gene (*hGDNF*) (Huang et al., 2013). Angiopep was used as the targeting ligand to mediate the BBB transport and cellular internalization of the nanoparticles via low-density lipoprotein receptor-related protein; while the biodegradable, cationic DGL was applied as the main gene vector. The angiopep-conjugated NPs exhibited higher cellular uptake and gene expression in brain when compared with the unmodified control. Behavioral study showed that multiple intravenous administrations of angiopep-modified NPs obtained improved locomotor activity and apparent recovery of dopaminergic neurons in rotenone-induced chronic rat model of PD. In another study by Peng et al., polyethylene imine (PEI)-grafted chitosan carrier was used for the delivery of GDNF gene (Peng et al., 2014), in which PEI was used to increase the water solubility of chitosan. Low toxicity and high transfection efficiency were achieved in in vitro experiments, while in vivo studies are needed to see its potential for the treatment of PD.

5.3 Nanotherapeutic strategies targeting oxidative stress

PD is associated with oxidative stress, presumably due to not only the high generation of ROS, but also the reduced activity of redox enzymes, catalase and superoxide dismutase, and other antioxidants (Ebadi et al., 1996; Ambani et al., 1975). In this regard, antioxidants have been investigated as potential drugs to relieve the oxidative stress of PD.

Haney et al. utilized the immune-privileged ability of exosomes to delivery catalase (Haney et al., 2015). The exosomes were isolated from cultured Raw 264.7 macrophages and incorporated with catalase (named as exoCAT). This formulation demonstrated high loading efficiency and sustained drug release. Following nasal administration, a considerable number of exosomes were found in the brain of PD model mouse and accumulated in neurons and microglial cells. Furthermore, in vitro and in vivo studies showed that exoCAT provided a significant neuroprotective effect. The antioxidative effects of polyphenols have also been studied in PD context. Da Rocha Lindner reported that resveratrol-loaded P-80-coated

PLA nanoparticles improved neuroprotective effects against MPTP-induced behavioral and neurochemical changes following intraperitoneal injection (Da Rocha Lindner et al., 2015).

5.4 Nanotherapeutic strategies targeting α-synclein production

For central role of α-synclein in PD, inhibition of its production via gene therapy has become a new frontier in the treatment of PD. Viral gene delivery systems exhibit limitations such as potent immunogenicity, mutagenesis, and carcinogenesis. These disadvantages can be avoided by replacing the viral vectors with nanoparticle-based gene delivery systems. Liu et al. synthesized PEG-polyethyleneimine (PEG-PEI) nanoparticles for α-synclein siRNA delivery (Liu et al., 2014). in vitro experiments on PC12 cells showed that PEG-PEI/siRNA achieved high transfection efficiency, significantly suppressed α-synclein mRNA expression, and protected cells from 1-methyl-4-phenylpyridinium (MPP+)-induced apoptosis. Furthermore, PEG-PEI/siRNA showed low cytotoxicity to PC12 cells. However, it is noteworthy that this study was rather preliminary and in vivo experiments are needed to validate the efficacy as well as confirm the safety of this gene therapy.

6 Conclusion and future perspectives

The potential use of nanotechnology for the treatment of AD and PD has been widely explored, based on the gradually uncovered understanding of their pathogenesis. However, several issues should be noted about nanotherapeutic strategies. For example, delivery efficiency of drug-loaded nanoparticles to cross BBB via strategies summarized here is far from satisfactory, and drugs with relatively high effective dose may not take effect. The combination of potential drugs and BBB-crossing strategies should be carefully chosen. Another issue is the safety concern. The toxicity of various nanoparticles in the brain and the clearance or degradation pathway of these nanoparticles have not been fully elucidated; hence, the relevant studies are needed. The selection of animal models is also noteworthy. Neurodegenerative diseases are very complex in pathogenesis and may present different pathological and clinical features in different disease stages. The current animal models for neurodegenerative diseases like AD and PD are not capable to fully mimic the disease pathology and staging in human. When using a specific pathogenesis-based therapy, a clear and comprehensive consideration on the animal models is necessary. Among all the issues that should be noted about nanotherapeutic strategies, the major one is the clinical translation. Many studies summarized here are still at the stage of animal model study and even only in vitro. How to translate these results into clinical application is still a big challenge.

Some of the therapies that are being designed for a specific neurodegenerative disease may potentially be applied to others, such as the antioxidants for both AD and PD treatment. Thus, nanotechnologies to facilitate the efficacy of these therapies could also benefit from each other. However, some of the nanotherapeutic strategies are especially designed for a certain type of neurodegenerative disease based on their unique pathogenesis, such as the rHDL and its multifunctional derivate for AD treatment. As more and more details on pathogenesis of neurodegenerative disease are revealed by epidemiological findings, pathological observations, and genetic discoveries, new therapeutic targets will be brought to light and nanotechnology may have more chance to show its strength.

References

Aguzzi, A., O'Connor, T., 2010. Protein aggregation diseases: pathogenicity and therapeutic perspectives. Nat. Rev. Drug Discov. 9, 237–248.

Ahyayauch, H., Raab, M., Busto, J.V., Andraka, N., Arrondo, J.L., Masserini, M., et al., 2012. Binding of beta-amyloid (1-42) peptide to negatively charged phospholipid membranes in the liquid-ordered state: modeling and experimental studies. Biophys. J. 103, 453–463.

Alvarez-Erviti, L., Rodriguez-Oroz, M.C., Cooper, J.M., Caballero, C., Ferrer, I., Obeso, J.A., et al., 2010. Chaperone-mediated autophagy markers in Parkinson disease brains. Arch. Neurol. 67, 1464–1472.

Alvarez-Erviti, L., Seow, Y., Yin, H., Betts, C., Lakhal, S., Wood, M.J.A., 2011. Delivery of siRNA to the mouse brain by systemic injection of targeted exosomes. Nat. Biotechnol. 29, 341–345.

Ambani, L.M., Van Woert, M.H., Murphy, S., 1975. Brain peroxidase and catalase in Parkinson disease. Arch. Neurol. 32, 114–118.

Athauda, D., Foltynie, T., 2015. The ongoing pursuit of neuroprotective therapies in Parkinson disease. Nat. Rev. Neurol. 11, 25–40.

Bana, L., Minniti, S., Salvati, E., Sesana, S., Zambelli, V., Cagnotto, A., et al., 2014. Liposomes bi-functionalized with phosphatidic acid and an ApoE-derived peptide affect Aβ aggregation features and cross the blood-brain-barrier: implications for therapy of Alzheimer disease. Nanomed. Nanotechnol. Biol. Med. 10, 1583–1590.

Banks, W.A., 2012. Drug delivery to the brain in Alzheimer's disease: consideration of the blood-brain barrier. Adv. Drug Deliv. Rev. 64, 629–639.

Barcia, E., Salama, A., Fernandez-Carballido, A., Negro, S., 2011. Protective effects of clioquinol on human neuronal-like cells: a new formulation of clioquinol-loaded PLGA microspheres for Alzheimer's disease. J. Drug Target. 19, 637–646.

Bard, F., Cannon, C., Barbour, R., Burke, R.L., Games, D., Grajeda, H., et al., 2000. Peripherally administered antibodies against amyloid β-peptide enter the central nervous system and reduce pathology in a mouse model of Alzheimer disease. Nat. Med. 6, 916–919.

Bartus, R.T., 2000. On neurodegenerative diseases, models, and treatment strategies: lessons learned and lessons forgotten a generation following the cholinergic hypothesis. Exp. Neurol. 163, 495–529.

Barua, N.U., Gill, S.S., Love, S., 2014. Convection-enhanced drug delivery to the brain: therapeutic potential and neuropathological considerations. Brain Pathol. 24, 117–127.

Barua, N.U., Miners, J.S., Bienemann, A.S., Wyatt, M.J., Welser, K., Tabor, A.B., et al., 2012. Convection-enhanced delivery of neprilysin: a novel amyloid-beta-degrading therapeutic strategy. J. Alzheimers Dis. 32, 43–56.

Baur, J.A., Sinclair, D.A., 2006. Therapeutic potential of resveratrol: the in vivo evidence. Nat. Rev. Drug Discov. 5, 493–506.

Berger, G., Kogan, T., Skutelsky, E., Ophir, D., 2005. Glycoconjugate expression in normal human inferior turbinate mucosa: a lectin histochemical study. Am. J. Rhinol. 19, 97–103.

Bhaskar, S., Tian, F., Stoeger, T., Kreyling, W., de la Fuente, J.M., Grazu, V., et al., 2010. Multifunctional nanocarriers for diagnostics, drug delivery and targeted treatment across blood-brain barrier: perspectives on tracking and neuroimaging. Part. Fibre Toxicol. 7, 3.

Blennow, K., de Leon, M.J., Zetterberg, H., 2006. Alzheimer's disease. Lancet 368, 387–403.

Bolognin, S., Messori, L., Drago, D., Gabbiani, C., Cendron, L., Zatta, P., 2011. Aluminum, copper, iron and zinc differentially alter amyloid-Abeta(1-42) aggregation and toxicity. Int. J. Biochem. Cell Biol. 43, 877–885.

Bricarello, D.A., Smilowitz, J.T., Zivkovic, A.M., German, J.B., Parikh, A.N., 2011. Reconstituted lipoprotein: a versatile class of biologically-inspired nanostructures. ACS Nano 5, 42–57.

Bush, A.I., 2003. The metallobiology of Alzheimer's disease. Trends Neurosci. 26, 207–214.

Camps, P., Munoz-Torrero, D., 2002. Cholinergic drugs in pharmacotherapy of Alzheimer's disease. Mini Rev. Med. Chem. 2, 11–25.

Camps, P., Muñoz-Torrero, D., 2002. Cholinergic drugs in pharmacotherapy of Alzheimer's disease. Mini Rev. Med. Chem. 2, 11–25.

Canovi, M., Markoutsa, E., Lazar, A.N., Pampalakis, G., Clemente, C., Re, F., et al., 2011. The binding affinity of anti-Abeta1-42 MAb-decorated nanoliposomes to Abeta1-42 peptides in vitro and to amyloid deposits in post-mortem tissue. Biomaterials 32, 5489–5497.

Carta, A.R., Pisanu, A., 2013. Modulating microglia activity with PPAR-gamma agonists: a promising therapy for Parkinson's disease? Neurotox. Res. 23, 112–123.

Castellano, J.M., Kim, J., Stewart, F.R., Jiang, H., DeMattos, R.B., Patterson, B.W., et al., 2011. Human apoE isoforms differentially regulate brain amyloid-beta peptide clearance. Sci. Transl. Med. 3, 89ra57.

Chan, S.L., Tan, E.K., 2017. Targeting LRRK2 in Parkinson's disease: an update on recent developments. Expert Opin. Ther. Targets 21, 601–610.

Chase, T.N., Baronti, F., Fabbrini, G., Heuser, I.J., Juncos, J.L., Mouradian, M.M., 1989. Rationale for continuous dopaminomimetic therapy of Parkinson's disease. Neurology 39, 7–10.

Cherny, R.A., Barnham, K.J., Lynch, T., Volitakis, I., Li, Q.X., McLean, C.A., et al., 2000. Chelation and intercalation: complementary properties in a compound for the treatment of Alzheimer's disease. J. Struct. Biol. 130, 209–216.

Churches, Q.I., Caine, J., Cavanagh, K., Epa, V.C., Waddington, L., Tranberg, C.E., et al., 2014. Naturally occurring polyphenolic inhibitors of amyloid beta aggregation. Bioorg. Med. Chem. Lett. 24, 3108–3112.

Conway, K.A., Harper, J.D., Lansbury, P.T., 1998. Accelerated in vitro fibril formation by a mutant alpha-synuclein linked to early-onset Parkinson disease. Nat. Med. 4, 1318–1320.

Cooper, O., Seo, H., Andrabi, S., Guardia-Laguarta, C., Graziotto, J., Sundberg, M., et al., 2012. Pharmacological rescue of mitochondrial deficits in iPSC-derived neural cells from patients with familial Parkinson's disease. Sci. Transl. Med. 4, 141ra90.

Cramer, P.E., Cirrito, J.R., Wesson, D.W., Lee, C.Y.D., Karlo, J.C., Zinn, A.E., et al., 2012. ApoE-directed therapeutics rapidly clear β-amyloid and reverse deficits in AD mouse models. Science 335, 1503–1506.

Cui, Z., Lockman, P.R., Atwood, C.S., Hsu, C.H., Gupte, A., Allen, D.D., et al., 2005. Novel D-penicillamine carrying nanoparticles for metal chelation therapy in Alzheimer's and other CNS diseases. Eur. J. Pharm. Biopharm. 59, 263–272.

Da Rocha Lindner, G., Bonfanti Santos, D., Colle, D., Gasnhar Moreira, E.L., Daniel Prediger, R., Farina, M., et al., 2015. Improved neuroprotective effects of resveratrol-loaded polysorbate 80-coated poly(lactide) nanoparticles in MPTP-induced Parkinsonism. Nanomedicine 10, 1127–1138.

DeMattos, R.B., Bales, K.R., Cummins, D.J., Dodart, J.C., Paul, S.M., Holtzman, D.M., 2001. Peripheral anti-Aβ antibody alters CNS and plasma Aβ clearance and decreases brain Aβ burden in a mouse model of Alzheimer's disease. Proc. Natl. Acad. Sci. USA 98, 8850–8855.

Dexter, D.T., Statton, S.A., Whitmore, C., Freinbichler, W., Weinberger, P., Tipton, K.F., et al., 2011. Clinically available iron chelators induce neuroprotection in the 6-OHDA model of Parkinson's disease after peripheral administration. J. Neural Transm. (Vienna) 118, 223–231.

Di Gioia, S., Trapani, A., Mandracchia, D., De Giglio, E., Cometa, S., Mangini, V., et al., 2015. Intranasal delivery of dopamine to the striatum using glycol chitosan/sulfobutylether-β-cyclodextrin based nanoparticles. Eur. J. Pharm. Biopharm. 94, 180–193.

Doherty, K.M., Silveira-Moriyama, L., Parkkinen, L., Healy, D.G., Farrell, M., Mencacci, N.E., et al., 2013. Parkin disease: a clinicopathologic entity? JAMA Neurol. 70, 571–579.

Dong, J., Atwood, C.S., Anderson, V.E., Siedlak, S.L., Smith, M.A., Perry, G., et al., 2003. Metal binding and oxidation of amyloid-beta within isolated senile plaque cores: Raman microscopic evidence. Biochemistry 42, 2768–2773.

Dorsey, E.R., Constantinescu, R., Thompson, J.P., Biglan, K.M., Holloway, R.G., Kieburtz, K., et al., 2007. Projected number of people with Parkinson disease in the most populous nations, 2005 through 2030. Neurology 68, 384–386.

Durairajan, S.S., Yuan, Q., Xie, L., Chan, W.S., Kum, W.F., Koo, I., et al., 2008. Salvianolic acid B inhibits Abeta fibril formation and disaggregates preformed fibrils and protects against Abeta-induced cytotoxicty. Neurochem. Int. 52, 741–750.

Duran, R., Mencacci, N.E., Angeli, A.V., Shoai, M., Deas, E., Houlden, H., et al., 2013. The glucocerobrosidase E326K variant predisposes to Parkinson's disease, but does not cause Gaucher's disease. Mov. Disord. 28, 232–236.

Ebadi, M., Srinivasan, S.K., Baxi, M.D., 1996. Oxidative stress and antioxidant therapy in Parkinson's disease. Progr. Neurobiol. 48, 1–19.

Ehmann, W.D., Markesbery, W.R., Alauddin, M., Hossain, T.I., Brubaker, E.H., 1986. Brain trace elements in Alzheimer's disease. Neurotoxicology 7, 195–206.

Fang, Y., Su, T., Qiu, X., Mao, P., Xu, Y., Hu, Z., et al., 2016. Protective effect of alpha-mangostin against oxidative stress induced-retinal cell death. Sci. Rep. 621018.

Ferguson, S.W., Nguyen, J., 2016. Exosomes as therapeutics: the implications of molecular composition and exosomal heterogeneity. J. Control. Release 228, 179–190.

Ferreira-Vieira, T.H., Guimaraes, I.M., Silva, F.R., Ribeiro, F.M., 2016. Alzheimer's disease: targeting the cholinergic system. Curr. Neuropharmacol. 14, 101–115.

Franceschelli, S., Pesce, M., Ferrone, A., Patruno, A., Pasqualone, L., Carlucci, G., et al., 2016. A novel biological role of alpha-mangostin in modulating inflammatory response through the activation of SIRT-1 signaling pathway. J. Cell. Physiol. 231, 2439–2451.

Francis, P.T., Palmer, A.M., Snape, M., Wilcock, G.K., 1999. The cholinergic hypothesis of Alzheimer's disease: a review of progress. J. Neurol. Neurosurg. Psychiatry 66, 137–147.

Frydman-Marom, A., Rechter, M., Shefler, I., Bram, Y., Shalev, D.E., Gazit, E., 2009. Cognitive-performance recovery of Alzheimer's disease model mice by modulation of early soluble amyloidal assemblies. Angew. Chem. Int. Ed. Engl. 48, 1981–1986.

Gabathuler, R., 2010. Approaches to transport therapeutic drugs across the blood-brain barrier to treat brain diseases. Neurobiol. Dis. 37, 48–57.

Gao, X., Chen, J., Tao, W., Zhu, J., Zhang, Q., Chen, H., et al., 2007a. UEA I-bearing nanoparticles for brain delivery following intranasal administration. Int. J. Pharm. 340, 207–215.

Gao, X., Tao, W., Lu, W., Zhang, Q., Zhang, Y., Jiang, X., et al., 2006. Lectin-conjugated PEG-PLA nanoparticles: preparation and brain delivery after intranasal administration. Biomaterials 27, 3482–3490.

Gao, X., Wu, B., Zhang, Q., Chen, J., Zhu, J., Zhang, W., et al., 2007b. Brain delivery of vasoactive intestinal peptide enhanced with the nanoparticles conjugated with wheat germ agglutinin following intranasal administration. J. Control. Release 121, 156–167.

Garbayo, E., Montero-Menei, C.N., Ansorena, E., Lanciego, J.L., Aymerich, M.S., Blanco-Prieto, M.J., 2009. Effective GDNF brain delivery using microspheres: a promising strategy for Parkinson's disease. J. Control. Release 135, 119–126.

Giasson, B.I., Lee, V.M., 2001. Parkin and the molecular pathways of Parkinson's disease. Neuron 31, 885–888.

Gobbi, M., Re, F., Canovi, M., Beeg, M., Gregori, M., Sesana, S., et al., 2010. Lipid-based nanoparticles with high binding affinity for amyloid-beta1-42 peptide. Biomaterials 31, 6519–6529.

Goedert, M., Eisenberg, D.S., Crowther, R.A., 2017. Propagation of tau aggregates and neurodegeneration. Annu. Rev. Neurosci. 40, 189–210.

Graham, W.V., Bonito-Oliva, A., Sakmar, T.P., 2017. Update on Alzheimer's disease therapy and prevention strategies. Annu. Rev. Med. 68, 413–430.

Gregori, M., Masserini, M., Mancini, S., 2015. Nanomedicine for the treatment of Alzheimer's disease. Nanomed. (Lond.) 10, 1203–1218.

Guan, Y., Li, M., Dong, K., Gao, N., Ren, J., Zheng, Y., et al., 2016. Ceria/POMs hybrid nanoparticles as a mimicking metallopeptidase for treatment of neurotoxicity of amyloid-β peptide. Biomaterials 98, 92–102.

Guerreiro, R., Wojtas, A., Bras, J., Carrasquillo, M., Rogaeva, E., Majounie, E., et al., 2013. TREM2 variants in Alzheimer's disease. N. Engl. J. Med. 368, 117–127.

Guzman, J.N., Sanchez-Padilla, J., Wokosin, D., Kondapalli, J., Ilijic, E., Schumacker, P.T., et al., 2010. Oxidant stress evoked by pacemaking in dopaminergic neurons is attenuated by DJ-1. Nature 468, 696–700.

Haass, C., Kaether, C., Thinakaran, G., Sisodia, S., 2012. Trafficking and proteolytic processing of APP. Cold Spring Harb. Perspect. Med. 2, a006270.

Hanafy, A.S., Farid, R.M., Helmy, M.W., ElGamal, S.S., 2016. Pharmacological, toxicological and neuronal localization assessment of galantamine/chitosan complex nanoparticles in rats: future potential contribution in Alzheimer's disease management. Drug Deliv. 23, 3111–3122.

Haney, M.J., Klyachko, N.L., Zhao, Y., Gupta, R., Plotnikova, E.G., He, Z., et al., 2015. Exosomes as drug delivery vehicles for Parkinson's disease therapy. J. Control. Release 207, 18–30.

Hardy, J., Selkoe, D.J., 2002. The amyloid hypothesis of Alzheimer's disease: progress and problems on the road to therapeutics. Science 297, 353–356.

Heffern, M.C., Velasco, P.T., Matosziuk, L.M., Coomes, J.L., Karras, C., Ratner, M.A., et al., 2014. Modulation of amyloid-beta aggregation by histidine-coordinating Cobalt(III) Schiff base complexes. ChemBioChem 15, 1584–1589.

Herskowitz, J.H., Seyfried, N.T., Gearing, M., Kahn, R.A., Peng, J., Levey, A.I., et al., 2011. Rho kinase II phosphorylation of the lipoprotein receptor LR11/SORLA alters amyloid-beta production. J. Biol. Chem. 286, 6117–6127.

Huang, J.L., Jiang, G., Song, Q.X., Gu, X., Hu, M., Wang, X.L., et al., 2017. Lipoprotein-biomimetic nanostructure enables efficient targeting delivery of siRNA to Ras-activated glioblastoma cells via macropinocytosis. Nat. Commun. 8, 15144.

Huang, M., Hu, M., Song, Q., Song, H., Huang, J., Gu, X., et al., 2015. GM1-modified lipoprotein-like nanoparticle: multifunctional nanoplatform for the combination therapy of Alzheimer's disease. ACS Nano 9, 10801–10816.

Huang, R., Ma, H., Guo, Y., Liu, S., Kuang, Y., Shao, K., et al., 2013. Angiopep-conjugated nanoparticles for targeted long-term gene therapy of parkinson's disease. Pharm. Res. 30, 2549–2559.

Hyman, B.T., 2011. Amyloid-dependent and amyloid-independent stages of alzheimer disease. Arch. Neurol. 68, 1062–1064.

Hynynen, K., McDannold, N., Vykhodtseva, N., Raymond, S., Weissleder, R., Jolesz, F.A., et al., 2006. Focal disruption of the blood-brain barrier due to 260-kHz ultrasound bursts: a method for molecular imaging and targeted drug delivery. J. Neurosurg. 105, 445–454.

Iadecola, C., 2010. The overlap between neurodegenerative and vascular factors in the pathogenesis of dementia. Acta Neuropathol. 120, 287–296.

Jafarieh, O., Md, S., Ali, M., Baboota, S., Sahni, J.K., Kumari, B., et al., 2015. Design, characterization, and evaluation of intranasal delivery of ropinirole-loaded mucoadhesive nanoparticles for brain targeting. Drug Dev. Ind. Pharm. 41, 1674–1681.

Jaruszewski, K.M., Ramakrishnan, S., Poduslo, J.F., Kandimalla, K.K., 2012. Chitosan enhances the stability and targeting of immuno-nanovehicles to cerebro-vascular deposits of Alzheimer's disease amyloid protein. Nanomed. Nanotechnol. Biol. Med. 8, 250–260.

Jonsson, T., Stefansson, H., Steinberg, S., Jonsdottir, I., Jonsson, P.V., Snaedal, J., et al., 2013. Variant of TREM2 associated with the risk of Alzheimer's disease. N. Engl. J. Med. 368, 107–116.

Kalia, L.V., Lang, A.E., 2015. Parkinson's disease. Lancet 386, 896–912.

Karakoti, A.S., Singh, S., Kumar, A., Malinska, M., Kuchibhatla, S.V., Wozniak, K., et al., 2009. PEGylated nanoceria as radical scavenger with tunable redox chemistry. J. Am. Chem. Soc. 131, 14144–14145.

Kean, T., Thanou, M., 2010. Biodegradation, biodistribution and toxicity of chitosan. Adv. Drug Deliv. Rev. 62, 3–11.

Khor, S.P., Hsu, A., 2007. The pharmacokinetics and pharmacodynamics of levodopa in the treatment of Parkinson's disease. Curr. Clin. Pharmacol. 2, 234–243.

Kinoshita, M., McDannold, N., Jolesz, F.A., Hynynen, K., 2006. Targeted delivery of antibodies through the blood-brain barrier by MRI-guided focused ultrasound. Biochem. Biophys. Res. Commun. 340, 1085–1090.

Kogan, M.J., Bastus, N.G., Amigo, R., Grillo-Bosch, D., Araya, E., Turiel, A., et al., 2006. Nanoparticle-mediated local and remote manipulation of protein aggregation. Nano Lett. 6, 110–115.

Kordower, J.H., Bjorklund, A., 2013. Trophic factor gene therapy for Parkinson's disease. Mov. Disord. 28, 96–109.

Kreuter, J., 2001. Nanoparticulate systems for brain delivery of drugs. Adv. Drug Deliv. Rev. 47, 65–81.

Kreuter, J., 2012. Nanoparticulate systems for brain delivery of drugs. Adv. Drug Deliv. Rev. 64, 213–222.

Kreuter, J., Shamenkov, D., Petrov, V., Ramge, P., Cychutek, K., Koch-Brandt, C., et al., 2002. Apolipoprotein-mediated transport of nanoparticle-bound drugs across the blood-brain barrier. J. Drug Target. 10, 317–325.

Kwon, H.J., Cha, M.Y., Kim, D., Kim, D.K., Soh, M., Shin, K., et al., 2016. Mitochondria-targeting ceria nanoparticles as antioxidants for Alzheimer's disease. ACS Nano 10, 2860–2870.

Lacalle-Aurioles, M., Mateos-Perez, J.M., Guzman-De-Villoria, J.A., Olazaran, J., Cruz-Orduna, I., Aleman-Gomez, Y., et al., 2014. Cerebral blood flow is an earlier indicator of perfusion abnormalities than cerebral blood volume in Alzheimer's disease. J. Cereb. Blood Flow Metab. 34, 654–659.

Lashuel, H.A., Overk, C.R., Oueslati, A., Masliah, E., 2013. The many faces of α-synuclein: from structure and toxicity to therapeutic target. Nat. Rev. Neurosci. 14, 38–48.

Li, M., Xu, C., Wu, L., Ren, J., Wang, E., Qu, X., 2013. Self-assembled peptide-polyoxometalate hybrid nanospheres: two in one enhances targeted inhibition of amyloid beta-peptide aggregation associated with Alzheimer's disease. Small 9, 3455–3461.

Lim, G.P., Chu, T., Yang, F., Beech, W., Frautschy, S.A., Cole, G.M., 2001. The curry spice curcumin reduces oxidative damage and amyloid pathology in an Alzheimer transgenic mouse. J. Neurosci. 21, 8370–8377.

Lin, L.F., Doherty, D.H., Lile, J.D., Bektesh, S., Collins, F., 1993a. GDNF: a glial cell line-derived neurotrophic factor for midbrain dopaminergic neurons. Science 260, 1130–1132.

Lin, L.H., Doherty, D.H., Lile, J.D., Bektesh, S., Collins, F., 1993b. GDNF: a glial cell line: derived neurotrophic factor for midbrain dopaminergic neurons. Science 260, 1130–1132.

Liu, G., Garrett, M.R., Men, P., Zhu, X., Perry, G., Smith, M.A., 2005. Nanoparticle and other metal chelation therapeutics in Alzheimer disease. Biochim. Biophys. Acta 1741, 246–252.

Liu, G., Men, P., Kudo, W., Perry, G., Smith, M.A., 2009a. Nanoparticle-chelator conjugates as inhibitors of amyloid-beta aggregation and neurotoxicity: a novel therapeutic approach for Alzheimer disease. Neurosci. Lett. 455, 187–190.

Liu, L., Xu, K., Wang, H., Tan, P.K., Fan, W., Venkatraman, S.S., et al., 2009b. Self-assembled cationic peptide nanoparticles as an efficient antimicrobial agent. Nat. Nanotechnol. 4, 457–463.

Liu, Y., An, S., Li, J., Kuang, Y., He, X., Guo, Y., et al., 2016. Brain-targeted co-delivery of therapeutic gene and peptide by multifunctional nanoparticles in Alzheimer's disease mice. Biomaterials 80, 33–45.

Liu, Y., Liu, Z., Wang, Y., Liang, Y.R., Wen, X., Hu, J., et al., 2013a. Investigation of the performance of PEG-PEI/ROCK-II-siRNA complexes for Alzheimer's disease in vitro. Brain Res. 1490, 43–51.

Liu, Y.H., Giunta, B., Zhou, H.D., Tan, J., Wang, Y.J., 2012. Immunotherapy for Alzheimer disease-the challenge of adverse effects. Nat. Rev. Neurol. 8, 465–469.

Liu, Y.Y., Yang, X.Y., Li, Z., Liu, Z.L., Cheng, D., Wang, Y., et al., 2014. Characterization of polyethylene glycol-polyethyleneimine as a vector for alpha-synuclein siRNA delivery to PC12 cells for Parkinson's disease. CNS Neurosci. Ther. 20, 76–85.

Liu, Z., Gao, X., Kang, T., Jiang, M., Miao, D., Gu, G., et al., 2013b. B6 peptide-modified PEG-PLA nanoparticles for enhanced brain delivery of neuroprotective peptide. Bioconjugate Chem. 24, 997–1007.

Liu, Z., Jiang, M., Kang, T., Miao, D., Gu, G., Song, Q., et al., 2013c. Lactoferrin-modified PEG-co-PCL nanoparticles for enhanced brain delivery of NAP peptide following intranasal administration. Biomaterials 34, 3870–3881.

Lockman, P.R., Koziara, J., Roder, K.E., Paulson, J., Abbruscato, T.J., Mumper, R.J., et al., 2003a. In vivo and in vitro assessment of baseline blood-brain barrier parameters in the presence of novel nanoparticles. Pharm. Res. 20, 705–713.

Lockman, P.R., Koziara, J.M., Mumper, R.J., Allen, D.D., 2004. Nanoparticle surface charges alter blood-brain barrier integrity and permeability. J. Drug Target. 12, 635–641.

Lockman, P.R., Oyewumi, M.O., Koziara, J.M., Roder, K.E., Mumper, R.J., Allen, D.D., 2003b. Brain uptake of thiamine-coated nanoparticles. J. Control. Release 93, 271–282.

Lonser, R.R., Sarntinoranont, M., Morrison, P.F., Oldfield, E.H., 2015. Convection-enhanced delivery to the central nervous system. J. Neurosurg. 122, 697–706.
Lotharius, J., Brundin, P., 2002. Pathogenesis of Parkinson's disease: dopamine, vesicles and alpha-synuclein. Nat. Rev. Neurosci. 3, 932–942.
Lu, X., Ji, C., Xu, H., Li, X., Ding, H., Ye, M., et al., 2009. Resveratrol-loaded polymeric micelles protect cells from Abeta-induced oxidative stress. Int. J. Pharm. 375, 89–96.
Luo, Y., Bolon, B., Kahn, S., Bennett, B.D., Babu-Khan, S., Denis, P., et al., 2001. Mice deficient in BACE1, the Alzheimer's beta-secretase, have normal phenotype and abolished beta-amyloid generation. Nat. Neurosci. 4, 231–232.
MacKay, J.A., Deen, D.F., Szoka Jr., F.C., 2005. Distribution in brain of liposomes after convection enhanced delivery; modulation by particle charge, particle diameter, and presence of steric coating. Brain Res. 1035, 139–153.
ManafiRad, A., Farzadfar, F., Habibi, L., Azhdarzadeh, M., Aghaverdi, H., Tehrani, K.H., et al., 2014. Is amyloid-beta an innocent bystander and marker in Alzheimer's disease? Is the liability of multivalent cation homeostasis and its influence on amyloid-beta function the real mechanism? J. Alzheimers Dis. 42, 69–85.
Mancini, S., Minniti, S., Gregori, M., Sancini, G., Cagnotto, A., Couraud, P.O., et al., 2016. The hunt for brain Aβ oligomers by peripherally circulating multi-functional nanoparticles: potential therapeutic approach for Alzheimer disease. Nanomed. Nanotechnol. Biol. Med. 12, 43–52.
Mancuso, C., Bates, T.E., Butterfield, D.A., Calafato, S., Cornelius, C., De Lorenzo, A., et al., 2007. Natural antioxidants in Alzheimer's disease. Expert Opin. Investig. Drugs 16, 1921–1931.
Mansoori, G.A., Nazem, A., 2014. Nanotechnology building blocks for intervention with Alzheimer's disease pathology: implications in disease modifying strategies. J. Bioanal. Biomed. 6, 9–14.
Marks Jr., W.J., Bartus, R.T., Siffert, J., Davis, C.S., Lozano, A., Boulis, N., et al., 2010. Gene delivery of AAV2-neurturin for Parkinson's disease: a double-blind, randomised, controlled trial. Lancet Neurol. 9, 1164–1172.
Martinez-Vicente, M., Talloczy, Z., Kaushik, S., Massey, A.C., Mazzulli, J., Mosharov, E.V., et al., 2008. Dopamine-modified alpha-synuclein blocks chaperone-mediated autophagy. J. Clin. Invest. 118, 777–788.
Masliah, E., Rockenstein, E., Adame, A., Alford, M., Crews, L., Hashimoto, M., et al., 2005. Effects of alpha-synuclein immunization in a mouse model of Parkinson's disease. Neuron 46, 857–868.
Masliah, E., Rockenstein, E., Mante, M., Crews, L., Spencer, B., Adame, A., et al., 2011. Passive immunization reduces behavioral and neuropathological deficits in an alpha-synuclein transgenic model of Lewy body disease. PLoS One 6, e19338.
Massaad, C.A., 2011. Neuronal and vascular oxidative stress in Alzheimer's disease. Curr. Neuropharmacol. 9, 662–673.
Mathew, A., Fukuda, T., Nagaoka, Y., Hasumura, T., Morimoto, H., Yoshida, Y., et al., 2012. Curcumin loaded-PLGA nanoparticles conjugated with Tet-1 peptide for potential use in Alzheimer's disease. PLoS ONE. 7.
Matsuoka, Y., Saito, M., LaFrancois, J., Saito, M., Gaynor, K., Olm, V., et al., 2003. Novel therapeutic approach for the treatment of Alzheimer's disease by peripheral administration of agents with an affinity to beta-amyloid. J. Neurosci. 23, 29–33.
Mawuenyega, K.G., Sigurdson, W., Ovod, V., Munsell, L., Kasten, T., Morris, J.C., et al., 2010. Decreased clearance of CNS β-amyloid in Alzheimer's disease. Science 330, 1774.

McDade, E., Kim, A., James, J., Sheu, L.K., Kuan, D.C., Minhas, D., et al., 2014. Cerebral perfusion alterations and cerebral amyloid in autosomal dominant Alzheimer disease. Neurology 83, 710–717.

Meng, F., Asghar, S., Gao, S., Su, Z., Song, J., Huo, M., et al., 2015. A novel LDL-mimic nanocarrier for the targeted delivery of curcumin into the brain to treat Alzheimer's disease. Colloids Surf. B: Biointerfaces 134, 88–97.

Misra, S., Chopra, K., Sinha, V.R., Medhi, B., 2016. Galantamine-loaded solid–lipid nanoparticles for enhanced brain delivery: preparation, characterization, in vitro and in vivo evaluations. Drug Deliv. 23, 1434–1443.

Mittal, D., Md, S., Hasan, Q., Fazil, M., Ali, A., Baboota, S., et al., 2016. Brain targeted nanoparticulate drug delivery system of rasagiline via intranasal route. Drug Deliv. 23, 130–139.

Mittal, G., Carswell, H., Brett, R., Currie, S., Kumar, M.N.V.R., 2011. Development and evaluation of polymer nanoparticles for oral delivery of estradiol to rat brain in a model of Alzheimer's pathology. J. Control. Release 150, 220–228.

Mondragon-Rodriguez, S., Perry, G., Zhu, X., Moreira, P.I., Acevedo-Aquino, M.C., Williams, S., 2013. Phosphorylation of tau protein as the link between oxidative stress, mitochondrial dysfunction, and connectivity failure: implications for Alzheimer's disease. Oxid. Med. Cell. Longev. 2013, 940603.

Morgan, D., Diamond, D.M., Gottschall, P.E., Ugen, K.E., Dickey, C., Hardy, J., et al., 2000. A beta peptide vaccination prevents memory loss in an animal model of Alzheimer's disease. Nature 408, 982–985.

Mourtas, S., Canovi, M., Zona, C., Aurilia, D., Niarakis, A., La Ferla, B., et al., 2011. Curcumin-decorated nanoliposomes with very high affinity for amyloid-β1-42 peptide. Biomaterials 32, 1635–1645.

Mourtas, S., Lazar, A.N., Markoutsa, E., Duyckaerts, C., Antimisiaris, S.G., 2014. Multifunctional nanoliposomes with curcumin–lipid derivative and brain targeting functionality with potential applications for Alzheimer disease. Eur. J. Med. Chem. 80, 175–183.

Nelson, A.R., Sweeney, M.D., Sagare, A.P., Zlokovic, B.V., 2016. Neurovascular dysfunction and neurodegeneration in dementia and Alzheimer's disease. Biochim. Biophys. Acta 1862, 887–900.

Noyce, A.J., Bestwick, J.P., Silveira-Moriyama, L., Hawkes, C.H., Giovannoni, G., Lees, A.J., et al., 2012. Meta-analysis of early nonmotor features and risk factors for Parkinson disease. Ann. Neurol. 72, 893–901.

Nutt, J.G., Burchiel, K.J., Comella, C.L., Jankovic, J., Lang, A.E., Laws Jr., E.R., et al., 2003. Randomized, double-blind trial of glial cell line-derived neurotrophic factor (GDNF) in PD. Neurology 60, 69–73.

Opazo, C., Huang, X., Cherny, R.A., Moir, R.D., Roher, A.E., White, A.R., et al., 2002. Metalloenzyme-like activity of Alzheimer's disease beta-amyloid. Cu-dependent catalytic conversion of dopamine, cholesterol, and biological reducing agents to neurotoxic H(2)O(2). J. Biol. Chem. 277, 40302–40308.

Padurariu, M., Ciobica, A., Lefter, R., Serban, I.L., Stefanescu, C., Chirita, R., 2013. The oxidative stress hypothesis in Alzheimer's disease. Psychiatr. Danub. 25, 401–409.

Pahuja, R., Seth, K., Shukla, A., Shukla, R.K., Bhatnagar, P., Chauhan, L.K.S., et al., 2015. Trans-blood brain barrier delivery of dopamine-loaded nanoparticles reverses functional deficits in parkinsonian rats. ACS Nano 9, 4850–4871.

Pardridge, W.M., 2003. Blood-brain barrier drug targeting: the future of brain drug development. Mol. Interv. 3, 90–105, 51.

Peng, K.A., Masliah, E., 2010. Lentivirus-expressed siRNA vectors against Alzheimer disease. Methods Mol. Biol. 614, 215–224.
Peng, Y.S., Lai, P.L., Peng, S., Wu, H.C., Yu, S., Tseng, T.Y., et al., 2014. Glial cell line-derived neurotrophic factor gene delivery via a polyethylene imine grafted chitosan carrier. Int. J. Nanomed. 9, 3163–3174.
Perlstein, B., Ram, Z., Daniels, D., Ocherashvilli, A., Roth, Y., Margel, S., et al., 2008. Convection-enhanced delivery of maghemite nanoparticles: Increased efficacy and MRI monitoring. Neuro Oncol. 10, 153–161.
Pilleri, M., Antonini, A., 2014. Novel levodopa formulations in the treatment of Parkinson's disease. Expert Rev. Neurother. 14, 143–149.
Prada, C.M., Garcia-Alloza, M., Betensky, R.A., Zhang-Nunes, S.X., Greenberg, S.M., Bacskai, B.J., et al., 2007. Antibody-mediated clearance of amyloid-β peptide from cerebral amyloid angiopathy revealed by quantitative in vivo imaging. J. Neurosci. 27, 1973–1980.
Re, F., Cambianica, I., Zona, C., Sesana, S., Gregori, M., Rigolio, R., et al., 2011. Functionalization of liposomes with ApoE-derived peptides at different density affects cellular uptake and drug transport across a blood-brain barrier model. Nanomed. Nanotechnol. Biol. Med. 7, 551–559.
Reinke, A.A., Gestwicki, J.E., 2007. Structure-activity relationships of amyloid beta-aggregation inhibitors based on curcumin: influence of linker length and flexibility. Chem. Biol. Drug Des. 70, 206–215.
Rezai-Zadeh, K., Shytle, D., Sun, N., Mori, T., Hou, H., Jeanniton, D., et al., 2005. Green tea epigallocatechin-3-gallate (EGCG) modulates amyloid precursor protein cleavage and reduces cerebral amyloidosis in Alzheimer transgenic mice. J. Neurosci. 25, 8807–8814.
Sardi, S.P., Clarke, J., Viel, C., Chan, M., Tamsett, T.J., Treleaven, C.M., et al., 2013. Augmenting CNS glucocerebrosidase activity as a therapeutic strategy for parkinsonism and other Gaucher-related synucleinopathies. Proc. Natl. Acad. Sci. U. S. A. 110, 3537–3542.
Schapira, A.H., Cooper, J.M., Dexter, D., Clark, J.B., Jenner, P., Marsden, C.D., 1990. Mitochondrial complex I deficiency in Parkinson's disease. J. Neurochem. 54, 823–827.
Schapira, A.H., Olanow, C.W., Greenamyre, J.T., Bezard, E., 2014. Slowing of neurodegeneration in Parkinson's disease and Huntington's disease: future therapeutic perspectives. Lancet 384, 545–555.
Scheltens, P., Blennow, K., Breteler, M.M., de Strooper, B., Frisoni, G.B., Salloway, S., et al., 2016. Alzheimer's disease. Lancet 388, 505–517.
Sharma, R.A., Gescher, A.J., Steward, W.P., 2005. Curcumin: the story so far. Eur. J. Cancer 41, 1955–1968.
Shen, Y., Yu, L.C., 2008. Potential protection of curcumin against hypoxia-induced decreases in beta-III tubulin content in rat prefrontal cortical neurons. Neurochem. Res. 33, 2112–2117.
Shyam, R., Ren, Y., Lee, J., Braunstein, K.E., Mao, H.Q., Wong, P.C., 2015. Intraventricular delivery of siRNA nanoparticles to the central nervous system. Mol. Ther. Nucleic Acids 4, e242.
Sian-Hulsmann, J., Mandel, S., Youdim, M.B., Riederer, P., 2011. The relevance of iron in the pathogenesis of Parkinson's disease. J. Neurochem. 118, 939–957.
Singh, A., Talekar, M., Tran, T.H., Samanta, A., Sundaram, R., Amiji, M., 2014. Combinatorial approach in the design of multifunctional polymeric nano-delivery systems for cancer therapy. J. Mater. Chem. B 2, 8069–8084.
Smith, A., Giunta, B., Bickford, P.C., Fountain, M., Tan, J., Shytle, R.D., 2010. Nanolipidic particles improve the bioavailability and α-secretase inducing ability of

epigallocatechin-3-gallate (EGCG) for the treatment of Alzheimer's disease. Int. J. Pharm. 389, 207–212.
Song, Q., Huang, M., Yao, L., Wang, X., Gu, X., Chen, J., et al., 2014. Lipoprotein-based nanoparticles rescue the memory loss of mice with alzheimer's disease by accelerating the clearance of amyloid-beta. ACS Nano 8, 2345–2359.
Song, Q., Song, H., Xu, J., Huang, J., Hu, M., Gu, X., et al., 2016. Biomimetic ApoE-reconstituted high density lipoprotein nanocarrier for blood-brain barrier penetration and amyloid beta-targeting drug delivery. Mol. Pharm. 13, 3976–3987.
Spillantini, M.G., Goedert, M., 2013. Tau pathology and neurodegeneration. Lancet Neurol. 12, 609–622.
Standridge, J.B., 2004. Pharmacotherapeutic approaches to the treatment of Alzheimer's disease. Clin. Ther. 26, 615–631.
Stanimirovic, D.B., Friedman, A., 2012. Pathophysiology of the neurovascular unit: disease cause or consequence? J. Cereb. Blood Flow Metab. 32, 1207–1221.
Storey, E., Cappai, R., 1999. The amyloid precursor protein of Alzheimer's disease and the Abeta peptide. Neuropathol. Appl. Neurobiol. 25, 81–97.
Surmeier, D.J., Schumacker, P.T., 2013. Calcium, bioenergetics, and neuronal vulnerability in Parkinson's disease. J. Biol. Chem. 288, 10736–10741.
Tardiff, D.F., Jui, N.T., Khurana, V., Tambe, M.A., Thompson, M.L., Chung, C.Y., et al., 2013. Yeast reveal a "druggable" Rsp5/Nedd4 network that ameliorates alpha-synuclein toxicity in neurons. Science 342, 979–983.
Taschenberger, G., Garrido, M., Tereshchenko, Y., Bahr, M., Zweckstetter, M., Kugler, S., 2012. Aggregation of alphaSynuclein promotes progressive in vivo neurotoxicity in adult rat dopaminergic neurons. Acta Neuropathol. 123, 671–683.
Taylor, M., Moore, S., Mourtas, S., Niarakis, A., Re, F., Zona, C., et al., 2011. Effect of curcumin-associated and lipid ligand-functionalized nanoliposomes on aggregation of the Alzheimer's Abeta peptide. Nanomedicine 7, 541–550.
Tjernberg, L.O., Naslund, J., Lindqvist, F., Johansson, J., Karlstrom, A.R., Thyberg, J., et al., 1996. Arrest of beta-amyloid fibril formation by a pentapeptide ligand. J. Biol. Chem. 271, 8545–8548.
Tofaris, G.K., Spillantini, M.G., 2007. Physiological and pathological properties of alpha-synuclein. Cell. Mol. Life Sci. 64, 2194–2201.
Tse, F.L.S., Laplanche, R., 1998. Absorption, metabolism, and disposition of [14C]SDZ ENA 713, an acetylcholinesterase inhibitor, in minipigs following oral, intravenous, and dermal administration. Pharm. Res. 15, 1614–1620.
Ungerstedt, U., Ljungberg, T., Steg, G., 1974. Behavioral, physiological, and neurochemical changes after 6-hydroxydopamine-induced degeneration of the nigro-striatal dopamine neurons. Adv Neurol. 5, 421–426.
Visanji, N.P., Brooks, P.L., Hazrati, L.N., Lang, A.E., 2013. The prion hypothesis in Parkinson's disease: braak to the future. Acta Neuropathol. Commun. 1, 2.
Wang, Y., Cella, M., Mallinson, K., Ulrich, J.D., Young, K.L., Robinette, M.L., et al., 2015. TREM2 lipid sensing sustains the microglial response in an Alzheimer's disease model. Cell 160, 1061–1071.
Wang, Y., Xia, Z., Xu, J.R., Wang, Y.X., Hou, L.N., Qiu, Y., et al., 2012. Alpha-mangostin, a polyphenolic xanthone derivative from mangosteen, attenuates beta-amyloid oligomers-induced neurotoxicity by inhibiting amyloid aggregation. Neuropharmacology 62, 871–881.
Wilson, B., Samanta, M.K., Santhi, K., Kumar, K.P.S., Paramakrishnan, N., Suresh, B., 2008a. Poly(n-butylcyanoacrylate) nanoparticles coated with polysorbate 80 for the targeted

delivery of rivastigmine into the brain to treat Alzheimer's disease. Brain Res. 1200, 159–168.
Wilson, B., Samanta, M.K., Santhi, K., Kumar, K.P.S., Paramakrishnan, N., Suresh, B., 2008b. Targeted delivery of tacrine into the brain with polysorbate 80-coated poly(n-butylcyanoacrylate) nanoparticles. Eur. J. Pharm. Biopharm. 70, 75–84.
Yanagisawa, K., Odaka, A., Suzuki, N., Ihara, Y., 1995. GM1 ganglioside-bound amyloid beta-protein (A beta): a possible form of preamyloid in Alzheimer's disease. Nat. Med. 1, 1062–1066.
Yang, P., Wen, H.Z., Zhang, J.H., 2010. Expression of a dominant-negative Rho-kinase promotes neurite outgrowth in a microenvironment mimicking injured central nervous system. Acta Pharmacol. Sin. 31, 531–539.
Yao, L., Gu, X., Song, Q., Wang, X., Huang, M., Hu, M., et al., 2016. Nanoformulated alpha-mangostin ameliorates Alzheimer's disease neuropathology by elevating LDLR expression and accelerating amyloid-beta clearance. J. Control. Release 226, 1–14.
Yao, L., Song, Q., Bai, W., Zhang, J., Miao, D., Jiang, M., et al., 2014. Facilitated brain delivery of poly (ethylene glycol)-poly (lactic acid) nanoparticles by microbubble-enhanced unfocused ultrasound. Biomaterials 35, 3384–3395.
Zensi, A., Begley, D., Pontikis, C., Legros, C., Mihoreanu, L., Wagner, S., et al., 2009. Albumin nanoparticles targeted with Apo E enter the CNS by transcytosis and are delivered to neurones. J. Control. Release 137, 78–86.
Zhang, C., Wan, X., Zheng, X., Shao, X., Liu, Q., Zhang, Q., et al., 2014a. Dual-functional nanoparticles targeting amyloid plaques in the brains of Alzheimer's disease mice. Biomaterials 35, 456–465.
Zhang, C., Zheng, X., Wan, X., Shao, X., Liu, Q., Zhang, Z., et al., 2014b. The potential use of H102 peptide-loaded dual-functional nanoparticles in the treatment of Alzheimer's disease. J. Control. Release 192, 317–324.
Zhang, Y., Chen, K., Sloan, S.A., Bennett, M.L., Scholze, A.R., O'Keeffe, S., et al., 2014c. An RNA-sequencing transcriptome and splicing database of glia, neurons, and vascular cells of the cerebral cortex. J. Neurosci. 34, 11929–11947.
Zheng, X., Zhang, C., Guo, Q., Wan, X., Shao, X., Liu, Q., et al., 2017. Dual-functional nanoparticles for precise drug delivery to Alzheimer's disease lesions: Targeting mechanisms, pharmacodynamics and safety. Int. J. Pharm. 525, 237–248.
Zlokovic, B.V., 2008. The blood-brain barrier in health and chronic neurodegenerative disorders. Neuron 57, 178–201.

Savaging brain ischemia by increasing brain uptake of neuroprotectants

14

Xiaojiao Ge, Cong Li
Key Laboratory of Smart Drug Delivery, Ministry of Education, School of Pharmacy, Fudan University, Shanghai, China

1 Introduction

Stroke is a devastating neurological condition that is the second leading cause of death and a major cause of disability all over the world (Donnan et al., 2008). Ischemic stroke has been estimated to account for 87% of all stroke cases. A cerebral ischemic event is characterized by the lack of an adequate blood supply to the brain. A transient or permanent reduction of cerebral blood flow (CBF) limits supply of oxygen and nutrients, which initiates an intercorrelated cascade of cellular events that ultimately lead to irreversible brain tissue injury and infarction (Mir et al., 2014). Brain ischemic region can be roughly divided by the infarct core and penumbra. Infarct core is the epicenter of brain ischemia and subjected to the severe damage. Neighboring territory of infract core known as the penumbra suffers functional impairment, but could be salvaged if reperfusion therapy and/or pharmacotherapy are offered timely (Leigh et al., 2017; McLeod et al., 2015). Timely restoration of blood flow, defined as reperfusion, can prevent a more extensive brain damage by rescuing the penumbra. The primary goal of ischemic stroke treatment is to salvage the penumbra as soon as possible and as early as possible to prevent the extension of the infarct core and progressive deterioration of the neurological outcomes.

Thrombolysis has been a standard treatment for ischemic stroke. The aim of thrombolysis is to break down the vascular occlusions, promote recanalization rate, and restore the CBF in time. Recombinant tissue plasminogen activator (rt-PA) is the only thrombolytic agent approved by US Food and Drug Administration (FDA) for acute ischemic stroke treatment. rt-PA catalyzes the conversion of plasminogen to plasmin, a major enzyme responsible for clot breakdown. However, the clinical application of rt-PA is severely limited by its short therapeutic time-window (3.0–4.5 h within onset of the stroke) and the side effects such as intracerebral hemorrhage and angioedema (Fugate et al., 2010). Therefore, most of ischemic stroke patients (95%–98%) cannot benefit from rt-PA treatment by missing the therapeutic time-window, which is caused by the low public awareness, poor recognition of symptoms, delay in emergency transport, and uncertainty to the onset of ischemic attack. Even endeavors such as penumbra selection(Robertson et al., 2015; An et al., 2015), hypothermia (Lee et al., 2017;

Brain Targeted Drug Delivery Systems. https://doi.org/10.1016/B978-0-12-814001-7.00014-7

Li et al., 2011; Liang et al., 2015), and dosage optimization(Meunier et al., 2011) had been tried to extend the time-window for thrombolytic intervention, the requirement of sophisticated imaging technologies and instrumental support prevents their wide applications. Therefore, there is a critical need for the development of novel approaches timely rescuing brain tissue after ischemic attack.

Brain depends exclusively on oxidative phosphorylation to produce energy and possesses a higher oxygen consumption than peripheral organs. Reduced perfusion of the brain initiates the ischemic cascade and results in a salvageable ischemic penumbra surrounding an irreversible infarct core. These cascade events include energy depletion, cell membrane depolarization, over-excitotoxicity, oxidative stress, cytoskeletal reorganization, protease activation, abnormal recruitment of inflammatory cells, neuron apoptosis, and finally the neuron damage and infarction (Fig. 1) (Kalogeris et al., 2016). The reduced blood flow results in failures of the mitochondrial electron transport chain and oxidative phosphorylation, ATP depletion, and up-regulated influx of sodium and calcium. The resulting anoxic depolarization leads to release of excitatory neurotransmitters such as glutamate leading to neuronal toxicity. Over-produced reactive oxygen species (ROS), arachidonic acid, nitric oxide, pro-inflammatory chemokines, and cytokines also cause tissue injury. Abovementioned ischemic cascade events do not necessarily occur sequentially and may instead follow a variable spatial and temporal course (Pandya et al., 2011). Neuroprotection aims to improve the survival of neurons by impeding the deleterious ischemic cascade events. In the past two decades, >1000 neuroprotective agents such as glutamate receptor inhibitors, neurotransmitter inhibitors, calcium channel

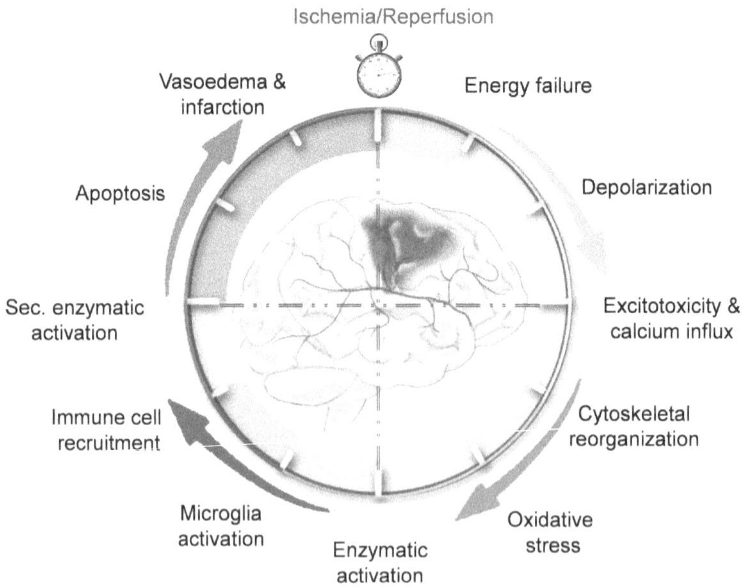

Fig. 1 Devastating cascade events after the onset of ischemic stroke.

blockers, free radical scavenges, and antiinflammatory agents had been developed. Even though part of them efficiently reduced infarct volume and improved functional outcome in animal models (Minnerup et al., 2012), few of them demonstrated unequivocal efficacy in clinical trials that fulfilled regulatory requirements for approval. Besides the limitations in experimental design, inadequate preclinical testing, and the animal models, the inefficient brain uptake of the neuroprotectant is likely, at least in part, caused by their incapability to circumvent the blood-brain barrier (BBB) that maintains brain homeostasis by shielding the brain from peripheral circulation. Strategies are desperately needed to block the disastrous ischemic cascade events by efficiently delivering the neuroprotectant into brain ischemia.

This chapter first summarized the dynamics of BBB structure and permeability as a function of time after the onset of ischemic stroke. Then strategies for delivering neuroprotective agents into brain ischemia by overcoming the BBB in ischemic region were introduced. At last, recent studies related to neuroprotectant brain delivery were briefly reviewed. Elucidating above knowledge is helpful to design drug delivery vectors to facilitate neuroprotective strategy with high efficiency and safety.

2 BBB dynamics after ischemic attack

BBB is a unique physiological structure in brain vasculature, which precisely regulates brain homeostasis by regulating the passage of molecules, ions, and cells at the blood-brain interface (Gao, 2016). The BBB is made up of components including brain capillary endothelial cells (BCECs), basal membrane, pericytes, and astrocyte end feet. BCECs are key compartment inducing the barrier property by forming intercellular tight junctions (TJs) and adhesion junctions (AJs). Due to the much higher electrical resistance (1000–2000 Ω/cm^2) and smaller paracellular pore size (0.4 nm) between the BCECs than that of peripheral capillaries (2–20 Ω/cm^2 and 6–7 nm), most of the blood-borne solutes cannot diffuse into brain parenchyma. Additionally, the BCECs show few fenestrations, smaller number of endocytotic vesicles, lower transcytosis rate, but higher expression levels of efflux transport proteins relative to peripheral endothelial cells (Gao et al., 2014). Therefore, brain drug delivery by crossing BBB via either para-endothelial diffusion or intra-endothelial transcytosis is restricted.

BBB dysfunction with increased permeability is widely observed in ischemic stroke. Early studies in murine models reported a biphasic course of BBB permeability after ischemia attack (Shi et al., 2016). The initial BBB hyper-permeability is observed as early as minutes after ischemic onset followed by a refractory period during which BBB permeability returns to the baseline. A second BBB permeability enhancement starts at 12–24 h after onset and lasts for days. However, recent animal (Bhattacharjee et al., 2001) and human (Chen et al., 2012) studies showed a continuous leakage of the BBB for weeks without evident refractory period after the starting of ischemic stroke. Therefore, understanding the dynamics of BBB permeability after ischemic attack is crucial in optimizing drug delivery strategies and enhancing the neuroprotective effect.

Even though BBB leakage was observed as early as 30 min after ischemia in mouse models, no convincing evidence showed that TJ disruption is responsive for the BBB leakage in the acute stage (< 6 h). Impressively, morphology and expression levels of TJ-associated proteins including claudin-5, occludin, and ZO-1 remain intact even at 24 h post the cerebral ischemia (Shi et al., 2016). Slight BBB leakage is found in the acute stage (<6 h) of ischemic stroke, which is explained by subtle and reversible TJ reorganization (Shi et al., 2016). Depletion of energy molecule and over-produced ROS after vascular occlusion trigger the polymerization of globular actin (G-actin) distributed throughout the BCECs as short filaments into linear stress fibrous actin (F-actin). This polymerization increases actomyosin contraction and cytoskeletal tension, resulting in morphological contraction, para-endothelial TJ disassembly and, eventually, para-endothelial diffusion. Notably, the TJ compromise in the acute stage after ischemic stroke is independent of matrix metalloproteinase (MMP) activities and does not accompany with obvious abnormalities within TJ strands. Different to the acute stage, transcellular transport is the main strategy taking advantage of the enhanced BBB permeability in the subacute stage (6–48 h) of ischemic stroke. In a transgenic mouse strain whose TJ integrity could be longitudinally monitored by in vivo fluorescence microscope, TJs remain intact within the infarct at least 24 h post-stroke, even though obvious BBB permeability enhancement was observed (Shi et al., 2016). Ultrastructural analysis observed that both the number of endocytotic vesicles and rate of endothelial transcytosis in ipsilateral cortex of stroke models increased remarkably compared to that in the contralateral cortex. In the chronic stage (>48 h), inflammatory mediators released by the injured neurons promote the expression of endothelial adhesion molecules such as intercellular adhesion molecule I (ICAM-1) and vascular cell adhesion molecule I (VCAM-1), which facilitate the recruitments of the circulating neutrophils, leukocytes, and macrophages into ischemic regions (Kim et al., 2014). The inflammation mediators secreted by the resident microglias and migrated immune cells perpetuate the positive-feedback loop of inflammation and exert irreversible damage to TJ proteins with the involvement of the MMPs. The aberrant TJ morphologies including gaps and protrusions were observed at 48 h after ischemic attack. The BBB breakdown results in uncontrollable leakage of water, albumin, or even erythrocytes through the injured TJs, which further aggravates the pathological symptoms including vasogenic edema, hemorrhage, and neuronal apoptosis. In summary, the BBB leakage in the acute stage of ischemic stroke is initiated by subtle but reversible TJ disassembly. The up-regulated intra-endothelial transcytosis is the predominated reason causing BBB hyper-permeability in the subacute stage. The amplified BBB leakage in the chronic stage is resulted from the irreversible TJ damage.

3 Brain delivery of neuroprotectant according to BBB dynamic after ischemic stroke

Even though BBB permeability enhancement was observed during all the stages after the onset of ischemic stroke, the efficacy of neuroprotective drugs to enter brain ischemia by taking advantage of the pathologically induced BBB hyper-permeability was not successful. For example, the clinical trial of brain-derived neurotrophic factor (BDNF, MW: 28kDa) as a neuroprotective drug for ischemic stroke treatment was failed owing to its poor intracerebral uptake (Béjot et al., 2011). Therefore, understanding BBB leakage magnitude as a function of time is important to develop strategies to enhance neuroprotectant uptake. Chen et al. studied the temporal profile of BBB disruption induced by transient focal cerebral ischemia via intravenous injection of fluorescence tracers with molecular weights of 3, 150, and 2000kDa (Fig. 2) (Shi et al., 2016). The leakage of Alexa555-dextran (3.0kDa) into the ischemic striatum was observed as early as 30min. The BBB compromise extended to whole striatum

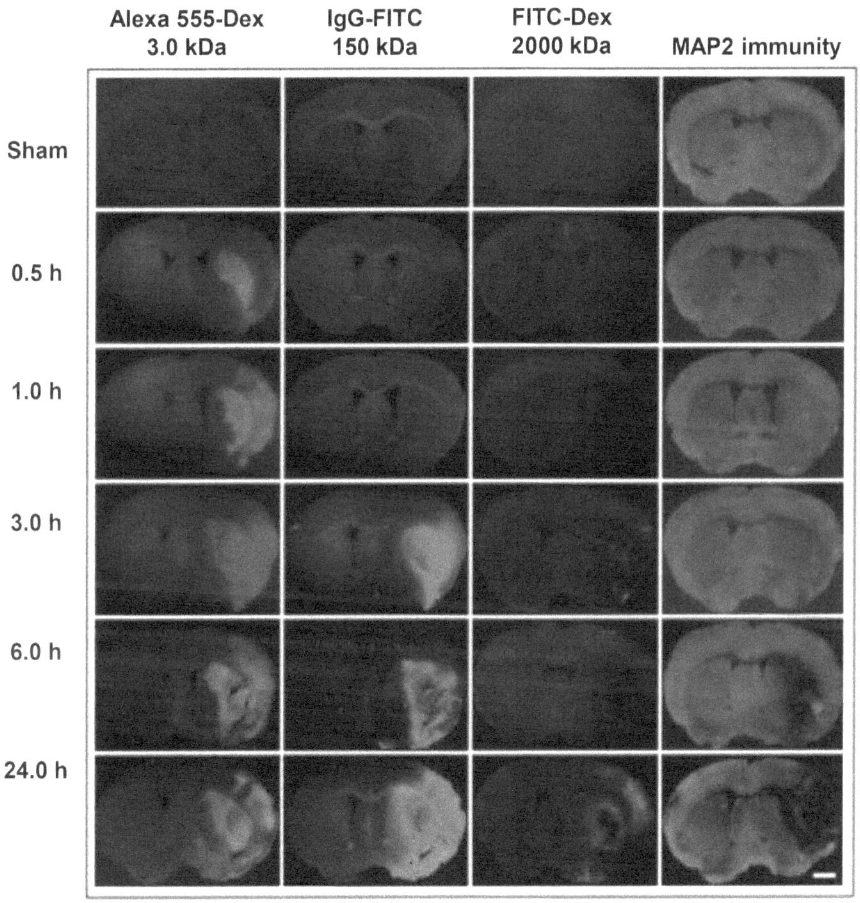

Fig. 2 BBB permeability of mouse brain as a function of time after the onset of ischemic stroke. Vascular leakage of Alexa555-dextran (3.0kDa) in the ischemic striatum was observed as early as 30min. Amplified BBB disruption was detected at 3h post ischemic onset with the presence of fluorophore labeled IgG (150kDa) in ischemic region. Continuous deterioration of BBB integrity was observed with the leakage of bulky FITC-dextran (2000kDa) at 24h post the stroke onset. MAP2 immunostaining was used to illustrate infarcts in the same brains. Scale bar, 1.0mm.

and the neighboring ischemic cortex within 1.0h. Amplified BBB disruption was detected at 3h post-ischemic onset with the presence of fluorophore-labeled IgG (150kDa) in ischemic striatum and partial cortex. Continuous deterioration of BBB integrity was observed with the leakage of bulky FITC-dextran (2000kDa) in striatum area at 24h post the stroke onset. Above study indicates that both magnitude and extension of BBB leakage in ischemic brain increased with the time after ischemic attack (Shi et al., 2016). Kassner et al. studied the dynamics of BBB permeability in ischemic stroke patients by using dynamic contrast-enhanced MRI (DCE-MRI) that noninvasively estimate BBB permeability by monitoring contrast agent exchange through the vasculatures (Kassner et al., 2011). BBB permeability elevated continually after the onset of ischemia and reached the maximal value at 6–48h (subacute stage). Both animal and human studies indicated that artificially tuning BBB permeability in ischemic region is required to achieve efficient brain uptake of the neuroprotective drugs in the acute stage.

Besides the TJs restricting the paracellular diffusion, transcellular barrier also plays an important role leading to the low BBB permeability with the evidence of limited endocytotic caveolae and a low transcytosis rate. Even though the enhanced transendothelial transport after ischemic stroke was observed >20years ago and believed as the initial response of vascular endothelium (Blum et al., 2012), this phenomenon is not been applied in brain drug delivery purpose. Nag et al. showed that both expression of caveolin1 (Cav1) and its phosphorylation state in caveolae increased as early as 2h after CNS injury, prior to disassembly of TJ complexes and BBB breakdown (Knowland et al., 2014). By developing a transgenic mouse strain whose endothelial TJ protein claudin-5 was coexpressed with eGFP, Agallie et al. showed that while the TJs didn't display pronounced defects within the infarct until 2days after ischemia, the transcytosis rate increased significantly as early as 6h (Knowland et al., 2014). Lawrence et al. also found the increased endothelial vesicles in ischemic region at both 4 and 24h poststroke in contrast to the barely compromised TJ structure (Yepes et al., 2000). Importantly, quantitatively assessment showed good correlation between endothelial vesicle number and BBB permeability in ischemic region. Therefore, increasing brain drug delivery by taking advantage of the enhanced endothelial transcytosis is feasible in the subacute stage of ischemic stroke.

Nutrients and metabolites are shuttled between the blood and the brain via multiple transcytosis pathways including carrier-mediated transport (CMT), adsorptive-mediated transport (AMT), and receptor-mediated transcytosis (RMT). CMT tends to ferry hydrophilic small molecular nutrients such as glucose, choline, and amino acids crossing the BBB. However, its application in brain drug delivery is limited due to its high selectivity to the size and steric conformation of the substrates. Even though enhanced brain delivery of small molecular drug conjugated to natural CMT ligand has been reported (Bhaskar et al., 2010; Alam et al., 2010), this strategy has not been successfully used for transport of bulky biologics. AMT occurs when the positively charged proteins interact with negatively charged domains on the luminal side of vascular endothelium. The association triggers endocytosis into the endothelial cells, subsequent intracellular vesicular transport, and eventual exocytosis into the brain parenchyma. Although AMT has been used to deliver a range of cationic vectors into the brain, its application for brain drug delivery is hindered by the inherent nonspecificity, which results in the undesirable drug accumulation into normal brain tissues. RMT is believed as the most promising strategy for delivering the therapeutics into the brain. The RMT process is made up of three steps including the association of circulating substrates to receptor expressed on the apical surface of brain capillaries, formation of membrane invagination followed intracellular vesicles containing receptor-substrate complex, and the traverse of the vesicles to basolateral endothelial surface where the exocytosis is happened. Compared to other transcytosis pathways, RMT shows advantages for delivery of cargoes including high specificity, loading capability, and velocity.

4 Strategies delivering neuroprotective drug by crossing the BBB

4.1 Paracellular diffusion

Due to the small number of endocytotic caveolae and a low transcytosis activity, temporarily compromising para-endothelial TJs is a feasible way to enhance BBB permeability in the acute stage after ischemic stroke. Multiple strategies have been used in increasing BBB permeability by compromising TJ integrity. Hypertonic agents such as mannitol were used to disrupt TJs by inducing osmotic pressure between the luminal and abluminal sides of the vessels (Neuwelt et al., 1979). However, the nonspecific BBB breakdown and slow TJ recovery rate lead to extravasation of blood-borne compartments, which results in severe side effects such as epileptic seizures and vasogenic edema (Bodor and Brewster, 1982; Gao et al., 2016). Microbubble-enhanced focused ultrasound (MB-FUS) was intensively investigated to disrupt BBB in a specific region by creating shear forces that disassemble the TJs. For example, Hynynen et al. showed that the anti-HER2 antibody Herceptin can be delivered into mouse brain through the MB-FUS-mediated BBB disruption (Kinoshita et al., 2006). Even though this strategy showed long-term safety in small animals and nonhuman primates (Burgess et al., 2012), it is hardly to facilitate ischemic stroke treatment due to the mechanic pressure-associated hemorrhage induced by the fragile ischemic vessels. Therefore, strategies tuning TJ tightness with high safety, efficiency. and specificity are crucially important for improving neuroprotective response of ischemic stroke in the acute stage.

Adenosine receptors (ARs) are a class of purinergic GPCRs with adenosine as endogenous agonist. Among the four subtypes of ARs that have been denoted adenosine A_1, A_{2A}, A_{2B}, and A_3 receptors, $A_{2A}R$ is highly distributed in cerebral striatum and olfactory bulb (Chen et al., 1999). Bynoe et al. showed that the $A_{2A}R$ played an active role in modulating BBB permeability in vivo. $A_{2A}R$ activation by its agonist enhanced brain uptakes of intravenously administered macromolecules including antibodies and dextrans with molecular weight above 70kDa (Kim and Bynoe, 2015). Importantly, the BBB opening period correlates with the half-life of the AR agonist. For example, the BBB opening time course after treatment of NECA is much longer than that of Lexiscan. To minimize the side effects of NECA that nonspecifically activates ARs, Li's group developed a series of nanoagonists, in which multiple copies of agonistic ligands were labeled on a G5 dendrimer (Fig. 3). Due to the prolonged circulation lifetime and amplified $A_{2A}R$-binding affinity via multivalent effect, these nanoagonists not only more efficiently increased BBB permeability than that of small molecular agonists, but also showed the flexibility to tune BBB opening time-window in range of 0.5–4.0h by changing the labeling degree of the agonistic ligands (Gao et al., 2014). By choosing a nanoagonist in which its BBB opening time-window matches the pharmacokinetics of a therapeutic agent, it is possible to maximize its brain uptake, but minimize the side effects induced by uncontrollable BBB leakage. Transmission electronic microscopy (TEM) studies clearly demonstrated the reversible disassembly of the para-endothelial TJs with an average width of 25 nm after intravenous administration of the dendrimer-based nanoagonist (Gao et al., 2016). In vivo dynamic contrast-enhanced magnetic resonance imaging (DCE-MRI) studies showed that globe brain uptake of small molecular model drug (500 Da) and macromolecule model drug (70 kDa) in normal mice with intact BBB increased 7 and 3 times, respectively, after the pre-administration of the nanoagonist. Importantly, timely restoration of BBB integrity and functionality was observed at 4 h post-nanoagonist administration (Zheng et al., 2015). While the pathological symptoms such as edema and neuronal apoptosis were observed after the treatment of mannitol, a clinically used hypertonic agent increased BBB permeability by enhancing osmotic pressure; the neurovascular unit (NVU) kept unspoiled and above symptoms were not observed after the nanoagonist treatment.

Li et al. developed a combined strategy to increase the therapeutic response of neuroprotective drug in the acute stage of ischemic stroke. In this strategy, a nanoagonist Den-RGD-CGS was first developed in which $A_{2A}R$ agonistic ligands and ischemic vasculature-targeted domains cyclic RGDyK peptides were labeled on a dendrimer (Fig. 3). This nanoagonist was injected at 4h post-establishment of ischemic stroke models and the vascular permeability in ipsilateral and contralateral hemispheres was determined by DCE-MRI. Compared to control group treated with PBS, the blood-to-tissue transfer constant (K_{trans}) of Gd^{3+}-DOTA in ipsilateral hemisphere increased 5.0 times after the pretreatment of Den-RGD-CGS. Additionally, Den-RGD-CGS showed high specificity to tune BBB permeability in ischemic region. Remarkable K_{trans} increase was only observed in ipsilateral hemisphere (1.48 and 0.79 mL/min/100 mL for Gd^{3+}-DOTA and Gd^{3+}-Den, respectively), but not in contralateral hemisphere (0.29 and 0.22 mL/min/100 mL for Gd^{3+}-DOTA and Gd^{3+}-Den, respectively) after Den-RGD-CGS treatment. Den-RGD-CGS also showed significantly higher K_{trans} ratio (5.1 for Gd^{3+}-DOTA and 3.6 for Gd^{3+}-Den) between the ipsilateral and contralateral hemispheres than that of nonspecific nanoparticle Den-CGS (2.2 for Gd^{3+}-DOTA and 2.3 for Gd^{3+}-Den), which indicates the feasibility to specifically up-regulate BBB permeability in brain ischemia for both small molecular and macromolecular drugs. When the vascular permeability was imaged to be high in brain ischemia and low in surrounding normal brain tissues after nanoagonist administration, superoxide dismutase (SOD), a free radical scavenger, was injected. Compared to ischemic stroke models injected with SOD alone, the combined treatment of

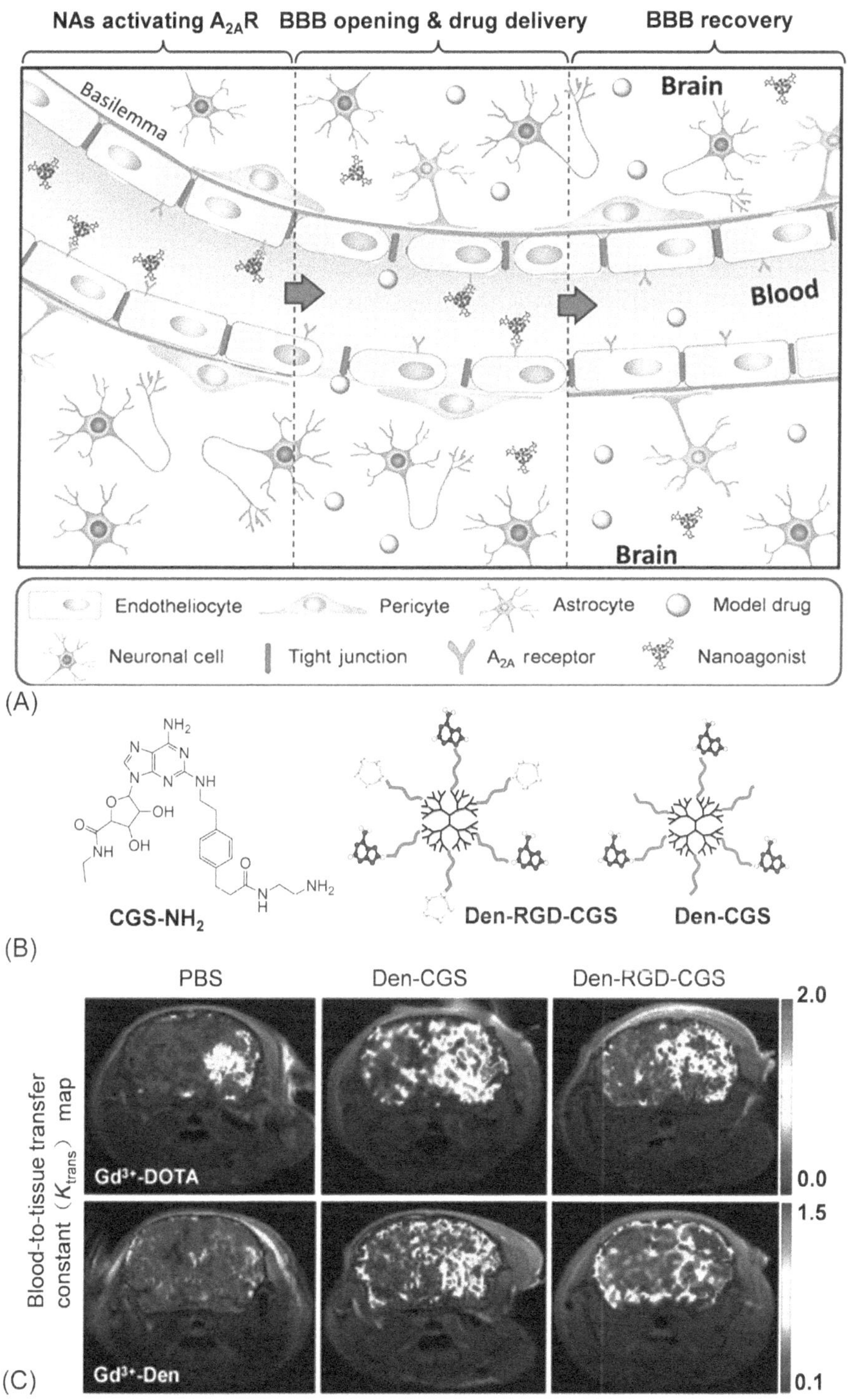

Fig. 3 See the legend on next page.

nanoagonist-followed SOD more efficiently eradicated the ROS in brain ischemia and reduced the volume of brain ischemia. The ischemic volumes at 4, 7, 10, and 14 days after above treatments were quantified by in vivo T2W-MRI. Remarkable ischemia salvaging efficiency with a 50.5% ischemic volume reduction was recorded at 4 day post a combined treatment of nanoagonist-followed SOD. In contrast, only 6.0% and 10.2% ischemic volume reductions were recorded after the treatment of PBS or SOD alone (Zheng et al., 2015).

To further simplify the therapeutic strategy, an agonistic micelle was reported in which the $A_{2A}R$ agonistic ligands were functionalized on the micelle surface and clinical-approved ROS scavenger edaravone was encapsulated with a high load in the internal cavity (Fig. 4). By this way, up-regulation of BBB permeability and enhanced brain uptake of the neuroprotectant can be achieved at the same time. At 14 days posttreatment, while only residual ischemia ($13.0 \pm 3.6\%$ of original ischemic volume) remained in the agonistic micelle treatment group, $67.1 \pm 3.1\%$ and $51.2 \pm 5.7\%$ original ischemic volumes were still presented after the treatment with PBS or free edaravone. Noninvasively, diffusion tensor imaging (DTI) observed the white matter fiber thickness and connectivity in the ipsilesional hemisphere increased remarkably after agonistic micelle treatment. Besides the improvement in structure abnormalities, animal models treated with agonistic micelle also showed the remarkable functional recovery. The modified neurological severity score (mNSS) that quantitatively determined the neurological functional deficits with respect to motor, sensory, reflex, and balance criteria was measured as 1.25 at 14 days post-agonistic micelle treatment, which is 3.7 and 3.4 times lower than that treated with PBS or edaravone alone. Agonistic micelle also substantially prolonged the survival of the ischemic stroke mouse models. The median survival of the models treated with the agonistic micelle was determined to be 42.9% at day 14 and was significantly higher than those treated with PBS (14.3%) or EDV (28.6%). Overall, the agonistic micelle more efficiently prolonged survival, improved axonal remodeling, and reduced behavioral deficits of the animal models by increasing brain uptake of neuroprotectant via temporarily compromising para-endothelial TJs (Qu et al., 2017).

4.2 Intracellular transcytosis

Transferrin receptor (TfR) is the most widely studied endothelial receptor for brain drug delivery via RMT approach (Qian et al., 2002). TfR plays an important role in mediating iron delivery to the brain via intracellular trafficking of the iron-binding

Fig. 3, Cont'd Specifically up-regulating BBB permeability in brain ischemia by signaling $A_{2A}R$. (A) Nanoagonist specifically activates $A_{2A}R$ on brain capillary endothelial cells. The intracellular signal transduction leads to TJ compromise. Drug is given when the BBB permeability is imaged to reach its maximum. (B) Chemical structure of nanoagonist Den-RGD-CGS and control nanoparticle Den-CGS without targeting specificity. (C) Representative K_{trans} maps of ischemic mouse brain when the small molecular (Gd^{3+}-DOTA, *upper panel*) or macromolecular (Gd^{3+}-Den, *below panel*) paramagnetic contrast agent was injected at 45 min PI of PBS or nanoagonist.

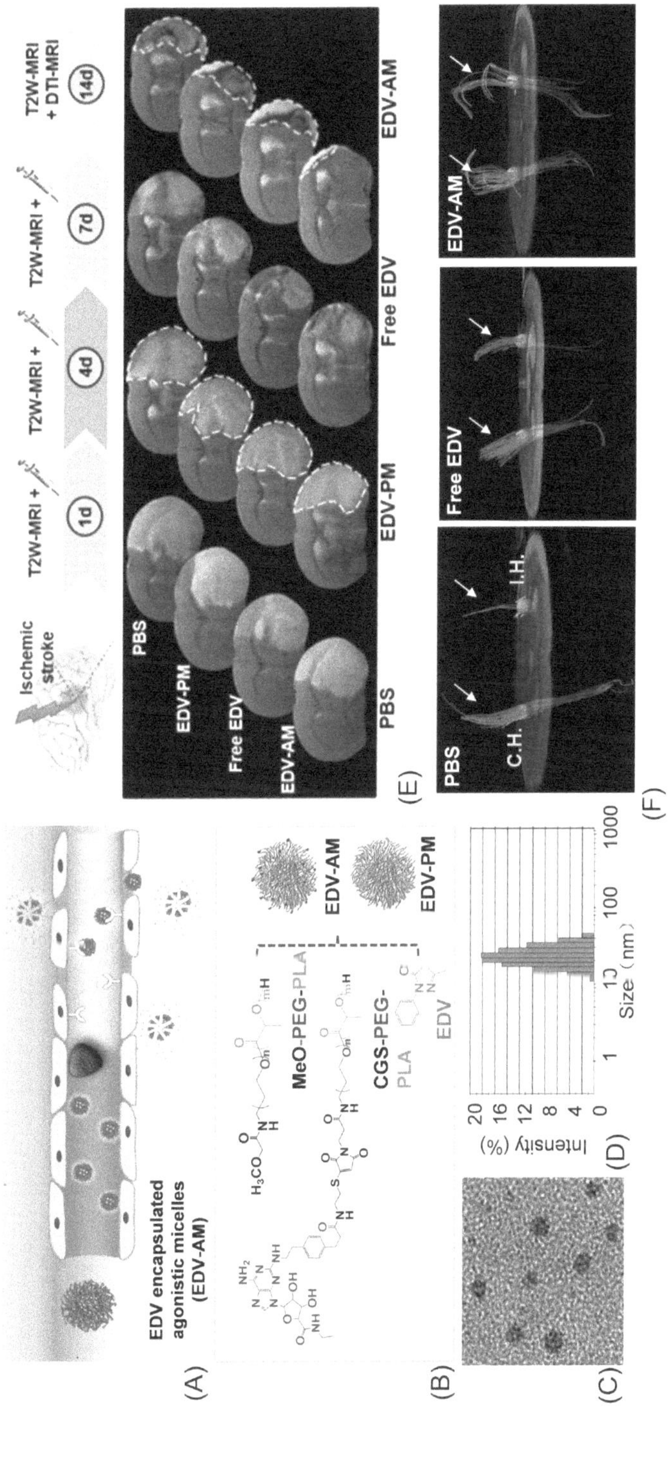

Fig. 4 Agonistic micelle savages brain ischemia by compromising para-endothelial tight junctions. (A) Agonistic micelle activates $A_{2A}R$, opens para-endothelial TJs, enters brain ischemia, releases the encapsulated edaravone and sustainably eradicates ROS. (B) Chemical structure of agonistic micelle EDV-PM. TEM image (C) and dynamic size distribution (D) of EDV-AM. (E) Representative in vivo T2W-MRI of the ischemic mouse brain at selected time PI of PBS, EDV-AM or EDV-PM with a same EDV dosage. (F) In vivo DTI demonstrated fiber tract integrity and orientation in the ipsilesional and contralateral inner capsule at 14 days post injection of PBS, free EDV, EDV-AM or EDV-PM with a same EDV dose.

protein transferrin (Tf) (Reyes-López et al., 2015). Numerous studies have shown that TfR-mediated RMT could significantly increase ischemic uptake of multiple types of neuroprotectants. For example, Pardridge et al. developed a conjugate in which brain-derived neurotrophic factor (BDNF) as a neuroprotectant was labeled with a monoclonal antibody (MAb) against the TfR (Zhang and Pardridge, 2006). Intravenous administration of this conjugate resulted in remarkable reduction in ischemic volume and a concomitantly parallel improvement in functional outcome. Pardridge's group further reported a BBB permeable fusion protein cTfR-MAb/TNFR in which the type II human TNF receptor (TNFR) was conjugated to each heavy chain of a genetically engineered chimeric monoclonal antibody (MAb) against the mouse TfR. At 7 days post the stroke model establishment, treatment of the cTfR-MAb/TNFR fusion protein caused a 45%, 48%, 42%, and 54% reduction in hemispheric, cortical, subcortical stroke volumes, and neural deficit, respectively (Sumbria et al., 2012). In another work, Glial cell line-derived neurotrophic factor (GDNF) as a neuroprotectant and type II tumor necrosis factor receptor (TNFR) decoy receptor as an anti-inflammatory agent were respectively fused to the heavy chain of a chimeric MAb against the mouse TfR. The combined treatment of cTfR-MAb/GDNF and cTfR-MAb/TNFR fusion proteins at 1.0 h post the onset of MCAO showed a synergistic effect and up to 69% reduction in stroke volume (Sumbria et al., 2013). Dalkara et al. reported two nanoparticles in which basic fibroblast growth factor (bFGF) protein as a neuroprotectant and small peptide z-DEVD-FMK as a caspase-3 inhibitor were loaded into dextran nanoparticle, respectively. Functionalization of TfR antibody on the dextran improved BBB permeability of these nanoparticles. Intravenous administration of bFGF- or z-DEVD-FMK-loaded NPs remarkably decreased the infarct volume in mouse brain after 2 h MCAO followed 22 h reperfusion (Yemisci et al., 2015). Significantly, coadministration of these two nanoparticles more efficiently reduced the infarct volume than either of the nanoparticle treated alone. Besides the TfR antibody, small peptides with specificity to TfR were also developed to up-regulate BBB permeability. Gu et al. reported a dual targeted liposome in which T7 peptide as TfR ligand and SHp peptide as ischemia homing domain were labeled on a liposome surface (Fig. 5). Meanwhile, ZL006, a small molecular neuroprotectant blocking the ischemic cascade, was encapsulated into liposomal cavity. This liposome not only efficiently delivered ZL006 into ipsilateral hemisphere than that in contralateral hemisphere of MCAO rats, but also significantly ameliorated infarct volume, neurological deficit, and histopathological severity of cerebral ischemia/reperfusion injury (Zhao et al., 2016). Low-density lipoprotein (LDL) receptor-related protein 1 (LRP1) is a scavenger receptor that participates in endocytosis and also acts as a signaling receptor to modulate numerous cellular processes. Intravenous administration of LRP1 ligand-conjugated immunoglobulin (IVIg), a purified plasma-derived human immunoglobulin for the treatment of neurological inflammatory disorders, showed improved neuroprotective efficacy for the ischemic stroke model by crossing the BBB (Lok et al., 2016).

Adsorption-mediated transport is mediated by the electrostatic interaction between the positive charge on the surface of the drug delivery system and the negative charge on the BBB membrane, which induces endocytosis transport of drugs into the brain.

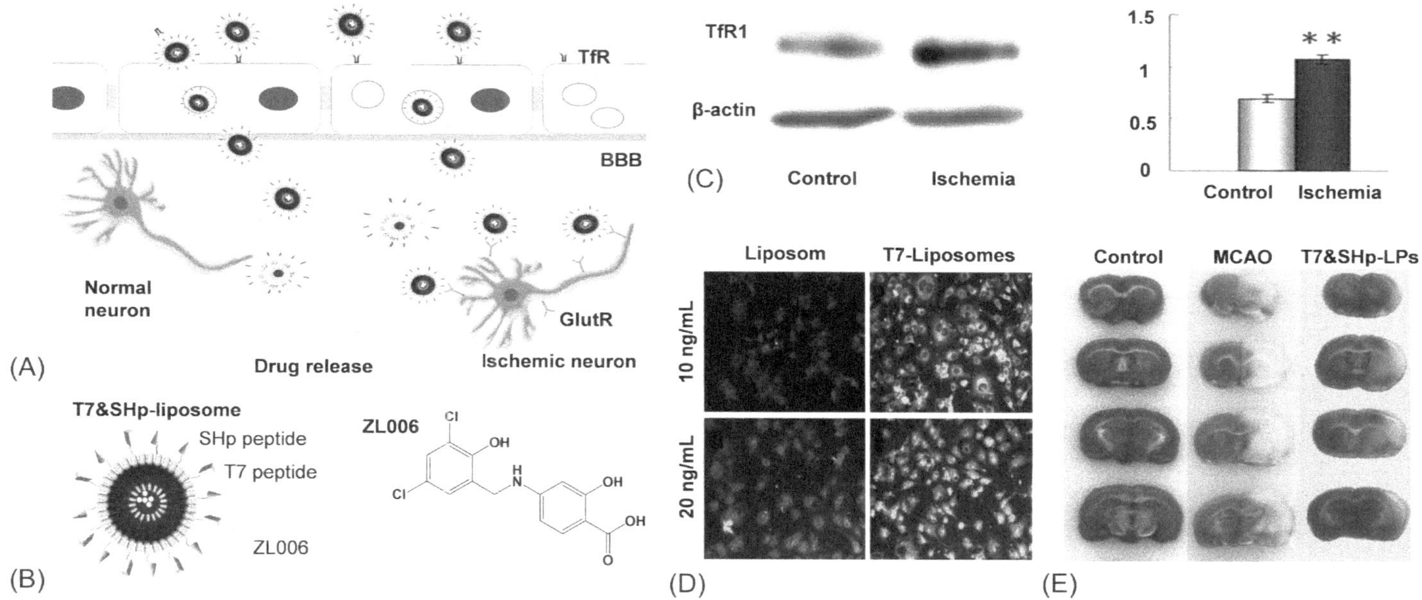

Fig. 5 Delivery of neuroprotectant into brain ischemia via receptor mediated transcytosis. (A) T7&SHp-Liposome traverses the BBB in brain ischemia via transferrin receptor (TfR) mediated transcytosis and then entered ischemic neurons via glutamate receptor (GlutR) mediated endocytosis. (B) Structure of T7&SHp-Liposome. T7 peptide as TfR ligand and SHp as ischemia homing peptide were labeled on the liposome surface. ROS scavenger ZL006 was encapsulated in the liposome. (C) Up-regulation of TfR in the endothelium after oxygen glucose deprivation treatment. (D) Endothelial uptake of T7&SHp-Liposome observed by fluorescent microscopy. (E) Representative TTC-stained brain sections of mouse brain treated with PBS, MCAO, MACO followed administration of ZL006 encapsulated T7&SHp-LP.

Tanshinone IIA (TIIA), one of the active ingredients of Salvia miltiorrhiza root, showed the capability to reduce brain infarct area in the ischemic hemisphere, suppress the expression of intercellular adhesion molecule-1 (ICAM-1) as well as matrix metalloproteinase-9 (MMP-9), and inhibit the degradation of tight junction proteins including zonula occludens-1 (ZO-1) and occludin (Tang et al., 2010). The surface embellishment of cationic bovine serum albumin (CBSA) on the TIIA-encapsulated nanoparticles (CBSA-TIIA-NPs) exhibited the up-regulated attachment to the negatively charged luminal side of the brain capillaries and the increased flux into the cerebrospinal fluid (Liu et al., 2013). Pharmacokinetic studies demonstrated that CBSA-TIIA-NP could significantly prolong circulation time and increase plasma concentration of TIIA compared to the intravenously administrated TIIA solution. Moreover, CBSA-TIIA-NP significantly suppressed the pro-inflammatory cytokines, but up-regulated the anti-inflammatory cytokines in brain ischemia. CBSA-TIIA-NP effectively reduced infarction volume, neurological dysfunctions, neutrophils infiltration, and neuronal apoptosis.

5 Stem cell-modulated neuroprotective therapy

Rehabilitation therapy is important for maximizing functional recovery in the chronic stage of ischemic stroke. Stem cell-based neuroprotective therapy is promising for accelerating neuron replacement and functional recovery after ischemic stroke. Mesenchymal stem cells (MSCs) are multipotent and can transdifferentiate into neurons (Lee et al., 2010). Moreover, MSCs secrete cytokines, growth, and trophic factors that improve neurological functions such as neurogenesis, angiogenesis, and synaptogenesis. Li et al. showed significant recovery of somatosensory behavior and neurological severity score ($P < .05$) in animals infused with 3×10^6 MSCs at 1 day and 7 days post the onset of ischemic stroke (Chen et al., 2001). The administrated MSCs homed to the ischemic region and part of them started to express markers of phenotypic neural cells (Chen et al., 2001). Kim et al. examined the neuroprotective effects of the implanted human umbilical cord-derived mesenchymal stem cells (hUC-MSCs) after ischemic attack (Koh et al., 2008). Twenty days after the induction of neuronal differentiation, about 77.4% of the inoculated hUC-MSCs displayed morphological features of neurons and expressed neuronal cell markers like TU-20, Trk A, NeuN, and NF-M. The cultured hUC-MSCs also produced granulocyte colony-stimulating factor, vascular endothelial growth factor, glial cell line-derived neurotrophic factor, and brain-derived neurotrophic factor. Implantation of the hUC-MSCs into the ipsilaternal hemisphere of ischemic stroke models improved neurobehavioral function and reduced infarct volume relative to the control animals. Three weeks after implantation, most of the implanted hUC-MSCs were present in the damaged hemisphere. Nestin expression level in the hippocampus was increased in the hUC-MSC-implanted group relative to the control group. Even though the hUC-MSCs were morphologically differentiated into neuronal cells and able to produce neurotrophic factors, no functionally active neuronal cells were observed. The improvement in neurobehavioral function and the reduction of infarct volume could be explained to the neuroprotective effects of hUC-MSCs rather than the formation of a new network between host neurons and the implanted hUC-MSCs (Koh et al., 2008). To evaluate the long-term safety and efficacy of the intravenous MSCs in ischemic stroke patients, an open-label, observer-blinded clinical trial of 85 patients with severe middle cerebral artery territory infarct was conducted (Lee et al., 2010). Significant side effects were not observed following MSC treatment and long-term safety and beneficial effects of autologous MSCs transplantation were observed. The occurrence of comorbidities including seizures and recurrent vascular episodes were kept similar between the groups. Compared to the control group, the follow-up-modified Rankin Scale (mRS) score was decreased, whereas the number of patients with mRS values in a range of 0–3 increased in the MSC group ($P = .046$). Clinical improvement in the MSC group was associated with serum levels of stromal cell-derived factor-1 and the degree of involvement of the subventricular region of the lateral ventricle. Above studies showed the benefit and safety of the autologous MSCs transplantation for ischemic stroke patients during long-term follow-up.

6 Conclusions

In the past decade, tremendous efforts were made for the development of strategies to efficiently deliver neuroprotective agents into brain ischemia by crossing the BBB. Even though the increased BBB permeability is observed at the different stages of the ischemic stroke, there is lack of systemic studies of the BBB structure, functionality, and permeability as a function of time after the onset of ischemic stroke. In this chapter, we summarized that temporarily increasing para-endothelial diffusion, taking advantage of the up-regulated intra-endothelial transcytosis, and attenuating the pro-inflammatory response are the feasible ways to increase drug delivery efficiency in the acute, subacute, and chronic stage, respectively. By reviewing recent work, we presented the feasible strategies to specifically deliver neuroprotectants into brain ischemia by traversing BBB via para-endothelial diffusion or inter-endothelial transcytosis. Overall, elucidating BBB dynamics after ischemic attack helps to design new drug delivery vectors to maximize neuroprotective response, but minimize the potential side-effects induced by the BBB leakage. Up-regulating neuroprotectant uptake in brain ischemia will benefit majority of ischemic stroke patients who lost the chance for thrombolytic treatment.

References

Alam, M.I., Beg, S., Samad, A., Baboota, S., Kohli, K., Ali, J., Ahuja, A., Akbar, M., 2010. Strategy for effective brain drug delivery. Eur. J. Pharm. Sci. 40, 385–403.

An, H., Ford, A.L., Chen, Y., Zhu, H., Ponisio, R., Kumar, G., Shanechi, A.M., Khoury, N., Vo, K.D., Williams, J., Derdeyn, C.P., Diringer, M.N., Panagos, P., Powers, W.J., Lee, J.-M., Lin, W., 2015. Defining the ischemic penumbra using magnetic resonance oxygen metabolic index. Stroke 46, 982–988.

Béjot, Y., Mossiat, C., Giroud, M., Prigent-Tessier, A., Marie, C., 2011. Circulating and brain BDNF levels in stroke rats. Relevance to clinical studies. PLoS One. 6. e29405.

Bhaskar, S., Tian, F., Stoeger, T., Kreyling, W., de la Fuente, J.M., Graz, V., Borm, P., Estrada, G., Ntziachristos, V., Razansky, D., 2010. Multifunctional nanocarriers for diagnostics, drug delivery and targeted treatment across blood-brain barrier: perspectives on tracking and neuroimaging. Part. Fibre Toxicol. 7, 3.

Bhattacharjee, A.K., Nagashima, T., Kondoh, T., Tamaki, N., 2001. Quantification of early blood-brain barrier disruption by in situ brain perfusion technique. Brain Res. Protocol 8, 126.

Blum, A., Vaispapir, V., Keinan-Boker, L., Soboh, S., Yehuda, H., Tamir, S., 2012. Endothelial dysfunction and procoagulant activity in acute ischemic stroke. J. Vasc. Interv. Neurol. 5, 33–39.

Bodor, N., Brewster, M.E., 1982. Problems of delivery of drugs to the brain. Pharmacol. Ther. 19, 337–386.

Burgess, A., Huang, Y., Querbes, W., Sah, D.W., Hynynen, K., 2012. Focused ultrasound for targeted delivery of siRNA and efficient knockdown of Htt expression. J. Control. Release 163, 125–129.

Chen, J., Li, Y., Wang, L., Zhang, Z., Lu, D., Lu, M., Chopp, M., 2001. Therapeutic benefit of intravenous administration of bone marrow stromal cells after cerebral ischemia in rats. Stroke 32, 1005–1011.

Chen, J.F., Huang, Z., Ma, J., Zhu, J., Moratalla, R., Standaert, D., Moskowitz, M.A., Fink, J.S., Schwarzschild, M.A., 1999. A(2A) adenosine receptor deficiency attenuates brain injury induced by transient focal ischemia in mice. J. Neurosci. 19, 9192–9200.

Chen, X., Threlkeld, S.W., Cummings, E.E., Juan, I., Makeyev, O., Besio, W.G., Gaitanis, J., Banks, W.A., Sadowska, G.B., Stonestreet, B.S., 2012. Ischemia-reperfusion impairs blood-brain barrier function and alters tight junction protein expression in the ovine fetus. Neuroscience 226, 89–100.

Donnan, G.A., Fisher, M., Macleod, M., Davis, S.M., 2008. Stroke. Lancet 371, 1612–1623.

Fugate, J.E., Giraldo, E.A., Rabinstein, A.A., 2010. Thrombolysis for cerebral ischemia. Front. Neurol. 1, 139.

Gao, H., 2016. Progress and perspectives on targeting nanoparticles for brain drug delivery. Acta Pharm. Sin. B 6, 268–286.

Gao, X., Qian, J., Zheng, S., Changyi, Y., Zhang, J., Ju, S., Zhu, J., Li, C., 2014. Overcoming the blood-brain barrier for delivering drugs into the brain by using adenosine receptor nanoagonist. ACS Nano 8, 3678–3689.

Gao, X., Wang, Y.-C., Liu, Y., Yue, Q., Liu, Z., Ke, M., Zhao, S., Li, C., 2016. Nanoagonist-mediated endothelial tight junction opening: a strategy for safely increasing brain drug delivery in mice. J. Cereb. Blood Flow Metab. 37, 1410–1424.

Kalogeris, T., Baines, C.P., Krenz, M., Korthuis, R.J., 2016. Ischemia/reperfusion. Compr. Physiol. 7, 113–170.

Kassner, A., Mandell, D.M., Mikulis, D.J., 2011. Measuring permeability in acute ischemic stroke. Neuroimaging Clin. N. Am. 21, 315–325.

Kim, D.G., Bynoe, M.S., 2015. A2A adenosine receptor regulates the human blood-brain barrier permeability. Mol. Neurobiol. 52, 664–678.

Kim, J.Y., Kawabori, M., Yenari, M.A., 2014. Innate inflammatory responses in stroke: mechanisms and potential therapeutic targets. Curr. Med. Chem. 21, 2076–2097.

Kinoshita, M., Mcdannold, N., Jolesz, F.A., Hynynen, K., 2006. Noninvasive localized delivery of herceptin to the mouse brain by MRI-guided focused ultrasound-induced blood–brain barrier disruption. Proc. Natl. Acad. Sci. U. S. A. 103, 11719.

Knowland, D., Arac, A., Sekiguchi, K.J., Hsu, M., Lutz, S.E., Perrino, J., Steinberg, G.K., Barres, B.A., Nimmerjahn, A., Agalliu, D., 2014. Stepwise recruitment of transcellular and paracellular pathways underlies blood-brain barrier breakdown in stroke. Neuron 82, 603–617.

Koh, S.-H., Kim, K.S., Choi, M.R., Jung, K.H., Park, K.S., Chai, Y.G., Roh, W., Hwang, S.J., Ko, H.-J., Huh, Y.-M., Kim, H.-T., Kim, S.H., 2008. Implantation of human umbilical cord-derived mesenchymal stem cells as a neuroprotective therapy for ischemic stroke in rats. Brain Res. 1229, 233–248.

Lee, J.H., Zhang, J., Yu, S.P., 2017. Neuroprotective mechanisms and translational potential of therapeutic hypothermia in the treatment of ischemic stroke. Neural Regen. Res. 12, 341–350.

Lee, J.S., Hong, J.M., Moon, G.J., Lee, P.H., Ahn, Y.H., Bang, O.Y., 2010. A long-term follow-up study of intravenous autologous mesenchymal stem cell transplantation in patients with ischemic stroke. Stem Cells 28, 1099–1106.

Leigh, R., Knutsson, L., Zhou, J., van Zijl, P.C.M., 2017. Imaging the physiological evolution of the ischemic penumbra in acute ischemic stroke. J. Cereb. Blood Flow Metab. 271678X17700913.

Li, J., Benashski, S., Mccullough, L.D., 2011. Post-stroke hypothermia provides neuroprotection through inhibition of AMP-activated protein kinase. J. Neurotrauma 28, 1281–1288.

Liang, J., Qi, Z., Liu, W., Wang, P., Shi, W., Dong, W., Ji, X., Luo, Y., Liu, K.J., 2015. Normobaric hyperoxia slows BBB damage and expands the therapeutic time window for tPA treatment in cerebral ischemia. Stroke 46, 1344–1351.

Liu, X., An, C., Jin, P., Liu, X., Wang, L., 2013. Protective effects of cationic bovine serum albumin-conjugated PEGylated tanshinone IIA nanoparticles on cerebral ischemia. Biomaterials 34, 817–830.

Lok, K.Z., Manzanero, S., Arumugam, T.V., 2016. Neuronal low-density lipoprotein receptor-related protein 1 (LRP1) enhances the anti-apoptotic effect of intravenous immunoglobulin (IVIg) in ischemic stroke. Brain Res. 1644, 192–202.

McLeod, D.D., Parsons, M.W., Hood, R., Hiles, B., Allen, J., Mccann, S.K., Murtha, L., Calford, M.B., Levi, C.R., Spratt, N.J., 2015. Perfusion computed tomography thresholds defining ischemic penumbra and infarct core: studies in a rat stroke model. Int. J. Stroke 10, 553–559.

Meunier, J.M., Holland, C.K., Porter, T.M., Lindsell, C.J., Shaw, G.J., 2011. Combination treatment with rt-PA is more effective than rt-PA alone in an in vitro human clot model. Curr. Neurovasc. Res. 8, 305–312.

Minnerup, J., Sutherland, B.A., Buchan, A.M., Kleinschnitz, C., 2012. Neuroprotection for stroke: current status and future perspectives. Int. J. Mol. Sci. 13, 11753–11772.

Mir, M., Albaradie, R., Alhassanavi, M., 2014. Pathophysiology of strokes. In: Recent Advances in Stroke Therapeutics. NOVA Science Publishers, USA.

Neuwelt, E.A., Frenkel, E.P., Diehl, J.T., Maravilla, K.R., Vu, L.H., Clark, W.K., Rapoport, S.I., Barnett, P.A., Hill, S.A., Lewis, S.E., Ehle, A.L., Beyer Jr., C.W., Moore, R.J., 1979. Osmotic blood-brain barrier disruption: a new means of increasing chemotherapeutic agent delivery. Trans. Am. Neurol. Assoc. 104, 256–260.

Pandya, R.S., Mao, L., Zhou, H., Zhou, S., Zeng, J., Popp, A.J., Wang, X., 2011. Central nervous system agents for ischemic stroke: neuroprotection mechanisms. Cent. Nerv. Syst. Agents Med. Chem. 11, 81–97.

Qian, Z.M., Li, H., Sun, H., Ho, K., 2002. Targeted drug delivery via the transferrin receptor-mediated endocytosis pathway. Pharmacol. Rev. 54, 561–587.

Qu, J., Yu, C., Li, S., Liu, H., Zhou, X., Lu, C., Gao, X., Qian, J., Zhang, J., Ju, S., 2017. Edaravone-encapsulated agonistic micelles rescue ischemic brain tissue by tuning blood-brain barrier permeability. Theranostics 7, 884–898.

Reyes-López, M., Piña-Vázquez, C., Serrano-Luna, J., 2015. Transferrin: endocytosis and cell signaling in parasitic protozoa. Biomed. Res. Int. 2015, 641392. https://doi.org/10.1155/2015/641392.

Robertson, C.A., Mccabe, C., Lopez-Gonzalez, M.R., Deuchar, G.A., Dani, K., Holmes, W.M., Muir, K.W., Santosh, C., Macrae, I.M., 2015. Detection of ischemic penumbra using combined perfusion and T2* oxygen challenge imaging. Int. J. Stroke 10, 42–50.

Shi, Y., Zhang, L., Pu, H., Mao, L., Hu, X., Jiang, X., Xu, N., Stetler, R.A., Zhang, F., Liu, X., Leak, R.K., Keep, R.F., Ji, X., Chen, J., 2016. Rapid endothelial cytoskeletal reorganization enables early blood–brain barrier disruption and long-term ischaemic reperfusion brain injury. Nat. Commun. 710523.

Sumbria, R.K., Boado, R.J., Pardridge, W.M., 2012. Brain protection from stroke with intravenous TNFα decoy receptor-trojan horse fusion protein. J. Cereb. Blood Flow Metab. 32, 1933–1938.

Sumbria, R.K., Boado, R.J., Pardridge, W.M., 2013. Combination stroke therapy in the mouse with blood–brain barrier penetrating IgG–GDNF and IgG–TNF decoy receptor fusion proteins. Brain Res. 1507, 91–96.

Tang, C., Xue, H., Bai, C., Fu, R., Wu, A., 2010. The effects of Tanshinone IIA on blood–brain barrier and brain edema after transient middle cerebral artery occlusion in rats. Phytomedicine 17, 1145–1149.

Yemisci, M., Caban, S., Gursoy-Ozdemir, Y., Lule, S., Novoa-Carballal, R., Riguera, R., Fernandez-Megia, E., Andrieux, K., Couvreur, P., Capan, Y., Dalkara, T., 2015. Systemically administered brain-targeted nanoparticles transport peptides across the blood-brain barrier and provide neuroprotection. J. Cereb. Blood Flow Metab. 35, 469–475.

Yepes, M., Sandkvist, M., Wong, M.K., Coleman, T.A., Smith, E., Cohan, S.L., Lawrence, D.A., 2000. Neuroserpin reduces cerebral infarct volume and protects neurons from ischemia-induced apoptosis. Blood 96, 569.

Zhang, Y., Pardridge, W.M., 2006. Blood–brain barrier targeting of BDNF improves motor function in rats with middle cerebral artery occlusion. Brain Res. 1111, 227–229.

Zhao, Y., Jiang, Y., Lv, W., Wang, Z., Lv, L., Wang, B., Liu, X., Liu, Y., Hu, Q., Sun, W., Xu, Q., Xin, H., Gu, Z., 2016. Dual targeted nanocarrier for brain ischemic stroke treatment. J. Control. Release 233, 64–71.

Zheng, S., Bai, Y.-Y., Liu, Y., Gao, X., Li, Y., Changyi, Y., Wang, Y., Chang, D., Ju, S., Li, C., 2015. Salvaging brain ischemia by increasing neuroprotectant uptake via nanoagonist mediated blood brain barrier permeability enhancement. Biomaterials 66, 9–20.

Part IV

Perspective and pitfalls of nanoparticles-based brain targeting delivery

Neurotoxicity concern about the brain targeting delivery systems

15

Yubin Li[*,†,‡], *Jiajun Fan*[*], *Dianwen Ju*[*]
[*]Department of Microbiological and Biochemical Pharmacy & The Key Laboratory of Smart Drug Delivery, Ministry of Education, School of Pharmacy, Fudan University, Shanghai, PR China, [†]Perelman School of Medicine, University of Pennsylvania, Philadelphia, PA, United States, [‡]Corporal Michael J. Crescenz VA Medical Center, Philadelphia, PA, United States

1 Introduction

Nanoparticles are the series of engineered structures whose diameter is less than 100nm and could be manufactured by numbers of different physicochemical processes depending on different types of properties and applications (De Jong and Borm, 2008; Boverhof et al., 2015). The exclusive characteristics of these nanoparticles such as unique structures, monodispersity, high surface to mass ratio, and effective cellular property to uptake and absorb genes, proteins, or small molecular chemical drugs make them suitable for various applications in the fields of biomedicine (Li et al., 2013; Wang and Wang, 2014; Zhang et al., 2013). Owing to their unique properties, nanoparticles have the capacity to enter the central nervous system (CNS) by passing the blood-brain barrier (BBB) (Saraiva et al., 2016; Upadhyay, 2014). However, there are also increased concerns about safety issues of brain-targeted drug delivery system usage. The toxicity, especially neurotoxicity triggered by nanoparticles, has become serious challenge during brain-targeted drug delivery, and their related mechanisms of nanoparticles-triggered neurotoxicity have been investigated (Masserini, 2013). This chapter introduces neurotoxicity concern about brain targeting drug delivery nanoparticles. It starts by presenting general neurotoxicity of the brain targeting drug delivery nanoparticles (metallic nanoparticles (silver, gold); metallic oxide nanoparticles (titanium dioxide; iron oxide); nonmetallic nanoparticles (silica, carbon); and polymers) in vitro (neurons; astrocytes; microglia; and other neuronal cells;) and in vivo. It then explains the related mechanisms of the brain targeting drug delivery nanoparticles-induced neurotoxicity, including physical mechanisms, cellular mechanisms, and molecular mechanisms. The physical mechanisms mainly include size, shape, and surface charge of nanoparticles; cellular mechanisms primarily focus on apoptosis, necrosis, autophagy, neutrophil extracellular traps (NETs)-mediated NETosis, pyroptosis, and cell cycle arrest; while molecular mechanisms are mainly involving reactive oxygen species, DNA damage, and signaling pathways. The related signaling pathways mainly include nuclear actor kappa-light-chain-enhancer of activated B cells (NF-kB), PI3K/Akt/mTOR, mitogen-activated protein kinase (MAPK), and transforming growth factor (TGF)-beta

Brain Targeted Drug Delivery Systems. https://doi.org/10.1016/B978-0-12-814001-7.00015-9

signaling pathway. There still have other potential complicated factors affecting neurotoxicity of nanoparticles that need to be further studied. The last part of the chapter briefly discusses current perspective to solve brain targeting delivery nanoparticles-induced neurotoxicity. The chapter highlighted nanoparticles-triggered neurotoxicity and its related physicochemical and biochemical mechanisms, which might be useful for evaluating neurotoxicity of drug delivery nanoparticles and developing novel biosafe brain-targeted drug delivery systems in the future.

2 Nanotoxicity of the brain targeting delivery systems

The central nervous system, consisting of brain, spinal cord, network of neurons, and the blood-brain barrier, is one of the most important microenvironments of the body (Wahl et al., 1988; Wong et al., 2013). Because of blood-brain barrier's tight junctions existing around the capillary tubes, central nervous system cannot directly receive blood through systemic circulation (Haddad-Tovolli et al., 2017; De Bock et al., 2014). Thus, most drugs cannot be used for brain disorders treatment due to their inability to pass through the blood-brain barrier (Pardridge, 2005). The nanoparticles translocation into the central nervous system without breaking the tight junction of the blood-brain barrier due to their unique properties leads to the development of diverse nanoparticles-based brain targeting delivery systems designed for brain disorders therapy (Kabanov and Gendelman, 2007; Morachis et al., 2012; Soni et al., 2016). However, considering the unique physicochemical properties and their potential release of these nanoparticles into the microenvironment and accumulation in human tissues, especially in central nervous system, it is urgent to figure out and analyze their nanotoxicity, especially neurotoxicity, through widely and well-designed experiments (Karmakar et al., 2014).

In general, neurotoxicity of nanoparticles is evaluated by using in vitro and in vivo models (Voigt et al., 2014). Organ-typical or dissociated cultures, cell lines, or stem cells are usually used as in vitro cell models, and the toxicity is measured by different types or doses of nanoparticles exposing to the in vitro cell models (Ivanov et al., 2015; Joris et al., 2016; Patil et al., 2015). The in vitro neurotoxicity of nanoparticles has been studied using different kinds of neuronal cells, such as neurons, astrocytes, microglia, and other neuronal cells (Yang et al., 2010). Besides, mostly, nonneural cells were also used to explore in vitro toxicity of nanoparticles, including dermal fibroblasts (Galandakova et al., 2016), vascular endothelial cells (Sun et al., 2017), bronchial epithelial cells (Ko et al., 2016), macrophages (Arai et al., 2015), and embryonic kidney cells (Wang et al., 2009). Neurotoxicity including nervous injury could also be assayed by behavioral and electrophysiological studies using in vivo model (Accardi et al., 2016). Behavioral studies were performed in a well-established animal model with a series of clinical signs of toxicity, including tremors, convulsions, salivation, nausea, vomiting, diarrhea, lethargy, and others (Voorhees et al., 2016). Furthermore, spatial learning ability and memory function related to hippocampus can be studied by examining the expression of related genes (Vanguilder and Freeman, 2011; Win-Shwe et al., 2008). Comparisons and analyses

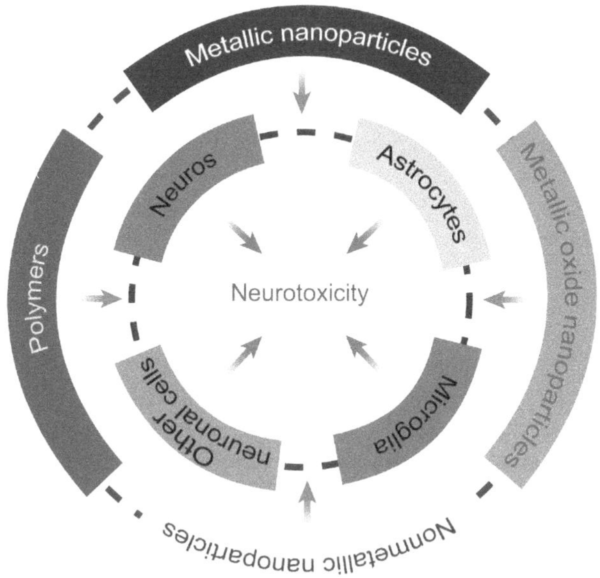

Fig. 1 Nanotoxicity of the brain targeting delivery systems.

of selected studies on nanoparticles-induced neurotoxicity in different cell and animal models are presented to illustrate the neurotoxicity of brain targeting delivery systems (Fig. 1).

2.1 *In vitro neurotoxicity of nanoparticles*

2.1.1 *Neurons*

Neurons are the cells within the nervous system that transmit information to other nerve cells, muscle, or gland cells and are major components of the brain and spinal cord of the central nervous systems.

Nyitrai et al. (2013) explored the early progression of polyamidoamine (PAMAM) generation 5 dendrimers action in brain tissues on neuronal and astroglial cells by detecting free intracellular Ca^{2+} and mitochondrial membrane potential changes and found that interaction of PAMAM dendrimers and plasma membrane led to robust activation of neurons, leading to mitochondrial depolarization and impaired mitochondrial oxidation in brain tissue: enhanced mitochondrial depolarization followed by impaired oxidative metabolism of neurons may be the primary basis of neurotoxicity induced by PAMAM dendrimers.

PC-12 cells are widely used in numbers of in vitro neurobiological studies due to their characteristics of dopaminergic neurons (Westerink and Ewing, 2008). Using PC-12 cell model, researchers examined the cell function affection after magnetic nanoparticles exposure and found that increasing concentrations of anionic magnetic nanoparticles resulted in a dose-dependent diminishing viability and capacity of PC12 cells to extend neuritis in response to their biological characteristics (Pisanic et al., 2007).

Apart from PC-12 cells, the neuroblastoma SH-SY5Y cell line was also widely used as an in vitro model, especially in Parkinson's disease research (Xicoy et al., 2017). Joris et al. (2016) used human and murine neuroblastoma cell line, neural progenitor cell line, and neural stem cells to evaluate the impact of cell type on in vitro neurotoxicity of nanoparticles (gold, silver, and iron oxide) by detecting reactive oxygen species production, calcium homeostasis mitochondrial integrity, and cell morphology; and reported that neural stem cells showed most acute nanotoxicity, while murine neuroblastoma cell line showed least neurotoxicity. Nanoparticles-induced cytotoxicity presented cell type- and species-specific responses (Joris et al., 2016).

To measure whether titanium dioxide nanoparticles could damage biological targeting brain through oxidative stress, brain cultures of immortalized mouse microglia BV-2, rat dopaminergic neurons N27, and primary cultures of embryonic rat striatum were incubated by commercial titanium dioxide nanoparticles. Mouse microglia BV-2 exposure immediately triggered prolonged release of reactive oxygen species, reduced Hoechst nuclear stain, and up-regulated inflammatory, apoptotic, and cell-cycling pathways. Titanium dioxide nanoparticles incubation increased intracellular ATP and caspase 3/7 activity in isolated rat dopaminergic neurons N27, while decreased immunohistochemically stained neurons in primary cultures of rat striatum (Long et al., 2007).

Besides rat dopaminergic neurons, different types of mouse brain neural cells were usually isolated and used as in vitro neurodegenerative disorder models. Using mouse neuron N2a cells, murine brain ALT astrocytes, and microglial BV-2 cells, scientists explored the inflammatory gene expression and neurodegenerative responses triggered by silver nanoparticles: Silver nanoparticles can be uptake by these neural cells and significantly increased secretion of interleukin-1 and C-X-C motif chemokine 13, macrophage receptor with collagenous structure, and glutathione synthetase gene expression and neutralized oxidative stress (Huang et al., 2015). Similarly, using cultured cerebral cortical neurons, Kim et al. also found that silver nanoparticles could suppress the cell viability in a dose- and time-dependent manner. Silver nanoparticles-induced cultured cerebral cortical neurons apoptotic death was confirmed by terminal deoxynucleotidyl transferase dUTP nick-end labeling (TUNEL), DNA fragmentation, and caspase-3 cleavage. These apoptotic effects were mediated by increasing intracellular reactive oxygen species production in cultured cortical neurons (Kim et al., 2015b).

2.1.2 Astrocytes

Astrocytes are characteristic star-shaped glial cells in the brain and spinal cord. They perform a lot of functions, including biochemical support of endothelial cells that form the blood-brain barrier, provision of nutrients to the nervous tissue, maintenance of extracellular ion balance, and the role in the repair and scarring process of the brain and spinal cord following traumatic injuries.

Amine-modified polystyrene nanoparticles induced human brain astrocytoma cells death through the mitochondria damage-mediated apoptotic mechanism. Cationic polystyrene nanoparticles treatment induced caspase 3/7, caspase 9, and poly (ADP-ribose) polymerase-1 cleavage. Apoptosis is followed by necrotic response together with rapid increase of reactive oxygen species in 1321N1 human brain astrocytoma cells during polystyrene exposure (Bexiga et al., 2011). Similarly, polyethyleneimine (PEI) polymers reduced the intracellular ATP activity, changed cell membrane integrity, and triggered direct necrosis and apoptosis during inhibiting cell viability in primary astrocytes (Newland et al., 2013).

Apart from polymers, metallic oxide nanoparticles also present neurotoxicity on astrocytes. Liu et al. (2013) studied the effect of different sized titanium dioxide nanoparticles in rat astrocytes, aiming to find the cytotoxicity of titanium dioxide nanoparticles, and found these nanoparticles could inhibit cell survival rates in a dose-dependent manner, with sparse arrangement changes, increscent cell spaces, intracellular particles increase, and cellular transparency decrease. Au studied the effects of a proprietary chemical formulation of iron oxide magnetic nanoparticles upon astrocytes in vitro at a specified concentration (175 μM) and also found significant effects upon mitochondrial function as well as decreased cell viability. Using cultured primary astrocytes, Wang et al. (2014a) reported that zinc oxide nanoparticles exposure could reduce astrocytes viability, increase lactate dehydrogenase release, stimulate intracellular reactive oxygen species generation, and activate caspase-3 cleavage. Cleavage of nuclear condensation and poly(ADP-ribose) polymerase-1, decrease in mitochondrial membrane potential, and increase in the expression of Bax/Bcl-2 ratio suggested that mitochondria was involved in zinc oxide nanoparticles-induced apoptosis.

2.1.3 Microglia

Microglia are a type of neuroglia located throughout the brain and spinal cord. As the resident macrophage cells, they act as the first and main form of active immune defense in the central nervous system and are key cells in overall brain maintenance.

Long et al. (2007) use Degussa P25, a commercially available titanium dioxide nanoparticle treating brain cultures of immortalized mouse microglia, rat dopaminergic neurons, and found BV2 microglia exposed to P25 responded with an immediate and prolonged release of reactive oxygen species; Hoechst nuclear stain was reduced after 24 h and 48 h exposure. P25-exposed BV2 microglia indicated up-regulation of inflammatory, apoptotic, and cell-cycling pathways and down-regulation of energy metabolism. P25 rapidly damages neurons at low concentrations in complex brain cultures; plausibly through microglial-generated reactive oxygen species. Besides, titanium dioxide nanoparticles and HAP nanoparticles also induced obvious iNOS expression, resulting in NO release from microglia. Titanium dioxide nanoparticles and HAP nanoparticles treatment upregulated the expression of MCP-1 and MIP-1 alpha, activated the transcription factor NF-kB, and increased secretion levels of tumor necrosis factor-alpha, interleukin-1 beta, and interleukin 6, suggesting that these nanoparticles activated microglia (Xue et al., 2012).

2.1.4 Other neuronal cells

Human brain microvascular endothelial cells are one of the most important cell types in the brain, which make up the blood vessels. Eldridge et al. (2017) compared the cytotoxic effects of multiwalled carbon nanotubes on tissue-mimicking cultures and monolayer cultures of human brain microvascular endothelial cells and reported that tissue-mimicking cultures were resistant to all types of nanoparticles than monolayer cultures of cells. Orlando et al. (2017) used human vascular endothelial cells and neurons to explore relations of mesoporous silica nanoparticles (size, dose, and exposure time) with cellular responses. Larger mesoporous silica nanoparticles showed higher toxicity due to mitochondrial activity, membrane integrity, autophagy, and nitric oxide production and suggested that mesoporous silica nanoparticles could influence endothelial functionality from outside of the cells. Anspach et al. (2016) exposed a series of different polymer-coated different-sized gold nanoparticles to human brain endothelial cells to evaluate their effects on cytotoxicity, pro-inflammatory mediators, barrier functions, and endoplasmic reticulum stress and found that exposure to gold nanoparticles increased pro-inflammatory markers in a time-dependent manner.

Apart from human brain-derived endothelial cells, endothelial cells isolated from mice and rat brain are also widely used for cytotoxic detection. Reduced grapheme oxide with/without polyethylene glycol modification both showed concentration-dependent toxicity in primary astrocytes and rat brain endothelial cells. The highest concentration of non-modified grapheme oxide had lower toxicity on cell viability, while polyethylene glycol-modified nanoparticles-induced deleterious effects and cell death (Mendonca et al., 2016). Trickler et al. (2010) isolated primary rat brain microvessel endothelial cells from adult Sprague-Dawley rats and used them as an in vitro blood-brain barrier model. Gold nanoparticles induced cytotoxicity at lower concentrations for smaller-sized nanoparticles. Larger gold nanoparticles induced obvious pro-inflammatory cytokines tumor necrosis factor-alpha secretion. These results suggested that gold nanoparticles interacted with the cerebral microvasculature secreting pro-inflammatory cytokines and further triggered neurotoxicity.

Embryonic neural stem cells from human and rat fetuses were used to determine whether nanoparticles are capable of causing neurotoxicity. Mitochondrial viability was substantially attenuated and LDH release was increased significantly in a dose-dependent manner after embryonic neural stem cells incubated with silver nanoparticles. Silver nanoparticles-induced neurotoxicity was further confirmed by up-regulated Bax protein expression, an increased number of TUNEL-positively stained cells, and elevated reactive oxygen species. Cell proliferation was also significantly decreased by silver nanoparticles; coadministration of antioxidant agent effectively blocked the adverse effects associated with silver nanoparticle exposure (Liu et al., 2015). Pongrac et al. (2016) investigated the mechanisms of neurotoxicity of superparamagnetic iron oxide nanoparticles on murine neural stem cells and showed that these nanoparticles depleted intracellular glutathione levels, altered activities of SOD and GPx, hyperpolarized mitochondrial membrane, dissipated cell-membrane potential, and increased DNA damage in murine neural stem cells.

2.2 *In vivo neurotoxicity of nanoparticles*

As previously mentioned, nanoparticles have the capacity to pass through the blood-brain barrier to enter the brain via series of mechanisms and pathways. Thus, it might have potential to influence brain physiology and trigger serious side effects. It is necessary to explore in vivo experiments investigating organ systems (including neuronal systems) to nanoparticles, which cannot be fully modeled in vitro.

For cationic polymers-induced neurotoxicity in vivo, scientists found that chitosan nanoparticles could enter into the brain and specially deposit in the frontal cortex and cerebellum after systemic injection. Seven days after exposure, apoptosis and necrosis of neurons, slight inflammatory response in frontal cortex, and decrease of astrocytes activation markers—glial fibrillary acidic protein—in cerebellum confirmed the neurotoxicity of chitosan nanoparticles (Yuan et al., 2015). Similar results were reported in PEI-induced acute brain toxicity, PEI-induced loss of gross tissue volume on brain tissues, and accumulated astrocytes (measured by GFAP, marker of the activation of astrocytes) and microglia (measured by microglia marker OX-42) during its induced neurotoxicity in adult Sprague-Dawley rats (Newland et al., 2013). Single dose of generation 4 PAMAM dendrimers intranasally administered to BALB/c mice could moderately activate immune competent cells of the CNS and alter related signaling pathways including serotonin-anxiety pathway, transforming growth factor-beta receptor signaling, prostaglandin synthesis regulation, complement coagulation cascades, chemokine signaling pathway, and nonodorant G protein-coupled receptor signaling pathway in brain tissues (Win-Shwe et al., 2014).

To evaluate the effects of grapheme oxide nanoparticles on the influence of blood-brain barrier, Mendonca et al. (2016) assessed hippocampal blood-brain barrier integrity in an in vivo rat model. The activation of astrocyte and the expression of the endothelial junction proteins (including tight junction and adherent junction) were detected. Obvious and progressive down-regulation of markers of astrocytes, endothelial junction, and basal lamina were presented 1 h to 7 days after nanoparticles injection. Besides, the formation of intracellular reactive oxygen species was also involved in nanoparticles-induced blood-brain barrier damage. Rat exposed to titanium dioxide nanoparticles showed destroyed blood-brain barrier, significantly increased the concentration of interleukin-1 beta, tumor necrosis factor-alpha, and interleukin-10 in brain tissues and necrosis, inflammation, and cellular edema in brain tissues (Liu et al., 2013). Nano-manganese dioxide was also found to cause dopaminergic neuronal dysfunction and astrocyte activation, thus affecting the learning abilities of rats (Li et al., 2014a). Zinc oxide nanoparticles intraperitoneal injection induced increased production of pro-inflammatory cytokines (interleukin 1 and interleukin 6) in the serum and the brain tissues. In the brain, increased oxidative stress level, impaired learning and memory abilities, and hippocampal pathological changes were presented after zinc oxide nanoparticles treatment. The contents of hippocampal cAMP response element binding protein, phosphorylated CREB, synapsin I, and cAMP were decreased in the mice injected by zinc oxide nanoparticles (Tian et al., 2015).

3 Physical chemical mechanisms of brain targeting delivery systems induced nanotoxicity

The neurotoxicity of brain targeting delivery nanoparticles could be modulated by their unique physicochemical characteristics, which include size, shape, charge, surface modification, crystal types, and so on (Song et al., 2015). Besides, dosage, types of administration, and exposure routes of nanoparticles are all the common factors affecting neurotoxicity (Feng et al., 2015) (Fig. 2).

3.1 Size

Plenty of research have been conducted as regard the effects of size of nanoparticles on neurotoxicity (Shim et al., 2014). Size has also been a major factor in crossing the blood-brain barrier leading to possible neurotoxicity, as smaller size nanoparticles are much easier to cross the blood-brain barrier compared with larger size nanoparticles (Simko and Mattsson, 2014; Shilo et al., 2015). For gold nanoparticles, only less than 50nm nanoparticles were able to pass through the blood-brain barrier in vivo; besides, only smallest nanoparticles were able to trigger nanotoxicity in primary rat brain microvessel endothelial cells and caused more serious toxicity than larger size gold particles when injected intravenously into mice (De Jong and Borm, 2008; Trickler et al., 2011). The reactivity of silver nanoparticles is also inversely proportional to the particle size (Christian et al., 2008). Existing evidence has indicated a tight relation between size and silver nanoparticles-induced toxicity: Higher cytotoxic potential of smaller silver nanoparticles has been proved in primary neuronal cultures when compared with larger silver nanoparticles exposure (Haase et al., 2012; Ivask et al., 2014). 5nm silver nanoparticles triggered more severe cell viability and cellular membrane

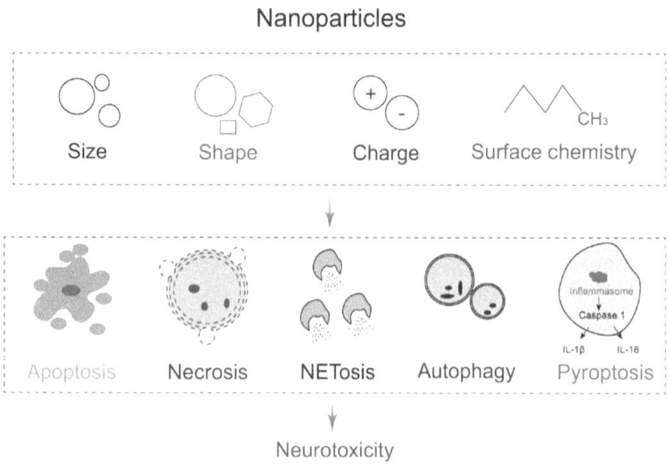

Fig. 2 Physical chemical mechanisms and cellular mechanisms of brain targeting delivery systems-induced nanotoxicity.

integrity change than 20 nm and 50 nm silver nanoparticles (Liu et al., 2010). Researchers also confirmed the size-dependent neurotoxicity of silver nanoparticles in an animal exposure model. When mice were treated with silver nanoparticles, small-sized silver nanoparticles were distributed to the organs including brain, while large-sized silver nanoparticles were not detected in these organs (Park et al., 2010); others also reported that 20–40 nm silver nanoparticles induced serious damage of brain cells than larger silver nanoparticles (Sharma et al., 2013). Data collected from current studies also compared the neurotoxicity of micro-TiO_2 with nano-TiO_2; only nano-TiO_2 but not micro-TiO_2 can be detected in the brain regions. Besides, TiO_2 nanoparticles showed moderately toxic effect on neuron cells, while the micron-sized TiO_2 did not exhibit any toxic response; these data suggested that nanoparticles were more toxic than micrometer-sized particles (Wu et al., 2010).

Besides metallic nanoparticles, similar results were also showed in non-metallic nanoparticles (such as silica nanoparticles)-triggered neurotoxicity. Zebrafish treated with 15 nm silica nanoparticles presents more apparent variation on advanced cognitive neurobehavioral patterns and acted on the retina and dopaminergic neurons when compared with 50 nm silica nanoparticles (Li et al., 2014a, b). Using the same size (15- and 50-nm) nanoparticles, scientists also found smaller silica nanoparticles did more harm in terms of the level of increased intracellular oxidative stress and thiobarbituric acid reactive species, as well as depleted GSH, suggesting that cytotoxicity triggered by silica nanoparticles is size-dependent (Kim et al., 2015b). Moreover, although cell viability was decreased in a size- and dose-dependent manner, together with the LDH activity, oxidative stress and mitochondrial damage significantly increased by both nano- and micro-scale silica particles. Nano-scale silica particles could induce mitochondrial damage and autophagy, but not micro-scale particles. Exposure to nano-scale silica particles rather than micro-scale particles could lead to autophagy dysfunction and impair cellular homeostasis (Li et al., 2016).

Although biomedically used PLGA nanoparticles did not exhibit obvious cytotoxic effects, 60 nm PLGA nanoparticles triggered the release of pro-inflammatory cytokines, whereas 200 nm PLGA nanoparticles did not trigger any negative response from cells (Xiong et al., 2013). The size-dependent cytotoxicity of nanoparticles could be smaller nanoparticles with larger specific surface area and could adsorb more biomolecules, and the ability to adsorb proteins might be the important paradigm to predict the in vitro toxicity of nanoparticles. However, different results were shown in PLL polymers-induced cytotoxicity. Researchers compared the cytotoxicity of PLL polymers of low molecular weight and high molecular weight through detecting mitochondrial membrane potential, cytochrome C release, and activation of caspase. Low-molecular-weight PLL polymers on mitochondria did not result in cytochrome C release or mitochondrial dysfunction when compared with high-molecular-weight PLL polymers (Symonds et al., 2015). Berit L. Strand also confirmed that the toxicity of PLL polymers was tightly associated with their molecular weight. PLL polymers with higher molecular weight (29.8 kDa) were more toxic than PLL polymers with lower molecular weight (4.0 kDa and 7.5 kDa). Thus, although nanoparticles-induced cytotoxicity was dependent on size of nanoparticles, it doesn't mean smaller sized nanoparticles were safer than larger ones; it also depends on the types of nanoparticles.

3.2 Shape

Neurotoxicity of nanoparticles is not only affected by the molecular weight (size), but also by the architecture of nanoparticles (shape).

Li et al. (2015a) systematically explored the acute nanotoxicity of different mesoporous silica nanoparticles with different aspect ratios via oral administration. Nanoparticles presented decreased in vivo biodegradation, systematic absorption, and excretion with the increase of aspect ratios, suggesting mesoporous silica nanoparticles induced nanotoxicity in a shape-dependent manner. Other groups also investigated short-rod mesoporous silica nanoparticles and long-rod mesoporous silica nanoparticles on bio-distribution, clearance, and biocompatibility in vivo. The clearance rate of nanoparticles was mainly dependent on the particle shape. Among them, short-rod nanoparticles showed more rapid clearance rate than long-rod ones (Huang et al., 2011; Hao et al., 2014).

In addition to non-metallic nanoparticles, the role of crystal structure of TiO_2 nanoparticles to the neurotoxicity was also investigated. The anatase TiO_2 nanoparticles displayed a dose-dependent behavior on decreasing cell viability, inducing apoptosis, disturbing cell cycle, and triggering JNK- and p53-mediated signaling pathway. In comparison to anatase TiO_2 nanoparticles, the rutile TiO_2 nanoparticles showed moderately toxic effect on neuron cells; thus, the anatase form was more toxic than the rutile (Wu et al., 2010). Scientists compared the antimicrobial activities of nano-sized silver on different shapes, including silver nanoplates, silver nanorods, and silver nanoparticles, and found that surface area of nanosilver shapes was the critical factor for controlling antimicrobial activity on Gram-positive and Gram-negative bacteria; silver nanoplates have best surface area and presented best antimicrobial activity.

For the shape influence on polymers, researchers compared the cytotoxicity and transfection efficiency of branched PEI and linear PEI in vitro. They found although branched PEI shows excellent transfection efficiency, its high toxicity to different cells limited its application; while linear PEI has been shown to be less toxic to cells (Wiseman et al., 2003). Using similar nanoparticles, other researchers also confirmed branched PEI could result in greater internalization and induce greater cytotoxicity (early and late apoptosis) than liner PEI by using Annexin V assay and DNA fragmentation analyses (Kafil and Omidi, 2011). Cai et al. (2011) explored the effects of chain length (short chain, medium-length chain, and long chain) on the cytotoxicity and endocytosis of linear polymers and found that, only for medium-length linear chains, the cytotoxicity is mainly due to the cooperative effect of membrane disruption and apoptosis and increased with the chain length and polymer concentration. For short and long-length chain polymers, the cytotoxicity is independent of the chain length. Besides, needle-shaped PLGA-PEG nanoparticles, but not the spherical-shaped nanoparticles, could induce obvious cytotoxicity through lysosome damage-mediated cell apoptosis, also suggesting that the cytotoxicity of nanoparticles depended on their shapes (Zhang et al., 2017).

3.3 Surface charge

Because of electrostatic attraction between cell membranes and positively charged nanoparticles, the surface charge of nanoparticles obviously influenced cellular uptake of these nanoparticles (Hsu et al., 2014). Nanoparticles with positively charged surfaces could be more easily attached on the cell membranes and accumulated inside the cells and could also lead to Ca^{2+} influx into cells and inhibit cell growth (Frohlich, 2012).

Researchers compared both positively and negatively charged gold nanoparticles for their toxicity and found that positively charged gold nanoparticles induced more DNA damage and were more toxic than negatively charged nanoparticles of the same size (Yao et al., 2015). Besides, the developmental nanotoxicity and bio-distribution of iron oxide nanoparticles with positive or negative charges were explored in pregnant CD-1 mice to evaluate the influence of surface charge on nanotoxicity. Both positively and negatively charged iron oxide nanoparticles could pass through the placenta and accumulate in the fetus, while positively charged iron oxide nanoparticles showed more serious bioaccumulation and toxicity (Di Bona et al., 2014). Xiao et al. (2011) evaluated the effect of surface charge on in vitro and in vivo toxicity of PEG-oligocholic acid-based micellar nanoparticles and reported that positively charged nanoparticles showed dose-dependent hemolytic activities and cytotoxicity in murine macrophages, whereas negatively charged nanoparticles showed no significant hemolytic and cytotoxic effects.

Previous studies have indicated that the toxicity of PAMAM dendrimers is obviously influenced by size and surface charge. Amine terminated dendrimers (G4 and G7) were safe only at doses lower than 10mg/kg. On the contrary, carboxyl and hydroxyl terminated dendrimers were safely administered at 50-fold or higher dose (Greish et al., 2012). Even different types of administration also showed similar influence of charge on PAMAM dendrimers-induced toxicity; negatively charged (G7-OH) PAMAM dendrimers presented oral toxicity until doses of 300mg/kg, while positively charged (G7-NH_2) PAMAM dendrimers presented toxicity only at doses of 30mg/kg, which is ten times less tolerated than negatively charged dendrimers (Thiagarajan et al., 2013). Similarly, surface charge of PLGA nanoparticle could also influence their in vitro genotoxicity, cytotoxicity, reactive oxygen species production, and endocytosis; compared with neutral and negative charged nanoparticles, positive charged nanoparticles were much more cytotoxic (Platel et al., 2016).

4 Cellular mechanisms of brain targeting delivery systems induced nanotoxicity

4.1 Apoptosis and necrosis

Apoptosis is one type of programmed cell death which occurs in multi-cellular organisms (Song et al., 2016). Apoptosis could be induced by the extrinsic death receptors or by the intrinsic mitochondrial pathway, as mitochondrion is the major regulator of cell death, especially for nanoparticle-triggered apoptotic cell death. Mitochondrial dysfunction associated with apoptosis is characterized as loss of mitochondrial membrane potential, release of cytochrome *c*, and activation of caspases. Necrosis is characterized by the rapid breakdown of cell membranes, which result in massive intracellular components released into the extracellular space. As a passive and uncontrolled process, necrosis could be initiated by series of factors such as infections, cellular stress, and toxins.

Terminal deoxynucleotidyl transferase dUTP nick-end labeling (TUNEL) experiments, DNA fragmentation, and increased caspase-3 cleavage confirmed that silver nanoparticles induced apoptotic cell death in cultured cerebral cortical neurons (Kim et al., 2014). 12 h and 24 h after zinc oxide nanoparticles exposure in human neuroblastoma, SH-SY-5Y cells reduced neuronal viability together with apoptotic injury (annexin V and caspase 3/7 activities increase); besides, typical necrotic characteristics, including swelling/loss of cell organelles and rupture of the cytosolic or nuclear membrane occurred during zinc oxide nanoparticles' incubation, suggested zinc oxide nanoparticles triggered apoptosis and necrosis during its induced neurotoxicity (Kim et al., 2015a, b). Using other cell models, researchers also investigated that zinc oxide nanoparticles caused a rapid induction of nuclear condensation, DNA fragmentation, and the formation of hypodiploid DNA nuclei and apoptotic bodies, thus induced necrosis and apoptosis in macrophages (Wilhelmi et al., 2013). Besides, exposure to titanium dioxide could induce apoptosis, necrosis, and possibly apoptosis-like and necrosis-like cell death types in human astrocytes-like astrocytoma U87 cells (Lai et al., 2008) and induced blood-brain barrier damage, cellular edema, and brain tissue necrosis in vivo.

In addition to metallic and metallic oxide nanoparticles, nonmetallic nanoparticles and polymers could also trigger apoptosis and necrosis during their induced neurotoxicity. Silica nanoparticles obviously decreased cell viability, increased cellular apoptosis, and elevated intracellular reactive oxygen species in human SK-N-SH and mouse neuro2a neuroblastoma cells (Yang et al., 2014). Amine-modified polystyrene nanoparticles increased cell membrane permeability of propidium iodide, induced activation of caspases 3/7/9, cleaved PARP-1, and induced an apoptotic followed by a secondary necrotic response in human brain astrocytoma cell lines (Bexiga et al., 2011). Poly(ethylenimine)-mediated cytotoxicity could be divided into necrosis in the early stage and apoptosis in the late stage, while poly-L-Lysine polymers-induced massive cell death was necrosis but not apoptosis (Moghimi et al., 2005; Strand et al., 2001).

4.2 Autophagy

Autophagy is the evolutionarily conserved process of degradation of cytoplasmic components such as dysfunctional organelles and misfolded protein within lysosomes under stress conditions (Xu et al., 2012). This process is different with endocytosis-mediated degradation and recycle of cytoplasmic components (Stern and Johnson, 2008). Autophagy triggered by nanoparticles during nanotoxicity might be an adaptive cellular response aiming to clear nanoparticles and could be harmful during cellular dysfunction (Stern et al., 2012; Feng et al., 2015).

Chang et al. (2014) found that nano-alumina could induce autophagy and mitochondria damage in primary cortical neuronal cells isolated from Wistar newborn rats, while the damaged mitochondria were removed by mitophagy. In addition, Manshian et al. (2015) treated murine neural progenitor cells with silver nanoparticles and found that LC3 fluorescent intensity was enhanced, which indicated that autophagy in murine neural progenitor cells was induced by silver nanoparticles. Afeseh Ngwa et al. (2011) reported that manganese nanoparticles treatment could effectively accumulate in N27 dopaminergic neuronal cells and induced changes of Beclin1 and LC3, which indicated manganese nanoparticles induced autophagy in dopaminergic neuronal cells.

In addition, autophagy triggered by polymers during their induced neurotoxicity was widely investigated. Kenzaoui et al. reported that amino PVA (poly(vinyl alcohol/vinylamine))-coated ultrasmall superparamagnetic iron oxide nanoparticles could induce autophagic vacuoles and LC3-II accumulation in human cerebral endothelial cells. Besides, the overexpression of cathepsin D protein also suggested that autophagy was activated in the cells (Halamoda Kenzaoui et al., 2012). Also, PAMAM dendrimers could induce autophagic flux in human glioma cells during their induced neurotoxicity. Suppression of autophagy could obviously protect against PAMAM dendrimers-induced neurotoxicity (Wang et al., 2014b). Similarly, results were also confirmed in other neuronal cell models and further suggested that PAMAM dendrimers-induced autophagy during their triggered neurotoxicity might be mediated by oxidative stress: suppression of reactive oxygen species impaired autophagic-related fluorescence and protein expression activated by PAMAM dendrimers (Li et al., 2015c).

4.3 NETosis

Polymorphonuclear neutrophil cells (PMNs) are the first type of leukocytes to migrate to the inflammatory sites during acute inflammation and have the ability to extrude their DNA (either mitochondrial or nuclear) along with microbiology and pathogen molecules, thus forming neutrophils extracellular traps (NETs) and releasing them into the extracellular environment(Delgado-Rizo et al., 2017; Qi et al., 2017). During sepsis-induced neuroinflammation or ischemic stroke, NK cells could promote neutrophil recruitment, pass through the blood-brain barrier, and enter into the brain (He et al., 2016; Perez-de-Puig et al., 2015; Bernardes-Silva et al., 2001).

A lot of literatures have confirmed that nanoparticles could activate neutrophils: Hedenborg reported that TiO_2 nanoparticles could trigger the production of reactive oxygen species in a concentration-dependent manner; the particle size and surface structures of the TiO_2 were also important factors determining the intensity of the response. Besides, incubated human primary neutrophils with increasing concentrations of polymethylmethacrylate nanoparticles could induce the release of lactate dehydrogenase, lysosome, and beta-glucuronidase in a dose-dependent manner (Goncalves et al., 2011). Exposure of neutrophils to TiO_2 nanoparticles induced an increased oxidative burst together with NETs release (Shah et al., 2017). Munoz et al. (2016) found that nanoparticles initiated self-limiting NETosis-driven inflammation in a size-dependent manner: 10- to 40-nm sized nanoparticles induced quick damage of plasma membrane and instability of the lysosomal compartment, leading to the immediate formation of NETs in various cell types, while particles sized 100–1000nm behaved rather slowly. Similarly, researchers in the same group reported that nanodiamonds also emerged as potent triggers for NETosis in cultured neutrophils, and the NETosis was depended by oxidative brust (Biermann et al., 2016). In contrast, Bartneck et al. (2010) thought that particle shape was not very important for the NETs formation, positive charges of the nanoparticles were the enhancer of this phenomenon, and the NETs formation after gold nanoparticles-stimulation worked as the physical barrier for the nanoparticles. But limited studies were involved in nanoparticles-induced NETosis during their triggered neurotoxicity, which might be a key mechanism during brain-targeted drug delivery systems-induced neurotoxicity and deserve deep investigation.

4.4 Pyroptosis

Pyroptosis is an inflammatory form of programmed cell death that occurs most frequently upon infection with intracellular pathogens (Le and Harton, 2013). In contrast to apoptosis and necrosis, pyroptosis requires the function of the enzyme caspase-1. Caspase-1 is activated during pyroptosis by a large supramolecular complex termed the pyroptosome (inflammasome) and subsequently mediates the maturation and secretion of interleukin-1 beta and interleukin-18 (Fernandes-Alnemri et al., 2007).

There have been massive studies regarding pyroptosis induced by infection with intracellular pathogens which were involved in various central nervous system diseases (Zhou et al., 2016); and a large set of nanoparticles could activate inflammasome and induce pyroptosis during their triggered nanotoxicity (Sun et al., 2013).

Exposure of macrophages (cell line or primary human macrophages) to carbon black nanoparticles resulted in inflammasome activation, cleavage of caspase-1 to its active form, and downstream interleukin-1 beta release. The cell death that occurred with carbon black nanoparticle exposure was identified as pyroptosis by the protective effect of a caspase 1 inhibitor and a pyroptosis inhibitor (Reisetter et al., 2011). Multiwalled carbon nanotube incubation could also induce NLR pyrin domain containing 3 (NLRP3) inflammasome-dependent pyroptosis in primary human bronchial epithelial cells (Hussain et al., 2014).

Song et al. (2013) reported that A549 cells stimulated with zinc oxide nanoparticles for 8h increased the activity of caspase-1 and the level of interleukin-1 beta, while at 24h exposure to zinc oxide nanoparticles, only levels of interleukin 1 beta treated by zinc oxide nanoparticles were significantly higher but not the activity of caspase-1. But Yazdi et al. (2010) found that only TiO_2 and SiO_2 nanoparticles, but not zinc oxide nanoparticles, could activate NLRP3 inflammasome, leading to interleukin-1 beta secretion during their induced pulmonary inflammation. Silver nanoparticles could also induce pyroptosome formation in human monocytes THP-1 cells and up-regulate the caspase-1 protein expression, indicating that pyroptosis in THP-1 was induced by silver nanoparticles (Song et al., 2016).

Apart from nonmetallic, metallic, and metallic oxide nanoparticles, polymers could also activate pyroptosis during their induced nanotoxicity. Lower size of chitosan, but not larger chitosan, provoked greater activity on NLRP3 inflammasome activation and mediated interleukin-1 beta secretion (Bueter et al., 2011). Besides, intraperitoneal poly(ethylenimine) injection could activate NLRP3 inflammasome, cleave caspase-1, and mediate pyroptosis in vivo (Wegmann et al., 2012). Amino-functionalized polystyrene nanoparticles could activate NLRP3 inflammasome and trigger the release of interleukin-1 beta much more effectively than carboxyl- and non-functionalized nanoparticles in human macrophages (Frohlich, 2012).

4.5 Cell cycle arrest

Cell cycle arrest is a stopping point in the cell cycle, where it is no longer involved in the processes surrounding duplication and division. Recent nanotoxicity studies have revealed that cell cycle arrest is an important mechanism during nanoparticles-induced cytotoxicity (Mahmoudi et al., 2011).

Panzarini et al. (2017) explored the interaction of glucose-capped silver nanoparticles and cells on cell cycle progression and found that cells were arrested at S and G2/M phases of the cell cycle and sub-G1 population increased when incubated with silver nanoparticles. Using other cell model, researchers also confirmed that silver nanoparticles mediated G2/M cycle arrest of renal epithelial cells; moreover, silver nanoparticles-induced cell cycle arrest was related with NRF2-GSH signals (Kang et al., 2012). Ramalingam et al. reported that biogenic gold nanoparticles induced cell cycle arrest at the G0/G2 phase through oxidative stress and sensitized mitochondrial membranes in A549 cells; after 24 h exposure, nanoparticles arrested the cell cycle at G2/M phase. Palladium nanoparticles-induced cytotoxicity was associated with a significant increase of cells within the G0/G1 phase and a significant reduction in S and G2/M phases. Meanwhile, cells incubated with palladium ions presented an obvious accumulation of these cell cycle alterations (Petrarca et al., 2014).

In addition to metallic nanoparticles, metallic oxide nanoparticles and polymers were also involved in cell cycle arrest during their induced cytotoxicity. Titanium dioxide nanoparticles could induce DNA double strand breaks and increase cell proportions, which are arrested in G2/M phase in a dose-dependent manner (Kansara et al., 2015); besides, reactive oxygen species-mediated JNK and P53 phosphorylation up-regulation was also involved in titanium dioxide nanoparticles-induced G2/M cell cycle arrest and apoptosis in neuron cells (Wu et al., 2010). Similarly, zinc oxide nanoparticles led to cell death and reactive oxygen species generation and were able to induce cell cycle arrest in S and G2/M phase with the higher uptake in G2/M phase compared with other phases (Patel et al., 2016). Although low dose of amino-modified polystyrene nanoparticles induced lower cell death, cell cycle was significantly arrested. Further studies suggested that nanoparticle uptake in the cells was affected by cell cycle arrest (Kim et al., 2013) (Fig. 3).

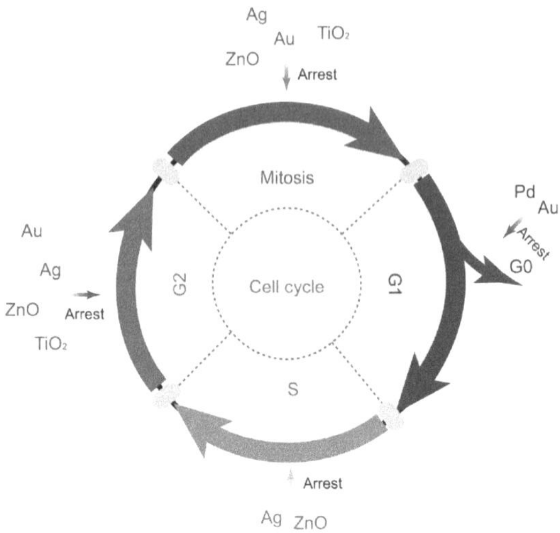

Fig. 3 Cell cycle arrest in brain targeting delivery systems-induced nanotoxicity.

5 Molecular mechanisms of brain targeting delivery systems induced nanotoxicity

5.1 Oxidative stress

An important mechanism of nanotoxicity is the generation of reactive oxygen species. Overproduction of reactive oxygen species can induce oxidative stress, resulting in imbalance between prooxidant and antioxidant levels in cells (Fu et al., 2014). Series of literatures have shown that oxidative stress could lead to neuronal apoptosis, DNA damage, and ion channels changes and has become the critical factor to acute brain injury-related disorders (Smith et al., 2013).

Yarjanli et al. (2017) reviewed recent studies on iron oxide nanoparticles threatening the cellular viability in the central nervous system and pointed out that iron contributed in Fenton's reaction and triggered reactive oxygen species production, and then caused damage to the macromolecules and organelles through oxidative stress. Researchers also reported that titanium dioxide could induce rapid and sustained reactive oxygen species release in BV2 brain microglia under the noncytotoxic concentrations (Long et al., 2006). Zinc oxide nanoparticles led to cellular morphological modification, mitochondrial dysfunction, superoxide dismutase reduction, glutathione depletion, and oxidative DNA damage during nanoparticles-elicited cell death (Guan et al., 2012). In addition, silica nanoparticles' exposure showed free radical generation, antioxidant enzymes activity depletion, and glutathione depletion, resulting in pro-inflammatory cytokines secretion and DNA damage during their induced cellular toxicity (Lehman et al., 2016).

In addition to nonmetallic and metallic oxide nanoparticles, polymers also presented activating oxidative stress properties. Polyethylenimine-poly(lactic-*co*-glycolic acid) (PLGA) nanoparticles could be endocytosed by the cells and triggered oxidative stress by inducing reactive oxygen species production, which in turn cause DNA damage without influencing cell viability (Calarco et al., 2013). Besides, cationic polystyrene nanoparticles could trigger mitochondria morphological changes and rapidly increase reactive oxygen species accumulation in human brain astrocytoma cells (Bexiga et al., 2011). PAMAM dendrimers could also evoke neuronal depolarization and induced cell death: PAMAM dendrimers could activate neurons and astroglial cells, resulting in mitochondrial depolarization and impaired oxidative metabolism of neurons (Nyitrai et al., 2013). Furthermore, different surface-modified PAMAM dendrimers showed different influence on the mitochondrial membrane potential and intracellular reactive oxygen species levels: Unmodified PAMAM dendrimers caused toxic response via reactive oxygen species generation and mitochondria damage, while pyrrolidone-modified dendrimers lacked the abilities on reactive oxygen species formation (Janaszewska et al., 2013).

5.2 DNA damage

As mentioned in the previous parts, nanoparticles-triggered oxidative stress is one of the most critical factors during their induced nanotoxicity (Fu et al., 2014). While all the molecules are vulnerable to oxidative stress by nanoparticles, DNA has received more attention. Large numbers of literatures have confirmed that nanoparticles could cause cellular toxicity via oxidative DNA damage (Rim et al., 2013) (Fig. 4).

Fpg comet assay is usually used for DNA damage detection (Matzenbacher et al., 2017). A significant concentration-dependent increase in DNA damage was observed in cells at different TiO_2 nanoparticles concentration (75 and 100 μg/mL) after 6 h exposure, as evident by the comet assay parameters. Besides, exposure to 75 and 100 μg/mL of TiO_2 nanoparticles significantly increased micronucleus formation, which is confirmed by cytokinesis-block micronucleus assays. Genomic and proteomic analyses confirmed that TiO_2 nanoparticles induced DNA double strand breaks during its induced toxicity (Kansara et al., 2015). Other groups reported that even at 1 μg/mL concentration, TiO_2 could also induce significant oxidative DNA damage by the Fpg-comet assay (Shukla et al., 2013). Moreover, mice orally exposed to TiO_2 nanoparticles for 14 consecutive days showed significant oxidative DNA damage, which could be attributed to oxidative stress (Shukla et al., 2014). Zinc oxide nanoparticles induced cytotoxicity through the induction of apoptosis, while apoptosis likely occurred as a consequence of DNA damage caused by increase in reactive oxygen species associated with loss of mitochondrial membrane potential (Han et al., 2016). Using alkaline comet assay and immunocytochemistry for gama-H2AX and 8-OHdG, researchers further confirmed that UVB exposure increased zinc oxide nanoparticles-mediated oxidative stress and oxidative DNA damage (Pal et al., 2016). Similarly, using other cell model, Wilhelmi et al. (2013) reported that zinc oxide nanoparticles caused DNA strand breakage and oxidative DNA damage in the RAW 264.7 cells as well as p47

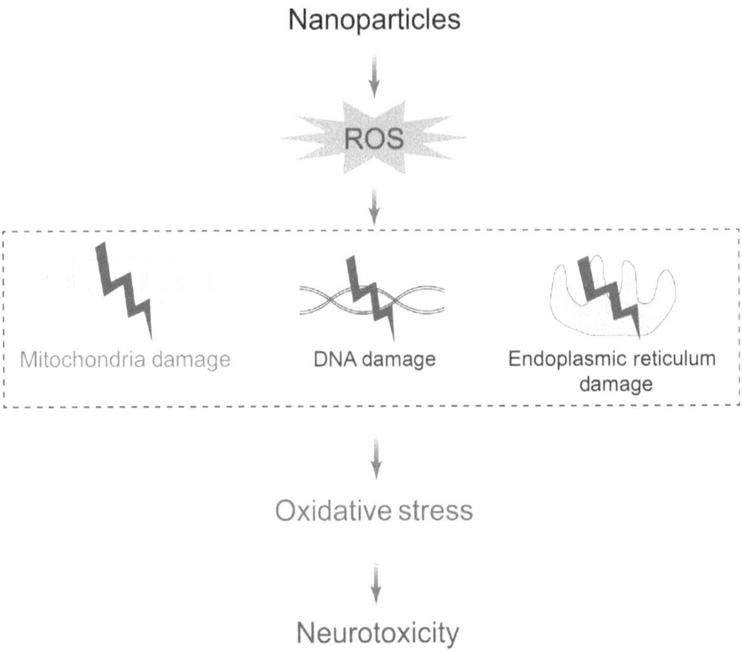

Fig. 4 Molecular mechanisms of brain targeting delivery systems-induced nanotoxicity.

(phox) NADPH oxidase-dependent superoxide generation in bone marrow-derived macrophages.

Besides, metallic nanoparticles could also induce genotoxicity via DNA damage during their triggered cytotoxicity. Palladium nanoparticles treatment not only suppression cell proliferation, but also induced apoptosis and cell cycle arrest at G2/M and S phase; moreover, oxidative stress and DNA damage were also obviously increased after palladium nanoparticles incubation (Alarifi et al., 2017). Silver nanoparticles orally-treated Sprague-Dawley rats obviously increased the induction of reactive oxygen species, numbers of structural chromosome aberrations, micronuclei formation, and damaged DNA (Patlolla et al., 2015). in vivo animal experiments also showed that gold nanoparticles could pass through the blood-brain barrier, accumulate in the brain, and induce DNA damage in the cerebral cortex of adult rats; chronic injection triggered more DNA damage than acute administration (Cardoso et al., 2014).

To explore the genotoxic effect of polymeric nanoparticles, Choi et al. (2010) evaluated cell death induced by polyethylenimine and PAMAM dendrimer via comet assay and cytokinesis-block micronucleus assay and found that polyethylenimine and PAMAM dendrimer treatment induced significant increases in DNA damage. PLGA-PEG nanoparticles could induce cytotoxicity via lysosome damage-mediated cell apoptotic signaling pathway and finally triggered DNA fragmentation and cell death (Zhang et al., 2017).

5.3 Signaling pathway

5.3.1 NF-kB

Researchers used different dose of titanium dioxide nanoparticles treating mice for 90 consecutive days and found neuroinflammation and spatial memory impairment occurred in mice. Nanoparticles obviously activated the expression of nucleic IkB kinase, NF-kB-inducible kinase, nucleic factor-kB, NF-kB2(p52), and RelA(p65) and significantly reduced IkB expression (Ze et al., 2014). Deng et al. (2011) explored that negatively charged poly(acrylic acid)-conjugated gold nanoparticles bind to and induce unfolding of fibrinogen, which could promote interaction with the integrin receptor, Mac-1. Mac-1 activation could increase the NF-kB signaling pathway and induce inflammatory cytokines release. Besides, silica dioxides nanoparticles could enter immune cells through caveolae-mediated endocytosis and activated NF-kB to stimulate immune cells activation (Wang et al., 2014a, b, c). These examples all suggested that NF-kB signal was involved in nanoparticles-induced cytotoxicity.

5.3.2 PI3K/Akt/mTOR signaling pathway

The phosphatidylinositol 3-kinase (PI3K)/Akt/mammalian target of rapamycin (mTOR) pathway played a key role in various cellular functions and has been widely investigated during nanoparticles-induced toxicity (Yu et al., 2015; Li et al., 2015a, b, c). As PI3K/Akt/mTOR signaling pathway is a major regulator of autophagy, series studies on the role of PI3K/Akt/mTOR in nanotoxicity was involved in nanoparticles-induced autophagy (Li et al., 2009).

Xie and Wu (2016) investigated the effect of silica nanoparticles on PC12 cells, a dopaminergic neuron-like cell line, and found that silica nanoparticles induced oxidative stress and alpha-synuclein aggregation by inhibiting the ubiquitin-proteasome system. Silica nanoparticles also induced autophagy through inhibiting phosphorylation of PI3K-Akt-mTOR signaling, which is known to negatively regulate autophagy. Similarly, using other cell models, researcher also confirmed that silica nanoparticles could induce autophagic vacuole accumulation and LC3 conversion, which means activation of autophagy, on endothelial cell homeostasis and angiogenesis, while PI3K/Akt/mTOR signaling pathway was involved in silica nanoparticles-induced toxicity (Duan et al., 2014). Antioxidant *N*-acetylcysteine could obviously attenuate silica nanoparticles-induced toxicity in human umbilical vein endothelial cells through suppression of autophagy via PI3K/Akt/mTOR signaling mediated by reactive oxygen species (Guo et al., 2016). Similar results were also confirmed in zinc oxide nanoparticles-induced macrophage cell death: Zinc oxide nanoparticles triggered autophagy that could further enhance apoptosis in macrophages. Autophagy was apparently caused by a significant decrease in phosphorylation of PI3K, Akt, and mTOR when exposed to zinc oxide nanoparticles, while inhibition of autophagy attenuated nanoparticle-induced apoptosis. Interestingly, both apoptotic and autophagic cell death could be impaired by antioxidant *N*-acetylcysteine (Roy et al., 2014). Besides nonmetallic and metallic nanoparticles, cationic polymers including polystyrene nanospheres and poly-amidoamine dendrimers could also induce autophagy via

PI3K/Akt/mTOR signaling pathway during their triggered cytotoxicity (Chiu et al., 2015; Wang et al., 2014a, b, c).

5.3.3 MAPK signaling pathway

The mitogen-activated protein kinases (MAPKs) including extracellular signaling-related kinase (ERK), c-Jun N-terminal kinase (JNK), and p38 mitogen-activated protein kinase (p38 MAPK) were tightly associated with reactive oxygen species production (Fu et al., 2014). Previous researches have suggested that MAPK signaling pathway was involved in nanoparticles-induced cytotoxicity.

Copper nanoparticles treatment increased phosphorylation of MAPKs, ERK, JNK, and p-38 in a dose-dependent manner in human bronchial epithelial cells when compared with untreated controls. MAPK inhibitors significantly decreased the phosphorylation of each MAPK, thus decreased mRNA expression and protein levels of pro-inflammatory mediators activated by copper nanoparticles (Ko et al., 2016). Using a murine asthma model, researchers investigated that copper oxide nanoparticles could induce airway inflammation and mucus secretion through increasing phosphorylation of the MAPKs including ERK, JNK, and p-38 (Park et al., 2016). Differently, although exposure-cultured primary astrocytes to zinc oxide nanoparticles increased phosphorylation of ERK, JNK, and p-38, only JNK inhibitor, but not ERK or p-38 MAPK inhibitors, could obviously impair zinc oxide nanoparticles-induced astrocytes PARP and caspase-3 cleavage, suggesting that JNK signal was involved in zinc oxide nanoparticles-induced apoptosis in primary astrocytes (Wang et al., 2014a, b, c). While for aluminum nanoparticles-treated mice, only ERK1 and p-38 MAPK protein expression, but not JNK, were activated in the brain after aluminum nanoparticles administration (Kwon et al., 2013). Besides, exposure to cerium oxide nanoparticles could also increase phosphorylation of p-38 MAPK, but diminish phosphorylation of ERK-1/2-MAPK (Rice et al., 2015).

5.3.4 TGF beta signaling pathway

Transforming growth factor (TGF)-beta signaling pathway plays critical roles in regulating various cellular activities including cell growth, cell differentiation, and cell development. Recent studies have shown that nanoparticles-induced cytotoxicity might be mediated by TGF-beta activation. Nickel oxide nanoparticles could induce pulmonary fibrosis through TGF-beta 1 activation in rats: nickel oxide nanoparticles' exposure increased TGF-beta 1 content expression and up-regulated TGF-beta signaling pathway-related genes expression, including TGF-beta 1, Smad2, and Smad4 (Chang et al., 2017). Titanium dioxide nanoparticles could also activate TGF-beta/Smads pathway in renal inflammation and fibration of mice (Hong et al., 2016) and may up-regulate TGF-beta to inhibit HSP70 (Shah et al., 2017). Besides, oral administration of small-sized silver nanoparticles, but not larger-sized nanoparticles, to mice could significantly increase TGF-beta level in serum during its triggered toxicity and inflammatory responses (Park et al., 2010). Similarly, only long multiwall carbon nanotubes, but not short nanotubes, could obviously activate macrophages

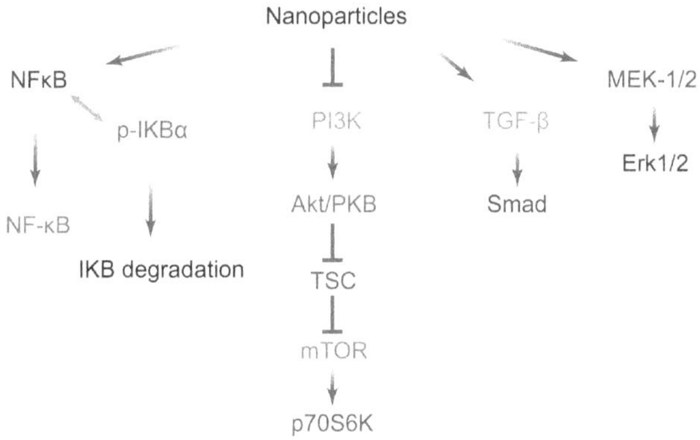

Fig. 5 Signaling pathways involved in brain targeting delivery systems-induced nanotoxicity.

and increase the production of TGF-beta, and then the activation of TGF-beta/Smads signaling pathway (Wang et al., 2015). The dispersal condition of multiwall carbon nanotubes could also influence these effects: well-dispersed multiwall carbon nanotubes could be rapidly taken up and triggered more TGF-beta than non-dispersed multiwall carbon nanotubes (Wang et al., 2011) (Fig. 5).

6 Conclusions and future directions

As nanoparticles possess unique physical structures and specific biological properties, a series of nanoparticles have been designed and developed as brain-targeted drug delivery systems over the past few decades. Although these nanoparticles-based brain-targeted drug delivery systems could be successfully used for gene carrier, drug delivery, and theranostic imaging, after passing through the blood-brain barrier and entering into brain, these nanoparticles might induce neurotoxicity and strongly limit their applications as brain-targeted drug delivery systems. Thus, it is an urgent need for scientists to address the concerns about neurotoxicity triggered by nanoparticles, and these researches could bring more benefits for designing and developing ideal nanoparticles for brain-targeted drug delivery systems. While evaluating the neurotoxicity of nanoparticles, the particle size, shape, surface charge, and surface chemistry are expected to play critical roles and should be carefully considered when the nanoparticles are designed. In addition, this chapter further highlighted the cellular and molecular mechanisms of nanoparticles-induced neurotoxicity. Cellular mechanisms included apoptosis, necrosis, NETosis, pyroptosis, and cell cycle arrest; while molecular mechanisms included oxidative stress, DNA damage, NF-kB signaling pathway, PI3K/Akt/mTOR signaling pathway, MAPK signaling pathway, and TGF-beta signaling pathway involved in nanoparticle-induced toxicity. These cellular and molecular mechanisms of nanotoxicity induced by nanoparticles could be helpful for designing, developing, and evaluating safety brain-targeted drug delivery systems in the future.

Acknowledgments

The contribution was supported by grants from the National Key Basic Research Program of China (2015CB931800, 2013CB932502) and the National Natural Science Foundation of China (81573332, 81773620). Dr. Yubin Li would like to thank his baby girl Charlotte (Qianxun) Li.

Conflict of interests

All the figures in "Neurotoxicity concern about the brain targeting delivery systems" are unpublished materials designed and prepared by Yubin Li and Dianwen Ju. The authors declared that there's no conflict of interests. Corresponding Author: Yubin Li, Email address: yubinli@upenn.edu; Dianwen Ju, Email address: dianwenju@fudan.edu.cn.

References

Accardi, M.V., Pugsley, M.K., Forster, R., Troncy, E., Huang, H., Authier, S., 2016. The emerging role of in vitro electrophysiological methods in CNS safety pharmacology. J. Pharmacol. Toxicol. Methods 81, 47–59.

Afeseh Ngwa, H., Kanthasamy, A., Gu, Y., Fang, N., Anantharam, V., Kanthasamy, A.G., 2011. Manganese nanoparticle activates mitochondrial-dependent apoptotic signaling and autophagy in dopaminergic neuronal cells. Toxicol. Appl. Pharmacol. 256, 227–240.

Alarifi, S., Ali, D., Alkahtani, S., Almeer, R.S., 2017. ROS-mediated apoptosis and genotoxicity induced by palladium nanoparticles in human skin malignant melanoma cells. Oxidative Med. Cell. Longev. 8439098. https://doi.org/10.1155/2017/8439098.

Anspach, L., Unger, R.E., Brochhausen, C., Gibson, M.I., Klok, H.A., Kirkpatrick, C.J., Freese, C., 2016. Impact of polymer-modified gold nanoparticles on brain endothelial cells: exclusion of endoplasmic reticulum stress as a potential risk factor. Nanotoxicology 10, 1341–1350.

Arai, Y., Miyayama, T., Hirano, S., 2015. Difference in the toxicity mechanism between ion and nanoparticle forms of silver in the mouse lung and in macrophages. Toxicology 328, 84–92.

Bartneck, M., Keul, H.A., Zwadlo-Klarwasser, G., Groll, J., 2010. Phagocytosis independent extracellular nanoparticle clearance by human immune cells. Nano Lett. 10, 59–63.

Bernardes-Silva, M., Anthony, D.C., Issekutz, A.C., Perry, V.H., 2001. Recruitment of neutrophils across the blood-brain barrier: the role of E- and P-selectins. J. Cereb. Blood Flow Metab. 21, 1115–1124.

Bexiga, M.G., Varela, J.A., Wang, F., Fenaroli, F., Salvati, A., Lynch, I., Simpson, J.C., Dawson, K.A., 2011. Cationic nanoparticles induce caspase 3-, 7- and 9-mediated cytotoxicity in a human astrocytoma cell line. Nanotoxicology 5, 557–567.

Biermann, M.H., Podolska, M.J., Knopf, J., Reinwald, C., Weidner, D., Maueroder, C., Hahn, J., Kienhofer, D., Barras, A., Boukherroub, R., Szunerits, S., Bilyy, R., Hoffmann, M., Zhao, Y., Schett, G., Herrmann, M., Munoz, L.E., 2016. Oxidative burst-dependent NETosis is implicated in the resolution of necrosis-associated sterile inflammation. Front. Immunol. 7(557).

Boverhof, D.R., Bramante, C.M., Butala, J.H., Clancy, S.F., Lafranconi, M., West, J., Gordon, S.C., 2015. Comparative assessment of nanomaterial definitions and safety evaluation considerations. Regul. Toxicol. Pharmacol. 73, 137–150.

Bueter, C.L., Lee, C.K., Rathinam, V.A., Healy, G.J., Taron, C.H., Specht, C.A., Levitz, S.M., 2011. Chitosan but not chitin activates the inflammasome by a mechanism dependent upon phagocytosis. J. Biol. Chem. 286, 35447–35455.

Cai, J., Yue, Y., Rui, D., Zhang, Y., Liu, S., Wu, C., 2011. Effect of chain length on cytotoxicity and endocytosis of cationic polymers. Macromolecules 44, 2050–2057.

Calarco, A., Bosetti, M., Margarucci, S., Fusaro, L., Nicoli, E., Petillo, O., Cannas, M., Galderisi, U., Peluso, G., 2013. The genotoxicity of PEI-based nanoparticles is reduced by acetylation of polyethylenimine amines in human primary cells. Toxicol. Lett. 218, 10–17.

Cardoso, E., Rezin, G.T., Zanoni, E.T., de Souza Notoya, F., Leffa, D.D., Damiani, A.P., Daumann, F., Rodriguez, J.C., Benavides, R., da Silva, L., Andrade, V.M., da Silva Paula, M.M., 2014. Acute and chronic administration of gold nanoparticles cause DNA damage in the cerebral cortex of adult rats. Mutat. Res. 766-767, 25–30.

Chang, L., Guo, W., Ge, C., Niu, Q., Zhang, Q., 2014. Effect of nano-alumina on mitophagy in primary cortical neuronal cells from wistar newborn rats. Chin. J. Pharmacol. Toxicol. 28, 737–742.

Chang, X.H., Zhu, A., Liu, F.F., Zou, L.Y., Su, L., Liu, S.K., Zhou, H.H., Sun, Y.Y., Han, A.J., Sun, Y.F., Li, S., Li, J., Sun, Y.B., 2017. Nickel oxide nanoparticles induced pulmonary fibrosis via TGF- beta1 activation in rats. Hum. Exp. Toxicol. 36, 802–812.

Chiu, H.W., Xia, T., Lee, Y.H., Chen, C.W., Tsai, J.C., Wang, Y.J., 2015. Cationic polystyrene nanospheres induce autophagic cell death through the induction of endoplasmic reticulum stress. Nano 7, 736–746.

Choi, Y.J., Kang, S.J., Kim, Y.J., Lim, Y.B., Chung, H.W., 2010. Comparative studies on the genotoxicity and cytotoxicity of polymeric gene carriers polyethylenimine (PEI) and polyamidoamine (PAMAM) dendrimer in Jurkat T-cells. Drug Chem. Toxicol. 33, 357–366.

Christian, P., Von der Kammer, F., Baalousha, M., Hofmann, T., 2008. Nanoparticles: structure, properties, preparation and behaviour in environmental media. Ecotoxicology 17, 326–343.

De Bock, M., Vandenbroucke, R.E., Decrock, E., Culot, M., Cecchelli, R., Leybaert, L., 2014. A new angle on blood-CNS interfaces: a role for connexins? FEBS Lett. 588, 1259–1270.

De Jong, W.H., Borm, P.J., 2008. Drug delivery and nanoparticles: applications and hazards. Int. J. Nanomedicine 3, 133–149.

Delgado-Rizo, V., Martinez-Guzman, M.A., Iniguez-Gutierrez, L., Garcia-Orozco, A., Alvarado-Navarro, A., Fafutis-Morris, M., 2017. Neutrophil extracellular traps and its implications in inflammation: an overview. Front. Immunol. 8(81).

Deng, Z.J., Liang, M., Monteiro, M., Toth, I., Minchin, R.F., 2011. Nanoparticle-induced unfolding of fibrinogen promotes Mac-1 receptor activation and inflammation. Nat. Nanotechnol. 6, 39–44.

Di Bona, K.R., Xu, Y., Ramirez, P.A., DeLaine, J., Parker, C., Bao, Y., Rasco, J.F., 2014. Surface charge and dosage dependent potential developmental toxicity and bio-distribution of iron oxide nanoparticles in pregnant CD-1 mice. Reprod. Toxicol. 50, 36–42.

Duan, J., Yu, Y., Yu, Y., Li, Y., Huang, P., Zhou, X., Peng, S., Sun, Z., 2014. Silica nanoparticles enhance autophagic activity, disturb endothelial cell homeostasis and impair angiogenesis. Part. Fibre Toxicol. 11(50).

Eldridge, B.N., Xing, F., Fahrenholtz, C.D., Singh, R.N., 2017. Evaluation of multiwalled carbon nanotube cytotoxicity in cultures of human brain microvascular endothelial cells grown on plastic or basement membrane. Toxicol. In Vitro 41, 223–231.

Feng, X., Chen, A., Zhang, Y., Wang, J., Shao, L., Wei, L., 2015. Central nervous system toxicity of metallic nanoparticles. Int. J. Nanomedicine 10, 4321–4340.

Fernandes-Alnemri, T., Wu, J., Yu, J.W., Datta, P., Miller, B., Jankowski, W., Rosenberg, S., Zhang, J., Alnemri, E.S., 2007. The pyroptosome: a supramolecular assembly of ASC dimers mediating inflammatory cell death via caspase-1 activation. Cell Death Differ. 14, 1590–1604.

Frohlich, E., 2012. The role of surface charge in cellular uptake and cytotoxicity of medical nanoparticles. Int. J. Nanomedicine 7, 5577–5591.

Fu, P.P., Xia, Q., Hwang, H.M., Ray, P.C., Yu, H., 2014. Mechanisms of nanotoxicity: generation of reactive oxygen species. J. Food Drug Anal. 22, 64–75.

Galandakova, A., Frankova, J., Ambrozova, N., Habartova, K., Pivodova, V., Zalesak, B., Safarova, K., Smekalova, M., Ulrichova, J., 2016. Effects of silver nanoparticles on human dermal fibroblasts and epidermal keratinocytes. Hum. Exp. Toxicol. 35, 946–957.

Goncalves, D.M., de Liz, R., Girard, D., 2011. Activation of neutrophils by nanoparticles. Sci. World J. 11, 1877–1885.

Greish, K., Thiagarajan, G., Herd, H., Price, R., Bauer, H., Hubbard, D., Burckle, A., Sadekar, S., Yu, T., Anwar, A., Ray, A., Ghandehari, H., 2012. Size and surface charge significantly influence the toxicity of silica and dendritic nanoparticles. Nanotoxicology 6, 713–723.

Guan, R., Kang, T., Lu, F., Zhang, Z., Shen, H., Liu, M., 2012. Cytotoxicity, oxidative stress, and genotoxicity in human hepatocyte and embryonic kidney cells exposed to ZnO nanoparticles. Nanoscale Res. Lett. 7, 602.

Guo, C., Yang, M., Jing, L., Wang, J., Yu, Y., Li, Y., Duan, J., Zhou, X., Li, Y., Sun, Z., 2016. Amorphous silica nanoparticles trigger vascular endothelial cell injury through apoptosis and autophagy via reactive oxygen species-mediated MAPK/Bcl-2 and PI3K/Akt/mTOR signaling. Int. J. Nanomedicine 11, 5257–5276.

Haase, A., Rott, S., Mantion, A., Graf, P., Plendl, J., Thunemann, A.F., Meier, W.P., Taubert, A., Luch, A., Reiser, G., 2012. Effects of silver nanoparticles on primary mixed neural cell cultures: uptake, oxidative stress and acute calcium responses. Toxicol. Sci. 126, 457–468.

Haddad-Tovolli, R., Dragano, N.R.V., Ramalho, A.F.S., Velloso, L.A., 2017. Development and function of the blood-brain barrier in the context of metabolic control. Front. Neurosci. 11 (224).

Halamoda Kenzaoui, B., Chapuis Bernasconi, C., Guney-Ayra, S., Juillerat-Jeanneret, L., 2012. Induction of oxidative stress, lysosome activation and autophagy by nanoparticles in human brain-derived endothelial cells. Biochem. J. 441, 813–821.

Han, Z., Yan, Q., Ge, W., Liu, Z.G., Gurunathan, S., De Felici, M., Shen, W., Zhang, X.F., 2016. Cytotoxic effects of ZnO nanoparticles on mouse testicular cells. Int. J. Nanomedicine 11, 5187–5203.

Hao, N., Li, L., Tang, F., 2014. Shape-mediated biological effects of mesoporous silica nanoparticles. J. Biomed. Nanotechnol. 10, 2508–2538.

He, H., Geng, T., Chen, P., Wang, M., Hu, J., Kang, L., Song, W., Tang, H., 2016. NK cells promote neutrophil recruitment in the brain during sepsis-induced neuroinflammation. Sci. Rep. 6(27711).

Hong, F., Wu, N., Ge, Y., Zhou, Y., Shen, T., Qiang, Q., Zhang, Q., Chen, M., Wang, Y., Wang, L., Hong, J., 2016. Nano-sized titanium dioxide resulted in the activation of TGF-beta/Smads/p38MAPK pathway in renal inflammation and fibration of mice. J. Biomed. Mater. Res. A 104, 1452–1461.

Hsu, E.W., Liu, S., Shrivats, A.R., Watt, A.C., McBride, S., Averick, S.E., Cho, H.Y., Matyjaszewski, K., Hollinger, J.O., 2014. Cationic nanostructured polymers for siRNA delivery in murine calvarial pre-osteoblasts. J. Biomed. Nanotechnol. 10, 1130–1136.

Huang, C.L., Hsiao, I.L., Lin, H.C., Wang, C.F., Huang, Y.J., Chuang, C.Y., 2015. Silver nanoparticles affect on gene expression of inflammatory and neurodegenerative responses in mouse brain neural cells. Environ. Res. 136, 253–263.

Huang, X., Li, L., Liu, T., Hao, N., Liu, H., Chen, D., Tang, F., 2011. The shape effect of mesoporous silica nanoparticles on bio-distribution, clearance, and biocompatibility in vivo. ACS Nano 5, 5390–5399.

Hussain, S., Sangtian, S., Anderson, S.M., Snyder, R.J., Marshburn, J.D., Rice, A.B., Bonner, J.C., Garantziotis, S., 2014. Inflammasome activation in airway epithelial cells after multiwalled carbon nanotube exposure mediates a profibrotic response in lung fibroblasts. Part. Fibre Toxicol. 11, 28.

Ivanov, D.P., Parker, T.L., Walker, D.A., Alexander, C., Ashford, M.B., Gellert, P.R., Garnett, M.C., 2015. In vitro co-culture model of medulloblastoma and human neural stem cells for drug delivery assessment. J. Biotechnol. 205, 3–13.

Ivask, A., Kurvet, I., Kasemets, K., Blinova, I., Aruoja, V., Suppi, S., Vija, H., Kakinen, A., Titma, T., Heinlaan, M., Visnapuu, M., Koller, D., Kisand, V., Kahru, A., 2014. Size-dependent toxicity of silver nanoparticles to bacteria, yeast, algae, crustaceans and mammalian cells in vitro. PLoS One. 9e102108.

Janaszewska, A., Ciolkowski, M., Wrobel, D., Petersen, J.F., Ficker, M., Christensen, J.B., Bryszewska, M., Klajnert, B., 2013. Modified PAMAM dendrimer with 4-carbomethoxypyrrolidone surface groups reveals negligible toxicity against three rodent cell-lines. Nanomedicine 9, 461–464.

Joris, F., Valdeperez, D., Pelaz, B., Soenen, S.J., Manshian, B.B., Parak, W.J., De Smedt, S.C., Raemdonck, K., 2016. The impact of species and cell type on the nanosafety profile of iron oxide nanoparticles in neural cells. J. Nanobiotechnol. 14(69).

Kabanov, A.V., Gendelman, H.E., 2007. Nanomedicine in the diagnosis and therapy of neurodegenerative disorders. Prog. Polym. Sci. 32, 1054–1082.

Kafil, V., Omidi, Y., 2011. Cytotoxic impacts of linear and branched polyethylenimine nanostructures in a431 cells. BioImpacts 1, 23–30.

Kang, S.J., Lee, Y.J., Lee, E.K., Kwak, M.K., 2012. Silver nanoparticles-mediated G2/M cycle arrest of renal epithelial cells is associated with NRF2-GSH signaling. Toxicol. Lett. 211, 334–341.

Kansara, K., Patel, P., Shah, D., Shukla, R.K., Singh, S., Kumar, A., Dhawan, A., 2015. TiO_2 nanoparticles induce DNA double strand breaks and cell cycle arrest in human alveolar cells. Environ. Mol. Mutagen. 56, 204–217.

Karmakar, A., Zhang, Q., Zhang, Y., 2014. Neurotoxicity of nanoscale materials. J. Food Drug Anal. 22, 147–160.

Kim, I.Y., Joachim, E., Choi, H., Kim, K., 2015b. Toxicity of silica nanoparticles depends on size, dose, and cell type. Nanomedicine 11, 1407–1416.

Kim, J.A., Aberg, C., de Carcer, G., Malumbres, M., Salvati, A., Dawson, K.A., 2013. Low dose of amino-modified nanoparticles induces cell cycle arrest. ACS Nano 7, 7483–7494.

Kim, J.H., Jeong, M.S., Kim, D.Y., Her, S., Wie, M.B., 2015a. Zinc oxide nanoparticles induce lipoxygenase-mediated apoptosis and necrosis in human neuroblastoma SH-SY5Y cells. Neurochem. Int. 90, 204–214.

Kim, S.H., Ko, J.W., Koh, S.K., Lee, I.C., Son, J.M., Moon, C., Kim, S.H., Shin, D.H., Kim, J.C., 2014. Silver nanoparticles induce apoptotic cell death in cultured cerebral cortical neurons. Mol. Cell. Toxicol. 10, 173–179.

Ko, J.W., Park, J.W., Shin, N.R., Kim, J.H., Cho, Y.K., Shin, D.H., Kim, J.C., Lee, I.C., Oh, S.R., Ahn, K.S., Shin, I.S., 2016. Copper oxide nanoparticle induces inflammatory

response and mucus production via MAPK signaling in human bronchial epithelial cells. Environ. Toxicol. Pharmacol. 43, 21–26.
Kwon, J.T., Seo, G.B., Jo, L.M., Kim, H.M., Shim, I., Lee, B.W., Yoon, B.I., Kim, P., Choi, K., 2013. Aluminum nanoparticles induce ERK and p38MAPK activation in rat brain. Toxicol. Res. 29, 181–185.
Lai, J.C., Lai, M.B., Jandhyam, S., Dukhande, V.V., Bhushan, A., Daniels, C.K., Leung, S.W., 2008. Exposure to titanium dioxide and other metallic oxide nanoparticles induces cytotoxicity on human neural cells and fibroblasts. Int. J. Nanomedicine 3, 533–545.
Le, H.T., Harton, J.A., 2013. Pyrin- and CARD-only proteins as regulators of NLR functions. Front. Immunol. 4(275).
Lehman, S.E., Morris, A.S., Mueller, P.S., Salem, A.K., Grassian, V.H., Larsen, S.C., 2016. Silica nanoparticle-generated ROS as a predictor of cellular toxicity: mechanistic insights and safety by design. Environ. Sci. Nano 3, 56–66.
Li, C., Liu, H., Sun, Y., Wang, H., Guo, F., Rao, S., Deng, J., Zhang, Y., Miao, Y., Guo, C., Meng, J., Chen, X., Li, L., Li, D., Xu, H., Wang, H., Li, B., Jiang, C., 2009. PAMAM nanoparticles promote acute lung injury by inducing autophagic cell death through the Akt-TSC2-mTOR signaling pathway. J. Mol. Cell Biol. 1, 37–45.
Li, J., Fan, C., Pei, H., Shi, J., Huang, Q., 2013. Smart drug delivery nanocarriers with self-assembled DNA nanostructures. Adv. Mater. 25, 4386–4396.
Li, L., Liu, T., Fu, C., Tan, L., Meng, X., Liu, H., 2015a. Biodistribution, excretion, and toxicity of mesoporous silica nanoparticles after oral administration depend on their shape. Nanomedicine 11, 1915–1924.
Li, Q., Hu, H., Jiang, L., Zou, Y., Duan, J., Sun, Z., 2016. Cytotoxicity and autophagy dysfunction induced by different sizes of silica particles in human bronchial epithelial BEAS-2B cells. Toxicol. Res. 5, 1216–1228.
Li, T., Shi, T., Li, X., Zeng, S., Yin, L., Pu, Y., 2014a. Effects of Nano-MnO_2 on dopaminergic neurons and the spatial learning capability of rats. Int. J. Environ. Res. Public Health 11, 7918–7930.
Li, Y., Wang, S., Wang, Z., Qian, X., Fan, J., Zeng, X., Sun, Y., Song, P., Feng, M., Ju, D., 2014b. Cationic poly(amidoamine) dendrimers induced cyto-protective autophagy in hepatocellular carcinoma cells. Nanotechnology. 25365101.
Li, Y., Zhu, H., Wang, S., Qian, X., Fan, J., Wang, Z., Song, P., Zhang, X., Lu, W., Ju, D., 2015c. Interplay of oxidative stress and autophagy in PAMAM dendrimers-induced neuronal cell death. Theranostics 5, 1363–1377.
Li, Y., Zeng, X., Wang, S., Sun, Y., Wang, Z., Fan, J., Song, P., Ju, D., 2015b. Inhibition of autophagy protects against PAMAM dendrimers-induced hepatotoxicity. Nanotoxicology 9, 344–355.
Liu, F., Mahmood, M., Xu, Y., Watanabe, F., Biris, A.S., Hansen, D.K., Inselman, A., Casciano, D., Patterson, T.A., Paule, M.G., Slikker Jr., W., Wang, C., 2015. Effects of silver nanoparticles on human and rat embryonic neural stem cells. Front. Neurosci. 9(115).
Liu, W., Wu, Y., Wang, C., Li, H.C., Wang, T., Liao, C.Y., Cui, L., Zhou, Q.F., Yan, B., Jiang, G.B., 2010. Impact of silver nanoparticles on human cells: effect of particle size. Nanotoxicology 4, 319–330.
Liu, Y., Xu, Z., Li, X., 2013. Cytotoxicity of titanium dioxide nanoparticles in rat neuroglia cells. Brain Inj. 27, 934–939.
Long, T.C., Saleh, N., Tilton, R.D., Lowry, G.V., Veronesi, B., 2006. Titanium dioxide (P25) produces reactive oxygen species in immortalized brain microglia (BV2): Implications for nanoparticle neurotoxicity. Environ. Sci. Technol. 40, 4346–4352.

Long, T.C., Tajuba, J., Sama, P., Saleh, N., Swartz, C., Parker, J., Hester, S., Lowry, G.V., Veronesi, B., 2007. Nanosize titanium dioxide stimulates reactive oxygen species in brain microglia and damages neurons in vitro. Environ. Health Perspect. 115, 1631–1637.

Mahmoudi, M., Azadmanesh, K., Shokrgozar, M.A., Journeay, W.S., Laurent, S., 2011. Effect of nanoparticles on the cell life cycle. Chem. Rev. 111, 3407–3432.

Manshian, B.B., Pfeiffer, C., Pelaz, B., Heimerl, T., Gallego, M., Moller, M., del Pino, P., Himmelreich, U., Parak, W.J., Soenen, S.J., 2015. High-content imaging and gene expression approaches to unravel the effect of surface functionality on cellular interactions of silver nanoparticles. ACS Nano 9, 10431–10444.

Masserini, M., 2013. Nanoparticles for brain drug delivery. ISRN Biochem. 238428. https://doi.org/10.1155/2013/238428.

Matzenbacher, C.A., Garcia, A.L., Dos Santos, M.S., Nicolau, C.C., Premoli, S., Correa, D.S., de Souza, C.T., Niekraszewicz, L., Dias, J.F., Delgado, T.V., Kalkreuth, W., Grivicich, I., da Silva, J., 2017. DNA damage induced by coal dust, fly and bottom ash from coal combustion evaluated using the micronucleus test and comet assay in vitro. J. Hazard. Mater. 324, 781–788.

Mendonca, M.C., Soares, E.S., de Jesus, M.B., Ceragioli, H.J., Batista, A.G., Nyul-Toth, A., Molnar, J., Wilhelm, I., Marostica Jr., M.R., Krizbai, I., da Cruz-Hofling, M.A., 2016. PEGylation of reduced graphene oxide induces toxicity in cells of the blood-brain barrier: an in vitro and in vivo study. Mol. Pharm. 13, 3913–3924.

Moghimi, S.M., Symonds, P., Murray, J.C., Hunter, A.C., Debska, G., Szewczyk, A., 2005. A two-stage poly(ethylenimine)-mediated cytotoxicity: implications for gene transfer/therapy. Mol. Ther. 11, 990–995.

Morachis, J.M., Mahmoud, E.A., Almutairi, A., 2012. Physical and chemical strategies for therapeutic delivery by using polymeric nanoparticles. Pharmacol. Rev. 64, 505–519.

Munoz, L.E., Bilyy, R., Biermann, M.H., Kienhofer, D., Maueroder, C., Hahn, J., Brauner, J.M., Weidner, D., Chen, J., Scharin-Mehlmann, M., Janko, C., Friedrich, R.P., Mielenz, D., Dumych, T., Lootsik, M.D., Schauer, C., Schett, G., Hoffmann, M., Zhao, Y., Herrmann, M., 2016. Nanoparticles size-dependently initiate self-limiting NETosis-driven inflammation. Proc. Natl. Acad. Sci. U. S. A. 113, E5856–E5865.

Newland, B., Moloney, T.C., Fontana, G., Browne, S., Abu-Rub, M.T., Dowd, E., Pandit, A.S., 2013. The neurotoxicity of gene vectors and its amelioration by packaging with collagen hollow spheres. Biomaterials 34, 2130–2141.

Nyitrai, G., Heja, L., Jablonkai, I., Pal, I., Visy, J., Kardos, J., 2013. Polyamidoamine dendrimer impairs mitochondrial oxidation in brain tissue. J. Nanobiotechnol. 11, 9.

Orlando, A., Cazzaniga, E., Tringali, M., Gullo, F., Becchetti, A., Minniti, S., Taraballi, F., Tasciotti, E., Re, F., 2017. Mesoporous silica nanoparticles trigger mitophagy in endothelial cells and perturb neuronal network activity in a size- and time-dependent manner. Int. J. Nanomedicine 12, 3547–3559.

Pal, A., Alam, S., Mittal, S., Arjaria, N., Shankar, J., Kumar, M., Singh, D., Pandey, A.K., Ansari, K.M., 2016. UVB irradiation-enhanced zinc oxide nanoparticles-induced DNA damage and cell death in mouse skin. Mutat. Rese. Genet. Toxicol. Environ. Mutagen. 807, 15–24.

Panzarini, E., Mariano, S., Vergallo, C., Carata, E., Fimia, G.M., Mura, F., Rossi, M., Vergaro, V., Ciccarella, G., Corazzari, M., Dini, L., 2017. Glucose capped silver nanoparticles induce cell cycle arrest in HeLa cells. Toxicol. In Vitro 41, 64–74.

Pardridge, W.M., 2005. The blood-brain barrier: bottleneck in brain drug development. NeuroRx 2, 3–14.

Park, E.J., Bae, E., Yi, J., Kim, Y., Choi, K., Lee, S.H., Yoon, J., Lee, B.C., Park, K., 2010. Repeated-dose toxicity and inflammatory responses in mice by oral administration of silver nanoparticles. Environ. Toxicol. Pharmacol. 30, 162–168.

Park, J.W., Lee, I.C., Shin, N.R., Jeon, C.M., Kwon, O.K., Ko, J.W., Kim, J.C., Oh, S.R., Shin, I.S., Ahn, K.S., 2016. Copper oxide nanoparticles aggravate airway inflammation and mucus production in asthmatic mice via MAPK signaling. Nanotoxicology 10, 445–452.

Patel, P., Kansara, K., Senapati, V.A., Shanker, R., Dhawan, A., Kumar, A., 2016. Cell cycle dependent cellular uptake of zinc oxide nanoparticles in human epidermal cells. Mutagenesis 31, 481–490.

Patil, U.S., Adireddy, S., Jaiswal, A., Mandava, S., Lee, B.R., Chrisey, D.B., 2015. In vitro/in vivo toxicity evaluation and quantification of Iron oxide nanoparticles. Int. J. Mol. Sci. 16, 24417–24450.

Patlolla, A.K., Hackett, D., Tchounwou, P.B., 2015. Genotoxicity study of silver nanoparticles in bone marrow cells of Sprague-Dawley rats. Food Chem. Toxicol. 85, 52–60.

Perez-de-Puig, I., Miro-Mur, F., Ferrer-Ferrer, M., Gelpi, E., Pedragosa, J., Justicia, C., Urra, X., Chamorro, A., Planas, A.M., 2015. Neutrophil recruitment to the brain in mouse and human ischemic stroke. Acta Neuropathol. 129, 239–257.

Petrarca, C., Clemente, E., Di Giampaolo, L., Mariani-Costantini, R., Leopold, K., Schindl, R., Lotti, L.V., Mangifesta, R., Sabbioni, E., Niu, Q., Bernardini, G., Di Gioacchino, M., 2014. Palladium nanoparticles induce disturbances in cell cycle entry and progression of peripheral blood mononuclear cells: paramount role of ions. J. Immunol. Res. 295092. https://doi.org/10.1155/2014/295092.

Pisanic 2nd., T.R., Blackwell, J.D., Shubayev, V.I., Finones, R.R., Jin, S., 2007. Nanotoxicity of iron oxide nanoparticle internalization in growing neurons. Biomaterials 28, 2572–2581.

Platel, A., Carpentier, R., Becart, E., Mordacq, G., Betbeder, D., Nesslany, F., 2016. Influence of the surface charge of PLGA nanoparticles on their in vitro genotoxicity, cytotoxicity, ROS production and endocytosis. J. Appl. Toxicol. 36, 434–444.

Pongrac, I.M., Pavicic, I., Milic, M., Brkic Ahmed, L., Babic, M., Horak, D., Vinkovic Vrcek, I., Gajovic, S., 2016. Oxidative stress response in neural stem cells exposed to different superparamagnetic iron oxide nanoparticles. Int. J. Nanomedicine 11, 1701–1715.

Qi, H., Yang, S., Zhang, L., 2017. Neutrophil extracellular traps and endothelial dysfunction in atherosclerosis and thrombosis. Front. Immunol. 8(928).

Reisetter, A.C., Stebounova, L.V., Baltrusaitis, J., Powers, L., Gupta, A., Grassian, V.H., Monick, M.M., 2011. Induction of inflammasome-dependent pyroptosis by carbon black nanoparticles. J. Biol. Chem. 286, 21844–21852.

Rice, K.M., Nalabotu, S.K., Manne, N.D., Kolli, M.B., Nandyala, G., Arvapalli, R., Ma, J.Y., Blough, E.R., 2015. Exposure to cerium oxide nanoparticles is associated with activation of mitogen-activated protein kinases signaling and apoptosis in rat lungs. J. Prev. Med. Public Health = Yebang Uihakhoe chi 48, 132–141.

Rim, K.T., Song, S.W., Kim, H.Y., 2013. Oxidative DNA damage from nanoparticle exposure and its application to workers' health: a literature review. Safety Health Work 4, 177–186.

Roy, R., Singh, S.K., Chauhan, L.K., Das, M., Tripathi, A., Dwivedi, P.D., 2014. Zinc oxide nanoparticles induce apoptosis by enhancement of autophagy via PI3K/Akt/mTOR inhibition. Toxicol. Lett. 227, 29–40.

Saraiva, C., Praca, C., Ferreira, R., Santos, T., Ferreira, L., Bernardino, L., 2016. Nanoparticle-mediated brain drug delivery: overcoming blood-brain barrier to treat neurodegenerative diseases. J. Control. Release 235, 34–47.

Shah, S.N., Shah, Z., Hussain, M., Khan, M., 2017. Hazardous effects of titanium dioxide nanoparticles in ecosystem. Bioinorg. Chem. Appl. 2017, 4101735.

Sharma, A., Muresanu, D.F., Patnaik, R., Sharma, H.S., 2013. Size- and age-dependent neurotoxicity of engineered metal nanoparticles in rats. Mol. Neurobiol. 48, 386–396.

Shilo, M., Sharon, A., Baranes, K., Motiei, M., Lellouche, J.P., Popovtzer, R., 2015. The effect of nanoparticle size on the probability to cross the blood-brain barrier: an in-vitro endothelial cell model. J. Nanobiotechnol. 13, 19.

Shim, K.H., Hulme, J., Maeng, E.H., Kim, M.K., An, S.S., 2014. Analysis of zinc oxide nanoparticles binding proteins in rat blood and brain homogenate. Int. J. Nanomed. 9 (Suppl 2), 217–224.

Shukla, R.K., Kumar, A., Gurbani, D., Pandey, A.K., Singh, S., Dhawan, A., 2013. TiO(2) nanoparticles induce oxidative DNA damage and apoptosis in human liver cells. Nanotoxicology 7, 48–60.

Shukla, R.K., Kumar, A., Vallabani, N.V., Pandey, A.K., Dhawan, A., 2014. Titanium dioxide nanoparticle-induced oxidative stress triggers DNA damage and hepatic injury in mice. Nanomedicine (Lond) 9, 1423–1434.

Simko, M., Mattsson, M.O., 2014. Interactions between nano-sized materials and the brain. Curr. Med. Chem. 21, 4200–4214.

Smith, J.A., Park, S., Krause, J.S., Banik, N.L., 2013. Oxidative stress, DNA damage, and the telomeric complex as therapeutic targets in acute neurodegeneration. Neurochem. Int. 62, 764–775.

Song, B., Liu, J., Feng, X., Wei, L., Shao, L., 2015. A review on potential neurotoxicity of titanium dioxide nanoparticles. Nanoscale Res. Lett. 10(1042).

Song, B., Zhou, T., Liu, J., Shao, L., 2016. Involvement of programmed cell death in neurotoxicity of metallic nanoparticles: recent advances and future perspectives. Nanoscale Res. Lett. 11(484).

Song, J., Du, L., Feng, Y., Wu, W., Yan, Z., 2013. Pyroptosis induced by zinc oxide nanoparticles in A549 cells. Wei sheng yan jiu = J. Hyg. Res. 42, 273–276.

Soni, S., Ruhela, R.K., Medhi, B., 2016. Nanomedicine in central nervous system (CNS) disorders: a present and future prospective. Adv. Pharm. Bull. 6, 319–335.

Stern, S.T., Johnson, D.N., 2008. Role for nanomaterial-autophagy interaction in neurodegenerative disease. Autophagy 4, 1097–1100.

Stern, S.T., Adiseshaiah, P.P., Crist, R.M., 2012. Autophagy and lysosomal dysfunction as emerging mechanisms of nanomaterial toxicity. Part. Fibre Toxicol. 9, 20.

Strand, B.L., Ryan, T.L., In't Veld, P., Kulseng, B., Rokstad, A.M., Skjak-Brek, G., Espevik, T., 2001. Poly-L-lysine induces fibrosis on alginate microcapsules via the induction of cytokines. Cell Transplant. 10, 263–275.

Sun, B., Wang, X., Ji, Z., Li, R., Xia, T., 2013. NLRP3 inflammasome activation induced by engineered nanomaterials. Small 9, 1595–1607.

Sun, X., Yang, Y., Shi, J., Wang, C., Yu, Z., Zhang, H., 2017. NOX4- and Nrf2-mediated oxidative stress induced by silver nanoparticles in vascular endothelial cells. J. Appl. Toxicol. 37, 1428–1437.

Symonds, P., Murray, J.C., Hunter, A.C., Debska, G., Szewczyk, A., Moghimi, S.M., 2015. Low and high molecular weight poly(L-lysine)s/poly(L-lysine)-DNA complexes initiate mitochondrial-mediated apoptosis differently. FEBS Lett. 27, 6191–6198.

Thiagarajan, G., Greish, K., Ghandehari, H., 2013. Charge affects the oral toxicity of poly(amidoamine) dendrimers. Eur. J. Pharm. Biopharm. 84, 330–334.

Tian, L., Lin, B., Wu, L., Li, K., Liu, H., Yan, J., Liu, X., Xi, Z., 2015. Neurotoxicity induced by zinc oxide nanoparticles: age-related differences and interaction. Sci. Rep. 5(16117).

Trickler, W.J., Lantz, S.M., Murdock, R.C., Schrand, A.M., Robinson, B.L., Newport, G.D., Schlager, J.J., Oldenburg, S.J., Paule, M.G., Slikker Jr., W., Hussain, S.M., Ali, S.F., 2010. Silver nanoparticle induced blood-brain barrier inflammation and increased permeability in primary rat brain microvessel endothelial cells. Toxicol. Sci. 118, 160–170.

Trickler, W.J., Lantz, S.M., Murdock, R.C., Schrand, A.M., Robinson, B.L., Newport, G.D., Schlager, J.J., Oldenburg, S.J., Paule, M.G., Slikker Jr., W., Hussain, S.M., Ali, S.F., 2011. Brain microvessel endothelial cells responses to gold nanoparticles: in vitro pro-inflammatory mediators and permeability. Nanotoxicology 5, 479–492.

Upadhyay, R.K., 2014. Drug delivery systems, CNS protection, and the blood brain barrier. Biomed. Res. Int. 869269 https://doi.org/10.1155/2014/869269.

Vanguilder, H.D., Freeman, W.M., 2011. The hippocampal neuroproteome with aging and cognitive decline: past progress and future directions. Front. Aging Neurosci. 3(8).

Voigt, N., Henrich-Noack, P., Kockentiedt, S., Hintz, W., Tomas, J., Sabel, B.A., 2014. Toxicity of polymeric nanoparticles in vivo and in vitro. J. Nanopart. Res. 16.

Voorhees, J.R., Rohlman, D.S., Lein, P.J., Pieper, A.A., 2016. Neurotoxicity in preclinical models of occupational exposure to organophosphorus compounds. Front. Neurosci. 10, 590.

Wahl, M., Unterberg, A., Baethmann, A., Schilling, L., 1988. Mediators of blood-brain barrier dysfunction and formation of vasogenic brain edema. J. Cereb. Blood Flow Metab. 8, 621–634.

Wang, E.C., Wang, A.Z., 2014. Nanoparticles and their applications in cell and molecular biology. Integr. Biol. 6, 9–26.

Wang, F., Gao, F., Lan, M., Yuan, H., Huang, Y., Liu, J., 2009. Oxidative stress contributes to silica nanoparticle-induced cytotoxicity in human embryonic kidney cells. Toxicol. In Vitro 23, 808–815.

Wang, J., Zhu, R., Gao, B., Wu, B., Li, K., Sun, X., Liu, H., Wang, S., 2014c. The enhanced immune response of hepatitis B virus DNA vaccine using SiO2@LDH nanoparticles as an adjuvant. Biomaterials 35, 466–478.

Wang, J., Deng, X., Zhang, F., Chen, D., Ding, W., 2014a. ZnO nanoparticle-induced oxidative stress triggers apoptosis by activating JNK signaling pathway in cultured primary astrocytes. Nanoscale Res. Lett. 9, 117.

Wang, P., Wang, Y., Nie, X., Braini, C., Bai, R., Chen, C., 2015. Multiwall carbon nanotubes directly promote fibroblast-myofibroblast and epithelial-mesenchymal transitions through the activation of the TGF-beta/Smad signaling pathway. Small 11, 446–455.

Wang, S., Li, Y., Fan, J., Wang, Z., Zeng, X., Sun, Y., Song, P., Ju, D., 2014b. The role of autophagy in the neurotoxicity of cationic PAMAM dendrimers. Biomaterials 35, 7588–7597.

Wang, X., Xia, T., Ntim, S.A., Ji, Z., Lin, S., Meng, H., Chung, C.H., George, S., Zhang, H., Wang, M., Li, N., Yang, Y., Castranova, V., Mitra, S., Bonner, J.C., Nel, A.E., 2011. Dispersal state of multiwalled carbon nanotubes elicits profibrogenic cellular responses that correlate with fibrogenesis biomarkers and fibrosis in the murine lung. ACS Nano 5, 9772–9787.

Wegmann, F., Gartlan, K.H., Harandi, A.M., Brinckmann, S.A., Coccia, M., Hillson, W.R., Kok, W.L., Cole, S., Ho, L.P., Lambe, T., Puthia, M., Svanborg, C., Scherer, E.M., Krashias, G., Williams, A., Blattman, J.N., Greenberg, P.D., Flavell, R.A., Moghaddam, A.E., Sheppard, N.C., Sattentau, Q.J., 2012. Polyethyleneimine is a potent mucosal adjuvant for viral glycoprotein antigens. Nat. Biotechnol. 30, 883–888.

Westerink, R.H., Ewing, A.G., 2008. The PC12 cell as model for neurosecretion. Acta Physiol. 192, 273–285.

Wilhelmi, V., Fischer, U., Weighardt, H., Schulze-Osthoff, K., Nickel, C., Stahlmecke, B., Kuhlbusch, T.A., Scherbart, A.M., Esser, C., Schins, R.P., Albrecht, C., 2013. Zinc oxide nanoparticles induce necrosis and apoptosis in macrophages in a p47phox- and Nrf2-independent manner. PLoS One. 8e65704.

Win-Shwe, T.T., Yamamoto, S., Fujitani, Y., Hirano, S., Fujimaki, H., 2008. Spatial learning and memory function-related gene expression in the hippocampus of mouse exposed to nanoparticle-rich diesel exhaust. Neurotoxicology 29, 940–947.

Win-Shwe, T.T., Sone, H., Kurokawa, Y., Zeng, Y., Zeng, Q., Nitta, H., Hirano, S., 2014. Effects of PAMAM dendrimers in the mouse brain after a single intranasal instillation. Toxicol. Lett. 228, 207–215.

Wiseman, J.W., Goddard, C.A., McLelland, D., Colledge, W.H., 2003. A comparison of linear and branched polyethylenimine (PEI) with DCChol/DOPE liposomes for gene delivery to epithelial cells in vitro and in vivo. Gene Ther. 10, 1654–1662.

Wong, A.D., Ye, M., Levy, A.F., Rothstein, J.D., Bergles, D.E., Searson, P.C., 2013. The blood-brain barrier: an engineering perspective. Front. Neuroeng. 6(7).

Wu, J., Sun, J., Xue, Y., 2010. Involvement of JNK and P53 activation in G2/M cell cycle arrest and apoptosis induced by titanium dioxide nanoparticles in neuron cells. Toxicol. Lett. 199, 269–276.

Xiao, K., Li, Y., Luo, J., Lee, J.S., Xiao, W., Gonik, A.M., Agarwal, R.G., Lam, K.S., 2011. The effect of surface charge on in vivo biodistribution of PEG-oligocholic acid-based micellar nanoparticles. Biomaterials 32, 3435–3446.

Xicoy, H., Wieringa, B., Martens, G.J., 2017. The SH-SY5Y cell line in Parkinson's disease research: a systematic review. Mol. Neurodegener. 12(10).

Xie, H., Wu, J., 2016. Silica nanoparticles induce alpha-synuclein induction and aggregation in PC12-cells. Chem. Biol. Interact. 258, 197–204.

Xiong, S., George, S., Yu, H., Damoiseaux, R., France, B., Ng, K.W., Loo, J.S., 2013. Size influences the cytotoxicity of poly (lactic-co-glycolic acid) (PLGA) and titanium dioxide (TiO (2)) nanoparticles. Arch. Toxicol. 87, 1075–1086.

Xu, J., Wang, Y., Tan, X., Jing, H., 2012. MicroRNAs in autophagy and their emerging roles in crosstalk with apoptosis. Autophagy 8, 873–882.

Xue, Y., Wu, J., Sun, J., 2012. Four types of inorganic nanoparticles stimulate the inflammatory reaction in brain microglia and damage neurons in vitro. Toxicol. Lett. 214, 91–98.

Yang, X., He, C., Li, J., Chen, H., Ma, Q., Sui, X., Tian, S., Ying, M., Zhang, Q., Luo, Y., Zhuang, Z., Liu, J., 2014. Uptake of silica nanoparticles: neurotoxicity and Alzheimer like pathology in human SK-N-SH and mouse neuro2a neuroblastoma cells. Toxicol. Lett. 229, 240–249.

Yang, Z., Liu, Z.W., Allaker, R.P., Reip, P., Oxford, J., Ahmad, Z., Ren, G., 2010. A review of nanoparticle functionality and toxicity on the central nervous system. J. R. Soc. Interface 7 (Suppl 4), S411–422.

Yao, X., Huang, C., Chen, X., Yi, Z., Sanche, L., 2015. Chemical radiosensitivity of DNA induced by gold nanoparticles. J. Biomed. Nanotechnol. 11, 478–485.

Yarjanli, Z., Ghaedi, K., Esmaeili, A., Rahgozar, S., Zarrabi, A., 2017. Iron oxide nanoparticles may damage to the neural tissue through iron accumulation, oxidative stress, and protein aggregation. BMC Neurosci. 18(51).

Yazdi, A.S., Guarda, G., Riteau, N., Drexler, S.K., Tardivel, A., Couillin, I., Tschopp, J., 2010. Nanoparticles activate the NLR pyrin domain containing 3 (Nlrp3) inflammasome and cause pulmonary inflammation through release of IL-1alpha and IL-1beta. Proc. Natl. Acad. Sci. U. S. A. 107, 19449–19454.

Yu, X., Long, Y.C., Shen, H.M., 2015. Differential regulatory functions of three classes of phosphatidylinositol and phosphoinositide 3-kinases in autophagy. Autophagy 11, 1711–1728.

Yuan, Z.Y., Hu, Y.L., Gao, J.Q., 2015. Brain localization and neurotoxicity evaluation of polysorbate 80-modified chitosan nanoparticles in rats. PLoS One. 10e0134722.

Ze, Y., Sheng, L., Zhao, X., Hong, J., Ze, X., Yu, X., Pan, X., Lin, A., Zhao, Y., Zhang, C., Zhou, Q., Wang, L., Hong, F., 2014. TiO_2 nanoparticles induced hippocampal neuroinflammation in mice. PLoS One. 9e92230.

Zhang, B., Sai Lung, P., Zhao, S., Chu, Z., Chrzanowski, W., Li, Q., 2017. Shape dependent cytotoxicity of PLGA-PEG nanoparticles on human cells. Sci. Rep. 7(7315).

Zhang, G., Zeng, X., Li, P., 2013. Nanomaterials in cancer-therapy drug delivery system. J. Biomed. Nanotechnol. 9, 741–750.

Zhou, K., Shi, L., Wang, Y., Chen, S., Zhang, J., 2016. Recent advances of the NLRP3 Inflammasome in central nervous system disorders. J. Immunol. Res. 2016, 9238290.

The intra-brain distribution of brain targeting delivery systems

16

*Xiaopeng Mo**,†, *Ergang Liu**,‡, *Yongzhuo Huang**
*Shanghai Institute of Materia Medica, Chinese Academy of Sciences, Shanghai, China, †Shanghai University College of Sciences, Shanghai, China, ‡School of Chemical Engineering and Technology, Tianjin University, Tianjin, China

1 Introduction

Brain is the most complex organ in all vertebrate systems. As the headquarter of life, the brain controls multiple physiological processes (motor, sensory, regulation, cognition, lateralization, etc.) that are critical in maintaining the functions of human body. On this account, the brain is the most energy-consuming organ, consuming 15% of cardiac output and up to 60% of blood glucose, in spite of its minimal body weight ratio (2%) (Berg et al., 2002). Brain diseases have been a real and growing threat for the global human society. The worldwide morbidity of central nervous system (CNS) disorders is continually rising, with an estimated rate of 20% in 2020 (Bedard et al., 2013).

Unfortunately, despite the global prevalence of CNS diseases, most of the currently applied medications fail to yield significant outcomes because of the poor permeation of CNS drugs across the blood-brain barrier (BBB). The brain has evolved the complicated mechanisms to protect itself from invasion of most exogenous stimuli. First, there is an impermeable membrane barrier between cerebrovascular and the brain. Unlike other kinds of blood vessels with the fenestrated endothelium (like in liver and kidney), the brain vessel endothelial cells are well-organized via "tight junctions", which strictly limit the penetration of blood solutes into the brain. Second, despite the rich blood perfusion, the uptake of blood nutrients by the brain is highly selective and strictly controlled by the active transportation processes. On one hand, it is critical in maintaining the homeostatic equilibrium in the brain and preventing fluctuations of blood solutes. On the other hand, this nature also largely rejects the efficient access of the therapeutic agents to the pathological sites in the brain. Generally, the BBB is only permeable for small lipid drugs with molecular weight no more than 400 Da and hydrogen bonds (with water) less than 8–10 (WM, 2012). Overall, it is reported that the BBB prevents 98% of small molecular drugs and almost 100% of macromolecular drugs from entering the brain via circulations (Pardridge, 2005), making the intra-brain delivery a formidable challenge for CNS disease treatment.

The rapidly developing nanotechnology provides a powerful tool for targeting delivery of various therapeutic/diagnostic agents, especially in the field of cancer therapy with the aid of active targeting technology and passive targeting method via EPR

Brain Targeted Drug Delivery Systems. https://doi.org/10.1016/B978-0-12-814001-7.00016-0

effect. Not only serving as drug carriers to preferentially deliver the encapsulated cargos to the pathological sites, the nanomaterials can also modulate the drug's physiochemical properties (e.g., solubility, lipophicity, and degradability by the enzymes). It thus improves the therapeutic index and the druggability of the candidate compounds. For the success in delivery of CNS drugs, it is dependent on: (1) the efficiency of the nano-sized vehicles to penetrate the BBB, and (2) the ability to overcome the heterogeneous environment in brain and reach the specific lesions.

In this chapter, the nanomaterials-based brain delivery is discussed, with a focus on the brain microenvironment, the blood and CSF circulation in brain, and the anatomic features of the BBB is described in details. Based on the understanding of these physiological features, the targeting strategies of nanomaterials for overcoming the BBB and the heterogeneous intra-brain delivery barriers are summarized, with a focus on brain cancer.

2 Anatomic characteristics of brain

Anatomically, human brain is mainly composed of four parts: cerebrum, cerebellum, brain stem, and the spinal cord. As a whole, the brain is surrounded by the calvarium. The subarachnoid space between the brain and the skull is filled with cerebrospinal fluid (CSF), which is originated from the cerebral blood in the choroid plexus. The newly formed CSF is then driven by the pressure gradient to flow from the ventricles into the cerebrospinal space, where it is either drained back into the venous network via arachnoid granulations, or be drained into the parenchyma and join the interstitial fluid. However, as the brain surface was covered by a layer of meninges, direct access of CSF into the parenchyma was confined at the Virchow-Robin space between the "flow-in" artery vassel and the surrounding astracytes.

At a cellular level, the brain parenchyma is composed of neurons and supporting glial cells, which are covered by the network of mircrocerebral vessels. The neurons and glial cells together make up the functional parts that occupy 70%–80% of the brain volume (Fisher et al., 2009). In comparison, cerebral vasculatures account for only 3% of the brain volume, and the average distance between the neighboring microcapplilaries is around 40 μm in normal brain (Fisher et al., 2009). The size of glial cells spans from several to tens of mironmeters, depending on the cell type and species, and therefore, every parenchymical cell is potentially accessed by a neighboring microvessel (Lange, 2014). The space between parenchymical cells and microvasculatures is filled with confluent fluids from the cells, cappillaries, and CSF.

2.1 Brain extracellular microenvironment (BEM)

The brain extracellular space (ECS), the interstitial fluid (ISF), and brain extracellular matrix (ECM), together constitute the BEM (Nicholson, 1993). Functionally, BEM can provide growth support to the neurons, glial cells, and vascular cells.

2.1.1 ECS

ECS is the unoccupied parenchyma volume and filled with ISF. ECS plays the key role in maintaining the stable electrical signal transmission between the brain cells, modulating the membrane iron channels and synaptic remodeling process (Syková and Nicholson, 2008; Nicholson, 2005).

Generally, ECS accounts for 20% of the brain volume, and the irregular interstitial gaps are in the range of 38–64 nm (Yao et al., 2008; Thorne and Nicholson, 2006; Depasquale et al., 1989). However, the width of the interstitial gaps varies in different regions, and even in the same region under different physiological conditions (Nicholson and Syková, 1998), potentially causing variation with regard to brain drug delivery in ECS (Vargovã and Sykovã, 2008).

2.1.2 ECM

ECM is composed of the soluble and insoluble biomacromolecules that are primarily secreted by the parenchyma cells (e.g., neurons and glial cells). ECM has been shown to be closely related with the emotional and cognitive processes, and the abnormal ECM may potentially cause psychiatric disorders (Hopkins et al., 2015).

The most common components of ECM are the long-chain glycosaminoglycans (e.g., hyaluronate), proteoglycans (e.g., chondroitin sulfate, heparan sulfate), and glycoproteins. Other ECM molecules include fibronectin, tendon protein, laminin, and tenascin (Kida et al., 1993). Moreover, during the development of CNS, the composition of ECM can be adapted in order to stimulate neurogenesis, gliogenesis, and axonal outgrowth (Fig. 1) (Bandtlow and Zimmermann, 2000; Soleman et al., 2013). Although ECMs are diverse in compositions, they have some physiochemical features in common, such as stickiness, negative charge, and abundance in hydrogen bonds. These features impose the diffusion barriers that limit the movement of molecules in the ECS (Nicholson et al., 2011).

2.2 Blood and lymphatics circulation

The oxygenated blood entered the brain via the internal carotid arteries and vertebrate arteries. The arteries then branch into small blood vessels and capillaries and distribute into different regions of the brain, delivering the blood oxygen and nutrients, and meanwhile exchanging with carbon dioxide and other metabolic wastes. The deoxygenated blood that carries metabolic wastes is then drained back through the venules and into the vein network, and exits the brain via jugular or spinal veins.

In comparison with the abundant blood perfusion, lymphatic vessels were conventionally believed to be absent in the brain (Földi et al., 1968), and the lymphatic drainage of brain interstitial fluid is mediated by CSF, which could be drained into the cervical lymphatics via the cranial nerves (Cserr et al., 1992). However, recent studies have revealed the existence of lymphatic network in the meninges of mouse brain (Aspelund et al., 2015; Bradstreet et al., 2015), which could serve as a potential path for the immunocytes or biomacromolecules to get out of the brain from CSF.

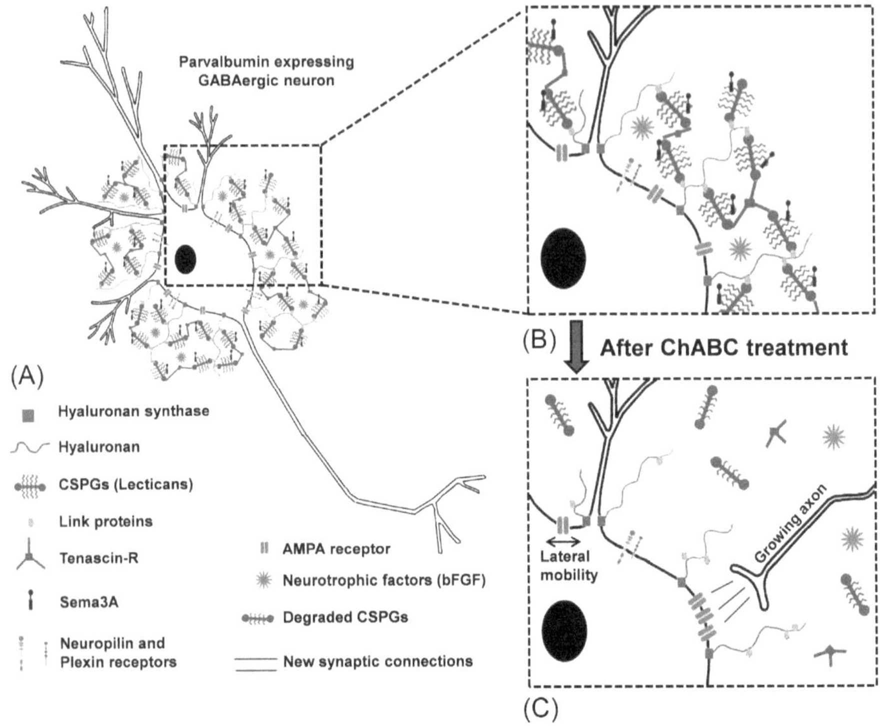

Fig. 1 Compositional variation of brain extracellular matrix in growing axons.
(A): Perineuronal nets formed around parvalbumin-expressing GABAergic neurons.
(B): Enlarged vision of (A), showing regeneration of growing axons is hindered by the ECM nets. (C): Axon growth can be restored by ChABC treatment to degrade the surrounding nets. Reproduced with permission from Soleman, S., Filippov, M.A., Dityatev, A., Fawcett, J.W., 2013. Targeting the neural extracellular matrix in neurological disorders. Neuroscience 253, 194–213.

2.2.1 CSF-ISF circulation

CSF is the extracellular fluid that is filled in the subarachnoid space between the brain and the skull. As the bathing buffer, CSF plays the dual roles in both protecting the brain from mechanical injuries and mediating nutrient and signaling exchange between the brain and the circulating system. Generally, there are four kinds of mass transfer in the brain:

(1) *CSF-blood exchange*: CSF is primarily produced via a two-step filtration process in the choroid plexus. Firstly, under pressure gradient, choroidal blood infiltrates through the leaky capillaries (different from capillaries with tight junctions in other parts of brain) and accumulates at the extravascular stroma of choroid plexus. The egressed blood is then selectively transported across the choroidal epithelium into the lateral ventricles and joins the bulk flow of CSF circulation. The selective transport of choroidal epithelium is a potential avenue for circulating immunocytes or biomacromolecules into the brain (Deczkowska et al., 2016).

(2) *CSF-ISF exchange*: Different from CSF, ISF is confined within the interstitial space of parenchyma, of which the surface is covered by pia matter that prevents the mass exchange between CSF and ISF. Alternatively, CSF must get into the interstitial space along with the "flow-in" arteries. Likewise, the ISF can be reversely drained out of the brain along the "flow-out" veins. The way of CSF in and out of brain parenchyma is termed as paravescular pathway.
(3) *CSF-lymph exchange*: Lymphatic vessels exist in brain (Louveau et al., 2015), and thus meningeal lymphatic vessels and olfactory/nasal lymphatics can drain CSF toward the cervical lymph nodes (CLNs). Through these channels, the brain and peripheral immune system can communicate effectively (Louveau et al., 2015; Sun et al., 2017).
(4) *ISF-blood exchange*: ISF-blood transfer is strictly confined by the BBB. The exchange of oxygen/nutrients and CO_2/metabolic wastes occurs at capillary interfaces.

2.3 Blood-brain and blood-CSF barriers

Mass exchange between the "flow-in" vasculature and the parenchyma is tightly controlled by the brain. Generally, there are two kinds of physiological barriers, the BBB and blood-CSF barrier (BCB), which define the membrane barriers between blood/ISF and blood/CSF, respectively (Fig. 2).

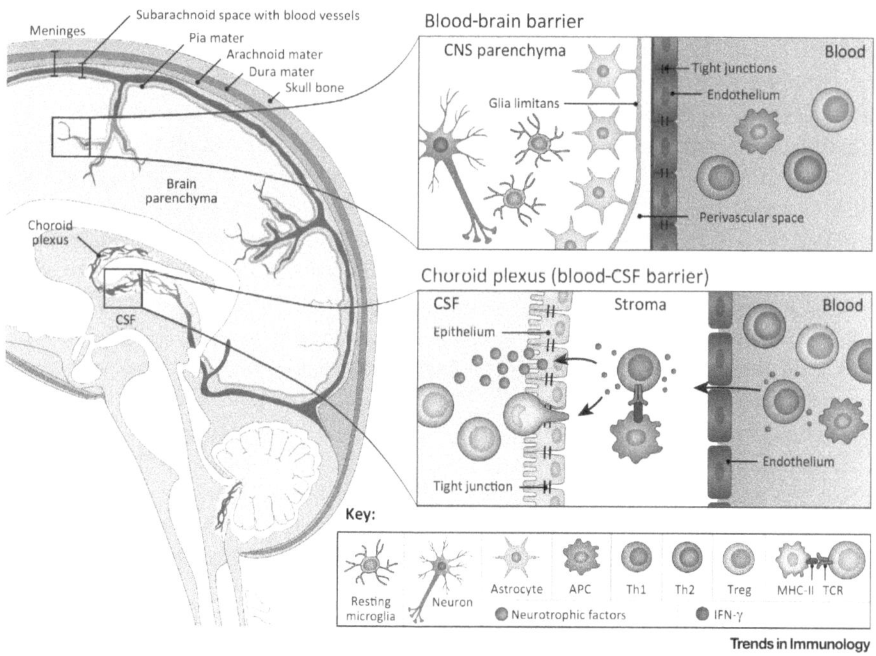

Fig. 2 Brain structure and blood-brain and blood-CSF barriers.
Reproduced with permission from Deczkowska, A., Baruch, K., Schwartz, M., 2016. Type I/II interferon balance in the regulation of brain physiology and pathology. Trends Immunol. 37, 181.

The BBB refers to the parenchyma vessels composed of an inner endothelium with tight junctions (TJ) and an outer layer of permeable basal membrane. The vessels are enclosed outside by a glial membrane composed of pericytes and astrocytes (Bandopadhyay et al., 2001). Functionally, the main barrier is defined from three different aspects (Abbott et al., 2006; Abbott, 2014):

(1) Physical barriers. Because of the tight junction between the endothelial cells, the paracellular access of soluble molecules is restricted.
(2) Transport barriers. There are many transport receptors expressed on the endothelial cells for mediating the transport and efflux of substances, maintaining the dynamic balance between the brain and blood. However, these transporters are substrate-specific, thereby limiting the vast majority of small molecule drugs and macromolecular drugs into the brain.
(3) Enzymatic barrier. There are the metabolic enzymes, which can metabolize the drug molecules and reduce their activity.

In comparison with the BBB, the BCB refers to the choroidal epithelium. Likewise, the BCB blocks the paracellular access of blood solutes into the lateral ventricle. The transportation of nutrients and immunocytes through the choroidal epithelium relies on an active transportation process.

2.4 Blood-brain tumor barrier (BBTB)

Between the blood and cancerous cells in the brain tumor, there is a separating endothelium, called the blood-brain tumor barrier (BBTB). A part of brain tumor vessels are temporally constructed under stimulation by tumor-secreted cytokines (Lorger et al., 2009; Guo et al., 2001). The newly formed neovasculatures can improve the blood perfusion and magnify nutrient supply to support the needs from rapid proliferating tumor. Meanwhile, the increased vascularization also carve out a way for blood solutes into brain tumor (Keunen and Klein, 2011). The BBTB remains intact at the early stage of brain tumors, and endothelial defects only appear at middle or late stages, which permit drugs and nanocarriers to penetrate the membrane via the paracellular way (Agarwal et al., 2011). However, it is worth noting that the EPR effect of the brain tumor neovasculatures is significantly diminished as compared with peripheral solid tumors (Susan et al., 1998). For example, the vascular pore size in the orthoptic U87MG glioma is less than 100 nm, whereas the pore diameter of subcutaneous tumor is much larger, ranging from 200 nm to 2000 nm (Susan et al., 1998).

In addition, high interstitial pressure within the tumor tissues also abates the EPR effect and reduces the intra-tumor penetration of drugs (Danhier et al., 2010; Iyer et al., 2006). Other ECM factors including fibrous matrices (Olive et al., 2009) and nonspecific phagocytosis by tumor-associated macrophages (Watters et al., 2005) also compromise the drug permeation in the BBTB. Generally, the physical distance between most tumor cells and neovascularization is longer than 100 μm. In comparison, drug diffusion within the tumor ECM is very slow, less than the range of 40–50 μm (Lu et al., 2012; Hambley and Hait, 2009; Ruoslahti et al., 2010; Primeau et al., 2005), thus the tumor ECM stands out as another impermeable barrier for brain drug delivery (Jiang et al., 2013).

3 Pathways for brain drug delivery

3.1 Invasive routes for brain delivery

Surgically administrated drugs can be directly given to the diseased sites inside the brain, which bypasses the BBB and provides an efficient way for delivering high dose of drugs without leading to systemic toxicities. Thus, intracerebral injection has gained wide applications in clinical treatment of a broad range of the brain diseases such as brain cancers (Cohen-Pfeffer et al., 2016). However, although intracerebral administration performs well in delivering drugs to the small lesions, its therapeutic potential for diseases with multiple or large lesions still relies on cerebral diffusion, which is concentration-dependent and decreases exponentially away from the injection site. For example, it will take about 3 days for a macromolecular drug to diffuse merely 1 mm (Lo et al., 2001). In comparison, though small drugs can diffuse faster than macromolecules, its elimination by the brain is rapid, and the drug concentration in the adjacent site can decrease to 10%, as compared to that at the injection site (Fung et al., 1996).

In order to improve the diffusion efficiency of the locally administrated brain drugs, convection-enhanced delivery (CED) has been explored. Unlike the concentration-dependent diffusion process, CED is driven by an infusion pump that produces pressure gradient, thus allowing the convective transport of drugs/nanoparticles irrespective of size/surface characters via the interstitial pathway. Of note, drug diffusion can be raised to a range of centimeters by CED, providing great potential for the treatment of brain tumor (Mehta et al., 2017). However, though intracerebral administration is an efficient way for brain drug delivery, surgical means are less tolerated and bring unpredictable risks such as infection and impairment of brain functions.

3.2 Noninvasive routes for brain delivery

The anatomic feature of brain capillary, brain cells, brain extracellular environment, as well as the directional fluid transfer together shape the potent transport pathways for brain drug delivery (Fig. 3). Generally, nonintracranial routes of brain drugs include nasal and systemic administration. For nasal delivery, the first physiological barrier is arachnoid membrane, which is also composed of lipid permeable epithelium. After crossing the nasal barrier, drugs reach CSF, then can follow the CSF flow into the ISF of brain parenchyma. Drugs in the ISF have to diffuse in the ECS before reaching the tumor site. As for systemic route, the circulating drugs must evade the opsonization-mediated RES elimination before entering the brain vasculatures, where the drugs can permeate into the tumor via three different ways. Since the tumors only account for a part of the parenchyma, a small fraction of circulating drugs may penetrate the BBTB and directly enter the tumor. In comparison, the main part of drugs in the brain vessels must overcome the BBB and BCB, and very limited drugs can pass these barriers and enter parenchyma and CSF, and further diffuse via the ECS path to reach the tumor site.

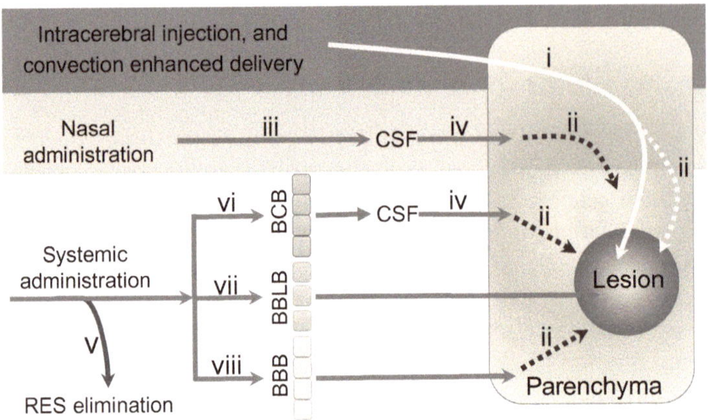

Fig. 3 The main routes for brain drug delivery. (i) Direct delivery of brain drugs via invasive intracerebral injection and convection-enhanced delivery; (ii) permeation in the parenchyma; (iii) arachnoid membrane; (iv) CSF-ISF circulation; (v) RES uptake and elimination; (vi) BCB permeation; (vii) blood-brain lesion barrier (BBLB) permeation; (viii) BBB permeation.

In the routes of drugs to brain tumor, there are a series of physiological barriers, which confine the intra-tumor transportation and diffusion process.

3.2.1 Systemic distribution and metabolism

The systemically administered drugs are indiscriminately delivered to all the organs via circulation, but the drug accumulation for a specific organ is more likely dependent on its uptake efficiency to the circulating agents. The RES organs (e.g., liver, spleen, and kidney) with the fenestrated endothelium are apt to take up the major portion of the administrated drugs, especially in a nanoparticulate form.

Drugs are subjected to metabolism either by serum enzymes or by cellular enzymes in the organs. Liver is the primary site for drug sequester and metabolism, and kidney for excretion of the drugs or their metabolites through urinary pathway. In addition, the blood components also influence the drug biofate. For example, serum proteins such as albumin are the natural surfactants, which can bind hydrophobic drugs and subsequently change their pharmacokinetic behaviors.

3.2.2 BBB & BCB permeation

Although paravascular permeation is restricted by the BBB and BCB, some serum solutes can pass through the BBB via the following pathways:

(1) *Passive diffusion*: Lipophilic molecules can diffuse through the BBB (Liu et al., 2004). However, the brain capillary endothelial cells highly express the ATP-binding cassette transporters (ABC transporters), which render the active efflux of the lipophilic molecules back to the blood and lead to insufficient drug accumulation and intracranial concentration for effective treatment (Begley, 2004a, b).

(2) *Carrier-mediated transport (CMT)*: The CNS needs a large supply of nutrients such as glucose, various amino acids, and phospholipids (Ohtsuki and Terasaki, 2007). However, the tight junctions between the brain capillary endothelial cells strictly restrict the paracellular diffusion. Therefore, the brain uptake of the water-soluble nutrients such as glucose and amino acids relies on the transporters (Zhang et al., 2002). A lot of transporters such as glucose transporter, amino acid transporter, nucleoside transporter, vitamin transporter, glutathione transporter and monocarboxylate transporter, organic anion transporters, and organic cation transporter are expressed by the brain capillary endothelial cells (Mittapalli et al., 2010). Drugs can be mediated to penetrate through the BBB via bioconjugation to the substrates of these transporters. However, the CMT pathway is generally effective for small molecule drugs, but has minor effect on macromolecules; the transport route is often inhibited due to the competitive binding of the endogenous substrates in the blood (Gynther et al., 2008).

(3) *Adsorptive-mediated transport (AMT)*: The cell membrane of the brain capillary endothelial cells presents negative charge, and the cationic substances are inclined to interact with the cell membrane and form hydrogen bonds, thus facilitating endocytosis (Sauer et al., 2005). The AMT pathway can effectively mediate the BBB penetration of cationic species (Hervé et al., 2008). However, the charge interaction is not specific, and the cationic compounds are ready to bind with the serum proteins and to be eliminated by the RES.

(4) *Receptor-mediated transport (RMT)*: In recent years, RMT-based drug systems have attracted much attention for achieving the specific and efficient brain drug delivery (Gaillard et al., 2005). RMT is an endocytosis initiated by the interaction of the substances and the specific receptors on the membrane and is mainly responsible for the transport of the macromolecules (Parkar et al., 2009). It is a concentration-independent transport. The commonly used RMT ligands include transferrin (Descamps et al., 1996a), lactoferrin (Fillebeen et al., 1999a), lipoproteins (Dehouck et al., 1996), insulin (Duffy and Pardridge, 1987), leptin (Golden et al., 1997), rabies virus glycoprotein (RVG) (Kumar et al., 2007), FC5 (Muruganandam et al., 2002), and angiopep-2 (Demeule et al., 2008a, b).

3.2.3 Diffusion in the CSF and ECS

Once passing through the BBB/BCB, the drugs reach the brain extracellular space or CSF, and then diffuse inside the brain parenchyma and finally accumulate at the target lesions. It should be noted that the drug in the CSF can follow the bulk flow of CSF into the interstitial space, which occurs rapidly, within a few hours (Iliff et al., 2012). Therefore, the limited-step is the diffusion process in the ECS, which is co-dictated by the particle character as well as the physiological features of the ECM.

3.2.3.1 Particle factors

(1) Size

The intracellular space of the EMC is reported to be 38–64 nm, which defines the mobility of floating nanomaterials by a "critical size" (Thorne and Nicholson, 2006). In this regard, the particles smaller than 60 nm are supposed to be able to move farther than the ones of larger scale. Below this range, the diffusion coefficient of particles increases with the decreasing size (Thorne and Nicholson, 2006). Interestingly, although the small particles can diffuse farther, the delivery efficiency may be compromised by the hyperactive particles. Therefore, there is an "effective size window" for nano-based delivery. As reported by Chan et al., the targeting efficiency of transferrin-modified and unmodified gold nanoparticles of different sizes were compared in a tumor-bearing mouse model (Sykes et al., 2014). Their results showed that only particles in the range of 30–60 nm manifested a targeting difference between transferrin-modified and unmodified nanoparticles. It suggested that the particle size should be carefully designed for specific applications.

(2) Zeta potential

The particles with high density of charges have been reported to be able to disrupt the integrity of BBB and thus gain access to the brain (Lockman et al., 2008). Once inside the ECM, the negatively charged extracellular matrix constitutes an electrostatic and steric barrier against the diffusion of nanoparticles. On this account, the surface charge of the nanomaterials plays another important role in the diffusion process, and the cationic particles with size comparable to ECM gaps will be slowed down by electrostatic interactions (Stylianopoulos et al., 2010).

(3) Surface PEGylation

PEGylation is an effective mean of preparing long circulating nano-vehicles. As a bio-inert polymer, the coating PEG can protect the enclosed nanoparticles from interactions with the blood components and cells. In the ECS, the densely coated PEG layer can promote the diffusion of the nanoparticles, resulting in a drastically increased mean square displacements (MSD) as compared with non-PEGylated particles (Nance et al., 2012). However, although PEGylation can promote ECM diffusion of nanoparticles, the PEG prevents the brain uptake of the nanoparticles at the same time. To address this problem, the ultrasound-mediated BBB opening technique was applied to deliver the PEGylated nanoparticles into the ECS, where the nanoparticles penetrated into the deep tissue and released the loading drugs, and thus gained improved therapeutic outcomes for CNS diseases (Nance et al., 2014).

3.2.3.2 ECM factors

Diffusion efficiency of drug/nanomaterial in the ECS is anisotropic (Vargovã and Sykovã, 2008), not only affected by particle features and diffusion regions, but also influenced by physiological variations including neurological activity, hormone level, and pathological disorders (Nicholson and Syková, 1998). Therefore, the diffusion process is collectively determined by the factors in two different aspects. One is the intrinsic characters of drugs/nanomaterials, defined as physiochemical properties including size, charge, shape, and structural issues. The other is the physiological features of the ECS. Accordingly, the limiting factors can be quantitatively assigned as ECM parameters including volumetric fraction α and tortuosity λ (Kilb et al., 2006); or codetermined parameters including the clearance constant k (Kilb et al., 2006) and diffusion coefficient D (Voříšek et al., 2002).

(1) Volumetric fraction, α

The volumetric fraction α refers to the limited volume of drug diffusion in the brain. It is defined as ECS volume/total brain tissue volume (Eq. 1). The total amount of drug retained in ECS is positively correlated with α value.

$$\alpha = V_{\text{ECS}} / V_{\text{Total}} \tag{1}$$

In normal brain, the volumetric fraction for most drugs is about 20%, but it could drop to 5% when global ischemia occurs (Syková and Nicholson, 2008). The decreased extracellular space is associated with the development of complex cell associations or certain pathological stimuli (Edgar et al., 2014). For example, during pathological conditions such as hypoxia/ischemia, the ion composition and content in ECS change rapidly, and dysfunction of Na^+-K^+ pump leads to the sharply increased concentration of K^+ and decreased Na^+ and Cl^- in the ECM. In addition, a large number of excitatory amino acids, especially glutamate, accumulate in ECS, which further drives the water influx from the extracellular space into the cells and leads to swelling of nerve and glial cells. On this account, it thus results in a significant reduction of α value 0.20–0.05 (Syková, 2004). In other conditions such as brain trauma and transplantation of dopaminergic neuronal, the increased expression of glial fibrillary acidic protein (GFAP) can be caused by hyperplasmic or hypertrophic astrocytes, resulting in an elevated α from 0.2 to 0.29 (Voříšek et al., 2002).

(2) Tortuosity, λ

The tortuosity, λ, is defined as the increased diffusion path of substances between two sites caused by various obstacles, such as nonspecific hindrances of drug/nanomaterials by membranes and glycoproteins in extracellular matrix. Tortuosity quantitatively defines the size of the diffusion barrier. For example, for small molecules and irons, the λ value of adult human brain is about 1.6, and the diffusion rate in the brain is about 2.6 times lower than that in free medium (Nicholson et al., 2011). However, as for macromolecules or nanoparticles, the size is significantly increased to the scale comparable to the extracellular gaps in the ECM, which leads to the increased contact frequency between the drugs and the channel walls consisting of the cells membranes and ECM molecules, thereby resulting in an increased λ (Thorne and Nicholson, 2006). There are two main influence factors for λ, presented as the geometric configuration and the composition of ECM. For instance, in the development of glioma, the lesion site grows due to the proliferation of glial cells and the highly secreted matrix molecules (e.g., the deposition of hyaluronic acid), so that the gaps between the cells become smaller (Vargová et al., 2003). As a result, the tortuosity λ increases and the diffusion rate reduces (Vargová et al., 2003).

(3) Clearance constant, k

The clearance constant, k, defines the rate of removal of drugs/nanomaterials from the ECS, which is caused by the reverse transportation across the BBB to the circulation and drainage out of the brain ECS. The main routes of the drugs/nanomaterials to be cleared from the brain ECS are via blood circulation, lymph circulation, and cerebrospinal fluid circulation (Nicholson, 2005). As described above, fluid transfer between ISF and CSF provides the main path for the egress of drugs/nanomaterials in the ISF, and they enter the subarachnoid space (SAS) and then are drained out of the brain by either cervical lymph node (Clapham et al., 2010) or intracranial venous system at the villi of SAS (Dickstein et al., 1999). The drainage of ISF in the white region of ECS must pass through the ependymal epithelium into the ventricles, where it follows the bulk flow of CSF and enters SAS (Clapham et al., 2010; Dickstein et al., 1999). The clearance constant k fluctuates between 3.3×10^{-3}/s and 6.3×10^{-3}/s during the course of brain development, and there are no significant differences between the cortical and white matter (Lehmenkühler et al., 1993).

(4) Diffusion coefficient, D

The diffusion coefficient D is defined as the range that the materials diffuse in a medium per unit time. It reflects the diffusion rate of matter in a medium and is the most intuitive parameter for the drug diffusion in the brain. As similar to other parameters, diffusion coefficient can be affected by many factors related to ECS and the drugs (Vořîšek et al., 2002; Vorisek and Sykova, 2009). The tortuosity and the regional spatial structure of the brain ECS are heterogeneous, thus leading to the anisotropic diffusion and the varied diffusion coefficient (Vorisek and Sykova, 2009). For example, when drugs/nanomaterials move along the axon in the corpus callosum, usually resulting in high diffusion coefficient. By contrast, the perpendicularly moving of the drugs/nanomaterials to the axon leads to a much decreased diffusion coefficient (Vorísek and Syková, 1997).

In conclusion, the volume fraction α and tortuosity λ are mainly affected by the spatial structure and composition of the brain ECM and the direction of the cell axons. The diffusion coefficient D and the clearance rate constant k are affected not only by the factors associated with the tortuosity λ, but also by the drug properties, such as structure, size, and polarity. Better understanding of the nature of these parameters and their influencing factors can help rational design of delivery systems. For example, the gap between the cells in the brain tissues is 38–64 nm (Yao et al., 2008; Thorne and Nicholson, 2006), suggesting that the nanocarriers smaller than this size range may achieve an increased diffusion coefficient. Besides, the negatively charged cell membrane and ECM may favor the inert nanomaterials that are electrically neutral, with reduced interaction with the extracellular matrix (Nance et al., 2012).

4 Designing nanomaterials for overcoming the brain barriers

Currently, the brain drug delivery is still a big challenge because of insufficient brain uptake, which is strictly confined by (1) the BBB, and (2) inefficient diffusion in the ECM. As a whole, the brain delivery efficiency of most systemically administrated drugs is below 0.1% (Kozlovskaya and Stepensky, 2013). To address the issues such as the BBB penetration, and cerebral diffusion, a number of technologies have been developed to improve the delivery efficiency of brain diseases.

4.1 Modulation of the BBB permeability

4.1.1 BBB modulation by HAV peptide

Delivery efficiency of brain drug can be significantly improved by increasing the BBB permeability. In clinical practice, the hyperosmotic mannitol solution (mannitol concentration up to 25%) can efficiently open the tight junctions of the BBB and promote the permeation of chemotherapeutics (Haluska and Anthony, 2004). However, defect of the BBB can potentially lead to serious adverse effects on the brain due to the invasion of blood solutes or even lymphocytes. Therefore, alternative reagents that can tailor the BBB permeability in a controllable manner are in need. On this account, Siahaan and coworkers synthesized a short E-cadherin-binding peptide called HAV peptide (sequence: Ac-SHAVSS-NH_2). The HAV can reversibly bind to E-cadherin, a major component of the tight junctions in the BBB, and lead to temporal opening of the tight junctions (On et al., 2014). By taking advantage of HAV, brain permeation of certain markers can be increased by 2–5 folds. Furthermore, HAV-induced tight-junction opening is temporal, and it could be restored within 1 h, thus reducing the potential adverse effects caused by long-term impairment of BBB functions.

4.1.2 Ultrasound-induced BBB opening

Ultrasound is a noninvasive physical method for BBB modulation. The cavitation effect of ultrasound can temporally disrupt the integrity of BBB and leads to a reversible opening of the barrier, thus facilitating the intra-brain transport of many drugs/nanomaterials (Hynynen et al., 2003). Importantly, combination of ultrasound and microbubbles can improve the potential of BBB modulation by focusing the cavitation site and reducing power of the applied ultrasound (Sheikov et al., 2004). Meanwhile, the bubble-forming lipids can be explored as drug loading materials, and thus microbubble-mediated BBB opening and drug delivery can be achieved simultaneously under externally applied ultrasound. By using this strategy, Aryal and coworkers successfully delivered Dox into the brain tumor of rats bearing 9L-glioma, which showed the significantly prolonged survival time (Aryal et al., 2013).

4.2 Receptor-mediated transportation (RMT) across the BBB

As described above, RMT is a main pathway for nutrient uptake in brain endothelium from circulation. Thereby, the overexpressed receptors on the endothelial membranes offer a feasible tool for the circulating drugs to penetrate the BBB and enter into the brain parenchyma (Zhou and Kopeček, 2013). Moreover, many receptors are also overexpressed by the tumor cells, thus achieving a dual-targeting effect. It is favorable to magnify the therapeutic response and decrease the side effects. RMT has been widely used in brain drug delivery. The commonly applied targeting ligands include transferrin (Descamps et al., 1996b), lactoferrin (Fillebeen et al., 1999a), lipoproteins (Dehouck et al., 1997), insulin (Duffy and Pardridge, 1987), leptin (Golden et al., 1997), angiopep-2 (Demeule et al., 2008c, d), Apo E (Sauer et al., 2005) etc.

4.2.1 LRP receptor-mediated delivery

Low-density lipoprotein receptor-related protein (LRP) is a family member of low-density lipoprotein (LDL) receptors, which can be specifically recognized by ligands such as lactoferrin (Fillebeen et al., 1999a) and receptor-related protein ligands (Pan et al., 2004), mediating transport of the ligands across the BBB via endocytosis. More importantly, LRP receptors are highly expressed not only on the brain capillary endothelial cells, but also on the glioma cells (Yamamoto et al., 1997; Maletínská et al., 2000; Bu et al., 1994). Therefore, the targeting LRP receptor can play dual roles in not only the BBB penetration, but also the glioma uptake.

Lactoferrin (Lf) is one of the most commonly used LRP ligands. Lf is a cationic glycoprotein present in mammals and belongs to the family of transferrin (Nuijens et al., 1996). Lf can enter the brain via the receptor-mediated endocytosis, and the transport process is one-way pattern without significant cross-cell degradation (Fillebeen et al., 1999a, b). By taking advantage of lactoferrin, Fang et al. prepared an Lf-modified polydiacetylene nanocarriers (PDNCs) for the treatment of brain tumor. Results showed that PDNCs modified with Lf displayed significantly improved cell uptake. Magnetism resonance imaging showed that Lf-PDNCs can efficiently deliver the loading drugs to the tumor region, and yielded significant tumor inhibition, showing that the tumor volume of rat treated with Lf-PDNCs was 1/3.5 of unmodified particles (Fang et al., 2016). Huang and coworkers using Lf-modified PAMAM significantly improved the pathological symptoms of rats with Alzheimer's disease and promoted growth of dopaminergic neurons in striatum and glaucoma, suggesting that Lf-modified nanoparticles were capable of intra-brain permeation into the diseased lesions (Huang et al., 2008, 2009).

Besides lactoferrin, Angiopep-2 is a short LRP-binding peptide consisting of 19 amino acid residues with a sequence of TFFYGGSRGKRNNFKTEEY. Angiopep-2 is a high potent brain targeting ligands; its brain permeation efficiency is reported to be 70 times that of transferrin (Demeule et al., 2008c, d). Xin et al. took the dual functional angiopep-2 (ANG) as surface ligands and prepared paclitaxel-loaded polyethylene glycol-polycaprolactone nanoparticles (ANG-NP-PTX). Results showed IC_{50} of ANG-NP-PTX on U87 cells was 1/3.4 and 1/3.8 of that obtained from Taxol and NP-PTX, respectively. Three-dimensional modeling of solid tumor showed that PEG-NP only accumulated around the surface of the tumor ball, whereas the ANG-NPs could be distributed inside the whole tumor, suggesting that the ANG modification could significantly promote penetration of nanoparticles into the tumor. in vivo antitumor assessment showed that the glioma bearing mice treated with ANG-NP-PTX manifested most alleviated tumor burdens and acquired extended survival time, indicating that ANG-modified target nanoparticles have a strong targeting ability for brain glioma (Xin et al., 2011).

4.2.2 Transferrin receptor (TfR)

Transferrin receptor (TfR) is a transmembrane glycoprotein which is widely expressed in various sites of human body with different levels. For example, TfR is highly expressed by red blood cells, brain endothelial cells, and several types of tumor cells. In comparison, TfR expression by the other kinds of cells is low. Consequently, the TfR level in brain tumor cell is reported to be 2–7 times that of normal cells, with its affinity to transferrin about 10–100 times to that of normal cells (Kawamoto et al., 2013; Zhang et al., 2012), thus is a potent target for brain drug delivery. However, it is worth noting that TfR can mediate bi-directional transport in and out of the brain endothelial cells. Meanwhile, the endogenous transferrin can compete with exogenously injected transferrin for tumor TfRs, both of which can diminish the targeting efficiency of nanocarriers for brain tumor.

With regard to the shortcomings of transferrin, researchers have screened out a novel kind of TfR-binding peptide via phage display. The new TfR-binding peptide, termed as T7 peptid, shows equivalent affinity to TfR, and its binding with the target cannot be inhibited by the endogenous transferrin, thus is superior to the original ligand in tumor drug delivery (Han et al., 2010). Bi et al. used T7 peptide as targeting moiety and penetration enhancer and found that T7 peptide can significantly improve the distribution in brain tumor, indicating the feasibility of T7 brain tumor delivery (Bi et al., 2016).

Antibody can also be utilized to mediate brain drug delivery. OX26, a monoclonal antibody from mouse anti-rat TfR, can bind with TfR at specific sites different from transferrin, thus can avoid competition of endogenous Tf. Pang et al. (2008) prepared neuropeptide-containing polymer vesicles modified with OX26 to treat Alzheimer's disease (AD). Results show that the OX26-modified polymer vesicles with dose of 1 ng/kg can significantly improve the AD, while the polymer vesicle without OX26 and free neuropeptide have no effect under the same dose.

4.2.3 NRP-1 receptor

As mentioned above, NRP-1 is also a receptor enriched in the tumor neovasculature and tumor cells (Nasarre et al., 2010). Likewise, NRP-1 receptor can mediate the transportation of NRP-1-modified nanomaterials from blood to brain tumors.

By utilizing the tLyp-1 (a kind of NRP-1 ligand) for surface modification, Hu et al. found that tLyp-1-modified nanoparticles could increase the uptake efficiency by tumor cells. in vivo experiments also showed that tLyp-1-modified nanoparticles could efficiently accumulate in the brain tumor and penetrate deep into the core of brain tumor (Hu et al., 2013a).

4.2.4 Heparan sulfate receptor

The heparan sulfate receptor is specifically expressed on the surface of Glioma neovasculature and glioma cells (Agemy et al., 2011), but not by normal tissue cells (Hoffman et al., 2003). Therefore, the short peptide ligand (CGKRK) for heparan sulfate receptor can be explored as tumor-selective cell-penetrating peptide that can promote BBB permeation of nanoparticles via heparin sulfate heparin receptor-mediated transportation (Agemy et al., 2011). Hu et al. reported that CGKRK-modified nanoparticles could penetrate deep into the tumor and achieve doubled payloads in brain tumor as compared with unmodified nanoparticles (Hu et al., 2013b).

4.2.5 N-Acetylcholine receptor (nAChR)

The *N*-acetylcholine receptor (nAChR) is widely expressed in brain tissue, including brain capillaries, containing the diseased cell of AD (Gotti and Clementi, 2004). It has been reported that rabies virus glycoprotein (RVG) can specifically bind to nAChR on neuronal cells to mediate RVG into neuronal cells (Liu et al., 2016a). They designed a RVG-modified nanoparticle to delivery drug to the lesion region of AD. The result shows that RVG-modified nanoparticles can improve the concentration of drugs in lesion region of AD.

4.2.6 Targeting to Aβ amyloid precipitation deposits

Alzheimer's disease (AD) is a common neurodegenerative disease. The etiology and pathogenesis of AD have not been elucidated, but it is generally believed that there are two characteristic pathological changes: First, Aβ amyloid protein deposition at brain parenchymal cells, due to the metabolic pathway disorders of β-secret enzyme (beta-site APP-cleaving enzyme 1, BACE 1) (Evin et al., 2010; Vassar et al., 2009); second, the hyperphosphorylation of tau-induced neurofibrillary tangles in nerve cells (Ward et al., 2012; Attems et al., 2012).

Utilizing the characteristics that a large number of Aβ amyloid precipitation deposits in the lesion region of AD, a target delivery system in the brain can be designed. Zhang et al. (2014) designed a dual-targeting delivery system that the first-level targeting functional groups are capable of selective affinity with BBB to facilitate the delivery of the system through BBB; the second-level targeting functional groups are able to affinity with the diseased tissue, to make more drugs further concentrate in the brain lesion region. Among them, author selects TNG (TGNYKALHPHNG) as the first-level targeting functional molecular and QSH (QSHYRHISPAQV) as the second-level targeting functional molecular. TNG peptides can improve selectivity of the delivery system to the blood-brain barrier. QSH peptides can specifically recognize and bind to senile plaques caused by Aβ amyloid protein (van Groen et al., 2009, 2008). The result shows that the nanoparticles modified with QSH and TNG were able to accumulate significantly in the lesion region.

Coincidentally, Yu et al. (2011) design a bispecific antibody (anti-TfR/BACE1) that can bind with TfR and enzyme β-secretase (BACE1) to realize the dual-targeting to brain region of AD. In this design, affinity of the antibody for TfR is low to enhance the quantity of antibody across the BBB into brain, rather than remaining in the BBB due to high affinity of antibody for TfR. Another domain of the antibody has high affinity to BACE1 to realize higher accumulation in the brain region with AD. The experiment shows that the mean bispecific antibody uptake is 4.75 times that of anti-BACE1 at 48 h, and the reduction of $A\beta_{1-40}$ treatment with anti-TfR/BACE1 is up to 50% in brain at 48 h with the dose of 50 mg/kg. Under the same conditions, the effect caused by anti-BACE1 is only 20%.

4.3 CPPs-mediated penetration across BBB

CPPs, also known as protein transduction domains, are a class of short peptides typically composed of no more than 30 amino acids and are able to carry various size of molecules (e.g., peptides, proteins, and nucleic acids) and nanoparticles to enter the cells (Zorko and Langel, 2005). At organ level, Dowdy and coworkers have firstly reported that cell-penetrating TAT can deliver β-galactosidase into the brain parenchyma via intraperitoneal injection. Of note, the molecular size of β-galactosidase is about 60 times larger than 11-amino acid TAT, which manifest the potent in brain drug delivery (Schwarze et al., 1999). Later, a number of pharmaceutical carriers including liposome, silica nanoparticle, quantum dots, etc. have been successfully delivered into the brain by CPPs (Farkhani et al., 2014). The collecting evidence from worldwide all approve CPPs as powerful tools in addressing the BBB challenge and mediating sufficient intra-brain delivery of drugs that is generally impermeable to the brain endothelium.

However, though CPPs are capable of intra-brain penetration, the CPP-mediated tissue penetration is nonspecific and can lead to indiscriminate distribution of cargos in the organs. Meanwhile, tumor cells are accompanied by many other cell types including microglia (Hanisch and Kettenmann, 2007), tumor-associated macrophages (Watters et al., 2005), astrocytes (Lee et al., 2006), and fibroblasts (Gallagher et al., 2005). These cells may compete with the tumor cells for the CPP-modified nanocarriers. Thus, additional designs have to be enclosed in order to improve brain targeting efficiency and selectivity of the pharmaceutical agent to the specific target.

4.4 Combining CPPs with targeting ligands for brain drug delivery

During cancerogenesis, tumor cells are originated from a series of genetic and epigenetic mutations. The mutated tumor cells then reshape the microenvironment in order to facilitate its proliferation and metastasis (Liotta and Kohn, 2001). On this account, tumor has distinguished itself from normal tissues in many ways, which can be explored to improve the targeting efficiency of nanocarriers. For example, tumor cells and the local neovasculature are rich in several kinds of nutrient transporters and receptor-mediated transporters to support its needs for nutrients and signal transductions, thus the overexpressed transporters and receptors can serve as potential target for drug delivery.

4.4.1 CPPs with nutrient transporter

Serum albumin is the most abundant protein in plasma and functions as an endogenous protein carrier for exogenous drugs. Meanwhile, albumin is also an important nutrient source for tissues and organs (Stehle et al., 1997; Wunder et al., 1997). Brain capillary endothelium and tumor cells are expressing high-level albumin-binding proteins, which approve its stronger affinity for the circulating albumin as compared with astrocytes and neutrons (Merlot et al., 2014). By conjugating albumin with CPPs,

Huang and coworkers found that the as-prepared BSA-LMWP can efficiently cross the BBB and be recognized by the albumin-binding protein that was highly expressed on both the BBB and glioma cells, called secreted protein acidic and rich in cysteine (SPARC) (Lin et al., 2016). The combination use of CPP significantly promoted the penetration efficiency of the nanoparticles across the BBB. Meanwhile, albumin in its nature further magnified its uptake by the glioma cells, thereby yielding an improved delivery efficiency and treatment efficacy for anti-glioma study.

4.4.2 CPPs with receptor-mediated transporter

4.4.2.1 Transferrin

As mentioned, Transferrin (Tf) can specifically bind with brain tumor-overexpressed TfR. Thus, in combination applications with CPP, Tf can serve as targeting ligands and improve selectivity of nanoparticles to the cancerous target. Moreover, CPP-mediated delivery does not require the ligand-receptor-specific binding, thus can help overcome the saturation effect of Tf (Torchilin and Levchenko, 2001).

Sharma et al. designed a poly-L-arginine/Tf co-modified cationic liposome system for dual-targeting delivery of pDNA (encoding β-gal) to brain tumors. The co-modified cationic liposomes showed the β-gal expression in the brain was 1.65 times higher than that of the Tf-modified liposomes. Moreover, the dual-targeted cationic liposomes did not cause significant adverse effects such as inflammation, necrosis, and edema on the major organs (Sharma et al., 2013).

4.4.2.2 RGD peptides

RGDs refer to a series of linear or cyclic peptides. The functional domain of RGD is composed of triple peptide RGD sequence that can specifically bind to tumor-overexpressed integrin $\alpha_v\beta_3$ (Zhan et al., 2010). RGDs are widely applied as targeting ligand that can efficiently improve tumor selectivity of various nanocarriers (Arosio and Casagrande, 2016). On this account, combining CPP with RGD peptide is supposed to simultaneously improve BBB permeation and tumor selectivity of the nanomateirals. Kibria et al. used R8 and cRGD to prepare a dual modified liposome, and the results showed that R8/cRGD-modified liposomes significantly improved the therapeutic efficacy in brain tumor (Kibria et al., 2011). Alternatively, CPP and RGD can be covalently connected for brain drug delivery. The as-synthesized tandem peptide integrated the functions of R8 and cRGD, with ability to improve both the targeting and permeability of drugs, thus is suitable for brain tumor delivery. The results showed tandem R8-RGD-modified liposomes was 2 and 30 times higher than that of the R8-liposomes and the cRGD-modified liposomes, respectively. In the in vitro BBB culture model, the R8-RGD-modified liposomes also exhibited significant penetration ability through the BBB and high accumulation in the tumor cells. in vivo imaging results further demonstrated the effective brain tumor targeting and accumulation of the R8-RGD-modified liposomes (Liu et al., 2014).

4.4.2.3 Neuropilin-1 (NRP-1) peptide

NRP-1 is a multifunctional receptor which involves in the signal transduction of many endogenous cytokines including vascular endothelial growth factor, heparin-binding protein, fibroblast growth factor, placental growth factor, platelet growth factor, fibronectin, and others. Functionally, NRP-1 participates in the regulation of several processes that are critical in tumor's growth, migration, and invasion (Prud'Homme and Glinka, 2012). Expression of NRP-1 is highly limited in tumor vessels and tumor tissues (Nasarre et al., 2010), which provides a specific address for tumor location. Structural analysis has identified the "CendR" domain, with a C-terminal R/K-X-X-R/K sequence (where X represents any amino acid), and can specifically bind to NRP-1 (Ruoslahti et al., 2010; Sugahara et al., 2009). Thus, "CendR" is often explored as tumor targeting peptides, which derives into different species such as LyP-1, F3, iRGD, and dGR (Teesalu et al., 2009; Haspel et al., 2011; Liu et al., 2016b).

Liu et al. designed a R8-dGR tandem peptide as a target ligand for brain tumor targeting. The dGP sequence can simultaneously target integrin $\alpha_v\beta_3$ and NRP-1. Besides, R8 sequence can induce the tissue penetration. Thus, the tandem peptide composed of R8 and dGR led to enhanced drug delivery by improving the targeting and permeability. Results from in vitro and in vivo studies demonstrated an increased delivery efficiency for brain tumor (Liu et al., 2016b).

4.5 Activatable cell-penetrating peptide-derived peptide

As mentioned, although CPP is a powerful tool in mediating cell uptake and tissue penetration of drugs and nanoparticles, its penetration-enhancing effect, however, lacked specificity. This nature of CPPs will generally lead to indiscriminate engulfment of CPP-seasoned drug/nanocarrier by all organs which may cause unfavorable side effects. Therefore, permeation-enhancing potential of CPP should be finely tamed to function specifically at the neoplastic target. On this account, CPP is always inactivated in a certain fashion, which can be reactivated by endogenous/exogenous stimuli, thus facilitating selectively enhanced penetration at the target organs.

4.5.1 Shielding effect by PEG

Pegylation is the most common way of acquiring long-circulating nanomaterials. Different from permeation-enhancing CPP, PEG is an inert hydrophilic polymer, which can decrease endocytosis of nanomaterials by cells. Furthermore, surface modification using PEG can efficiently protect nanomaterials from opsonization and nonspecific uptake by the RES organs. On this account, PEG can be explored as efficient shelters to temporally neutralize the permeability of CPPs.

We previously developed a protease activatable system for delivering the anticancer CPP-drug conjugate (Fig. 4) (Chen et al., 2017). The system was composed of series connected trichosanthin (TCS), low molecular weight protamine (LMWP), MMP-2 (matrix metalloproteinase-2) substrate peptides (MSP), PEG (MW: 5000 Da), and lactoferrin (Lf). Among them, TCS is a kind of potential anticancer protein, which lacked sufficient means to enter the cell (Walsh et al., 2013; Ng et al., 2010), thereby

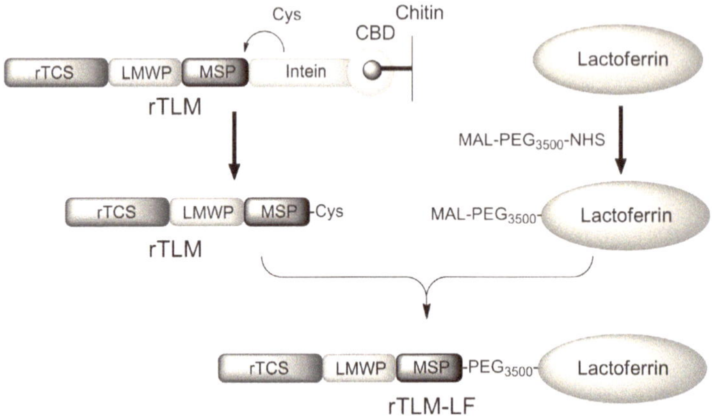

Fig. 4 The construction of rTLM-LF.
Reproduced with permission from Chen, Y.Z., Zhang, M., Jin, H.Y., Li, D.D., Xu, F., Wu, A.H., et al., 2017. Glioma dual-targeting nanohybrid protein toxin constructed by intein-mediated site-specific ligation for multistage booster delivery. Theranostics 7, 3489–3503.

its covalent form with CPP magnified the ribosome inactivating potency against several types of cancer in vitro. However, nonspecific penetration of the cell toxic TCS-CPP would lead to adverse effect to the normal organs. In order to shield the cell-penetrating potential of CPP, TCS-CPP was covalently tethered with PEG by an MMP-2 substrate peptide, which could be cleaved by the tumor overexpressing MMP-2 (Chaudhary et al., 2013), thus facilitating the on-site CPP activation. Moreover, TCS-CPP-MSP-PEG was further modified by a brain tumor targeting protein lactoferrin (Lf) to further improve its selectivity to the tumor tissue via LRP-1 receptor (low-density lipoprotein receptor-related protein-1) (Alexander et al., 2012; Yu et al., 2012; Somani et al., 2015; Gao et al., 2014; Wei et al., 2014). By taking advantage of this system, it was found that active TCS-CPP could be efficiently delivered to the brain tumor and significantly promoted survival of mice bearing brain tumors.

4.5.2 Shielding effect by negative charge

Apart from PEG-mediated shielding strategy, permeation-enhancing effect of CPP can be directly inhibited in a compromising way. Since the permeation functions of CPP rely on its structural and physiochemical properties, changes of these features would significantly compromise the penetrating ability of CPP.

Based on this, Gao and coworkers covalently connected cell-penetrating octa-polyarginine (R8, polycationic) with octa-glutamic acid (E8, polyanionic) via a short MMP-2 substrate peptide (PLGLAG) as internal spacer (Fig. 5) (Gao et al., 2014). The resulting sequence would form a hairpin structure (called ACP) due to the strong electrostatic force between E8 and R8. As the permeation capacity of R8 was dependent on its polycationic property, which had been blocked by the polyanionic E8, the as-formed hairpin structure could function as inactivated pro-CPP, whose penetrating

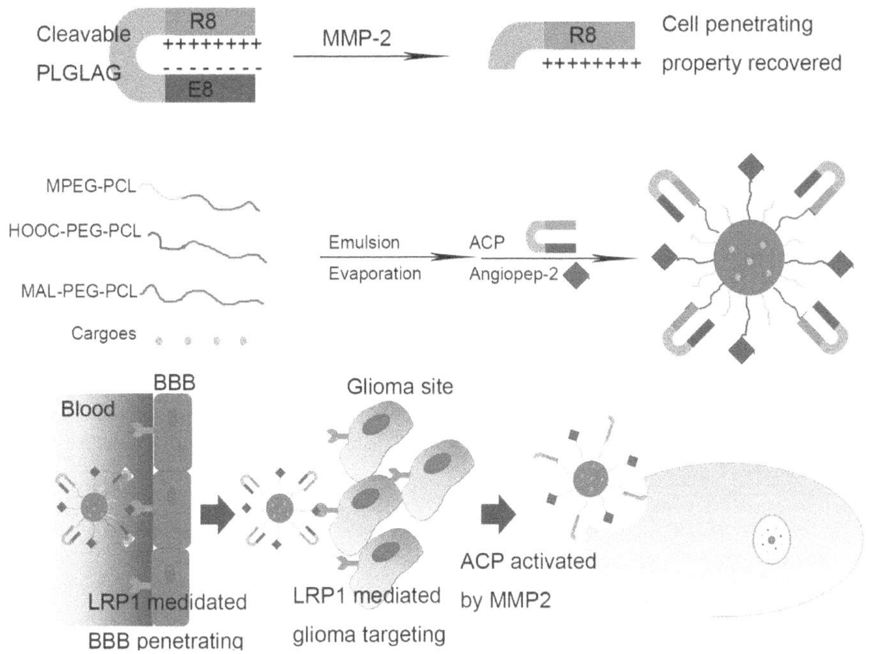

Fig. 5 Schematic design of brain targeting drug delivery system.
Reproduced with permission from Gao, H., Zhang, S., Cao, S., Yang, Z., Pang, Z., Jiang, X., 2014. Angiopep-2 and activatable cell-penetrating peptide dual-functionalized nanoparticles for systemic glioma-targeting delivery. Mol. Pharm. 11, 2755-2763

ability could be restored by the tumor overexpressing MMP-2 (Jiang et al., 2004). Gao and coworkers then grafted the pro-CPP (ACP) and angiopep-2 (a LRP-1 targeting ligand) on the surface of PEG-PCL micelles, producing a dual functionalized system for brain drug delivery. The in vitro experiments showed that pro-CPP could only be activated and promote cellular uptake of nanoparticles in the presence of MMP-2. The in vivo results manifested that the dual functional micelle could efficiently pass through BBB and accumulate in brain tumor, thereby producing more pronounced therapeutic outcomes than either single modified nanoparticle and significantly prolonged the median survival time of the tumor-bearing mice.

5 Conclusions

Brain is a very complicated organ. When drugs are delivered to the brain, they usually encounter two major obstacles: blood-brain barrier and brain cell microenvironment barrier. Due to the high complexity and heterogeneity of the spatial configuration and matrix composition of brain cell microenvironment, the diffusion of drugs in the brain is very slow and has been eliminated by non-targeted cells. Therefore, it is necessary to study the differences of cells and microenvironment between brain lesions and normal brain tissue. Combined with the development of current biology and chemical technologies, it is a promising development direction to design drug delivery system to directly achieve the accumulation of drugs through the blood-brain barrier to the lesion. But subject to current biological level, we need to continue to investigate the differences in cell and microenvironment in brain lesions and search for more efficient targeting strategies or target molecules.

References

Abbott, N., Ronnback, L., Hansson, E., 2006. Astrocyte-endothelial interactions at the blood-brain barrier. Nat. Rev. Neurosci. 7, 41–53.

Abbott, N.J., 2014. Anatomy and Physiology of the Blood-Brain Barriers. Springer, New York.

Agarwal, S., Sane, R., Oberoi, R., Ohlfest, J.R., Elmquist, W., 2011. Delivery of molecularly targeted therapy to malignant glioma, a disease of the whole brain. Expert Rev. Mol. Med. 13.

Agemy, L., Friedmann-Morvinski, D., Kotamraju, V.R., Roth, L., Sugahara, K.N., Girard, O.M., et al., 2011. Targeted nanoparticle enhanced proapoptotic peptide as potential therapy for glioblastoma. Proc. Natl. Acad. Sci. 108, 17450–17455.

Alexander, D.B., Iigo, M., Yamauchi, K., Suzui, M., Tsuda, H., 2012. Lactoferrin: an alternative view of its role in human biological fluids 1 1 this article is part of a special issue entitled Lactoferrin and has undergone the Journal's usual peer review process. Biochem. Cell Biol. 90, 279–306.

Arosio, D., Casagrande, C., 2016. Advancement in integrin facilitated drug delivery. Adv. Drug Deliv. Rev. 97, 111–143.

Aryal, M., Vykhodtseva, N., Zhang, Y.Z., Park, J., Mcdannold, N., 2013. Multiple treatments with liposomal doxorubicin and ultrasound-induced disruption of blood-tumor and blood-brain barriers improve outcomes in a rat glioma model. J. Control. Release 169, 103.

Aspelund, A., Antila, S., Proulx, S.T., Karlsen, T.V., Karaman, S., Detmar, M., et al., 2015. A dural lymphatic vascular system that drains brain interstitial fluid and macromolecules. J. Exp. Med. 212, 991.

Attems, J., Thal, D.R., Jellinger, K.A., 2012. The relationship between subcortical tau pathology and Alzheimer's disease. Biochem. Soc. Trans. 40 (4), 711–715.

Bandopadhyay, R., Orte, C., Lawrenson, J.G., Reid, A.R., Silva, S.D., Allt, G., 2001. Contractile proteins in pericytes at the blood-brain and blood-retinal barriers. J. Neurocytol. 30, 35–44.

Bandtlow, C.E., Zimmermann, D.R., 2000. Proteoglycans in the developing brain: new conceptual insights for old proteins. Physiol. Rev. 80, 1267.

Bedard, P.L., Hansen, A.R., Ratain, M.J., Siu, L.L., 2013. Tumour heterogeneity in the clinic. Nature 501, 355–364.

Begley, D.J., 2004a. Delivery of therapeutic agents to the central nervous system: the problems and the possibilities. Pharmacol. Ther. 104, 29–45.

Begley, D.J., 2004b. ABC transporters and the blood-brain barrier. Curr. Pharm. Des. 10, 1295–1312.

Berg, J.M., Tymoczko, J.L., Stryer, L., 2002. Biochemistry, 5th ed. W. H. Freeman Publishing, New York, pp. 93–126.

Bi, Y., Liu, L., Lu, Y., Sun, T., Shen, C., Chen, X., et al., 2016. T7 peptide-functionalized PEG-PLGA micelles loaded with Carmustine for targeting therapy of glioma. ACS Appl. Mater. Interfaces 8, 27465–27473.

Bradstreet, J.J., Ruggiero, M., Pacini, S., 2015. Commentary: structural and functional features of central nervous system lymphatic vessels. Front. Neurosci. 9.

Bu, G., Maksymovitch, E.A., Geuze, H., Schwartz, A.L., 1994. Subcellular localization and endocytic function of low density lipoprotein receptor-related protein in human glioblastoma cells. J. Biol. Chem. 269, 29874–29882.

Chaudhary, A.K., Pandya, S., Ghosh, K., Nadkarni, A., 2013. Matrix metalloproteinase and its drug targets therapy in solid and hematological malignancies: an overview. Mutat. Res. Rev. Mutat. Res. 753, 7–23.

Chen, Y.Z., Zhang, M., Jin, H.Y., Li, D.D., Xu, F., Wu, A.H., et al., 2017. Glioma dual-targeting nanohybrid protein toxin constructed by intein-mediated site-specific ligation for multistage booster delivery. Theranostics 7, 3489–3503.

Clapham, R., O'Sullivan, E., Weller, R.O., Carare, R.O., 2010. Cervical lymph nodes are found in direct relationship with the internal carotid artery: significance for the lymphatic drainage of the brain. Clin. Anat. 23, 43–47.

Cohen-Pfeffer, J.L., Gururangan, S., Lester, T., Lim, D.A., Shaywitz, A.J., Westphal, M., et al., 2016. Intracerebroventricular delivery as a safe, long-term route of administration. Pediatr. Neurol. 67, 23–35.

Cserr, H.F., Harlingberg, C.J., Knopf, P.M., 1992. Drainage of brain extracellular fluid into blood and deep cervical lymph and its immunological significance. Brain Pathol. 2, 269–276.

Danhier, F., Feron, O., Préat, V., 2010. To exploit the tumor microenvironment: passive and active tumor targeting of nanocarriers for anti-cancer drug delivery. J. Control. Release 148, 135–146.

Deczkowska, A., Baruch, K., Schwartz, M., 2016. Type I/II interferon balance in the regulation of brain physiology and pathology. Trends Immunol. 37, 181.

Dehouck, B., Dehouck, M.P., Fruchart, J.C., Cecchelli, R., 1996. A New Function for the LDL Receptor: Transcytosis of LDL Through the Blood-Brain Barrier. Springer, USA.

Dehouck, B., Fenart, L., Dehouck, M.-P., Pierce, A., Torpier, G., Cecchelli, R., 1997. A new function for the LDL receptor: transcytosis of LDL across the blood-brain barrier. J. Cell Biol. 138, 877–889.

Demeule, M., Currie, J.C., Bertrand, Y., Ché, C., Nguyen, T., Régina, A., et al., 2008a. Involvement of the low-density lipoprotein receptor-related protein in the transcytosis of the brain delivery vector angiopep-2. J. Neurochem. 106, 1534–1544.

Demeule, M., Régina, A., Ché, C., Poirier, J., Nguyen, T., Gabathuler, R., et al., 2008b. Identification and design of peptides as a new drug delivery system for the brain. J. Pharmacol. Exp. Ther. 324, 1064–1072.

Depasquale, M., Patlak, C.S., Cserr, H.F., 1989. Brain ion and volume regulation during acute hypernatremia in Brattleboro rats. Am. J. Phys. 256, F1059.

Descamps, L., Dehouck, M.P., Torpier, G., Cecchelli, R., 1996. Receptor-mediated transcytosis of transferrin through blood-brain barrier endothelial cells. Am. J. Physiol. 270, H1149–H1158.

Dickstein, J.B., Moldofsky, H., Lue, F.A., Hay, J.B., 1999. Intracerebroventricular injection of TNF-alpha promotes sleep and is recovered in cervical lymph. Am. J. Phys. 276, 1018–1022.

Duffy, K.R., Pardridge, W.M., 1987. Blood-brain barrier transcytosis of insulin in developing rabbits. Brain Res. 420, 32–38.

Edgar, L.T., Underwood, C.J., Guilkey, J.E., Hoying, J.B., Weiss, J.A., 2014. Extracellular matrix density regulates the rate of neovessel growth and branching in sprouting angiogenesis. PLoS One. 9e85178.

Evin, G., Barakat, A., Masters, C.L., 2010. BACE: therapeutic target and potential biomarker for Alzheimer's disease. Int. J. Biochem. Cell Biol. 42, 1923–1926.

Fang, J.H., Chiu, T.L., Huang, W.C., Lai, Y.H., Hu, S.H., Chen, Y.Y., et al., 2016. Dual-targeting Lactoferrin-conjugated polymerized magnetic Polydiacetylene-assembled Nanocarriers with self-responsive fluorescence/magnetic resonance imaging for in vivo brain tumor therapy. Adv. Healthcare Mater. 5, 688–695.

Farkhani, S.M., Valizadeh, A., Karami, H., Mohammadi, S., Sohrabi, N., Badrzadeh, F., 2014. Cell penetrating peptides: efficient vectors for delivery of nanoparticles, nanocarriers, therapeutic and diagnostic molecules. Peptides 57, 78.

Fillebeen, C., Dehouck, B., Benaïssa, M., Dhennin-Duthille, I., Cecchelli, R., Pierce, A., 1999b. Tumor necrosis factor-α increases lactoferrin transcytosis through the blood-brain barrier. J. Neurochem. 73, 2491–2500.

Fillebeen, C., Descamps, L., Dehouck, M.-P., Fenart, L., Benaïssa, M., Spik, G., et al., 1999a. Receptor-mediated transcytosis of lactoferrin through the blood-brain barrier. J. Biol. Chem. 274, 7011–7017.

Fisher, M., Feuerstein, G., Howells, D.W., Hurn, P.D., Kent, T.A., Savitz, S.I., et al., 2009. Update of the stroke therapy academic industry roundtable preclinical recommendations. Stroke 40, 2244–2250.

Földi, M., Csillik, B., Zoltán, O.T., 1968. Lymphatic drainage of the brain. Experientia 24, 1283.

Fung, L.K., Shin, M., Tyler, B., Brem, H., Saltzman, W.M., 1996. Chemotherapeutic drugs released from polymers: distribution of 1,3-bis(2-chloroethyl)-l-nitrosourea in the rat brain. Pharm. Res. 13, 671.

Gaillard, P.J., Visser, C.C., Boer, A.G.D., 2005. Targeted delivery across the blood-brain barrier. Expert Opin. Drug Deliv. 2, 299–309.

Gallagher, P.G., Bao, Y., Prorock, A., Zigrino, P., Nischt, R., Politi, V., et al., 2005. Gene expression profiling reveals cross-talk between melanoma and fibroblasts: implications for host-tumor interactions in metastasis. Cancer Res. 65, 4134–4146.

Gao, H., Zhang, S., Cao, S., Yang, Z., Pang, Z., Jiang, X., 2014. Angiopep-2 and activatable cell-penetrating peptide dual-functionalized nanoparticles for systemic glioma-targeting delivery. Mol. Pharm. 11, 2755–2763.

Golden, P.L., Maccagnan, T.J., Pardridge, W.M., 1997. Human blood-brain barrier leptin receptor. Binding and endocytosis in isolated human brain microvessels. J. Clin. Investig. 99, 14–18.

Gotti, C., Clementi, F., 2004. Neuronal nicotinic receptors: from structure to pathology. Prog. Neurobiol. 74, 363–396.

Guo, P., Xu, L., Pan, S., Brekken, R.A., Yang, S.T., Whitaker, G.B., et al., 2001. Vascular endothelial growth factor isoforms display distinct activities in promoting tumor angiogenesis at different anatomic sites. Cancer Res. 61, 8569–8577.

Gynther, M., Laine, K., Ropponen, J., Leppänen, J., Mannila, A., Nevalainen, T., et al., 2008. Large neutral amino acid transporter enables brain drug delivery via Prodrugs. J. Med. Chem. 51, 932–936.

Haluska, M., Anthony, M.L., 2004. Osmotic blood-brain barrier modification for the treatment of malignant brain tumors. Clin. J. Oncol. Nurs. 8, 263.

Hambley, T.W., Hait, W.N., 2009. Is anticancer drug development heading in the right direction? Cancer Res. 69, 1259–1262.

Han, L., Huang, R., Liu, S., Huang, S., Jiang, C., 2010. Peptide-conjugated PAMAM for targeted doxorubicin delivery to transferrin receptor overexpressed tumors. Mol. Pharm. 7, 2156.

Hanisch, U.K., Kettenmann, H., 2007. Microglia: active sensor and versatile effector cells in the normal and pathologic brain. Nat. Neurosci. 10, 1387.

Haspel, N., Zanuy, D., Nussinov, R., Teesalu, T., Ruoslahti, E., Aleman, C., 2011. Binding of a C-end rule peptide to the neuropilin-1 receptor: a molecular modeling approach. Biochemistry 50, 1755–1762.

Hervé, F., Ghinea, N., Scherrmann, J.M., 2008. CNS delivery via adsorptive transcytosis. AAPS J. 10, 455–472.

Hoffman, J.A., Giraudo, E., Singh, M., Zhang, L., Inoue, M., Porkka, K., et al., 2003. Progressive vascular changes in a transgenic mouse model of squamous cell carcinoma. Cancer Cell 4, 383–391.

Hopkins, A.M., DeSimone, E., Chwalek, K., Kaplan, D.L., 2015. 3D in vitro modeling of the central nervous system. Prog. Neurobiol. 125, 1–25.

Hu, Q., Gao, X., Gu, G., Kang, T., Tu, Y., Liu, Z., et al., 2013a. Glioma therapy using tumor homing and penetrating peptide-functionalized PEG–PLA nanoparticles loaded with paclitaxel. Biomaterials 34, 5640–5650.

Hu, Q., Gao, X., Kang, T., Feng, X., Jiang, D., Tu, Y., et al., 2013b. CGKRK-modified nanoparticles for dual-targeting drug delivery to tumor cells and angiogenic blood vessels. Biomaterials 34, 9496–9508.

Huang, R., Han, L., Li, J., Ren, F., Ke, W., Jiang, C., et al., 2009. Neuroprotection in a 6-hydroxydopamine-lesioned Parkinson model using lactoferrin-modified nanoparticles. J. Gene Med. 11, 754–763.

Huang, R., Ke, W., Liu, Y., Jiang, C., Pei, Y., 2008. The use of lactoferrin as a ligand for targeting the polyamidoamine-based gene delivery system to the brain. Biomaterials 29, 238–246.

Hynynen, K., Mcdannold, N., Vykhodtseva, N., Jolesz, F.A., 2003. Non-invasive opening of BBB by focused ultrasound. Acta Neurochir. Suppl. 86, 555.

Iliff, J.J., Wang, M., Liao, Y., Plogg, B.A., Peng, W., Gundersen, G.A., et al., 2012. A paravascular pathway facilitates CSF flow through the brain parenchyma and the clearance of interstitial solutes, including amyloid β. Sci. Transl. Med. 4147ra11.

Iyer, A.K., Khaled, G., Fang, J., Maeda, H., 2006. Exploiting the enhanced permeability and retention effect for tumor targeting. Drug Discov. Today 11, 812.

Jiang, T., Olson, E.S., Nguyen, Q.T., Roy, M., Jennings, P.A., Tsien, R.Y., 2004. Tumor imaging by means of proteolytic activation of cell-penetrating peptides. Proc. Natl. Acad. Sci. U. S. A. 101, 17867–17872.

Jiang, X., Xin, H., Gu, J., Xu, X., Xia, W., Chen, S., et al., 2013. Solid tumor penetration by integrin-mediated pegylated poly(trimethylene carbonate) nanoparticles loaded with paclitaxel. Biomaterials 34, 1739–1746.

Kawamoto, M., Kohno, M., Horibe, T., Kawakami, K., 2013. Immunogenicity and toxicity of transferrin receptor-targeted hybrid peptide as a potent anticancer agent. Cancer Chemother. Pharmacol. 71, 799–807.

Keunen, O., Klein, G., 2011. Anti-VEGF treatment reduces blood supply and increases tumor cell invasion in glioblastoma. Proc. Natl. Acad. Sci. U. S. A. 108, 3749–3754.

Kibria, G., Hatakeyama, H., Ohga, N., Hida, K., Harashima, H., 2011. Dual-ligand modification of PEGylated liposomes shows better cell selectivity and efficient gene delivery. J. Control. Release 153, 141–148.

Kida, S., Steart, P.V., Zhang, E.T., Weller, R.O., 1993. Perivascular cells act as scavengers in the cerebral perivascular spaces and remain distinct from pericytes, microglia and macrophages. Acta Neuropathol. 85, 646–652.

Kilb, W., Dierkes, P.W., Syková, E., Vargová, L., Luhmann, H.J., 2006. Hypoosmolar conditions reduce extracellular volume fraction and enhance epileptiform activity in the CA3 region of the immature rat hippocampus. J. Neurosci. Res. 84, 119–129.

Kozlovskaya, L., Stepensky, D., 2013. Quantitative analysis of the brain-targeted delivery of drugs and model compounds using nano-delivery systems. J. Control. Release 171, 17–23.

Kumar, P., Wu, H., Mcbride, J.L., Jung, K.E., Kim, M.H., Davidson, B.L., et al., 2007. Transvascular delivery of small interfering RNA to the central nervous system. Nature 448, 39.

Lange, E.D., 2014. Drug Delivery to the Brain: Physiological Concepts, Methodologies, and Approaches. Springer, New York.

Lee, S.G., Su, Z.Z., Emdad, L., Sarkar, D., Fisher, P.B., 2006. Astrocyte elevated gene-1 (AEG-1) is a target gene of oncogenic Ha-ras requiring phosphatidylinositol 3-kinase and c-Myc. Proc. Natl. Acad. Sci. U. S. A. 103, 17390.

Lehmenkühler, A., Syková, E., Svoboda, J., Zilles, K., Nicholson, C., 1993. Extracellular space parameters in the rat neocortex and subcortical white matter during postnatal development determined by diffusion analysis. Neuroscience 55, 339–351.

Lin, T., Zhao, P., Jiang, Y., Tang, Y., Jin, H., Pan, Z., et al., 2016. Blood-brain-barrier-penetrating albumin nanoparticles for biomimetic drug delivery via albumin-binding protein pathways for antiglioma therapy. ACS Nano 10, 9999.

Liotta, L.A., Kohn, E.C., 2001. The microenvironment of the tumour-host interface. Nature 411, 375.

Liu, X., Tu, M., Kelly, R.S., Chen, C., Smith, B.J., 2004. Development of a computational approach to predict blood-brain barrier permeability. Drug Metab. Dispos. 32, 132.

Liu, Y., An, S., Li, J., Kuang, Y., He, X., Guo, Y., et al., 2016a. Brain-targeted co-delivery of therapeutic gene and peptide by multifunctional nanoparticles in Alzheimer's disease mice. Biomaterials 80, 33–45.

Liu, Y., Mei, L., Xu, C., Yu, Q., Shi, K., Zhang, L., et al., 2016b. Dual receptor recognizing cell penetrating peptide for selective targeting, efficient intratumoral diffusion and synthesized anti-glioma therapy. Theranostics 12, 177–191.

Liu, Y., Ran, R., Chen, J., Kuang, Q., Tang, J., Mei, L., et al., 2014. Paclitaxel loaded liposomes decorated with a multifunctional tandem peptide for glioma targeting. Biomaterials 35, 4835–4847.

Lo, E.H., Singhal, A.B., Torchilin, V.P., Abbott, N.J., 2001. Drug delivery to damaged brain. Brain Res. Rev. 38, 140–148.

Lockman, P.R., Koziara, J.M., Mumper, R.J., Allen, D.D., 2008. Nanoparticle surface charges alter blood-brain barrier integrity and permeability. J. Drug Target. 12, 635–641.

Lorger, M., Krueger, J.S., O'Neal, M., Staflin, K., Feldinghabermann, B., 2009. Activation of tumor cell integrin alphavbeta3 controls angiogenesis and metastatic growth in the brain. Proc. Natl. Acad. Sci. U. S. A. 106, 10666.

Louveau, A., Smirnov, I., Keyes, T.J., Eccles, J.D., Rouhani, S.J., Peske, J.D., et al., 2015. Structural and functional features of central nervous system lymphatic vessels. Nature 523, 337–341.

Lu, W., Xiong, C., Zhang, R., Shi, L., Huang, M., Zhang, G., et al., 2012. Receptor-mediated transcytosis: a mechanism for active extravascular transport of nanoparticles in solid tumors. J. Control. Release 161, 959–966.

Maletínská, L., Blakely, E.A., Bjornstad, K.A., Deen, D.F., Knoff, L.J., Forte, T.M., 2000. Human glioblastoma cell lines: levels of low-density lipoprotein receptor and low-density lipoprotein receptor-related protein. Cancer Res. 60, 2300–2303.

Mehta, A.M., Sonabend, A.M., Bruce, J.N., 2017. Convection-enhanced delivery. Neurotherapeutics 14, 358–371.

Merlot, A.M., Kalinowski, D.S., Richardson, D.R., 2014. Unraveling the mysteries of serum albumin—more than just a serum protein. Front. Physiol. 5, 299.

Mittapalli, R.K., Manda, V.K., Adkins, C.E., Geldenhuys, W.J., Lockman, P.R., 2010. Exploiting nutrient transporters at the blood-brain barrier to improve brain distribution of small molecules. Ther. Deliv. 1, 775–784.

Muruganandam, A., Tanha, J., Narang, S., Stanimirovic, D., 2002. Selection of phage-displayed llama single-domain antibodies that transmigrate across human blood-brain barrier endothelium. J. Inequal. Appl. 16, 240.

Nance, E., Timbie, K., Miller, G.W., Song, J., Louttit, C., Klibanov, A.L., et al., 2014. Non-invasive delivery of stealth, brain-penetrating nanoparticles across the blood-brain barrier using MRI-guided focused ultrasound. J. Control. Release 189, 123–132.

Nance, E.A., Woodworth, G.F., Sailor, K.A., Shih, T.Y., Xu, Q., Swaminathan, G., et al., 2012. A dense poly(ethylene glycol) coating improves penetration of large polymeric nanoparticles within brain tissue. Sci. Transl. Med. 4149ra19.

Nasarre, C., Roth, M., Jacob, L., Roth, L., Koncina, E., Thien, A., et al., 2010. Peptide-based interference of the transmembrane domain of neuropilin-1 inhibits glioma growth in vivo. Oncogene 29, 2381.

Ng, T.B., Wong, J.H., Wang, H., 2010. Recent progress in research on ribosome inactivating proteins. Curr. Protein Pept. Sci. 11, 37–53.

Nicholson, C., 1993. Ion-selective microelectrodes and diffusion measurements as tools to explore the brain cell microenvironment. J. Neurosci. Methods 48, 199–213.

Nicholson, C., 2005. Factors governing diffusing molecular signals in brain extracellular space. J. Neural Transm. 112, 29–44.

Nicholson, C., Kamalizare, P., Tao, L., 2011. Brain extracellular space as a diffusion barrier. Comput. Vis. Sci. 14, 309–325.

Nicholson, C., Syková, E., 1998. Extracellular space structure revealed by diffusion analysis. Trends Neurosci. 21, 207–215.

Nuijens, J.H., van Berkel, P.H., Schanbacher, F.L., 1996. Structure and biological actions of lactoferrin. J. Mammary Gland Biol. Neoplasia 1, 285–295.

Ohtsuki, S., Terasaki, T., 2007. Contribution of carrier-mediated transport systems to the blood-brain barrier as a supporting and protecting interface for the brain; importance for CNS drug discovery and development. Pharm. Res. 24, 1745–1758.

Olive, K.P., Jacobetz, M.A., Davidson, C.J., Gopinathan, A., Mcintyre, D., Honess, D., et al., 2009. Inhibition of hedgehog signaling enhances delivery of chemotherapy in a mouse model of pancreatic cancer. Science 324, 1457–1461.

On, N.H., Kiptoo, P., Siahaan, T.J., Miller, D.W., 2014. Modulation of blood-brain barrier permeability in mice using synthetic E-cadherin peptide. Mol. Pharm. 11, 974.

Pan, W., Kastin, A.J., Zankel, T.C., van Kerkhof, P., Terasaki, T., Bu, G., 2004. Efficient transfer of receptor-associated protein (RAP) across the blood-brain barrier. J. Cell Sci. 117, 5071–5078.

Pang, Z., Lu, W., Gao, H., Hu, K., Chen, J., Zhang, C., et al., 2008. Preparation and brain delivery property of biodegradable polymersomes conjugated with OX26. J. Control. Release 128, 120.

Pardridge, W.M., 2005. The blood-brain barrier: bottleneck in brain drug development. Neurorx J. Am. Soc. Exp. Neurother. 2, 3–14.

Parkar, N.S., Akpa, B.S., Nitsche, L.C., Wedgewood, L.E., Place, A.T., Sverdlov, M.S., et al., 2009. Vesicle formation and endocytosis: function, machinery, mechanisms, and modeling. Antioxid. Redox Signal. 11, 1301–1312.

Primeau, A.J., Rendon, A., Hedley, D., Lilge, L., Tannock, I.F., 2005. The distribution of the anticancer drug doxorubicin in relation to blood vessels in solid tumors. Clin. Cancer Res. 11, 8782–8788.

Prud'Homme, G.J., Glinka, Y., 2012. Neuropilins are multifunctional coreceptors involved in tumor initiation, growth, metastasis and immunity. Oncotarget 3, 921.

Ruoslahti, E., Bhatia, S.N., Sailor, M.J., 2010. Targeting of drugs and nanoparticles to tumors. J. Cell Biol. 188, 759.

Sauer, I., Dunay, I.R., Weisgraber, K., Bienert, M., Dathe, M., 2005. An apolipoprotein E-derived peptide mediates uptake of sterically stabilized liposomes into brain capillary endothelial cells. Biochemistry 44, 2021.

Schwarze, S.R., Ho, A., Voceroakbani, A., Dowdy, S.F., 1999. In vivo protein transduction: delivery of a biologically active protein into the mouse. Science 285, 1569–1572.

Sharma, G., Modgil, A., Layek, B., Arora, K., Sun, C., Law, B., et al., 2013. Cell penetrating peptide tethered bi-ligand liposomes for delivery to brain in vivo: biodistribution and transfection. J. Control. Release 167, 1–10.

Sheikov, N., Mcdannold, N., Vykhodtseva, N., Jolesz, F., Hynynen, K., 2004. Cellular mechanisms of the blood-brain barrier opening induced by ultrasound in presence of microbubbles. Ultrasound Med. Biol. 30, 979.

Soleman, S., Filippov, M.A., Dityatev, A., Fawcett, J.W., 2013. Targeting the neural extracellular matrix in neurological disorders. Neuroscience 253, 194–213.

Somani, S., Robb, G., Pickard, B.S., Dufès, C., 2015. Enhanced gene expression in the brain following intravenous administration of lactoferrin-bearing polypropylenimine dendriplex. J. Control. Release 217, 235–242.

Stehle, G., Sinn, H., Wunder, A., Schrenk, H.H., Stewart, J.C., Hartung, G., et al., 1997. Plasma protein (albumin) catabolism by the tumor itself-implications for tumor metabolism and the genesis of cachexia. Crit. Rev. Oncol. Hematol. 26, 77–100.

Stylianopoulos, T., Poh, M.Z., Insin, N., Bawendi, M.G., Dai, F., Munn, L.L., et al., 2010. Diffusion of particles in the extracellular matrix: the effect of repulsive electrostatic interactions. Biophys. J. 99, 1342.

Sugahara, K.N., Teesalu, T., Karmali, P.P., Kotamraju, V.R., Agemy, L., Girard, O.M., et al., 2009. Tissue-penetrating delivery of compounds and nanoparticles into tumors. Cancer Cell 16, 510.

Sun, B.L., Wang, L.H., Yang, T., Mao, L.L., Sun, J.Y., Yang, M.F., et al., 2017. Lymphatic drainage system of the brain: a novel target for intervention of neurological diseases. Prog. Neurobiol.

Susan, K., Hobbs, W.L.M., Fan Yuan, W., Roberts, G., Griffith, L., Torchilin, V.P., Jain, R.K., 1998. Regulation of transport pathways in tumor vessels: role of tumor type and microenvironment. Proc. Natl. Acad. Sci. USA 95, 4607–4612.

Sykes, E.A., Chen, J., Zheng, G., Chan, W.C., 2014. Investigating the impact of nanoparticle size on active and passive tumor targeting efficiency. ACS Nano 8, 5696.

Syková, E., 2004. Diffusion properties of the brain in health and disease. Neurochem. Int. 45, 453–466.

Syková, E., Nicholson, C., 2008. Diffusion in brain extracellular space. Physiol. Rev. 88, 1277–1340.

Teesalu, T., Sugahara, K.N., Kotamraju, V.R., Ruoslahti, E., 2009. C-end rule peptides mediate neuropilin-1-dependent cell, vascular, and tissue penetration. Proc. Natl. Acad. Sci. U. S. A. 106, 16157.

Thorne, R.G., Nicholson, C., 2006. In vivo diffusion analysis with quantum dots and dextrans predicts the width of brain extracellular space. Proc. Natl. Acad. Sci. U. S. A. 103, 5567.

Torchilin, V.P., Levchenko, T.S., 2001. TAT peptide on the surface of liposomes affords their efficient intracellular delivery even at low temperature and in the presence of metabolic inhibitors. Proc. Natl. Acad. Sci. U. S. A. 98, 8786–8791.

van Groen, T., Kadish, I., Wiesehan, K., Funke, S.A., Willbold, D., 2009. In vitro and in vivo staining characteristics of small, fluorescent, Aβ42-binding D-enantiomeric peptides in transgenic AD mouse models. ChemMedChem 4, 276–282.

Van Groen, T., Wiesehan, K., Funke, S.A., Kadish, I., Nagel-Steger, L., Willbold, D., 2008. Reduction of Alzheimer's disease amyloid plaque load in transgenic mice by D3, a D-enantiomeric peptide identified by mirror image phage display. ChemMedChem 3, 1848–1852.

Vargová, L., Homola, A., Zámecník, J., Tichý, M., Benes, V., Syková, E., 2003. Diffusion parameters of the extracellular space in human gliomas. Glia 42, 77.

Vargovã, L., Sykovã, E., 2008. Extracellular space diffusion and extrasynaptic transmission. Physiol. Res. 57, S89.

Vassar, R., Kovacs, D.M., Yan, R., Wong, P.C., 2009. The β-secretase enzyme BACE in health and Alzheimer's disease: regulation, cell biology, function, and therapeutic potential. J. Neurosci. 29, 12787–12794.

Voříšek, I., Hajek, M., Tintěra, J., Nicolay, K., Syková, E., 2002. Water ADC, extracellular space volume, and tortuosity in the rat cortex after traumatic injury. Magn. Reson. Med. 48, 994–1003.

Vorísek, I., Syková, E., 1997. Evolution of anisotropic diffusion in the developing rat corpus callosum. J. Neurophysiol. 78, 912–919.

Vorisek, I., Sykova, E., 2009. Measuring diffusion parameters in the brain: comparing the real-time iontophoretic method and diffusion-weighted magnetic resonance. Acta Physiol. 195, 101–110.

Walsh, M.J., Dodd, J.E., Hautbergue, G.M., 2013. Ribosome-inactivating proteins: potent poisons and molecular tools. Virulence 4, 774–784.

Ward, S.M., Himmelstein, D.S., Lancia, J.K., Binder, L.I., 2012. Tau oligomers and tau toxicity in neurodegenerative disease. Biochem. Soc. Trans. 40 (4), 667–671.

Watters, J.J., Schartner, J.M., Badie, B., 2005. Microglia function in brain tumors. J. Neurosci. Res. 81, 447.

Wei, X., Zhan, C., Chen, X., Hou, J., Xie, C., Lu, W., 2014. Retro-inverso isomer of Angiopep-2: a stable d-peptide ligand inspires brain-targeted drug delivery. Mol. Pharm. 11, 3261–3268.

WM, P., 2012. Drug transport across the blood-brain barrier. J. Cereb. Blood Flow Metab. 32, 1959–1972.

Wunder, A., Stehle, G., Sinn, H., Schrenk, H., Hoffbiederbeck, D., Bader, F., et al., 1997. Enhanced albumin uptake by rat tumors. Int. J. Oncol. 11, 497–507.

Xin, H., Jiang, X., Gu, J., Sha, X., Chen, L., Law, K., et al., 2011. Angiopep-conjugated poly (ethylene glycol)-co-poly (ε-caprolactone) nanoparticles as dual-targeting drug delivery system for brain glioma. Biomaterials 32, 4293–4305.

Yamamoto, M., Ikeda, K., Ohshima, K., Tsugu, H., Kimura, H., Tomonaga, M., 1997. Increased expression of low density lipoprotein receptor-related protein/α2-macroglobulin receptor in human malignant astrocytomas. Cancer Res. 57, 2799–2805.

Yao, X., Hrabětová, S., Nicholson, C., Manley, G.T., 2008. Aquaporin-4 deficient mice have increased extracellular space without tortuosity change. J. Neurosci. 28, 5460–5464.

Yu, Y., Pang, Z., Lu, W., Yin, Q., Gao, H., Jiang, X., 2012. Self-assembled polymersomes conjugated with lactoferrin as novel drug carrier for brain delivery. Pharm. Res. 29, 83–96.

Yu, Y.J., Zhang, Y., Kenrick, M., Hoyte, K., Luk, W., Lu, Y., et al., 2011. Boosting brain uptake of a therapeutic antibody by reducing its affinity for a transcytosis target. Sci. Transl. Med. 384ra44.

Zhan, C., Gu, B., Xie, C., Li, J., Liu, Y., Lu, W., 2010. Cyclic RGD conjugated poly (ethylene glycol)-co-poly (lactic acid) micelle enhances paclitaxel anti-glioblastoma effect. J. Control. Release 143, 136–142.

Zhang, C., Wan, X., Zheng, X., Shao, X., Liu, Q., Zhang, Q., et al., 2014. Dual-functional nanoparticles targeting amyloid plaques in the brains of Alzheimer's disease mice. Biomaterials 35, 456–465.

Zhang, E.Y., Knipp, G.T., Ekins, S., Swaan, P.W., 2002. Structural biology and function of solute transporters: implications for identifying and designing substrates. Drug Metab. Rev. 34, 709–750.

Zhang, M.-Z., Yu, R.-N., Chen, J., Ma, Z.-Y., Zhao, Y.-D., 2012. Targeted quantum dots fluorescence probes functionalized with aptamer and peptide for transferrin receptor on tumor cells. Nanotechnology. 23485104.

Zhou, Y., Kopeček, J., 2013. Biological rationale for the design of polymeric anti-cancer nanomedicines. J. Drug Target. 21, 1–26.

Zorko, M., Langel, U., 2005. Cell-penetrating peptides: mechanism and kinetics of cargo delivery. Adv. Drug Deliv. Rev. 57, 529–545.

The elimination of brain-targeted nanomaterials

17

Xiao Gu, Xiuxiu Hao, Xiaoyu Shen, Hualin Wang, Yuyan Zhang, Xiaoling Gao
Department of Pharmacology and Chemical Biology, Faculty of Basic Medicine, Shanghai Jiao Tong University School of Medicine, Shanghai, China

1 Introduction

Brain drug delivery is made difficult by the presence of the blood-brain barrier (BBB), which excludes 100% of large-molecule neurotherapeutics and >98% of all small-molecule drugs (Pardridge, 2005). Finding ways to get diagnostic and therapeutic agents to the brain effectively, safely, and conveniently is of great interest and importance. With the vast progress of nanotechnology in the past few decades, nanoparticles (NPs) have been extensively explored as a promising new-generation drug loading and delivery system for brain drug delivery.

The nanocarriers that have been applied for brain drug delivery range from polymeric nanoparticles, solid lipid nanoparticles, liposomes, metallic nanoparticles, micelles, dendrimers, nanogels, nanoemulsions to nanosuspensions and have demonstrated early preclinical success for the management of central nervous system (CNS) diseases such as brain tumors, Alzheimer's disease, Parkinson disease, HIV encephalopathy, and acute ischemic stroke (Wong et al., 2012). Although it has been well-acknowledged that the application of certain nanoparticulate drug delivery systems can increase the amount of drug delivered to the brain, the mechanism of cerebral metabolism and excretion of NPs is poorly understood, given the fact that few preclinical data are available regarding the fate of NPs in the brain. Therefore, the retention time of NPs in the target site as well as the amount of drug that can be delivered remain unknown. In addition, NPs' clearance is uncontrolled in the peripheral circulation, especially via macrophage; multiple dose of NPs may need to be injected into the host for maintaining effective drug concentration amount in plasma, whereas the cytotoxicity of nanoparticles and/or their degradation/metabolic products remains a major concern.

Due to their high surface volume ratio, NPs accumulated in the CNS might also interact with nontargeted cells and extracellular enzymes, induce neurotoxic effects, and disturb the biological environment of the CNS, particularly those difficult or unable to be degraded. Several physicochemical features of NPs like particle size, shape, and zeta potential have been shown to play an important role in determining their interaction with the biological system. Surface modification which can improve the half-life and targeting capacity of NPs might also pose additional cytotoxic effects. Besides, long-term NPs exposure may induce changes in cell viability by activating

Brain Targeted Drug Delivery Systems. https://doi.org/10.1016/B978-0-12-814001-7.00017-2

multiple cellular pathways that regulate cytotoxicity. For example, 8 weeks of intraperitoneal administration of zinc oxide NPs in Wistar rats damaged the spatial learning and memory ability of the animals by altering the synaptic plasticity (Han et al., 2011). Intragastric administration of TiO_2 NPs for 2 months led to TiO_2 NPs accumulation in the mouse hippocampus and induced hippocampal apoptosis and impairment of spatial recognition memory (Hu et al., 2011). Therefore, to ensure the safety of future applications, there is an urgent need to understand the biofate of NPs, especially in the CNS.

Nonbiodegradable NPs pose higher risks to human health than biodegradable ones because of their long-term accumulation. For example, after cellular internalization, imidazole-stabilized gold nanoparticles were found to accumulate within the endosome/lysosomes and induced neuron apoptosis both in vitro and in vivo (Imperatore et al., 2015). Therefore, the development of biodegradable NPs is of increasing interest. But for those biocompatible and biodegradable nanoparticulate drug delivery systems such as liposomes, polymersomes, and micelles, understanding the mechanism of cerebral metabolism and excretion of NPs is also important as it could help in the rational design of NPs by modulating their retention time at the target site as well as the amount of drug that can be delivered.

The current chapter summarized the systems for the clearance of nanomaterials both in the brain and in the peripheral circulation, highlighted the recent researches about the elimination of brain-targeted nanoparticulate drug delivery systems, and discussed the related factors.

2 The clearance systems for nanoparticulate drug delivery systems

2.1 Brain clearance systems

Three routes are likely involved in the brain clearance of nanoparticles: (a) degradation in the brain, (b) entering cerebrospinal fluid (CSF) circulation mediated by the convective bulk flow, and then cleared from the CNS to the bloodstream or the cervical lymphatics, and (c) brain-to-blood efflux.

2.1.1 Degradation in the brain

Enzyme-mediated degradation including extracellular and intracellular degradation is one of the major mechanisms for the brain clearance of exogenous substances. Metabolic enzymes like aminopeptidase and hyaluronidases that exist in the extracellular space of the brain parenchyma could account for the extracellular degradation of nanoparticles such as PEGylated hyaluronic acid nanocarrier (Choi et al., 2011). Nanomaterials can also be taken up from the extracellular space to be degraded intracellularly in neurons or glia, including phagocytic microglia and astrocytes. Microglia, serving as the gatekeeper of the CNS, could be the major cell type that mediates the intracellular degradation of nanomaterials in the CNS. Intracellular degradation occurs via the ubiquitin-proteasome pathway, the autophagy-lysosome pathway, and the endosome-lysosome pathway (Tarasoff-Conway et al., 2015). As the terminal organelle in the cellular degradation systems, lysosomes degrade an array of biological substances under normal conditions, including proteins, nucleic acids, and lipids. In addition, they also usually take the responsibility for the intracellular degradation of the different kinds of internalized NPs. However, due to aging or certain diseases, lysosomes are not always completely efficient to degrade the substances that are not needed. On the other hand, nondegradable nanocarriers such as carboxylated polystyrene NPs can also be internalized by the brain endothelia and accumulate within lysosomes without degradation (Raghnaill et al., 2014). More attention should be paid to reveal how these NPs be cleared after cellular internalization in the brain.

2.1.2 Entering CSF circulation mediated by the convective bulk flow

Interstitial fluid (ISF) metabolites and waste products can also be cleared directly into the CSF via ISF bulk flow that enters the CSF circulation through the paravascular space. The paravascular circulation hypothesis was proposed by Iliff et al. and confirmed in both animals and human beings (Gaberel et al., 2014; Iliff et al., 2012). CSF circulation was found to act like the lymphatic system. It flushes out interstitial substances in a process facilitated by glial cells, through the so-called glymphatic system (Fig. 1). Driven by a combination of arterial pulsatility, respiration, slow

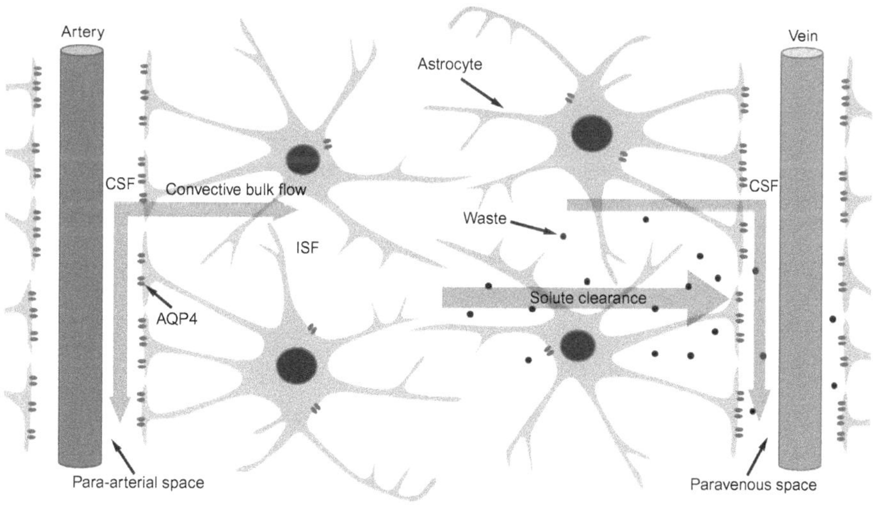

Fig. 1 The glymphatic pathway. Cerebrospinal fluid (CSF) enters the brain along para-arterial routes, whereas ISF is cleared from the brain along paravenous routes. Aquaporin-4 (AQP-4)-dependent astroglial water flux mediates the convective bulk ISF flow and drives the clearance of metabolites and waste products from the brain parenchyma.

vasomotion, and CSF pressure gradients, CSF flows into the periarterial Virchow-Robin space from the subarachnoid space and enters the brain parenchyma to drive convective ISF fluxes to the perivenous space from where CSF drains out of the brain (Jessen et al., 2015). Astroglial aquaporin-4 (AQP-4) channels mediate CSF transport from the para-arterial space across the pial-glial membrane into the interstitium, where it mixes with ISF and drives the clearance of metabolites and waste products from the brain parenchyma (Iliff et al., 2012). A recent work by Ma et al. elucidated a complex flow pattern of CSF after ventricular infusion of tracers in mice and found that perineural lymphatic outflow to the mandibular and deep cervical lymph nodes was the major outflow route for CSF (Ma et al., 2017). In addition, functional lymphatic vessels are also found in the CNS lining the dural sinuses, being able to carry both fluid and immune cells from the CSF and connecting to the deep cervical lymph nodes (Louveau et al., 2015). Collectively, following clearance from the ISF into the CSF, metabolites and waste products can be cleared from the brain. Such CSF circulation system could also be a pathway that mediated the clearance of nanomaterials from brain.

2.1.3 Brain-to-blood efflux

Interstitial substances can also be cleared from the brain into the blood directly via specialized transport systems located in the brain endothelium (Tarasoff-Conway et al., 2015). BBB actually acts as a CNS detoxifying system for both endogenous substrates and xenobiotics in the brain (Terasaki and Ohtsuki, 2005). It has been reported that large hydrophilic molecules, such as IgG, apo-transferrin, and amyloid-beta peptide, are susceptible to brain-to-blood efflux transport via Fc receptor, transferrin receptor, and low density lipoprotein receptor-related protein 1, respectively. The multidrug resistance transporter P-glycoprotein (P-gp), an ATP-dependent efflux pump, plays an important role in the efflux of undesirable substances such as amyloid-beta from the brain into the blood as well as many drugs such as anticancer drugs (Ueno et al., 2010). As receptor or transporter-mediated transcytosis can mediate blood-to-brain delivery of NPs, it is also very much possible that these transport systems can facilitate the brain-to-blood clearance of NPs.

2.2 Systemic clearance pathways

In general, after entering the blood circulation, NPs will encounter blood cells, platelets, coagulation factors, plasma proteins, and other components in the vascular compartment depending on their physicochemial properties. They may undergo adsorption or opsonization by serum proteins, which is an important factor affecting their clearance process (Longmire et al., 2008; Yu and Zheng, 2015). The NPs will then interact with various cells, some of which may be able to reach their targets and some may never be able to get to the intended site. Generally, NPs in the circulatory system can be cleared through two major pathways, the renal clearance pathway and the hepatic clearance pathway.

2.2.1 Renal clearance pathway

Systemically administered nanoparticles NPs travel along blood circulation and get into organs with abundant vasculatures. The kidney can rapidly eliminate intravascular agents with little cellular internalization/metabolism, and therefore, renal excretion represents a desirable pathway for NPs elimination with minimal catabolism or degradation from the human body to avoid the unexpected side effects (Longmire et al., 2008). Circulating NPs enter the glomerular capillary bed via the afferent arteriole. The glomerular capillary wall is composed of three layers: fenestrated endothelium, the highly negatively charged glomerular basement membrane (GBM), and podocyte extensions of glomerular epithelial cells. Glomerular filtration flows through fenestrate, across GBM, and through filtration silts formed by podocyte extensions. The filtration slit has a physiologic pore size of 4.5–5 nm. Therefore, filtration of NPs through the glomerular capillary wall is highly dependent on molecule size. Nanoparticles <6 nm can easily be filtrated, while filtration of nanoparticles between 6 and 8 nm is dependent on charge interactions between particles and the negatively charged GBM. Generally, positively charged particles are easily filtrated than same-sized negatively charged particles (Longmire et al., 2008).

2.2.2 Hepatic clearance pathway

The hepatic clearance is more complex than renal clearance. Like renal clearance, hepatic clearance involves filtering of the blood. Small-molecule drugs, viruses, bacteria or nanoparticles in the blood can be taken up by sinusoidal endothelial cells, hepatocytes, and Kupffer cells in the liver (Zhang et al., 2016). Kupffer cells and hepatocytes are the two kinds of cells that play important roles in the hepatic clearance. Phagocytic Kupffer cells have ciliated borders and stellate branches that serve as highly adapted mechanical traps for the removal of unwanted substances from the blood. They possess numerous receptors (receptors for complement proteins and for the Fc part of IgG) for selective endocytosis of opsonized particles. Particles processed by Kupffer cells are mostly degraded intracellularly, while those that are not broken down by intracellular processes will likely remain within the cells and will therefore be retained in the body for a long time. Hepatocytes typically metabolize small-molecule drugs and release the metabolized products either back into the bloodstream or into the bile. Like Kupffer cells, hepatocytes can also endocytose NPs, but at a much lower efficiency, and is only seen when a large amount of NPs have been given (Liu et al., 2015) or when macrophages have been depleted (Zhang et al., 2016). Once processed by hepatocytes, these NPs are cleared through bile and into the feces.

3 Pharmaceutical factors that influence the elimination profiles of NPs

3.1 Size

Size plays an important role in determining the kinetics and biodistribution of NPs. In the development of therapeutics against CNS diseases, 20 nm, large enough to escape renal glomerular filtration, is thought to be a sufficiently small size (Jo et al., 2015). Generally, smaller NPs enter the brain more easily than larger ones. For example, Gao compared the brain drug delivery efficiency of polysorbate 80-coated polybutylcyanoacrylate nanoparticles, finding that nanoparticles at 70 nm delivered more drugs into brain, while no significant difference was observed among those at 170, 220, and 345 nm (Gao and Jiang, 2006). Tang et al. investigated the distribution and accumulation of subcutaneously administrated silver nanoparticles (SNPs) and silver microparticles (SMPs) in rats, finding that SNPs can translocate to the brain while SMPs cannot (Tang et al., 2009).

The diffusion of nanoparticles in the brain tissue extracellular space (ECS) was also size-dependent. Using the minimally adhesive poly(ethylene glycol) (PEG)-coated particles, it was estimated that human brain tissue ECS has some pores larger than 200 nm, and that more than one-quarter of all pores are $\geq$100 nm, and 40- and 100-nm, but not 200-nm, nanoparticles spread rapidly within brain tissue, only if densely coated with PEG. Similar results were observed in rat brain tissue with paclitaxel-loaded biodegradable nanoparticles of similar size (85 nm) and surface properties (Nance et al., 2012).

The size of NPs may influence the microscopic distribution of different sizes of NPs in the brain, but not their macroscopic distribution. For example, Chen et al. observed that 17 and 37 nm AuNPs injected intraperitoneally could both pass through the BBB and their macroscopic biodistributions within the brain and were indistinguishable. Interestingly, the 17 nm AuNPs could be internalized by pyramidal cells and be located in cytoplasm in the hippocampus CA region, while the 37 nm AuNPs did not enter the neurons (Chen et al., 2010). Another interesting example is the design of a hybrid nanodrug (AuM) that can block only excessive pathological activation of *N*-methyl-D-aspartate receptors (NMDARs), but preserve physiological role of synaptic NMDARs (sNMDARs). AuM ($\sim$35 nm) is designed to be larger than synaptic cleft ($\sim$25 nm) by attaching memantine, NMDAR antagonist, via polymer linkers to a gold nanoparticle. It efficiently and selectively block only excessive pathological activation of NMDARs by inhibiting the overactivated extrasynaptic NMDARs (eNMDARs), while having no effect on synaptic NMDARs (sNMDARs) and synaptic transmission (Savchenko et al., 2016).

Besides influencing the brain distribution profile, size might also affect the elimination of NPs in brain. Previous work demonstrated that dextran with lower molecular weight were cleared via the CSF flow quicker than those with higher molecular weight (Iliff et al., 2012). Therefore, it's very possible that the CSF-mediated clearance of NPs would also be size-dependent.

3.2 Shape

The shape of NPs influences the affinity of NPs with the target organs or cells, and therefore, affects the clearance. For example, Kolhar et al. demonstrated that intracellular adhesion molecule-1 (ICAM-1)-conjugated nanorods were taken up by endothelial cells in a higher degree than nanospheres. And, in vivo studies in mice showed that, compared with nanospheres, intravascular-administered nanorods got a higher concentration in the brain endothelium (Kolhar et al., 2013). Agarwal et al. studied the influence of nanoscale geometry on the NPs uptake in mammalian cells and found that nanodiscs were taken up most efficiently, followed by nanorods, and then nanospheres. This phenomenon can be explained by different energy requirements for folding the membrane near the NPs with the different shape (Agarwal et al., 2013).

Shape may also have an impact on the inflammatory response induced by NPs, which could eventually affect the biofate of the NPs. For instance, intranasal administration of AuNPs with different shapes and modification of PEG or cetyl trimethylammonium bromide (CTAB) on mice showed different abilities to activate microglia in the brain. Spherical AuNPs induced a small but detectable activation of microglia after 24 h of administration and this activity lasted for 1 week. Rod AuNPs caused a biphasic microglia activation with one early peak at 24 h and the other after 7 days. In contrast, PEGylated urchin AuNPs did not significantly induce microglia activation, while CTAB-conjugated urchin AuNPs induced a temporary activity which disappeared after 1 week (Hutter et al., 2010). Different inflammatory response of microglia induced by the different shapes of NPs would also influence the brain clearance of NPs.

3.3 Matrix materials

Deformability and biodegradability are the key factors determining the particle stability in the biological system, which also definitely affect the elimination of nanomaterials in the CNS.

3.3.1 Biodegradable nanomaterials

For deformable micelle (Sonali Agrawal et al., 2016), biodegradable liposome (Boado and Pardridge, 2011), reconstituted lipoproteins (Huang et al., 2015; Song et al., 2014), poly(butyl cyanoacrylate) (PBCA) or poly(isohexyl cyanoacrylate) (PIHCA), poly(lactic acid) (PLA) or its *co*polymer (lactide-co-glycolide) (PLGA), and human serum albumin (HSA), in situ deformation or degradation can be a key mechanism for their elimination. Therefore, any chemical component factors that affect the interaction between NPs and brain extracellular matrix or cerebral cells would influence the brain elimination of NPs. For example, Albertazzi et al. investigated the behavior of different PAMAM dendrimers in the brain, finding that G4 PAMAM could diffuse into the CSF and get into the brain parenchyma across the ependymal cell border, whereas G4-C12 PAMAM dendrimers were almost obstructed in the injection site. The researchers believed that C12 lipid chains on the G4-C12 dendrimers increased their hydrophobicity and induced a stronger interaction with the surrounding extracellular matrix and cell membranes, and therefore, decreased the diffusion ability of G4-C12 PAMAM (Albertazzi et al., 2013).

3.3.2 Nondegradable and hardly degradable nanomaterials

In contrast, nondegradable or hardly degradable nanomaterials such as gold nanoparticles, SNPs (van der Zande et al., 2012), cerium oxide particles (Geraets et al., 2014), and quantum dots (QDs) seem to retain longer in the brain. Semiconductor

QDs, nanometer-sized particles with unique optical and electrical characteristics, have been widely applied for molecular imaging in various biological systems. Minami et al. found that QDs could be selectively taken up by microglia when incubated with mixed primary cortical cell cultures or stereotaxic injected into the brain of healthy mouse. The specific uptake by microglia is through a clathrin-mediated endocytosis following their binding to two microglia-specific receptors, macrophage scavenger receptor-1 and mannose receptor. The in vivo study performed in mice showed that QDs targeted microglia with high efficiency and remained there for at least 1 month, indicating its slow metabolism and clearance from microglia (Minami et al., 2012). However, even for inorganic NPs, chemical structures also affect their distribution and elimination in the brain. For instance, following intranasal administration, the concentration of SiO_2 NPs in different brain regions from high to low was olfactory bulb, striatum, hippocampus, brain stem, cerebellum, and frontal cortex (Wu et al., 2011), while that of TiO_2 NPs was hippocampus, olfactory bulb, cerebellum, and cerebral cortex (Wang et al., 2008).

3.4 Surface properties

3.4.1 Surface charge

The surface charge of NPs poses an important role in determining their biodistribution and elimination in the brain. Shcharbin et al. found that dendrimers with positive surface charge are cleared rapidly from circulatory system, whereas dendriplex (complexes of PAMAM dendrimers and nucleic acids) exhibits a longer retention time in blood circulation (Shcharbin et al., 2014). Xu et al. evaluated the brain delivery and systemic pharmacokinetics of cationic bovine serum albumin (CBSA)-conjugated poly(ethylene glycol)-poly(D,L-lactide-*co*-glycolide) (PEG-PLGA) nanoparticle (CBSA-NP), finding a preferential localization of CBSA-NP in the CNS. Specifically, the concentration of CBSA-NP in brain tissue was nearly 2.31-fold over that of the unmodified NP. Besides, compared with unmodified NP, CBSA-NP achieved significantly higher AUC in the brain, but a lower AUC and quicker clearance from the systemic circulation (Xu et al., 2009).

3.4.2 PEGylation

If NPs in the circulatory system are slowly eliminated, their chances to get into the brain through the BBB increase. Polyethylene glycols (PEG) modification is a common strategy which can increase the circulatory time of NPs by avoiding the clearance by the mononuclear phagocytic system. In addition, PEGylation can also stabilize the NPs by avoiding agglomeration. Lindqvist et al. showed that just PEGylation on the liposomes without using a specific brain targeting ligand could increase the brain concentration of drug that has been encapsulated (Lindqvist et al., 2016). However, literature reports of ligand-targeted PEGylated nanoparticles have not consistently shown successful results. Stefanick et al. found that when targeting peptides were tethered to nanoparticles with a PEG2000 linker, their cellular uptake was not enhanced compared to nontargeted versions regardless of the liposomal PEG coating used. Conversely, reduction of the liposomal PEG to PEG350 and the peptide linker to

EG12 dramatically enhanced cellular uptake by ~9-fold and ~100-fold in the breast cancer and multiple myeloma cells, respectively. Uptake efficiency reached a maximum and a plateau with ~2% peptide density in both disease models. These evidences indicated that long and dense PEG chains conjugated on the surface of NPs may hinder the interaction between the NPs and the target cells, thereby reducing their efficiency (Stefanick et al., 2013). Xie et al. compared the brain targeting ability of glucose-conjugated liposomes modified with different chain lengths of PEG (PEG200, PEG400-LIP, PEG1000-LIP, and PEG2000), finding that the glucose-conjugated liposomes with medium chain length PEG (PEG1000) demonstrated the highest efficiency to get into the brain (Xie et al., 2012).

3.4.3 Protein corona

NPs in the biological media like serum may adsorb proteins and other biomolecules which is termed as "corona" on the NPs surface, unless fabricated to avoid adsorption. It confers a new identity on the NPs. The composition of corona is not unalterable; on the contrary, it is time-dependent and will be influenced by the physiological environment. The highest activity proteins will adhere to the NPs first and are replaced gradually by proteins with less activity but a higher affinity for the NPs surface (Casals et al., 2010). In addition, different physical conditions of human body, like those of diabetic, aged, or infected patients, will change the plasma proteins concentrations and types, therefore influencing the components and stability of the corona of NPs (Cupaioli et al., 2014). The corona of NPs plays a very important role in the targeting ability and elimination of NPs both in the CNS and peripheral circulatory system. Wang et al. found that the corona was strong enough to be attached on the NPs, even when the NPs were internalized into cells and transported into the lysosomes. Then the corona might be degraded in the lysosomes and the bare NPs could then induce lysosomal damage and apoptosis of cells ultimately (Wang et al., 2013). The results suggested that the kinetics of corona formation and degradation should be taken into consideration when assessing the metabolism and toxicity of NPs.

3.4.4 Targeting ligands

Targeting ligands conjugated with NPs have an enormous impact on the biofate of NPs in the brain. Wiley et al. reported that following intravenous administration, transferrin (Tf)-conjugated gold NPs distributed into the brain parenchyma, and their brain accumulation is dependent on the avidity to Tf receptor. NPs with more Tf and higher avidity to Tf receptor were captured by brain endothelial cells, whereas those with less Tf were easier to detach from the BBB and then got into the brain parenchyma (Wiley et al., 2013). Zensi et al. developed apolipoprotein E (ApoE)-functionalized albumin nanoparticles and witnessed their distribution in brain capillary endothelial cells and neurons after intravenous injection. In contrast, following intravenous administration, the concentration of unmodified albumin nanoparticles was undetectable in the brain (Zensi et al., 2009).

Cell-penetrating peptides (CPPs), such as Tat, are cationic peptides that can be conjugated to the nanoparticles to enhance their cellular uptake. Kanazawa et al.

synthesized Tat analog-modified methoxy poly(ethylene glycol) (MPEG)/poly (ε-caprolactone) (PCL) amphiphilic block copolymers (MPEG-PCL-Tat) and evaluated the brain distribution of coumarin-loaded MPEG-PCL and MPEG-PCL-Tat micelles after intranasal administration, finding that, at 4 h after administration, the brain amount of coumarin in those rats administered with MPEG-PCL-Tat micelles was significantly higher than that in those animals given MPEG-PCL micelles (Kanazawa et al., 2011). Sharma et al. developed bi-ligand (transferrin-poly-L-arginine, Tf-PR) liposomes for brain gene delivery. These bi-ligand liposomes combine the benefits of the targeting ability of Tf and the enhanced cell penetration ability of poly-L-arginine, achieving greater brain penetration and longer in vivo retention time than the single-ligand (Tf) or plain liposomes (Sharma et al., 2013).

3.4.5 Cell-mediated NPs delivery system

For some CNS diseases, we hope that NPs can specifically accumulate and retain at the lesion sites to exert their therapeutic effects. Mooney et al. demonstrated that tumor-tropic neural stem cells (NSCs)-coupled polystyrene NPs (~800 nm) had a significantly improved tumor-selective distribution and retention in the xenografted glioma of mouse brain, compared to free-NPs. In this study, NSC-coupled NPs were injected near to an intracerebral glioma, into the contralateral hemisphere or intravenously. At 4 days after injection, all three in vivo injection strategies showed significantly improved tumor-selective distribution and retention of NPs. These results suggested that NSCs can be used as a tool to slow the NPs clearance rate from the disease area of the CNS (Mooney et al., 2014).

3.5 Administration routes

The route of administration determines the brain distribution of NPs as well. For example, Balasubramanian et al. studied the effect of different administration routes on the brain accumulations of gold NPs (AuNPs) in rats, finding that, at 1 day, 1 week, 1 month, and 2 months after a single intravenous (i.v.) injection, no accumulation of Au was detected in the brain (Balasubramanian et al., 2010). In contrast, through inhalation, AuNPs accumulation was found in the brain areas including olfactory bulb, hippocampus, striatum, frontal cortex, entorhinal cortex, septum, and cerebellum. In addition, the AuNPs' accumulation in the brain after inhalation was size-dependent. For example, the concentration of 7 nm AuNPs in olfactory bulb was twofolds of that of 20 nm AuNPs (Balasubramanian et al., 2013). Wu et al. intranasally instilled Fe_3O_4-NPs (~30 nm) to rat for consecutive 7 days and found that Fe_3O_4-NPs specifically deposited in the striatum and hippocampus of rat brain. Even at 14 days after administration, more than half of the NPs stayed in the striatum. In addition, these NPs in the striatum caused oxidative damage. This study indicated that intranasal administration of NPs might render their distribution to certain specific brain regions and these NPs are not easy to be cleared (Wu et al., 2013).

4 Physiological conditions that influence the metabolism and excretion of NPs

Three routes are likely involved in the brain clearance of nanoparticles, in situ degradation, CSF circulation, and brain-to-blood efflux. Therefore, any physiological conditions that can influence the above routes are likely to affect the brain clearance of NPs.

4.1 Conscious state

Sleep has a critical function in ensuring metabolic homeostasis. Natural sleep or anesthesia has been shown to associate with a 60% increase in the interstitial space and results in a striking increase in convective exchange of CSF with ISF (Xie et al., 2013). It has been found that sleep and anesthesia increased the rate of amyloid-beta and lactate clearance (Lundgaard et al., 2017). Thus, it is very possible that sleep and anesthesia also accelerate the brain clearance of nanomaterials.

4.2 Brian regional distribution

The brain regional distribution of membrane-bound pyroglutamate aminopeptidase was not homogeneous: a 10-fold difference was observed between regions. The highest activity was detected in olfactory bulb, while the lowest was in the cervical part of spinal cord. The differential distribution of this enzyme is consistent with the hypothesis that it is responsible for extracellular degradation of neuroactive peptides (Vargas et al., 1987). Such site-specific distribution profile of metabolic enzyme in the brain could also induce site-specific degradation of certain NPs.

4.3 Disease conditions

4.3.1 Brain tumors

Metabolic enzymes such as hyaluronidases are known to increase various malignant tumors including brain tumors. Thus, the degradation of poly(ethylene glycol) (PEG)-conjugated hyaluronic acid nanoparticles occurred at the tumor site, and this unique degradation pathway for hyaluronic acid allows its application as an enzyme-sensitive nanocarrier for tumor-targeting drug delivery (Choi et al., 2011).

4.3.2 Stroke

Activation of microglia and astrocytes occurs within hours following the onset of ischemia, which produced and secreted several pro- and anti-inflammatory cytokines. These cytokines contribute to leukocyte infiltration in the damaged tissue. Infiltration of leukocytes from bloodstream into brain tissue further results in release of additional cytokines and chemokines, ultimately leading to excessive oxidative stress and activation of the matrix metalloproteinases (MMPs). The MMPs activation contributes to breakdown of the extracellular matrix that comprises the basal lamina and, thus, directly causes enhanced BBB disruption, leading to further inflammatory cell recruitment and associated inflammation (Ronaldson and Davis, 2012). This cascade is likely to suppress CSF circulation and brain-to-blood efflux and inhibit NPs clearance. In contrast, the activated glial cells are likely to take up more NPs for intracellular degradation.

4.3.3 Neurodegenerative diseases

Neurodegenerative diseases greatly influence the metabolism and excretion of the brain. Study has shown that glymphatic transport, defined as CSF periarterial inflow into brain and ISF clearance, is reduced in the aging brain and people having Alzheimer's disease (Peng et al., 2016). The metabolism and excretion of NPs in the brain would also be reduced due to the neurodegenerative diseases.

4.3.4 Hydrocephalus

Hydrocephalus is a disease with an abnormal accumulation of CSF in the brain that results in cognitive and physical impairments. Krishnamurthy et al. found that the hydrocephalus delayed the ventricular clearance of normal macromolecular. They compared the transport and clearance rate of intraventricularly injected 10 kDa dextran between the normal and the hydrocephalic rat brain in vivo. The results showed that the dextran transport was delayed in the hydrocephalic state (Krishnamurthy et al., 2018). Therefore, we postulate that the hydrocephalus might also reduce the brain clearance rate of certain nanomaterials.

5 Conclusion and perspective

Nanomaterials possess the powerful potential to be developed as the drug delivery systems for CNS diseases therapy or diagnosis. In recent years, a great amount of studies have been done to improve the brain targeting ability of nanoparticulate drug delivery systems; however, little attention has been paid to the metabolism and excretion of these nanomaterials in the CNS. Also, limited work have been conducted to investigate the factors affecting the brain clearance of NPs. Studies have shown that certain NPs in the brain could induce the neurotoxicity and other side effects. Accordingly, there is an urgent requirement to investigate the metabolism and excretion of nanomaterials which can cross the BBB. Here, we briefly introduced the clearance systems of nanomaterials both in the brain and the peripheral circulation, highlighted the recent researches about the elimination of brain-targeted nanoparticulate drug delivery systems, and discussed the related factors. Most work in this field just detected the nanomaterials' concentrations in the brain at different time periods, while the mechanisms under these distribution and clearance characteristics were not discussed. We claimed that for the safe and efficient application of nanotechnology in medicine, especially for the treatment of brain disorders, more investigations on the biofate of NPs in brain should be conducted.

References

Agarwal, R., Singh, V., Jurney, P., Shi, L., Sreenivasan, S.V., Roy, K., 2013. Mammalian cells preferentially internalize hydrogel nanodiscs over nanorods and use shape-specific uptake mechanisms. Proc. Natl. Acad. Sci. U. S. A. 110 (43), 17247–17252.

Albertazzi, L., Gherardini, L., Brondi, M., Sulis, S.S., Bifone, A., Pizzorusso, T., et al., 2013. In vivo distribution and toxicity of PAMAM dendrimers in the central nervous system depend on their surface chemistry. Mol. Pharm. 10 (1), 249–260.

Balasubramanian, S.K., Jittiwat, J., Manikandan, J., Ong, C.N., Yu, L.E., Ong, W.Y., 2010. Biodistribution of gold nanoparticles and gene expression changes in the liver and spleen after intravenous administration in rats. Biomaterials 31 (8), 2034–2042.

Balasubramanian, S.K., Poh, K.W., Ong, C.N., Kreyling, W.G., Ong, W.Y., Yu, L.E., 2013. The effect of primary particle size on biodistribution of inhaled gold nano-agglomerates. Biomaterials 34 (22), 5439–5452.

Boado, R.J., Pardridge, W.M., 2011. The Trojan horse liposome technology for nonviral gene transfer across the blood-brain barrier. J. Drug Deliv. 2011296151.

Casals, E., Pfaller, T., Duschl, A., Oostingh, G.J., Puntes, V., 2010. Time evolution of the nanoparticle protein corona. ACS Nano 4 (7), 3623–3632.

Chen, Y.S., Hung, Y.C., Lin, L.W., Liau, I., Hong, M.Y., Huang, G.S., 2010. Size-dependent impairment of cognition in mice caused by the injection of gold nanoparticles. Nanotechnology. 21(48)485102.

Choi, K.Y., Yoon, H.Y., Kim, J.H., Bae, S.M., Park, R.W., Kang, Y.M., et al., 2011. Smart nanocarrier based on PEGylated hyaluronic acid for cancer therapy. ACS Nano 5 (11), 8591–8599.

Cupaioli, F.A., Zucca, F.A., Boraschi, D., Zecca, L., 2014. Engineered nanoparticles. How brain friendly is this new guest? Prog. Neurobiol. 119-120, 20–38.

Gaberel, T., Gakuba, C., Goulay, R., Martinez, D.L.S., Hanouz, J.L., Emery, E., et al., 2014. Impaired glymphatic perfusion after strokes revealed by contrast-enhanced MRI: a new target for fibrinolysis? Stroke 45 (10), 3092–3096.

Gao, K., Jiang, X., 2006. Influence of particle size on transport of methotrexate across blood brain barrier by polysorbate 80-coated polybutylcyanoacrylate nanoparticles. Int. J. Pharm. 310 (1–2), 213–219.

Geraets, L., Oomen, A.G., Krystek, P., Jacobsen, N.R., Wallin, H., Laurentie, M., et al., 2014. Tissue distribution and elimination after oral and intravenous administration of different titanium dioxide nanoparticles in rats. Part. Fibre Toxicol. 11, 30.

Han, D., Tian, Y., Zhang, T., Ren, G., Yang, Z., 2011. Nano-zinc oxide damages spatial cognition capability via over-enhanced long-term potentiation in hippocampus of Wistar rats. Int. J. Nanomed. 6, 1453–1461.

Hu, R., Zheng, L., Zhang, T., Gao, G., Cui, Y., Cheng, Z., et al., 2011. Molecular mechanism of hippocampal apoptosis of mice following exposure to titanium dioxide nanoparticles. J. Hazard. Mater. 191 (1–3), 32–40.

Huang, M., Hu, M., Song, Q., Song, H., Huang, J., Gu, X., et al., 2015. GM1-modified lipoprotein-like nanoparticle: multifunctional nanoplatform for the combination therapy of Alzheimer's disease. ACS Nano 9 (11), 10801–10816.

Hutter, E., Boridy, S., Labrecque, S., Lalancette-Hebert, M., Kriz, J., Winnik, F.M., et al., 2010. Microglial response to gold nanoparticles. ACS Nano 4 (5), 2595–2606.

Iliff, J.J., Wang, M., Liao, Y., Plogg, B.A., Peng, W., Gundersen, G.A., et al., 2012. A paravascular pathway facilitates CSF flow through the brain parenchyma and the clearance of interstitial solutes, including amyloid beta. Sci. Transl. Med. 4 (147), 111r–147r.

Imperatore, R., Carotenuto, G., Di Grazia, M.A., Ferrandino, I., Palomba, L., Mariotti, R., et al., 2015. Imidazole-stabilized gold nanoparticles induce neuronal apoptosis: an in vitro and in vivo study. J. Biomed. Mater. Res. A 103 (4), 1436–1446.

Jessen, N.A., Munk, A.S., Lundgaard, I., Nedergaard, M., 2015. The glymphatic system: a beginner's guide. Neurochem. Res. 40 (12), 2583–2599.

Jo, D.H., Kim, J.H., Lee, T.G., Kim, J.H., 2015. Size, surface charge, and shape determine therapeutic effects of nanoparticles on brain and retinal diseases. Nanomedicine 11 (7), 1603–1611.

Kanazawa, T., Taki, H., Tanaka, K., Takashima, Y., Okada, H., 2011. Cell-penetrating peptide-modified block copolymer micelles promote direct brain delivery via intranasal administration. Pharm. Res. 28 (9), 2130–2139.

Kolhar, P., Anselmo, A.C., Gupta, V., Pant, K., Prabhakarpandian, B., Ruoslahti, E., et al., 2013. Using shape effects to target antibody-coated nanoparticles to lung and brain endothelium. Proc. Natl. Acad. Sci. U. S. A. 110 (26), 10753–10758.

Krishnamurthy, S., Li, J., Shen, Y., Duncan, T.M., Jenrow, K.A., Haacke, E.M., 2018. Normal macromolecular clearance out of the ventricles is delayed in hydrocephalus. Brain Res. 1678, 337–355.

Lindqvist, A., Rip, J., van Kregten, J., Gaillard, P.J., Hammarlund-Udenaes, M., 2016. In vivo functional evaluation of increased brain delivery of the opioid peptide DAMGO by glutathione-PEGylated liposomes. Pharm. Res. 33 (1), 177–185.

Liu, T., Choi, H., Zhou, R., Chen, I.W., 2015. RES blockade: a strategy for boosting efficiency of nanoparticle drug. Nano Today 10 (1), 11–21.

Longmire, M., Choyke, P.L., Kobayashi, H., 2008. Clearance properties of nano-sized particles and molecules as imaging agents: considerations and caveats. Nanomedicine (London) 3 (5), 703–717.

Louveau, A., Smirnov, I., Keyes, T.J., Eccles, J.D., Rouhani, S.J., Peske, J.D., et al., 2015. Structural and functional features of central nervous system lymphatic vessels. Nature 523 (7560), 337–341.

Lundgaard, I., Lu, M.L., Yang, E., Peng, W., Mestre, H., Hitomi, E., et al., 2017. Glymphatic clearance controls state-dependent changes in brain lactate concentration. J. Cereb. Blood Flow Metab. 37 (6), 2112–2124.

Ma, Q., Ineichen, B.V., Detmar, M., Proulx, S.T., 2017. Outflow of cerebrospinal fluid is predominantly through lymphatic vessels and is reduced in aged mice. Nat. Commun. 8 (1), 1434.

Minami, S.S., Sun, B., Popat, K., Kauppinen, T., Pleiss, M., Zhou, Y., et al., 2012. Selective targeting of microglia by quantum dots. J. Neuroinflammat. 9, 22.

Mooney, R., Weng, Y., Tirughana-Sambandan, R., Valenzuela, V., Aramburo, S., Garcia, E., et al., 2014. Neural stem cells improve intracranial nanoparticle retention and tumor-selective distribution. Future Oncol. 10 (3), 401–415.

Nance, E.A., Woodworth, G.F., Sailor, K.A., Shih, T.Y., Xu, Q., Swaminathan, G., et al., 2012. A dense poly(ethylene glycol) coating improves penetration of large polymeric nanoparticles within brain tissue. Sci. Transl. Med. 4 (149), 119r–149r.

Pardridge, W.M., 2005. The blood-brain barrier: bottleneck in brain drug development. NeuroRx 2 (1), 3–14.

Peng, W., Achariyar, T.M., Li, B., Liao, Y., Mestre, H., Hitomi, E., et al., 2016. Suppression of glymphatic fluid transport in a mouse model of Alzheimer's disease. Neurobiol. Dis. 93, 215–225.

Raghnaill, M.N., Bramini, M., Ye, D., Couraud, P.O., Romero, I.A., Weksler, B., et al., 2014. Paracrine signalling of inflammatory cytokines from an in vitro blood brain barrier model upon exposure to polymeric nanoparticles. Analyst 139 (5), 923–930.

Ronaldson, P.T., Davis, T.P., 2012. Blood-brain barrier integrity and glial support: mechanisms that can be targeted for novel therapeutic approaches in stroke. Curr. Pharm. Des. 18 (25), 3624–3644.

Savchenko, A., Braun, G.B., Molokanova, E., 2016. Nanostructured antagonist of extrasynaptic NMDA receptors. Nano Lett. 16 (9), 5495–5502.

Sharma, G., Modgil, A., Layek, B., Arora, K., Sun, C., Law, B., et al., 2013. Cell penetrating peptide tethered bi-ligand liposomes for delivery to brain in vivo: biodistribution and transfection. J. Control. Release 167 (1), 1–10.

Shcharbin, D., Janaszewska, A., Klajnert-Maculewicz, B., Ziemba, B., Dzmitruk, V., Halets, I., et al., 2014. How to study dendrimers and dendriplexes III. Biodistribution, pharmacokinetics and toxicity in vivo. J. Control. Release 181, 40–52.

Sonali Agrawal, P., Singh, R.P., Rajesh, C.V., Singh, S., Vijayakumar, M.R., et al., 2016. Transferrin receptor-targeted vitamin E TPGS micelles for brain cancer therapy: preparation, characterization and brain distribution in rats. Drug Deliv. 23 (5), 1788–1798.

Song, Q., Huang, M., Yao, L., Wang, X., Gu, X., Chen, J., et al., 2014. Lipoprotein-based nanoparticles rescue the memory loss of mice with Alzheimer's disease by accelerating the clearance of amyloid-beta. ACS Nano 8 (3), 2345–2359.

Stefanick, J.F., Ashley, J.D., Kiziltepe, T., Bilgicer, B., 2013. A systematic analysis of peptide linker length and liposomal polyethylene glycol coating on cellular uptake of peptide-targeted liposomes. ACS Nano 7 (4), 2935–2947.

Tang, J., Xiong, L., Wang, S., Wang, J., Liu, L., Li, J., et al., 2009. Distribution, translocation and accumulation of silver nanoparticles in rats. J. Nanosci. Nanotechnol. 9 (8), 4924–4932.

Tarasoff-Conway, J.M., Carare, R.O., Osorio, R.S., Glodzik, L., Butler, T., Fieremans, E., et al., 2015. Clearance systems in the brain-implications for Alzheimer disease. Nat. Rev. Neurol. 11 (8), 457–470.

Terasaki, T., Ohtsuki, S., 2005. Brain-to-blood transporters for endogenous substrates and xenobiotics at the blood-brain barrier: an overview of biology and methodology. NeuroRx 2 (1), 63–72.

Ueno, M., Nakagawa, T., Wu, B., Onodera, M., Huang, C.L., Kusaka, T., et al., 2010. Transporters in the brain endothelial barrier. Curr. Med. Chem. 17 (12), 1125–1138.

van der Zande, M., Vandebriel, R.J., Van Doren, E., Kramer, E., Herrera, R.Z., Serrano-Rojero, C.S., et al., 2012. Distribution, elimination, and toxicity of silver nanoparticles and silver ions in rats after 28-day oral exposure. ACS Nano 6 (8), 7427–7442.

Vargas, M., Mendez, M., Cisneros, M., Joseph-Bravo, P., Charli, J.L., 1987. Regional distribution of the membrane-bound pyroglutamate amino peptidase-degrading thyrotropin-releasing hormone in rat brain. Neurosci. Lett. 79 (3), 311–314.

Wang, F., Yu, L., Monopoli, M.P., Sandin, P., Mahon, E., Salvati, A., et al., 2013. The biomolecular corona is retained during nanoparticle uptake and protects the cells from the damage induced by cationic nanoparticles until degraded in the lysosomes. Nanomedicine 9 (8), 1159–1168.

Wang, J., Liu, Y., Jiao, F., Lao, F., Li, W., Gu, Y., et al., 2008. Time-dependent translocation and potential impairment on central nervous system by intranasally instilled TiO_2 nanoparticles. Toxicology 254 (1–2), 82–90.

Wiley, D.T., Webster, P., Gale, A., Davis, M.E., 2013. Transcytosis and brain uptake of transferrin-containing nanoparticles by tuning avidity to transferrin receptor. Proc. Natl. Acad. Sci. U. S. A. 110 (21), 8662–8667.

Wong, H.L., Wu, X.Y., Bendayan, R., 2012. Nanotechnological advances for the delivery of CNS therapeutics. Adv. Drug Deliv. Rev. 64 (7), 686–700.

Wu, J., Ding, T., Sun, J., 2013. Neurotoxic potential of iron oxide nanoparticles in the rat brain striatum and hippocampus. NeuroToxicology 34, 243–253.

Wu, J., Wang, C., Sun, J., Xue, Y., 2011. Neurotoxicity of silica nanoparticles: brain localization and dopaminergic neurons damage pathways. ACS Nano 5 (6), 4476–4489.

Xie, F., Yao, N., Qin, Y., Zhang, Q., Chen, H., Yuan, M., et al., 2012. Investigation of glucose-modified liposomes using polyethylene glycols with different chain lengths as the linkers for brain targeting. Int. J. Nanomedicine 7, 163–175.

Xie, L., Kang, H., Xu, Q., Chen, M.J., Liao, Y., Thiyagarajan, M., et al., 2013. Sleep drives metabolite clearance from the adult brain. Science 342 (6156), 373–377.

Xu, F., Lu, W., Wu, H., Fan, L., Gao, X., Jiang, X., 2009. Brain delivery and systemic effect of cationic albumin conjugated PLGA nanoparticles. J. Drug Target. 17 (6), 423–434.

Yu, M., Zheng, J., 2015. Clearance pathways and tumor targeting of imaging nanoparticles. ACS Nano 9 (7), 6655–6674.

Zensi, A., Begley, D., Pontikis, C., Legros, C., Mihoreanu, L., Wagner, S., et al., 2009. Albumin nanoparticles targeted with Apo E enter the CNS by transcytosis and are delivered to neurones. J. Control. Release 137 (1), 78–86.

Zhang, Y.N., Poon, W., Tavares, A.J., Mcgilvray, I.D., Chan, W., 2016. Nanoparticle-liver interactions: cellular uptake and hepatobiliary elimination. J. Control. Release 240, 332–348.

Perspective on brain targeting drug delivery systems

18

Huile Gao
Key Laboratory of Drug Targeting and Drug Delivery Systems, West China School of Pharmacy, Sichuan University, Chengdu, China

1 Introduction

Brain, a most important organ of human being, is carefully protected by blood brain barrier (BBB) to avoid access of harmful compounds from blood circulation. However, the BBB also greatly hinders brain access of drugs for central nervous system (CNS) disorders, making treatment of CNS disorders the most difficult task for doctors and pharmaceutists. Therefore, many researchers have been trying to overcome the barrier and solve this task. In Chapters 5–16 of this book, the current developed brain targeting drug delivery systems (DDS) are reviewed and categorized by diseases and targeting mechanisms. Using "brain targeting drug delivery" as keyword to search in PubMed, we could see that the number of papers in this area shows an exponentially growth in the past decade (Fig. 1), suggesting the brain targeting drug delivery has been gaining increasing attention.

Although great progress has been made in brain targeting drug delivery, the treatment of CNS disorders is still far away from satisfactory. Until 2017, only several nanoparticles (NPs) are under clinical evaluation for glioma treatment, but no nanoformulation was developed for other CNS disorders. Even worse, the percentage injected dose per gram brain (%ID/g brain) could only achieve several percentages even lower than 1%. The drug delivery efficiency is far from satisfactory. Therefore, in-depth discussion was required to elucidate the problems faced in brain targeting drug delivery, and the potential directions were also discussed.

2 The targeting specificity of DDS

The targeting specificity is a mandatory requirement for targeting DDS. Although unselected cell-penetrating peptide modification showed the ability to improve brain targeting drug delivery, the distribution in other organs was increased correspondingly (Qin et al., 2011), which was not good news for diagnostic and therapeutic application. Therefore, researchers have devoted to find ligands that can specifically target BBB. There are many receptors and transporters overexpressed on BBB (Gao, 2016), including transferrin receptor (TfR) (Qian et al., 2002), insulin receptor (Guo et al., 2012), low-density lipoprotein receptor-related protein (Ito et al., 2006), nicotinic acetylcholine receptor (Kumar et al., 2007), insulin-like growth factor receptor

Brain Targeted Drug Delivery Systems. https://doi.org/10.1016/B978-0-12-814001-7.00018-4

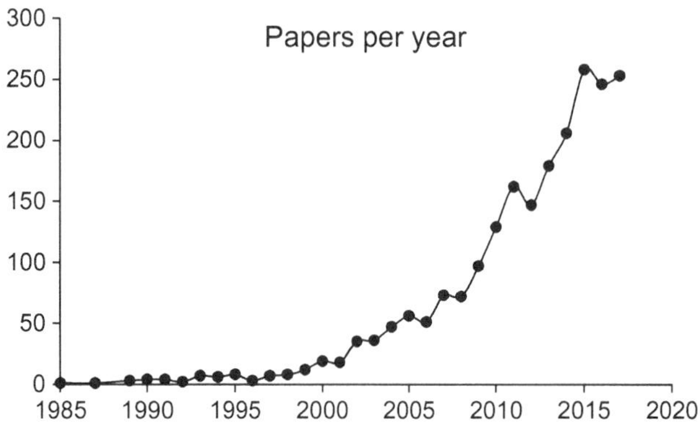

Fig. 1 Papers published every year in the topic of "brain targeting drug delivery." The numbers were obtained from PubMed at Dec. 12, 2017.

(Guo et al., 2012), diphtheria toxin receptor (Guo et al., 2012), scavenger receptor call B type (Pardridge, 2007), leptin receptor (Guo et al., 2012), neonatal Fc receptor (Zhang et al., 2016), adenosine triphosphate-binding cassette (ABC) transporter, subfamily B, member 1 (P-glycoprotein) (Cannon et al., 2012), ABC transporter, subfamily C (Guo et al., 2012), ABC transporter, subfamily G, member 2 (Pardridge, 2007), organic anion transporter (Guo et al., 2012), organic anion-transporting polypeptide (Pardridge, 2007), glutamic acid, amino acid transporter (Hsu et al., 2010), taurine transporter (Pardridge, 2007), glucose transporter, member 1 (Gorin et al., 2004), large neutral amino acid transporter, member 1 (Li et al., 2016), cationic amino acid transporter, member 1 (Guo et al., 2012), monocarboxylic acid transporter, member 1 (Guo et al., 2012), concentrative nucleoside transporter (Guo et al., 2012), Choline transporter (Geldenhuys and Allen, 2012), nucleobase transporter (Pardridge, 2007), etc. The corresponding ligands could be served for brain targeting drug delivery. At the beginning, endogenous ligands of these receptors and transporters were utilized for constructing brain targeting DDS; however, the competition binding of free endogenous ligands impelled researchers to find alternative ligands. For this purpose, two methods were widely used, i.e., redesigned the existent ligands and selected ligands from a random library.

Redesign the ligands may provide new ligands with higher binding affinity and specificity compared with the initial ligands. For example, a 16-residue peptide CDX was derived from the loop II region of the snake neurotoxin candoxin, which showed high binding affinity to nicotine acetylcholine receptor (Zhan et al., 2011). Wei et al. (2015) further designed ^{D}CDX, a retro–inverso isomer of L-formed CDX (^{L}CDX). The half inhibition concentration (IC_{50}) of ^{D}CDX was 84.5 nm, which was approximately five times lower than that of ^{L}CDX (441.6 nm). Both in vitro and in vivo, ^{D}CDX-decorated liposomes showed higher BBB penetration and brain accumulation than ^{L}CDX-modified liposomes (Fig. 2). Different from redesign the ligands, the de novo selected ligands may have good specificity through several rounds screening against target and negative control. Until now, several peptides, antibody

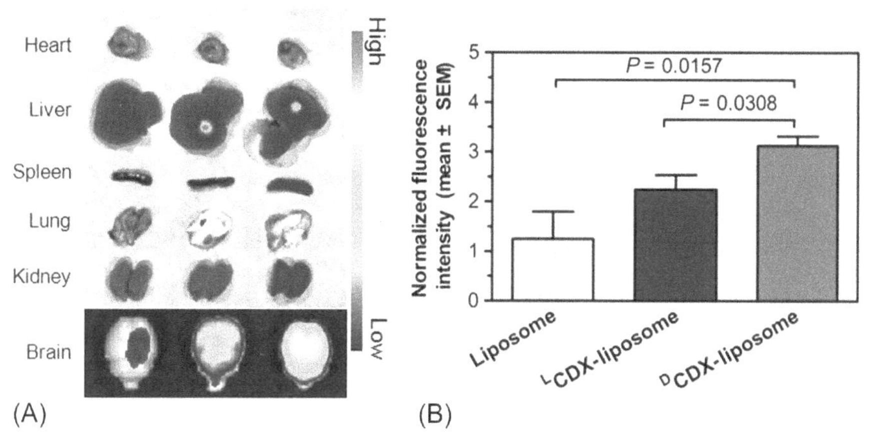

Fig. 2 In vivo biodistribution of rhodamine B-labeled ^{D}CDX-liposomes, ^{L}CDX-liposomes, and plain liposomes. (A) ex vivo imaging of dissected tissues including brains and other organs of mice 8h after injection. Organs from left to right are from mice administrated with plain liposomes, ^{L}CDX-liposomes, and ^{D}CDX-liposomes. (B) Normalized fluorescence intensity of brain in each group. Mean ± SD, $n=3$.
Reprinted from Wei, X., Zhan, C., Shen, Q., Fu, W., Xie, C., Gao, J., Peng, C., Zheng, P., Lu, W., 2015. A D-peptide ligand of nicotine acetylcholine receptors for brain-targeted drug delivery. Angew Chem. Int. Ed. Engl. 54(10), 3023–3027, with permission of the copyright holder John Wiley and Sons.

single-chain variable fragments, and aptamers were selected with good brain targeting capacity (Diaz-Perlas et al., 2017; Li et al., 2011; Sakamoto et al., 2017; Thom et al., 2018). However, most of them still target the already known receptors. For example, T7 peptide (HAIYPRH) targets transferrin receptor (Lee et al., 2001), L57 peptide (TWPKHFDKHTFYSILKLGKH-OH) targets cluster 4 (Ser3332-Asp3779) of low-density lipoprotein receptor-related protein 1 (Sakamoto et al., 2017), and AS1411 aptamer targets nucleon receptor (Mongelard and Bouvet, 2010). The novel ligands may provide an opportunity to further improve the brain targeting delivery specificity and efficiency.

3 Off-target potential of DDS

The foundation of ligand-modified NPs for brain targeting delivery is that the ligands could specifically bind with corresponding receptors or transporters on the BBB and then mediated transportation. Unfortunately, the protein corona would form as soon as the NPs were introduced into biological milieu (Nel et al., 2009). The corona would greatly influence the in vivo biodistribution and cellular uptake of NPs (Gao and He, 2014). In addition, the protein corona may cover the targeting ligand, thus hindered the specific reaction between ligands and its target. For example, the protein corona could shield the specific binding between transferrin on NPs and free TfR or receptor on cells (Salvati et al., 2013), resulting in decreased cellular uptake by target cells. To attenuate the shield effect of protein corona, several methods were developed, including PEG backfilling (Dai et al., 2014), specifically exposure ligand in target site by de-shielding PEG cover (Sun et al., 2015), optimizing the nanomaterials for preparing NPs (Kang et al., 2015), selecting ligands that could inhibit protein adsorption (Garcia et al., 2015), and changing the surface cover of NPs from PEG to lipid (Xu et al., 2016). Although these methods showed somewhat improvement in specific targeting, they could not totally overcome the influence by protein corona. Therefore, it is important to evaluate the protein corona formation and the influence on brain targeting capacity of DDS and to optimize the composition of NPs to minimize the influence of protein corona.

Apart from the protein corona, the wide expression of receptors in other tissues could also lead to off-target. Unfortunately, most, if not all, of the receptors used for brain targeting were expressed also on normal cells, some even with high level. For example, TfR overexpressed on BBB and brain tumor cells, but it almost expressed on all cells with various level, while high levels were expressed in immature erythroid cells, placental tissue, and rapidly dividing cells (Ponka and Lok, 1999). Thus, the transferrin-modified NPs would be inevitably distributed in the corresponding tissues and cells. To avoid the unintended distribution, labeling target cells with exogenous ligand as a target showed promising results. 9-Azido sialic acid could be labeled onto brain cells because the metabolism of brain cells required high level of sialic acid. Then the intravenous-injected alkyne-functionalized biotin probe could be labeled onto brain cells due to azide-alkyne click reaction, resulting in specific imaging of brain sialoglycans in living animals (Xie et al., 2016).

4 BBB penetration capacity of DDS

For the brain targeting drug delivery, DDS should penetrate through the BBB. BBB is such an intact barrier that particles could penetrate only through transcytosis rather than paracellular pathway. Traditionally, a transcytosis procedure includes recognizing by the cell membrane, internalizing into endosomes, escaping from endosomes, and then exocytosis from cells. Although many publications suggested the NPs could be internalized into endothelial cells of BBB by receptor-, carrier-, and adsorptive-mediated endocytosis (Guo et al., 2012), recent research indicated most of the particles were trapped in the cells, while only less than 5% pass BBB after even 48 h (Bramini et al., 2014). The exocytosis of NPs is influenced by particle size, shape, and surface chemistry (Kim et al., 2014; Oh and Park, 2014), while the penetration through BBB, requiring one-way exocytosis, was rarely discussed.

To improve the penetration through BBB, Yu et al. (2011) designed anti-TfR antibodies with different binding affinities. The anti-TfR with high binding affinity only showed modest brain uptake, while anti-TfR with low binding affinity showed increased uptake. For example, the IC_{50} of anti-TfR^{A} and anti-TfR^{D} to TfR was 1.7 and 111 nM, respectively, while the %ID/g brain of anti-TfR^{A} and anti-TfR^{D} at

24 h was about 0.2 and 0.6, respectively. According to the results, Yu et al. provided a potential mechanism. Under nonsaturating concentration, low binding affinity led to low internalization and transcytosis. While under therapeutic dose (normally much higher than serum concentration of transferrin), luminal TfR would be saturated by antibodies regardless of their binding affinity, resulting in similar internalization. However, low binding affinity would lead to higher brain accumulation through easy dissociation from TfR and release to brain. Additionally, low binding affinity would also reduce the probability of receptor-mediated efflux from the brain because the concentration in parenchyma was lower than saturation. Based on this hypothesis, Clark and Davis (2015) modified transferrin onto gold NPs with an acid-cleavable linkage between the transferrin and the NP core to facilitate NP dissociation from TfR after internalization. In in vitro BBB model, about 0.75% of 200Tf-C (200 transferrin per particle, through cleavable bond) cross the BBB after 8 h, which was 10-fold higher than the noncleavable control particles. In vivo, the 200Tf-C also showed highest accumulation in mice brain.

5 Intra-brain distribution and brain cell type selectivity of DDS

As the main and first barrier for brain targeting delivery, many strategies were developed to overcome BBB, bypass BBB, or temporarily open BBB (Gao, 2016). After entering the brain, a critical concern is the intra-brain distribution. Although these DDS improved overall drug concentrations in the brain, their lack of selective distribution or poor cell type selectivity in the brain has emerged as an increasing concern as the drugs distributed in the healthy part of brain may cause serious drug-oriented side effect. Therefore, how to reduce the distribution in normal brain as well as increase the distribution in diseased site and cells? To partially answer this question, the concept of dual targeting drug delivery was proposed that can first penetrate through BBB and then specifically target diseased brain regions or cells (Du et al., 2009; Gao et al., 2011). According to this concept, many novel DDS were constructed with promising drug delivery efficiency and treatment outcome in the past half-decade. Basically, the dual targeting delivery strategy is established by modifying nanoparticles with two ligands, one is to penetrate through or bypass the BBB (first barrier) and another is to specifically target diseased cells in brain (second barrier) (Fig. 3). However, during the development, DDS with one ligand that can conquer two barriers were also named with dual targeting drug delivery.

Brain tumor gained much attention for dual targeting drug delivery (Gao, 2017). TGN peptide (TGNYKALHPHNG) is a 12-mer peptide that showed high BBB targeting efficiency (Li et al., 2011), while AS1411 aptamer can specifically bind with nucleon that is overexpressed on brain tumor cells (Bates et al., 2009). Our group functionalized these two ligands onto NPs to construct brain tumor dual targeting DDS, AsTNPs (Gao et al., 2012). In vivo, the distribution of AsTNPs in the brain tumor region was 4.91-fold higher than that of unmodified NPs. To evaluate the brain tumor selectivity, an index was introduced that named with T/N ratio (the intensity

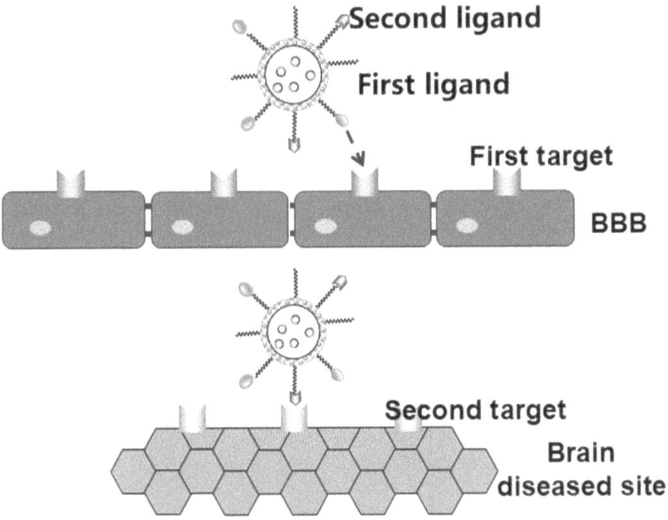

Fig. 3 Concept of dual targeting drug delivery systems.

ratio of brain tumor to normal brain). Although TGN modification could enhance BBB penetration, the T/N ratio of TGN-modified NPs was only 1.2, while T/N ratio of AsTNPs was as high as 2.6, suggesting dual modification could indeed improve the selectivity of particles in the brain. Consequently, 6mg/kg of docetaxel-loaded AsTNPs (every 3 days for three times) could significantly prolong the median survival time of brain tumor bearing mice (32 days), which was much longer than other groups. The study clearly demonstrated that the dual targeting DDS was superior to traditional brain targeting DDS. Some receptors, such as TfR and low-density lipoprotein-related protein-1, were overexpressed on both BBB and brain tumor cells, thus the corresponding ligands, transferrin and angiopep-2, respectively, could be served as a ligand with dual functions. The angiopep-2-modified NPs (AnNPs) showed good BBB penetration and brain tumor-targeted accumulation (Ruan et al., 2015; Xin et al., 2011). Huang et al. (2017) designed an apolipoprotein E3-reconstituted high-density lipoprotein (ApoE-rHDL). To load with siRNA, the ApoE-rHDL was fabricated with a calcium phosphate (CaP) core. The obtained CaP-ApoE-rHDL could effectively penetrate through BBB mediated by low-density lipoprotein receptor, and then target and be internalized by brain tumor cells through Ras-mediated macropinocytosis. Compared with CaP-loaded lipid nanocarrier (CaP-LNC), the CaP-ApoE-rHDL showed about threefold higher accumulation in brain tumor and much higher internalization in brain tumor cells, which can be specifically inhibited by ethylisopropylamiloride, an inhibitor of micropinocytosis.

Later, the dual targeting drug delivery strategy was utilized for Alzheimer's disease (AD) and stroke. As a dominant characteristic of AD, amyloid plaque is formed by aggregation of Aβ, in which 96% is $A\beta_{1-42}$ (Allaman et al., 2010).

Thus, Zhang et al. conjugated QSH (QSHYRHISPAQV) and TGN onto NPs (TQNPs) for dual targeting delivery to amyloid plaque of AD mice because QSH showed high binding affinity with $A\beta_{1-42}$ (van Groen et al., 2009; Zhang et al., 2014a). In the brain hippocampus where the $A\beta_{1-42}$ is located, TQNPs delivered 1.84-fold higher amount of therapeutic H102 peptide than TGN-modified NPs, while the concentration of H102 peptide in cerebrum and cerebellum (normal part of brain) of TQNPs group was similar to the TGN-modified NPs, suggesting the dual modification could further improve selective distribution in Aβ-positive part, while do not elevate concentration in normal brain (Zhang et al., 2014b). Zheng et al. (2017a) further modified CGN peptide (d-CGNHPHLAKYNGT) and QSH onto NPs (CQNPs) to deliver therapeutic siRNA into AD bearing mice. After intravenous injection, the BACE1 mRNA expression in the hippocampi was reduced to 63.58% compared to the sham control, while CGN-modified NPs only reduced to over 95% mRNA expression (Zheng et al., 2017b). Consequently, the amyloid plaques, tau protein phosphorylation, and synaptic loss in AD mice were significantly reduced, the spatial learning and memory of the AD mice in the siRNA-loaded CQNPs group were significantly improved compared with the AD control group and other NPs groups. Another system, ApoE-rHDL, could not only penetrate through BBB, but also showed with high binding affinity with Aβ (Song et al., 2014). One hour after injection, 0.4% ID/g of ApoE3-rHDL gained access to the brain, displaying excellent AD treatment effect by accelerating the microglial, astroglial, and liver cell degradation of Aβ. To dual target brain ischemic stroke, Zhao et al. (2016) modified NPs with T7 peptide (HAIYPRH) for BBB penetration and SHp (CLEVSRKNC) for stroke targeting. The dual modification significantly enhanced the accumulation of particles in ischemic part of brain, resulting in decreased infarct volume.

Although the dual targeting delivery strategy enhanced the distribution in diseased region or cells, we have to be aware that the strategy could not reduce the distribution in normal brain. The superiority of the dual targeting drug delivery strategy is that lower dose could be used when a certain therapeutic concentration in diseased site needs to be achieved. At same therapeutic response, the dual targeting drug delivery strategy would show lower concentration in normal brain accompanied with lower drug-oriented side effect. Unfortunately, this strategy did not satisfy the initial problem, how to reduce the distribution in normal brain? From best of our knowledge, the answer may be hidden behind the difference between the BBB in normal brain and BBB in diseased region. Selectively targeting and penetration through BBB in diseased region would deliver therapeutics directly into their target. Recently, Mann et al. (2017) identified a cyclic peptide (CDAGRKQKC, termed as DAG) that can recognize cerebrovascular changes in AD mice (Fig. 4). It was found that the receptor of DAG was connective tissue growth factor (CTGF), a matricellular protein that is highly expressed in the brain of individuals with AD and in mouse models (Ueberham et al., 2003). Therefore, the DAG could be served as an AD brain-specific targeting ligand for iron oxide NPs delivery. Results showed the DAG-modified iron oxide NPs could specifically accumulate in AD-positive region, while no NPs were observed in normal brain (Mann et al., 2017).

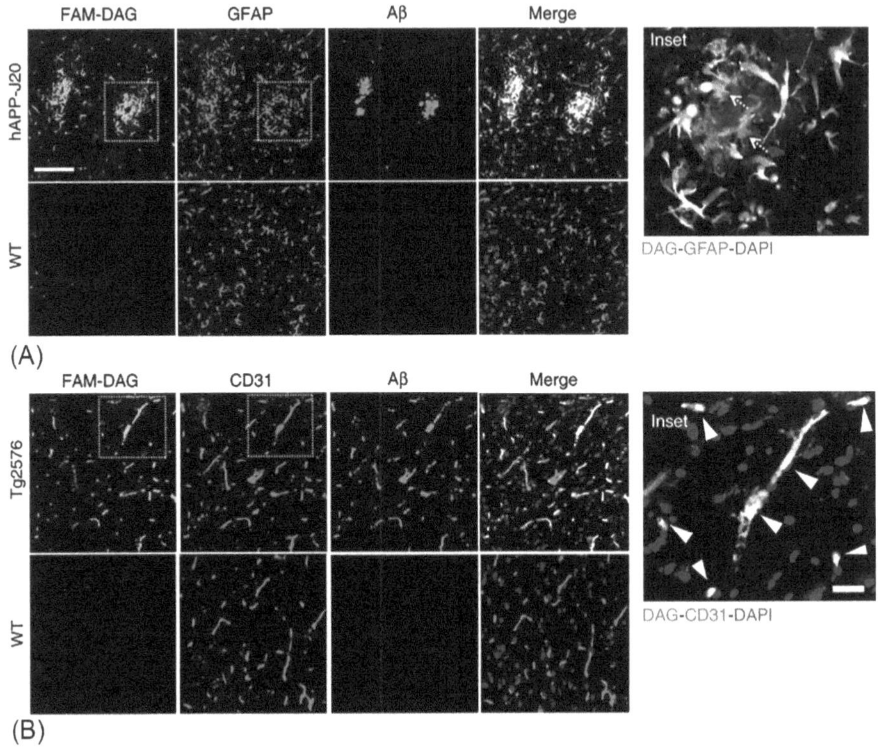

Fig. 4 Homing of DAG peptide to the brains of AD model mice. (A) DAG targets activated astrocytes in AD mouse brain. (A) FAM-DAG was intravenously injected to 9-month-old hAPP-J20 and WT mice and allowed to circulate for 30 min. The mice were perfused, and the brains were fixed, sectioned, and stained for FAM in DAG *(first panel from left)*, GFAP *(second panel)*, and Aβ *(third panel)*. The region shown is the hippocampus. The *inset* shows co-localization between DAG and GFAP, and also DAG^+ and $GFAP^-$ regions *(arrows)*. (B) DAG targets vessels positive for Aβ in Tg mice (B). DAG was injected intravenously to 20-month-old Tg2576 WT mice, and processed as in panel (A). The brain sections were stained for FAM *(first panel from left)*, CD31 *(second panel)*, and Aβ *(third panel)*. The region shown is the cortex. The *inset* shows co-localization of DAG and CD31 *(yellow, white arrowheads)*. *Scale bars*, 50 μm (A and B), 20 μm *(insets)*.
Reprinted from Mann, A.P., Scodeller, P., Hussain, S., Braun, G.B., Molder, T., Toome, K., Ambasudhan, R., Teesalu, T., Lipton, S.A., Ruoslahti, E., 2017. Identification of a peptide recognizing cerebrovascular changes in mouse models of Alzheimer's disease. *Nat. Commun.* 8 (1), 1403, with permission of the copyright holder.

6 Neurotoxicity of DDS

When we try our best to improve the brain targeting drug delivery efficiency, we must take potential neurotoxicity of the DDS into consideration. In a recent book edited by Jiang and Gao (2016), the neurotoxicity potential and mechanism of most widely used NPs were discussed, such as metal NPs, carbon nanotubes, and cationic polymers.

These NPs shared similar mechanism behind their neurotoxicity. As reviewed by Li et al. in Chapter 15 of this book, the NPs could cause oxidative stress and DNA damage and alter signal pathway, leading to cell apoptosis, necrosis, autophagy, and cell cycle arrest, and finally resulting in toxicity to almost all kinds of cells in brain. Therefore, researchers should pay particular attention to reduce potential neurotoxicity when designing brain targeting DDS (Gao and Jiang, 2016a). And neurotoxicity evaluation should be always performed in the evaluation of brain targeting DDS.

The toxicity is influenced by the intrinsic composition as well as the particle size, shape, surface charge, and other properties of the NPs. Although inorganic NPs, especially heavy metal containing NPs attracted great attention as novel platform for drug delivery, thermotherapy, photodynamic therapy, and theranostics, the intrinsic toxicity of these NPs hindered the application in clinical translated DDS. Especially, most inorganic NPs are non-biodegradable, thus the long-term accumulation of these NPs would lead to high risk to human health. At present, most promising DDS for CNS disorder treatment were still based on lipids, degradable polymers, and proteins (Bobo et al., 2016). For example, glutathione PEGylated liposomes successfully delivered approximately 1.5-fold higher doxorubicin to brain than PEGylated liposomes, resulting in significantly prolonged mice survival time with acceptable safety (Gaillard et al., 2014). Now the doxorubicin-loaded glutathione PEGylated liposomes (2B3-101) were under a clinical phase I/IIa study in patients with recurrent glioma or brain metastases of solid tumors (clinicaltrials.gov NCT01386580, NCT01818713) (Rip et al., 2014). Albumin is another successful example. Paclitaxel-loaded albumin NPs are approved for clinical use by FDA in 2005 due to their high safety and tolerance dose (Gao and Jiang, 2016b). Our data suggested the albumin NPs could effectively target and accumulate in brain tumor and deliver 0.08%ID/g tissue of lapatinib to glioma, resulting in prolonged survival time of glioma bearing mice (Gao et al., 2014). Lin et al. (2016) further modified albumin NPs with cell-penetrating peptide LMWP. The LMWP-modified albumin nanoparticles can penetrate the BBB and target glioma cells via the mechanism of SPARC- and gp60-mediated biomimetic transport, delivering more paclitaxel and fenretinide into glioma and resulting in significant better anti-glioma effect. In addition, ultrasmall inorganic NPs or hybridized NPs, such as ultrasmall iron oxide NPs and gold nanoclusters, also gained increasing attention because these particles could be directly excreted from body through kidney, leading to low accumulation in body and good safety (Liu et al., 2013; Luo et al., 2015).

7 Conclusion

In the past decades, brain targeting drug delivery has made great progress, and many kinds of brain targeting DDS were developed to enhance the brain distribution of drugs and improve the therapeutic outcomes of CNS disorders. Unfortunately, the drug delivery efficiency is far from satisfactory, and several key factors need further evaluation, including the targeting specificity, off-target potential, BBB penetration capacity, intra-brain distribution, and neurotoxicity of brain targeting DDS. The fundamental elucidation of these concerns may pave a new way to improve brain targeting drug delivery, and finally, provide clinical translationable DDS to improve the CNS disorder treatment.

References

Allaman, I., Gavillet, M., Belanger, M., Laroche, T., Viertl, D., Lashuel, H.A., Magistretti, P.J., 2010. Amyloid-beta aggregates cause alterations of astrocytic metabolic phenotype: impact on neuronal viability. J. Neurosci. 30 (9), 3326–3338.

Bates, P.J., Laber, D.A., Miller, D.M., Thomas, S.D., Trent, J.O., 2009. Discovery and development of the G-rich oligonucleotide AS1411 as a novel treatment for cancer. Exp. Mol. Pathol. 86 (3), 151–164.

Bobo, D., Robinson, K.J., Islam, J., Thurecht, K.J., Corrie, S.R., 2016. Nanoparticle-based medicines: a review of FDA-approved materials and clinical trials to date. Pharm. Res. 33 (10), 2373–2387.

Bramini, M., Ye, D., Hallerbach, A., Nic, R.M., Salvati, A., Aberg, C., Dawson, K.A., 2014. Imaging approach to mechanistic study of nanoparticle interactions with the blood-brain barrier. ACS Nano 8 (5), 4304–4312.

Cannon, R.E., Peart, J.C., Hawkins, B.T., Campos, C.R., Miller, D.S., 2012. Targeting blood-brain barrier sphingolipid signaling reduces basal P-glycoprotein activity and improves drug delivery to the brain. Proc. Natl. Acad. Sci. U. S. A. 109 (39), 15930–15935.

Clark, A.J., Davis, M.E., 2015. Increased brain uptake of targeted nanoparticles by adding an acid-cleavable linkage between transferrin and the nanoparticle core. Proc. Natl. Acad. Sci. U. S. A. 112 (40), 12486–12491.

Dai, Q., Walkey, C., Chan, W.C., 2014. Polyethylene glycol backfilling mitigates the negative impact of the protein corona on nanoparticle cell targeting. Angew Chem. Int. Ed. Engl. 53 (20), 5093–5096.

Diaz-Perlas, C., Sanchez-Navarro, M., Oller-Salvia, B., Moreno, M., Teixido, M., Giralt, E., 2017. Phage display as a tool to discover blood-brain barrier (BBB)-shuttle peptides: panning against a human BBB cellular model. Biopolymers. 108(1), e22928.

Du, J., Lu, W.L., Ying, X., Liu, Y., Du, P., Tian, W., Men, Y., Guo, J., Zhang, Y., Li, R.J., Zhou, J., Lou, J.N., Wang, J.C., Zhang, X., Zhang, Q., 2009. Dual-targeting topotecan liposomes modified with tamoxifen and wheat germ agglutinin significantly improve drug transport across the blood-brain barrier and survival of brain tumor-bearing animals. Mol. Pharm. 6 (3), 905–917.

Gaillard, P.J., Appeldoorn, C.C., Dorland, R., van Kregten, J., Manca, F., Vugts, D.J., Windhorst, B., van Dongen, G.A., de Vries, H.E., Maussang, D., van Tellingen, O., 2014. Pharmacokinetics, brain delivery, and efficacy in brain tumor-bearing mice of glutathione pegylated liposomal doxorubicin (2B3-101). PLoS One. 9(1)e82331.

Gao, H., 2016. Progress and perspectives on targeting nanoparticles for brain drug delivery. Acta Pharm. Sin. B 6 (4), 268–286.

Gao, H., 2017. Perspectives on dual targeting delivery systems for brain tumors. J. Neuroimmune Pharmacol. 12 (1), 6–16.

Gao, H., He, Q., 2014. The interaction of nanoparticles with plasma proteins and the consequent influence on nanoparticles behavior. Expert Opin. Drug Deliv. 11 (3), 409–420.

Gao, H., Jiang, X., 2016a. Chapter 13 Perspective on strategies to reduce the neurotoxicity of nanomaterials and nanomedicines. In: Neurotoxicity of Nanomaterials and Nanomedicine. Academic Press, Singapore, pp. 331–336.

Gao, H., Jiang, X., 2016b. The development of novel tumor targeting delivery strategy. Acta Pharm. Sin. 51 (02), 272–280.

Gao, H., Pan, S., Yang, Z., Cao, S., Chen, C., Jiang, X., Shen, S., Pang, Z., Hu, Y., 2011. A cascade targeting strategy for brain neuroglial cells employing nanoparticles modified with angiopep-2 peptide and EGFP-EGF1 protein. Biomaterials 32 (33), 8669–8675.

Gao, H., Qian, J., Cao, S., Yang, Z., Pang, Z., Pan, S., Fan, L., Xi, Z., Jiang, X., Zhang, Q., 2012. Precise glioma targeting of and penetration by aptamer and peptide dual-functioned nanoparticles. Biomaterials 33 (20), 5115–5123.

Gao, H., Wang, Y., Chen, C., Chen, J., We, Y., Cao, S., Jiang, X., 2014. Incorporation of lapatinib into core-shell nanoparticles improves both the solubility and anti-glioma effects of the drug. Int. J. Pharm. 461 (1–2), 478–488.

Garcia, I., Sanchez-Iglesias, A., Henriksen-Lacey, M., Grzelczak, M., Penades, S., Liz-Marzan, L.M., 2015. Glycans as biofunctional ligands for gold nanorods: stability and targeting in protein-rich media. J. Am. Chem. Soc. 137 (10), 3686–3692.

Geldenhuys, W.J., Allen, D.D., 2012. The blood-brain barrier choline transporter. Cent. Nerv. Syst. Agents Med. Chem. 12 (2), 95–99.

Gorin, F., Harley, W., Schnier, J., Lyeth, B., Jue, T., 2004. Perinecrotic glioma proliferation and metabolic profile within an intracerebral tumor xenograft. Acta Neuropathol. 107 (3), 235–244.

Guo, L., Ren, J., Jiang, X., 2012. Perspectives on brain-targeting drug delivery systems. Curr. Pharm. Biotechnol. 13 (12), 2310–2318.

Hsu, S.H., Wen, C.J., Al-Suwayeh, S.A., Chang, H.W., Yen, T.C., Fang, J.Y., 2010. Physicochemical characterization and in vivo bioluminescence imaging of nanostructured lipid carriers for targeting the brain: apomorphine as a model drug. Nanotechnology 21 (40), 405101.

Huang, J.L., Jiang, G., Song, Q.X., Gu, X., Hu, M., Wang, X.L., Song, H.H., Chen, L.P., Lin, Y.Y., Jiang, D., Chen, J., Feng, J.F., Qiu, Y.M., Jiang, J.Y., Jiang, X.G., Chen, H.Z., Gao, X.L., 2017. Lipoprotein-biomimetic nanostructure enables efficient targeting delivery of siRNA to Ras-activated glioblastoma cells via macropinocytosis. Nat. Commun. 8, 15144.

Ito, S., Ohtsuki, S., Terasaki, T., 2006. Functional characterization of the brain-to-blood efflux clearance of human amyloid-beta peptide (1-40) across the rat blood-brain barrier. Neurosci. Res. 56 (3), 246–252.

Jiang, X., Gao, H. (Eds.), 2016. Neurotoxicity of Nanomaterials and Nanomedicine. Academic Press, Singapore.

Kang, B., Okwieka, P., Schottler, S., Winzen, S., Langhanki, J., Mohr, K., Opatz, T., Mailander, V., Landfester, K., Wurm, F.R., 2015. Carbohydrate-based nanocarriers exhibiting specific cell targeting with minimum influence from the protein corona. Angew Chem. Int. Ed. Engl. 54 (25), 7436–7440.

Kim, C.S., Le, N.D., Xing, Y., Yan, B., Tonga, G.Y., Kim, C., Vachet, R.W., Rotello, V.M., 2014. The role of surface functionality in nanoparticle exocytosis. Adv. Healthc. Mater. 3 (8), 1200–1202.

Kumar, P., Wu, H., McBride, J.L., Jung, K.E., Kim, M.H., Davidson, B.L., Lee, S.K., Shankar, P., Manjunath, N., 2007. Transvascular delivery of small interfering RNA to the central nervous system. Nature 448 (7149), 39–43.

Lee, J.H., Engler, J.A., Collawn, J.F., Moore, B.A., 2001. Receptor mediated uptake of peptides that bind the human transferrin receptor. Eur. J. Biochem. 268 (7), 2004–2012.

Li, J., Feng, L., Fan, L., Zha, Y., Guo, L., Zhang, Q., Chen, J., Pang, Z., Wang, Y., Jiang, X., Yang, V.C., Wen, L., 2011. Targeting the brain with PEG-PLGA nanoparticles modified with phage-displayed peptides. Biomaterials 32 (21), 4943–4950.

Li, L., Di, X., Zhang, S., Kan, Q., Liu, H., Lu, T., Wang, Y., Fu, Q., Sun, J., He, Z., 2016. Large amino acid transporter 1 mediated glutamate modified docetaxel-loaded liposomes for glioma targeting. Colloids Surf. B Biointerfaces 141, 260–267.

Lin, T., Zhao, P., Jiang, Y., Tang, Y., Jin, H., Pan, Z., He, H., Yang, V.C., Huang, Y., 2016. Blood-brain-barrier-penetrating albumin nanoparticles for biomimetic drug delivery via

albumin-binding protein pathways for antiglioma therapy. ACS Nano 10 (11), 9999–10012.
Liu, J., Yu, M., Zhou, C., Yang, S., Ning, X., Zheng, J., 2013. Passive tumor targeting of renal-clearable luminescent gold nanoparticles: long tumor retention and fast normal tissue clearance. J. Am. Chem. Soc. 135 (13), 4978–4981.
Luo, Y., Yang, J., Yan, Y., Li, J., Shen, M., Zhang, G., Mignani, S., Shi, X., 2015. RGD-functionalized ultrasmall iron oxide nanoparticles for targeted T(1)-weighted MR imaging of gliomas. Nanoscale 7 (34), 14538–14546.
Mann, A.P., Scodeller, P., Hussain, S., Braun, G.B., Molder, T., Toome, K., Ambasudhan, R., Teesalu, T., Lipton, S.A., Ruoslahti, E., 2017. Identification of a peptide recognizing cerebrovascular changes in mouse models of Alzheimer's disease. Nat. Commun. 8 (1), 1403.
Mongelard, F., Bouvet, P., 2010. AS-1411, a guanosine-rich oligonucleotide aptamer targeting nucleolin for the potential treatment of cancer, including acute myeloid leukemia. Curr. Opin. Mol. Ther. 12 (1), 107–114.
Nel, A.E., Madler, L., Velegol, D., Xia, T., Hoek, E.M., Somasundaran, P., Klaessig, F., Castranova, V., Thompson, M., 2009. Understanding biophysicochemical interactions at the nano-bio interface. Nat. Mater. 8 (7), 543–557.
Oh, N., Park, J.H., 2014. Surface chemistry of gold nanoparticles mediates their exocytosis in macrophages. ACS Nano 8 (6), 6232–6241.
Pardridge, W.M., 2007. Blood-brain barrier delivery. Drug Discov. Today 12 (1–2), 54–61.
Ponka, P., Lok, C.N., 1999. The transferrin receptor: role in health and disease. Int. J. Biochem. Cell Biol. 31 (10), 1111–1137.
Qian, Z.M., Li, H., Sun, H., Ho, K., 2002. Targeted drug delivery via the transferrin receptor-mediated endocytosis pathway. Pharmacol. Rev. 54 (4), 561–587.
Qin, Y., Chen, H., Yuan, W., Kuai, R., Zhang, Q., Xie, F., Zhang, L., Zhang, Z., Liu, J., He, Q., 2011. Liposome formulated with TAT-modified cholesterol for enhancing the brain delivery. Int. J. Pharm. 419 (1–2), 85–95.
Rip, J., Chen, L., Hartman, R., van den Heuvel, A., Reijerkerk, A., van Kregten, J., van der Boom, B., Appeldoorn, C., de Boer, M., Maussang, D., de Lange, E.C., Gaillard, P.J., 2014. Glutathione PEGylated liposomes: pharmacokinetics and delivery of cargo across the blood-brain barrier in rats. J. Drug Target. 22 (5), 460–467.
Ruan, S., Yuan, M., Zhang, L., Hu, G., Chen, J., Cun, X., Zhang, Q., Yang, Y., He, Q., Gao, H., 2015. Tumor microenvironment sensitive doxorubicin delivery and release to glioma using angiopep-2 decorated gold nanoparticles. Biomaterials 37, 425–435.
Sakamoto, K., Shinohara, T., Adachi, Y., Asami, T., Ohtaki, T., 2017. A novel LRP1-binding peptide L57 that crosses the blood brain barrier. Biochem. Biophys. Rep. 12, 135–139.
Salvati, A., Pitek, A.S., Monopoli, M.P., Prapainop, K., Bombelli, F.B., Hristov, D.R., Kelly, P.M., Aberg, C., Mahon, E., Dawson, K.A., 2013. Transferrin-functionalized nanoparticles lose their targeting capabilities when a biomolecule corona adsorbs on the surface. Nat. Nanotechnol. 8 (2), 137–143.
Song, Q., Huang, M., Yao, L., Wang, X., Gu, X., Chen, J., Chen, J., Huang, J., Hu, Q., Kang, T., Rong, Z., Qi, H., Zheng, G., Chen, H., Gao, X., 2014. Lipoprotein-based nanoparticles rescue the memory loss of mice with Alzheimer's disease by accelerating the clearance of amyloid-Beta. ACS Nano 8 (3), 2345–2359.
Sun, C.Y., Shen, S., Xu, C.F., Li, H.J., Liu, Y., Cao, Z.T., Yang, X.Z., Xia, J.X., Wang, J., 2015. Tumor acidity-sensitive polymeric vector for active targeted siRNA delivery. J. Am. Chem. Soc. 137 (48), 15217–15224.
Thom, G., Hatcher, J., Hearn, A., Paterson, J., Rodrigo, N., Gurrell, A., Webster, C., 2018. Isolation of blood-brain barrier-crossing antibodies from a phage display library by

competitive elution and their ability to penetrate the central nervous system. MABS-AUSTIN 10 (2), 304–314.

Ueberham, U., Ueberham, E., Gruschka, H., Arendt, T., 2003. Connective tissue growth factor in Alzheimer's disease. Neuroscience 116 (1), 1–6.

van Groen, T., Kadish, I., Wiesehan, K., Funke, S.A., Willbold, D., 2009. In vitro and in vivo staining characteristics of small, fluorescent, Abeta42-binding D-enantiomeric peptides in transgenic AD mouse models. ChemMedChem 4 (2), 276–282.

Wei, X., Zhan, C., Shen, Q., Fu, W., Xie, C., Gao, J., Peng, C., Zheng, P., Lu, W., 2015. A D-peptide ligand of nicotine acetylcholine receptors for brain-targeted drug delivery. Angew Chem. Int. Ed. Engl. 54 (10), 3023–3027.

Xie, R., Dong, L., Du, Y., Zhu, Y., Hua, R., Zhang, C., Chen, X., 2016. In vivo metabolic labeling of sialoglycans in the mouse brain by using a liposome-assisted bioorthogonal reporter strategy. Proc. Natl. Acad. Sci. U. S. A. 113 (19), 5173–5178.

Xin, H., Jiang, X., Gu, J., Sha, X., Chen, L., Law, K., Chen, Y., Wang, X., Jiang, Y., Fang, X., 2011. Angiopep-conjugated poly(ethylene glycol)-co-poly(epsilon-caprolactone) nanoparticles as dual-targeting drug delivery system for brain glioma. Biomaterials 32 (18), 4293–4305.

Xu, F., Reiser, M., Yu, X., Gummuluru, S., Wetzler, L., Reinhard, B.M., 2016. Lipid-mediated targeting with membrane-wrapped nanoparticles in the presence of corona formation. ACS Nano 10 (1), 1189–1200.

Yu, Y.J., Zhang, Y., Kenrick, M., Hoyte, K., Luk, W., Lu, Y., Atwal, J., Elliott, J.M., Prabhu, S., Watts, R.J., Dennis, M.S., 2011. Boosting brain uptake of a therapeutic antibody by reducing its affinity for a transcytosis target. Sci. Transl. Med. 3 (84), 44r–84r.

Zhan, C., Li, B., Hu, L., Wei, X., Feng, L., Fu, W., Lu, W., 2011. Micelle-based brain-targeted drug delivery enabled by a nicotine acetylcholine receptor ligand. Angew Chem. Int. Ed. Engl. 50 (24), 5482–5485.

Zhang, C., Wan, X., Zheng, X., Shao, X., Liu, Q., Zhang, Q., Qian, Y., 2014a. Dual-functional nanoparticles targeting amyloid plaques in the brains of Alzheimer's disease mice. Biomaterials 35 (1), 456–465.

Zhang, C., Zheng, X., Wan, X., Shao, X., Liu, Q., Zhang, Z., Zhang, Q., 2014b. The potential use of H102 peptide-loaded dual-functional nanoparticles in the treatment of Alzheimer's disease. J. Control. Release 192, 317–324.

Zhang, T., Li, W., Meng, G., Wang, P., Liao, W., 2016. Strategies for transporting nanoparticles across the blood-brain barrier. Biomater. Sci. 4, 219–229.

Zhao, Y., Jiang, Y., Lv, W., Wang, Z., Lv, L., Wang, B., Liu, X., Liu, Y., Hu, Q., Sun, W., Xu, Q., Xin, H., Gu, Z., 2016. Dual targeted nanocarrier for brain ischemic stroke treatment. J. Control. Release 233, 64–71.

Zheng, X., Pang, X., Yang, P., Wan, X., Wei, Y., Guo, Q., Zhang, Q., Jiang, X., 2017a. A hybrid siRNA delivery complex for enhanced brain penetration and precise amyloid plaque targeting in Alzheimer's disease mice. Acta Biomater. 49, 388–401.

Zheng, X., Zhang, C., Guo, Q., Wan, X., Shao, X., Liu, Q., Zhang, Q., 2017b. Dual-functional nanoparticles for precise drug delivery to Alzheimer's disease lesions: targeting mechanisms, pharmacodynamics and safety. Int. J. Pharm. 525 (1), 237–248.

Index

Note: Page numbers followed by *f* indicate figures and *t* indicate tables.

B

I

J

L

Kolibri 360 GmbH
Ferdinand-Jühlke-Straße 7
99095 Erfurt, Deutschland
produktsicherheit@kolibri360.de